# Hybrid PET/CT and SPECT/CT Imaging

Dominique Delbeke · Ora Israel
Editors

# Hybrid PET/CT and SPECT/CT Imaging

A Teaching File

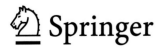 Springer

*Editors*

Dominique Delbeke
Department of Radiology
  and Radiological Sciences
Vanderbilt University Medical Center
1161 21st Ave. S. & Garland
Nashville TN 37232-2675
USA
dominique.delbeke@vanderbilt.edu

Ora Israel
Department of Nuclear Medicine
Rambam Health Care Campus
Bat-Galim
35 254 Haifa
Israel
o_israel@rambam.health.gov.il

ISBN 978-0-387-92819-7     e-ISBN 978-0-387-92820-3
DOI 10.1007/978-0-387-92820-3
Springer New York Dordrecht Heidelberg London

Library of Congress Control Number: 2009930385

Printed on acid-free paper

Springer is part of Springer Science+Business Media (www.springer.com)

*To my children: Cerine and Cedric Jeanty.*
Dominique Delbeke

*In loving memory of my parents.*
*To my husband, Stefan,*
*To Dalit, Yair, Harel and Rani.*
Ora Israel

# Preface

Our profession has progressed tremendously over the last decade. A few years ago one of us (DD) was the senior editor of *FDG Imaging: A Teaching File*, a book that proved to be a reference source of FDG image cases obtained both on dedicated PET tomographs and hybrid scintillation gamma cameras. This was followed by *Nuclear Cardiology and Correlative Imaging: A Teaching File*, a text already providing important insights into the complementarity of SPECT and PET cardiac imaging with cardiovascular CT and MRI. These two books were modeled after *Nuclear Medicine Imaging: A Teaching File*, recently updated with the second edition and designed as a manual of nuclear medicine cases, including studies that were performed with both SPECT and PET tracers.

Today, following the continuing development of new imaging devices and of our understanding of molecular processes, we found an unmet need for presenting and discussing cases that demonstrate the role of hybrid imaging with SPECT/CT and PET/CT with a variety of radiopharmaceuticals used in daily practice.

With clinical cases related to multiple clinical entities presented in depth, *Hybrid PET/CT and SPECT/CT Imaging: A Teaching File* is designed to be a teaching manual and everyday companion for our colleagues working in private practice, for residents training in nuclear medicine or radiology, for medical students, and for physicians whose specialties carry over into molecular imaging with radiopharmaceuticals.

The first two chapters cover the technical aspects of hybrid imaging and a historical perspective of the development of this technology. Recommendations for patient preparation and acquisition protocols, with special emphasis on physiologic variants, pitfalls, and artifacts follow. The next 15 chapters are devoted to clinical applications in oncology, according to specific malignant diseases and patient populations. The final three chapters present relatively new clinical applications of hybrid imaging in the field of cardiology, skeletal, and infectious diseases.

Each chapter begins with a succinct summary of the recent literature for the specific clinical application. This is followed by a series of case presentations ranging from the simple to the more complex in an attempt to simulate clinical practice. Images are presented in PET/SPECT stand-alone, CT stand-alone, and fused-images format in order to highlight the advantages and incremental value of the hybrid technology in the cases selected. At the end of each chapter, up-to-date references allow the reader to follow in greater depth the rapidly expanding volume of knowledge.

We sincerely hope that this text will provide nuclear physicians, radiologists, trainees, and those with an interest in hybrid imaging with a reference text that will enhance their practice of nuclear medicine. We also believe that this book will be used by our colleagues, the referring clinicians, interested in learning more about how this new medical imaging technology can be applied to their patients.

Over the past decade, the two editors of this book have had the opportunity to work together on multiple projects related to novel technological developments and their implementation in the clinical routine. The teams at Vanderbilt, in Nashville, Tennessee, and Rambam, in Haifa, Israel, were separated geographically by thousands of miles, but together they developed a vast clinical experience with both SPECT/CT and PET/CT, exploring new clinical indications for the hybrid technology in what has since become standard practice in cancer patients and beyond.

It was a natural sequence of events that led from common work and research to a wonderful professional and personal friendship. We have worked together with great mentors, Dr Martin Sandler and the late Dr Dov Front, who have taught us to think, ask tough questions, search for answers, and never give up. We have been fortunate to work with wonderful teams, including physicians, technical and administrative staff, and physicists. Our research involving hybrid imaging has been successful because we have all joined forces and have developed a good working relationship with our colleagues, the engineers and scientists in the industry.

We are grateful to our valued contributors whom we know and appreciate for their expertise, knowledge, dedication, and contributions to the field of hybrid imaging for many years. This book is a collaborative effort of numerous teams in multiple centers all over the world.

Most of all, our families have always been there for us, not only with words, but with acts of encouragement and understanding, making our journey through Hybrid Imaging a great experience.

Nashville, Tennessee                                    Dominique Delbeke, MD, PhD
Haifa, Israel                                            Ora Israel, MD

# Acknowledgments

We wish to express our gratitude to the staff of the Departments of Nuclear Medicine – physicians, physicists, technologists, and administrative assistants – at Vanderbilt and Rambam, for their support, encouragement, and specifically their outstanding technical assistance during our work on this project. We would like to thank all contributors, authors, and publishers who granted permission to reproduce their illustrations. We acknowledge the work of the staff at Springer for their highly professional expertise, tireless assistance, and commitment to this text, as well as the work of the staff at Hermes Medical Solutions for their contribution to producing the DVD.

# Contents

# Expanded Chapter Contents

# Contributors

**Rachel Bar-Shalom, MD** Department of Nuclear Medicine, Rambam Health Care Campus, B. and R. Rappaport School of Medicine, Technion—Israel Institute of Technology, Haifa, Israel

**Simona Ben-Haim, MD, DSc** Institute of Nuclear Medicine, University College London Hospital NHS Trust, London, UK

**Arye Blachar, MD** Department of Radiology, Sackler School of Medicine, Tel Aviv Sourasky Medical Center, Tel Aviv University, Tel Aviv, Israel

**Angela T. Byrne, MB, MRCPI, FFRRCSI** Department of Radiology, British Columbia Children's Hospital, Vancouver, British Columbia, Canada

**Marcelo Daitzchman, MD** Department of Diagnostic Imaging, Rambam Health Care Campus, Haifa, Israel

**Farrokh Dehdashti, MD** Mallinckrodt Institute of Radiology, Washington University School of Medicine, St. Louis, MO, USA

**Dominique Delbeke, MD, PhD** Department of Radiology and Radiological Sciences, Vanderbilt University Medical Center, Nashville, TN, USA

**Marcelo F. Di Carli, MD, FACC** Department of Medicine and Radiology, Division of Nuclear Medicine-PET, Brigham and Women's Hospital, Boston, MA, USA

**Sharmila Dorbala, MBBS** Department of Radiology and Medicine, Brigham and Women's Hospital, Harvard University, Boston, MA, USA

**Einat Even-Sapir, MD, PhD** Department of Nuclear Medicine, Tel-Aviv Sourasky Medical Center, Tel Aviv University, Tel Aviv, Israel

**Gideon Flusser, MD** Department of Radiology, Tel Aviv Sourasky Medical Center, Tel Aviv, Israel

**Sibyll Goetze, MD** Department of Radiology, Division of Nuclear Medicine/PET, The University of Alabama at Birmingham, Birmingham, AL, USA

**Arie Gordin, MD** Department of Otolaryngology, Head and Neck Surgery, The Hospital for Sick Children, Toronto, ON, Canada

**Ludmila Guralnik, MD** Departments of Diagnostic Imaging, Rambam Health Care Campus, Haifa, Israel

**Ora Israel, MD**   Rambam Health Care Campus, B. and R. Rappaport School of Medicine, Technion, Israel Institute of Technology, Haifa, Israel

**Heather A. Jacene, MD**   Division of Nuclear Medicine/PET, Russell H. Morgan Department of Radiology and Radiological Science, Johns Hopkins University School of Medicine, Baltimore, MD, USA

**Aaron C. Jessop, MD**   Department of Radiology and Radiological Sciences, Vanderbilt University Medical Center, Nashville, TN, USA

**Laurie B. Jones-Jackson, MD**   Department of Radiology and Radiological Sciences, Vanderbilt University Medical Center, Nashville, TN, USA

**Zohar Keidar, MD, PhD**   Department of Nuclear Medicine, B. and R. Rappaport School of Medicine, Rambam Health Care Campus, Haifa, Israel

**Martine Klein, MD**   Department of Biophysics and Nuclear Medicine, Hadassah Hebrew University Medical Center, Jerusalem, Israel

**Yodphat Krausz, MD**   Department of Medical Biophysics and Nuclear Medicine, Hadassah Hebrew University Medical Center, Jerusalem, Israel

**Hedva Lerman, MD**   Department of Nuclear Medicine, Tel Aviv Sourasky Medical Center, Tel Aviv, Israel

**Charito Love, MD**   Division of Nuclear Medicine and Molecular Imaging, North Shore Long Island Jewish Health System, Manhasset and New Hyde Park, NY, USA

**Helen R. Nadel, MD, FRCPC**   Division of Nuclear Medicine, Department of Radiology, British Columbia Children's Hospital, University of British Columbia, Vancouver, BC, Canada

**Marina Orevi, MD**   Department of Biophysics and Nuclear Medicine, Hadassah Medical Center, Jerusalem, Israel

**Christopher J. Palestro, MD**   Albert Einstein College of Medicine of Yeshiva University, Bronx, NY, USA; Division of Nuclear Medicine and Molecular Imaging, North Shore Long Island Jewish Health System, Manhasset and New Hyde Park, NY, USA

**James A. Patton, PhD**   Department of Radiology and Radiological Sciences, Vanderbilt University Medical Center, Nashville, TN, USA

**Vineet Prakash, MBChB, MRCP, FRCR**   Institute of Nuclear Medicine, University College London Hospital NHS Trust, London, UK

**Barry A. Siegel, MD**   Division of Nuclear Medicine, Edward Mallinckrodt Institute of Radiology and the Alvin J. Siteman Cancer Center Washington University School of Medicine, Saint Louis, MO, USA

**Gabriel Vorobiof, MD**   Department of Cardiovascular Imaging, Yale University, New Haven, CT, USA

**Richard L. Wahl, MD**   Russell H. Morgan Department of Radiology and Radiological Science, Division of Nuclear Medicine/PET, Johns Hopkins University School of Medicine, Baltimore, MD, USA

**Ronald C. Walker, MD** Department of Radiology and Radiological Sciences, Vanderbilt University Medical Center, Nashville, TN, USA

**Michal Weiler-Sagie, MD, PhD** Department of Nuclear Medicine, Rambam Health Care Campus, Haifa, Israel

# Chapter I.1
# History and Principles of Hybrid Imaging

James A. Patton

## Introduction

Positron emission tomography (PET) and single photon emission computed tomography (SPECT) systems are used to image distribution of radiopharmaceuticals in order to provide physicians with physiological information for diagnostic and therapeutic purposes. However, these images often lack sufficient anatomical detail, a fact that has triggered the development of a new technology termed hybrid imaging. Hybrid imaging is a term that is now being used to describe the combination of x-ray computed tomography (CT) systems with nuclear medicine imaging devices (PET and SPECT systems) in order to provide the technology for acquiring images of anatomy and function in a registered format during a single imaging session with the patient positioned on a common imaging table. There are two primary advantages to this technology. First, the x-ray transmission images acquired with CT can be used to perform attenuation correction of the PET and SPECT emission data. In addition, the CT anatomical images can be fused with the PET and SPECT functional images to provide precise anatomical localization of regions of questionable uptake of radiopharmaceuticals. This chapter will provide a review of SPECT, PET, and CT instrumentation and then discuss the technology involved in combining these systems to provide the capabilities for hybrid imaging.

## Single Photon Emission Computed Tomography

For many years, nuclear medicine procedures have been performed using a scintillation camera. Originally, multiple planar projections were acquired to provide diagnostic information, but, more recently, the techniques of SPECT have been utilized. During this time, the scintillation camera has evolved to a high-quality imaging device, and much of this evolution is due to the integration of digital technology into every aspect of the data acquisition, processing, and display processes.

Conventional planar images generally suffered from poor contrast due to the presence of overlying and underlying activity that interferes with imaging of the region of interest. This is caused by the superposition of depth information into single data points collected from

J.A. Patton (✉)
Department of Radiology and Radiological Sciences, Vanderbilt University Medical Center, Nashville, TN, USA
e-mail: jim.patton@vanderbilt.edu

D. Delbeke, O. Israel (eds.), *Hybrid PET/CT and SPECT/CT Imaging*, DOI 10.1007/978-0-387-92820-3_1, © Springer Science+Business Media, LLC 2010

perpendicular or angled lines of travel of photons from the distribution being studied into the holes of the parallel hole collimator fitted to the scintillation camera. The resulting planar image is low in contrast due to the effect of the superposition of depth information. This effect can be reduced by collecting images from multiple positions around the distribution and producing an image of a transverse slice through the distribution. The resulting tomographic image is of higher contrast than the planar image due to the elimination of contributions of activity above and below the region of interest. This is the goal of SPECT, i.e., to provide images of slices of radionuclide distributions with image contrast that is higher than that provided by conventional techniques.

## Data Acquisition

### Instrumentation

The introduction of the scintillation camera by Anger and Rosenthal in 1959[1] and its ultimate evolution into the imaging system of choice for routine nuclear medicine imaging applications resulted in a great deal of effort being expended toward the extension of the scintillation camera as a tomographic imaging device. In the early 1960s, Kuhl and Edwards established the fundamentals for SPECT using multi-detector scanning systems to acquire cross-sectional images of radionuclide distributions.[2-4] In the 1970s, Muehllehner,[5] Keyes and colleagues[6] and Jaszczak and colleagues[7] adapted this technology to a rotating scintillation camera. The result of these efforts along with the integration of computer systems was the development of the modern day SPECT system as a scintillation camera/computer system with one, two, or three heads and tomographic imaging capability. The scintillation camera collects tomographic data by rotating around the region of interest and acquiring multiple planar projection images during its rotation. It is imperative that the region of interest is included in every projection image. If this is not the case, the resulting truncation of the images will produce artifacts in the final reconstructed images. The camera may move in a continuous motion during acquisition but typically remains stationary during the acquisition of each projection image before advancing to the next position in a "step and shoot" mode of operation. A complete 360° rotation of a scintillation camera with a rectangular field of view will completely sample a cylindrical region of interest. Originally, camera systems were only capable of circular orbits; however, modern day systems have elliptical orbit capability. This is accomplished by equipping the collimators with sensors that detect the presence of the patient and maintain the camera head(s) in close proximity to the patient as the orbit is completed. Since the spatial resolution of collimators used with the scintillation camera degrades with distance from the collimator face, the optimum resolution is obtained in each projection image when the camera is as close to the patient as possible.

Initial SPECT applications were performed with a single-head scintillation camera acquiring data from a 360° orbit as shown in Fig. I.1.1A. When interest in imaging the myocardium became prominent, experimental work demonstrated that acceptable images could be obtained using a 180° orbit (right anterior oblique to left posterior oblique).[8,9] Although this results in an incomplete sampling of the region of interest, this lies in the near field of view of the camera throughout the partial orbit where the spatial resolution is optimum, and images of acceptable quality are obtained. Early in the evolution of SPECT imaging, it became evident that optimum counting statistics for many applications could not be obtained

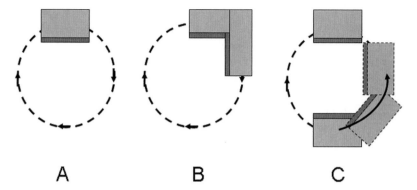

**Fig. I.1.1** Scintillation cameras for nuclear medicine applications have evolved from single-head (**A**) to dual-head, fixed 90° geometry (**B**), and finally to dual-head, variable-angle multipurpose cameras (**C**) (Reprinted with permission of Springer Science + Business Media from Vitola J, Delbeke D, eds. *Nuclear Cardiology and Correlative* Imaging: A Teaching File. New York: Springer-Verlag, 2004.)

in a reasonable time frame that could be tolerated by patients. This situation was remedied by the development of multi-head scintillation cameras. The first system to evolve was a dual-head camera in a fixed 180° geometry permitting a 360° acquisition with only a 180° rotation of the gantry. This development provided a twofold increase in sensitivity for SPECT applications. However, this increase in sensitivity was not available for cardiac applications using 180° acquisitions. To address this problem, special purpose, dual-head cameras were developed with the camera heads fixed in a 90° geometry as shown in Fig. I.1.1B. This made the twofold increase in sensitivity also available for cardiac imaging, and the acquisition of projections through 180° could be acquired with a 90° rotation of the dual-head gantry. Since many scintillation cameras must serve multiple purposes in nuclear medicine departments, the next step was the development of dual-head, variable-angle scintillation cameras as shown in Fig. I.1.1C. These cameras can acquire images with the heads in a 180° geometry for routine 360° applications, and one head can be moved into a 90° geometry with the other head for 180° cardiac applications. The two latter configurations are presently considered the cameras of choice for cardiac imaging.

**Acquisition Parameters**

Collimation

SPECT applications typically make use of parallel hole collimators in order to establish an orthogonal detection geometry with the crystal detectors. Imaging of low-energy radio-nuclides is generally limited to the use of general purpose, parallel hole collimators.

The resulting images typically exhibited poor spatial resolution. The emergence of multi-head cameras and the resulting increase in sensitivity have made it possible to improve spatial resolution by the use of high-resolution collimators, and these collimators are now the choice for most imaging applications.

Matrix Size

For most SPECT applications, the acquisition matrix size for acquiring planar projection images is typically a 64 × 64 data point array. The decision is based on the size of the smallest object to be imaged in the distribution being studied. Sampling theory states that in order to resolve frequencies (objects) up to a maximum frequency (smallest object) at least two measurements must be made across one cycle (the object). This maximum frequency is referred to as the Nyquist frequency. For example, using a camera with a 540-mm field of view, a zoom factor of 1.4 and a 64 × 64 acquisition matrix size would result in a pixel size of 6 mm, making it possible to image structures of 1.2 cm or larger. This is generally considered sufficient for most SPECT applications. The one exception is bone SPECT where a 128 × 128 matrix may be used to take advantage of the higher counting statistics to improve spatial resolution.

### Arc of Rotation

As previously stated, a 180° acquisition is acceptable (right anterior oblique position to left posterior oblique position) for cardiac imaging since the myocardium is always in the near field of the detector(s). Photons traveling in a posterior direction from the myocardium must travel significant distances through tissue and, therefore, spatial resolution and sensitivity (due to attenuation) are degraded in posterior and right posterior oblique views. Thus, the data from the omitted projections are considered to be of poor quality and generally not acquired. For most applications, however, a 360° acquisition is required in order to obtain a complete set of projections for acceptable image reconstructions.

### Projections per Arc of Rotation

The same sampling theory previously described also applies to the determination of the number of projection views that should be acquired throughout an arc of rotation. With current instrumentation, 120 views are typically obtained with a 360° acquisition, and, therefore, 60 views are generally acquired with a 180° acquisition.

### Time per Projection

In general, SPECT techniques require the acquisition of as many photon events as possible in order to produce high-quality images. However, the limiting factor is typically the time that a patient can remain motionless during the acquisition. This is typically a period of 15–30 min and results in imaging times of 15–30 s for each projection when 120 projections are acquired in a 360° rotation. For cardiac applications, the imaging time is typically reduced to 10–15 min.

## *SPECT Image Formation*

SPECT data are acquired in the form of multiple projection images as the scintillation camera heads rotate about the region of interest. Each acquired image is actually a set of count profiles measured from different views with the number of count profiles determined by the number of rows of pixels in the acquisition matrix (e.g., 64 for a 64 × 64 matrix size). Using parallel hole collimators, each pixel is the sum of measured photon events traveling along a perpendicular ray and interacting at a point in the detector crystal represented by the pixel location. For a 360° acquisition with 120 acquired projection arrays, 120 count profiles are acquired at 3° increments around the region of interest for each transaxial slice through the radionuclide distribution.

**Image Reconstruction**

An image of a transaxial slice through the distribution can be generated by sequentially projecting the data in each count profile collected from the selected slice back along the rays from which the data were collected and adding the data to previously backprojected rays. The mathematical term for this process is the linear superposition of backprojections. Since there is no a priori knowledge of the origin of photons along each ray, the value of each pixel in the count profile is placed in each data cell of the reconstructed image along the ray. Representations of the images resulting from this process are shown in Fig. I.1.2. It should be noted that uniform projections are used in Fig. I.1.2 to illustrate the backprojection principle. In fact, the rays at the periphery of the sphere are of less intensity than at the middle. The classic "star effect" blur pattern inherent in backprojection images is also evident in these images with each ray of the star corresponding to one projection view. The importance of collecting the appropriate number of projections is evident from this diagram. Increasing the number of projections enhances the image contrast and reduces the potential for artifacts from the "star effect." This can be seen in Fig. I.1.2D, where two additional sets of data at 45° and 135° are projected back into the image.

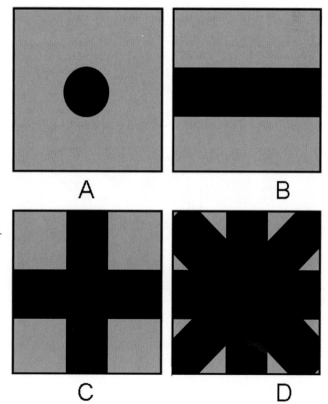

**Fig. I.1.2 A–D** Examples of two filtered count profiles of data acquired at 90° from a spherical source and the resulting image distribution after backprojection of the filtered profiles (Reprinted with permission of Springer Science + Business Media from Vitola J, Delbeke D, eds. *Nuclear Cardiology and Correlative Imaging: A Teaching File*. New York: Springer-Verlag, 2004.)

It is apparent from the data in Fig. I.1.2 that the blur pattern inherent in backprojection results in a significant background that reduces image contrast. To reduce these effects and also to reduce the statistical effects of noise in the images, the mathematical technique of filtering is applied to the count profiles in the projection data before backprojection is performed. A filter is a mathematical function that is defined to perform specific enhancements to the profile data. In general, filters enhance edges (sharpen images) and reduce background. The effects of a simple edge enhancement filter are shown in Fig. I.1.3. In the application of this filter, each data point in the profile is replaced by a mathematical relationship between its value and those of adjacent data points. This relationship is designed such that negative values are added to the count profiles. Figure I.1.3 shows the backprojection of the filtered count profile at 0° added to the filtered backprojected count profile at 90°. It can be observed that the negative data at the edges of one profile cancel unwanted data from other profiles. This effect is shown diagrammatically in Fig. I.1.3B, C. As the number of projections is increased, this effect becomes more pronounced as shown in Fig. I.1.3D, where the filtered backprojections at 45° and 135° are added to the image. The final step is to set to zero each pixel in the reconstructed image that has a negative value as shown in Fig. I.1.3E. The figure shows that the scanned object is now visible in the image but many non-zero pixels remain. The addition of multiple projections will remove

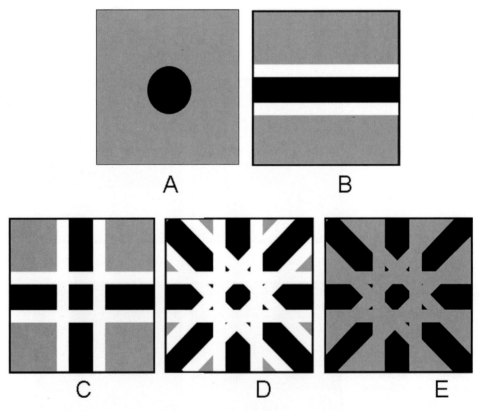

**Fig. I.1.3** Demonstration of the blur pattern from a spherical source (**A**) resulting from filtered backprojection of a single view (**B**), two views at 0 and 90° (**C**), and 0, 45, 90, and 135° (**D**). In the final image (**E**) the negative values have been set to zero (Reprinted with permission of Springer Science + Business Media from Vitola J, Delbeke D, eds. *Nuclear Cardiology and Correlative Imaging: A Teaching File.* New York: Springer-Verlag, 2004.)

these artifacts and further enhance the image of the actual measured distribution. This technique of linear superposition of filtered backprojections has been the image reconstruction algorithm of choice throughout most of the history of SPECT. Figure I.1.3 also demonstrates the need to select an appropriate filter for each imaging application. If too many negative numbers are added to the image (over-filtering), valuable image data will be removed. If not enough negative numbers are added to the image (under-filtering), unwanted data will remain in the image resulting in artifacts. The selection of the appropriate filter is probably the most significant factor in producing a high-quality image reconstruction. The effect of over-filtering and under-filtering is shown in the single reconstructed slice of the myocardium of a patient in Fig. I.1.4.

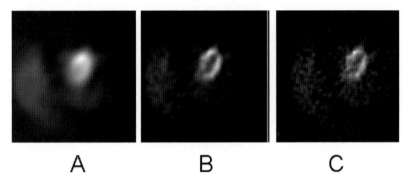

**Fig. I.1.4** Single short axis view of the myocardium with $^{99m}$Tc Sestamibi demonstrating over-filtering (**A**), under-filtering (**C**), and optimal filtering (**B**) (Reprinted with permission of Springer Science + Business Media from Vitola J, Delbeke D, eds. *Nuclear Cardiology and Correlative Imaging: A Teaching File*. New York: Springer-Verlag, 2004.)

The techniques previously discussed were illustrated using data for a single transverse slice. In practice, it is possible to reconstruct as many transverse slices as there are rows in the acquisition matrix. For example, a $64 \times 64$ matrix provides 64 rows of data that can be used to reconstruct 64 slices. However, because the slice thickness of a single slice often exceeds the spatial resolution of the camera and the data in a single slice are often statistically limited, it is common practice to add two or more adjacent slices in order to reconstruct thicker slices with improved statistics. The final result of the reconstruction process is a set of transverse slices. Images of sagittal and coronal slices can easily be generated from this data set by simply reformatting the data. For the special case of the heart where its orientation is not in the traditional x, y, z orientation of the human body, it is necessary to re-orient the axes to correspond to the long and short axes of the left ventricle. This is a straightforward procedure that can be accomplished automatically or manually under software control.

### Filters

Routine methods for characterizing nuclear medicine images and data sets relate to the number of counts in a pixel. When data are referred to using this terminology, the data are defined as being in the *spatial domain* and the simple filter previously used to illustrate the effects of filtering on image reconstruction was a *spatial filter*. In practice, filtering of projection data in the spatial domain is often cumbersome and time consuming. This problem can be overcome by working in the *frequency domain*. Here, the projection data may be expressed as a series of sine waves, and a frequency filter may be used to modify the data. The conversion of the projection data into the frequency domain is accomplished by the application of a mathematical function, the Fourier transform, and the result is that the projection data are represented as a frequency spectrum plotting the amplitude of each frequency in the data as shown in Fig. I.1.5A. In SPECT, this frequency spectrum has three distinct components. Background data (including the data from the star effect previously described) typically have very low frequencies and therefore are the main components of the low-frequency portion of the spectrum. Statistical fluctuations in the data (noise) generally have high frequencies and therefore dominate the high frequencies of the spectrum. True source data lie somewhere in the

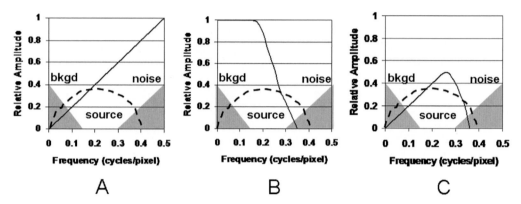

**Fig. I.1.5** In the frequency domain, image data can be represented as a series of sine waves, and the data can be plotted as a frequency spectrum showing the amplitude of each frequency. Image data have three major components: background, source information, and noise. A ramp filter is used to eliminate or reduce the contribution of background to the reconstructed image (**A**). A low-pass filter reduces the contribution of noise to the image (**B**). Combining the two filters (**C**) creates a window or band-pass filter that accepts frequencies primarily from the source distribution (Reprinted with permission of Springer Science + Business Media from Vitola J, Delbeke D, eds. *Nuclear Cardiology and Correlative Imaging: A Teaching File*. New York: Springer-Verlag, 2004.)

middle while overlapping the background and noise components of the spectrum. Thus, the challenge in filtering SPECT data is clearly demonstrated in Fig. I.1.5A. The goal is to eliminate background and noise from the data while preserving as much of the source data as possible. It should also be noted that the frequency data in the figure are plotted as a function of cycles/pixel. In the discussion of matrix size previously presented, the concept of the Nyquist frequency was introduced. In the frequency domain, the highest frequency in a data set occurs when one complete cycle covers two pixels. Frequencies higher than this value cannot be imaged. This fact translates into a frequency of 0.5 cycles/pixel as the frequency limit and is defined as the Nyquist frequency. This is why the plot in Fig. I.1.5A terminates at 0.5 cycles/pixel. The pixel size used in a particular application can be introduced into this definition so that the Nyquist frequency for the application can be determined. For example, a pixel size of 0.5 cm would define a Nyquist frequency of 1.0 cycles/cm. And the smallest object size that could possibly be resolved in an image would be 1 cm.

The first step in filtering is to design a filter to remove or reduce the background. This typically is a ramp filter as shown in Fig. I.1.5A, a high-pass filter that reduces only the amplitudes of low-frequency data while having no effect on the mid-range and high-frequency data which contain the detail in the source (and also the noise). The second step is to define a filter to remove or reduce the noise while preserving the detail in the source data. This is accomplished using a low-pass filter as shown in Fig. I.1.5B, which accepts selected frequencies up to a certain value. There are a number of low-pass filters that are available for processing SPECT data. Some have fixed characteristics, and others have flexibility in choosing the cutoff frequency and/or the slope of the filter. Some filters are optimized for image data with excellent counting statistics, and others provide the capability for filtering data with poor statistics. Also, the amount of detail in an image and the object sizes to be resolved (spatial resolution) are important factors to be considered in the selection of a filter. In practice, the low-pass filter may be applied first to reduce the effects of noise, and then the ramp filter is applied to reduce background. The two filters may be combined as shown in Fig. I.1.5C to function as a band-pass filter. It can be seen in the latter figure that appropriate selection of the cutoff frequency will eliminate much of the noise, and selecting an appropriate filter shape will preserve most of the source data. The terms under-filtering and over-filtering were previously referenced, and examples were shown in Fig. I.1.4. From Fig. I.1.5C, it can be observed that, when a cutoff frequency is chosen that is too low, some of the source data will be excluded from the final image, and this situation is referred to as over-filtering. Similarly, when too high a cutoff frequency is chosen, excessive noise will be included in the final image, and this is referred to as under-filtering. In clinical applications, most imaging systems provide the capability for trying different filters and filter parameters on a single slice of image data in order to select the appropriate processing algorithm for a specific patient study. Technologists and physicians in the clinical setting often prefer this method of trial and error.

**Iterative Reconstruction**

Filtered backprojection amplifies statistical noise, which adversely affects image quality. To address this problem, Shepp and Vardi introduced an iterative reconstruction technique in 1982[10] based on the theory of expectation maximization (EM), which has a proven theoretical convergence to an estimate of the actual image distribution that has a maximum likelihood of having projections most similar to the acquired projections. The initial implementation of these algorithms was very time consuming, with several iterations being required to reach a solution, and extensive computer power was required. Since that time, much effort has been expended in improving and testing algorithms based on this concept. Significant improvements in speed and signal-to-noise and reconstruction accuracy have resulted from these efforts. In 1994, Hudson and Larkin[11] developed the technique of ordered sets EM (OS-EM) for image reconstruction from 2D projection data. This algorithm was based on the concept of dividing the projection data into small subsets (e.g., paired opposite projections in SPECT data) and performing the EM algorithm on each subset. The solution of each subset was used as the starting point for the next subset, with subsequent subsets being selected to provide the maximum information (e.g., chose the second subset of data to be orthogonal to the first subset). The advantage of this technique is that, at the end of the first pass, the entire data set has been processed one time, but $n$ successive approximations to the final solution have been made where $n$ is the number of subsets. Thus, OS-EM is $n$ times faster than the original EM algorithm. Typically, only two to three passes through the data set (iterations) are required for the reconstructed image to converge to a final value that is essentially unchanged by further iterations. Correction for scatter and attenuation effects (topics that will be discussed later) can be performed on the acquired projection data during the reconstruction process. The advantage of this technique is that the star effect inherent in filtered backprojection is virtually eliminated since the acquired data are distributed within the body contour. Because of this result, signal-to-noise is generally improved. Filtering of the data can also be performed to further enhance the reconstructed images.

**Attenuation Correction**

One of the primary factors affecting image quality in SPECT is photon attenuation. Photons are attenuated in the body due to photoelectric absorption and Compton scatter, with Compton scattering being the most predominant interaction in the diagnostic energy range. The probability of Compton scattering decreases with increasing energy. The effects of attenuation are significant, with approximately 62% of 70 keV photons and 54% of 140 keV photons being attenuated in 5 cm of tissue. Photoelectric absorption results in a complete removal of the photon from the radiation field, while Compton scattering results in a change in direction with loss of photon energy, the magnitude of the loss being determined by the angle of scatter. Thus, Compton scattered photons enter the camera crystal with minimal or no information on their origins due to their change in direction within the patient. Pulse height analysis is used to prevent the counting of photons that have scattered through large angles (greater loss of energy), but small angle scattered photons are counted. The use of a 20% window at 70 keV permits the acceptance of photons that have scattered through 0–79°. At 140 keV, a 20% window permits the acceptance of photons that have scattered through 0–53° and a 15% window accepts photons scattered through 0–45°.

Correction of images for attenuation effects are complicated by the broad range of tissue types (lung, soft tissue, muscle, and bone) that may reside in the region of interest resulting in a non-uniform attenuation medium. A commercial approach to attenuation correction that has been used in the past used line sources of $^{153}$Gd as shown in Fig. I.1.6. These sources provide beams of 100 keV photons and are scanned in the longitudinal direction at each step of the SPECT acquisition to provide transmission maps of the region under study. Emission and transmission scans at each step can be acquired sequentially or simultaneously using

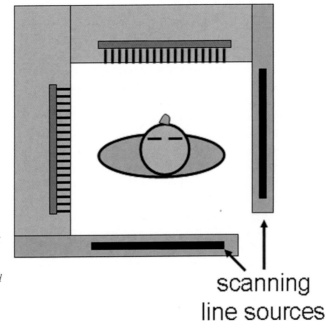

**Fig. I.1.6** Scanning line sources mounted on a dual-head, 90° geometry scintillation camera for attenuation correction measurements (Reprinted with permission of Springer Science + Business Media from Vitola J, Delbeke D, eds. *Nuclear Cardiology and Correlative Imaging: A Teaching File*. New York: Springer-Verlag, 2004.)

scanning
line sources

synchronized energy windows that move with the sources to acquire the transmission data. These are then used to correct the projection data prior to SPECT image reconstruction.

Correction methods tend to overcorrect for attenuation, and it is generally accepted that a scatter correction must also be performed. One solution to this problem is the simultaneous acquisition of a second set of planar projections using a scatter window positioned just below the photopeak energy being measured. This window is used to determine correction factors for the acquired planar projections prior to image reconstruction.

## Positron Emission Tomography

Previous discussions have been related to the imaging of single photon emitting radionuclides using conventional scintillation camera systems. Another classification of radionuclides that have applications in nuclear medicine is positron emitters that can be imaged using specially designed PET systems optimized for the unique decay properties of these radionuclides. Anger and Rosenthal[1] originally proposed the use of the scintillation camera for this application, and throughout the years numerous attempts have been made to use this instrument for this application.[12,13] However, these approaches suffered from deficiencies in the efficiency of NaI(Tl). Robertson and coworkers[14] and Brownell and Burnham[15,16] developed special purpose positron imaging systems in the early 1970s, but the modern day PET scanner began to evolve in 1975[17] with the work of Phelps and his associates producing a system of detectors operating in coincidence mode and surrounding the patient to provide transverse section imaging capabilities.[18–22] Positron emitting radionuclides are distinguished by the unique method by which they are detected. The positron is a positively charged electron. When emitted from a radioactive nucleus, it travels only a very short distance before losing all of its energy and coming to rest. At that instant, it combines with a negatively charged electron, and the masses of the two particles are completely converted into energy in the form of two 511 keV photons. This process is termed *annihilation*. The two annihilation photons leave the site of their production at 180° from each other. This process can be detected as shown in Fig. I.1.7 by using small, dual-opposed detectors connected by a timing circuit, termed a *coincidence* circuit, to simultaneously detect the presence of the two annihilation photons, a signature of the positron decay process.

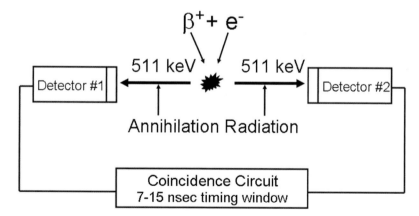

**Fig. I.1.7** Block diagram of a two-detector grouping with a coincidence timing window used to simultaneously detect the two photons resulting from the annihilation of a positron–electron pair using the technique of coincidence counting (Reprinted with permission of Springer Science + Business Media from Vitola J, Delbeke D, eds. *Nuclear Cardiology and Correlative Imaging: A Teaching File.* New York: Springer-Verlag, 2004.)

The timing window must be small, 7–15 ns, in order to reduce the possibility of detecting photons from two separate decay processes, i.e., random events. The spatial resolution of the imaging system is primarily determined by the size of the detectors, combined with the uncertainty due to the travel of the positron before annihilation which is typically less than 0.5 mm in tissue. In clinical imaging systems, many small detectors are used in multiple rings to provide high sensitivity for detection in the region being examined as shown in Fig. I.1.8.

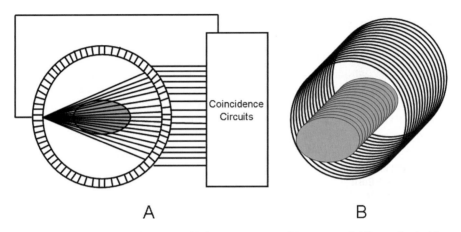

A                                                                  B

**Fig. I.1.8** One ring of detectors from a multi-ring PET system. Many potential lines of coincidence are possible for each detector in the ring (**A**). Multiple rings of detectors are used to extend the axial field of view (**B**) (Reprinted with permission of Springer Science + Business Media from Vitola J, Delbeke D, eds. *Nuclear Cardiology and Correlative Imaging: A Teaching File.* New York: Springer-Verlag, 2004.)

## PET Detectors

For many years, the scintillation detector of choice for PET imaging has been bismuth germanate (BGO) instead of NaI(Tl), which is used in other nuclear medicine imaging devices. BGO is used because of its high-density and high effective atomic number, which results in a high intrinsic detection efficiency for 511 keV photons. A 30-mm thick crystal of BGO has an intrinsic detection efficiency of approximately 90% at 511 keV. When two detectors are used in coincidence to simultaneously detect two 511 keV photons, the coincidence detection efficiency is the product of the efficiencies of the two detectors or approximately 81%. Recently, a new scintillation material, lutetium oxyorthosilicate (LSO), has been introduced as a possible replacement for BGO. Although currently more expensive than BGO, LSO has the advantage of greater light output (factor of 6) and faster decay time (factor of 7.5), and these improvements can be used to advantage in increasing the count rate capabilities of modern day systems. PET systems using LSO are now available from one manufacturer (Siemens-CTI). More recently, another new scintillation detector material, gadolinium oxyorthosilicate (GSO) has been introduced with similar characteristics to those of LSO, but with improved energy resolution. PET systems using GSO detectors are now available from another manufacturer (Philips Medical Systems).

The high spatial resolution of these systems is accomplished by using a unique combination of small crystals and photomultiplier tubes. An example of this technology is shown in Fig. I.1.9. A rectangular solid crystal of detector material is modified by the addition of vertical and

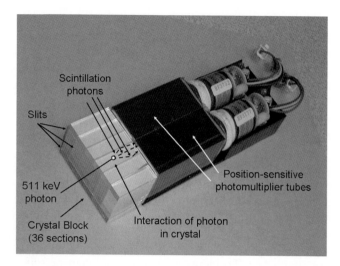

**Fig. I.1.9** For high-resolution imaging, a block of crystal (BGO in this example) is segmented into many small discrete detectors (32 in this example). Two position-sensitive photomultiplier tubes positioned at the back of the crystal block determine the detector in which an interaction occurs (Reprinted with permission of Springer Science + Business Media from Vitola J, Delbeke D, eds. *Nuclear Cardiology and Correlative Imaging: A Teaching File.* New York: Springer-Verlag, 2004.)

horizontal grooves partially through the volume to effectively create a block of many small discrete detectors (36 in the figure). Some manufactures actually separate the discrete crystals entirely, creating pixilated detectors as in the figure. A photon interaction in one of the discrete crystals will result in scintillations localized primarily in that crystal. The crystal in which the interaction occurred is then identified by photomultiplier tubes using conventional Anger logic and mounted on the base of the crystal block or by using position-sensitive photomultiplier tubes. In the detector block shown in Fig. I.1.10, the discrete crystals are

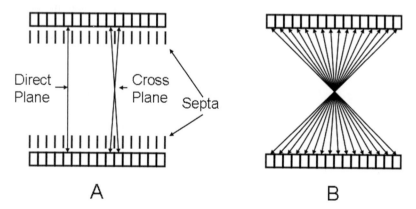

**Fig. I.1.10** The use of septa collimators permit 2D acquisition by limiting the detection of coincidence events to detectors within a single ring (direct planes) and detectors in adjacent rings (cross planes) (**A**). When the septa are withdrawn, 3D acquisition is established by permitting the measurement of a coincidence event in two detectors in any two rings of the system (**B**) (Reprinted with permission of Springer Science + Business Media from Vitola J, Delbeke D, eds. *Nuclear Cardiology and Correlative Imaging: A Teaching File.* New York: Springer-Verlag, 2004.)

4 mm × 8 mm × 30 mm deep, resulting in a transaxial spatial resolution of 4.6 mm. Current systems have 18–32 rings of detectors providing axial fields of view of 15–18 cm (Fig. I.1.8). Thus, the imaging of sections of the body greater than 15 cm in the axial direction requires multiple acquisitions obtained by indexing the patient through the system using a movable imaging table under precise computer control.

## 2D Versus 3D Imaging

It is possible to reduce the effects of scatter and the possibility of random events by adding thin 1D collimators, termed septa, between adjacent rings of detectors to shield the detection of events in the axial direction as shown in Fig. I.1.10A. These septa are typically constructed from tungsten with a thickness of 1 mm and spacing to match the axial width of each discrete crystal. They have the effect of creating 2D slices from which events can be accepted in any transaxial direction. Thus, for a system with 18 rings of detectors, 18 direct imaging planes are established. To increase sensitivity, coincidence circuitry can also be used to record interactions occurring in two detectors in adjacent rings, resulting in the addition of a new acquisition plane positioned midway between the adjacent detector rings. Thus, in an 18-ring system, 17 new cross imaging planes can be added for a total of 35 imaging planes in this example. Additional sensitivity is obtainable by adding adjacent planes to this process. For example, three or five planes of detectors may be electronically grouped so that coincidence events may be measured in any two detectors within these groupings. The localization of the coincidence event in a transaxial imaging plane is typically determined by averaging the axial positions of the two detectors. The length of the septa limits the axial separation of any two rings that can actually be used in the measurement of the activity in a 2D plane.

With the septa retracted or in systems using only 3D technology, detector rings are opened to photons traveling in all directions, and a 3D imaging geometry is established as shown in Fig. I.1.10B. This increases the system sensitivity by a factor of 3–5 over that of 2D imaging. However, the randoms rate and scatter fraction are increased with this geometry, which may reduce contrast. It is possible to limit the acceptance angle in the axial direction to reduce the effects of randoms and scatter, but this process results in a reduction in sensitivity.

## Data Acquisition and Image Reconstruction

As previously described, a coincidence event is recorded when two photons are simultaneously measured in two separate detectors. Thus, the coordinates of the two detectors determine the line of response (LOR) defined by the coincidence detection of the two photons as shown in Fig. I.1.11A. These coordinates are captured by calculating the perpendicular distance from the center of the scan field to the LOR (r) and measuring the angle between this line and the vertical axis ($\phi$). These coordinates are then recorded as a data point in an (r,$\phi$) plot or sinogram as shown in Fig. I.1.11B. Each unit in the final sinogram will consist of the total number of coincidence events recorded by a two-detector pair. The sinogram method of storage is used because it is more efficient than the storing of list mode data that record individual coordinates of detector pairs. In 2D image acquisition, there will be (2n − 1) sinograms recorded, one for each direct plane

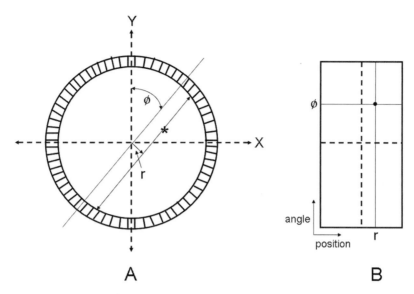

**Fig. I.1.11.** The coordinates of the two detectors involved in a coincidence measurement are captured by calculating the perpendicular distance from the center of the scan field to a line connecting the two detectors (r) and measuring the angle between this line and the vertical axis (φ) (**A**). These coordinates are then recorded as a data point in an (r,φ) plot or sinogram (**B**). Each unit in the final sinogram will consist of the total number of coincidence events recorded by a two-detector pair (Reprinted with permission of Springer Science + Business Media from Vitola J, Delbeke D, eds. *Nuclear Cardiology and Correlative Imaging: A Teaching File.* New York: Springer-Verlag, 2004.)

and one for each cross plane, where n is the number of detector rings in the PET system. When the two detectors are in different detector rings, the event is recorded in the sinogram corresponding to the average axial position of the two rings as previously stated.

   Image reconstruction of the 2D data is accomplished by first converting each sinogram of data into a set of planar projections. This can be accomplished in a straightforward manner from the sinograms since each horizontal row of data in a sinogram represents events recorded at one angular position. It should also be noted that the events from each two-detector pair are uniformly spread across the sinogram. As described in the section on SPECT reconstruction, a filtering algorithm is applied to each projection, after which the data are projected back along the lines from which they were acquired to generate the final image (i.e., filtered backprojection). Each sinogram of data is used in this fashion to generate an image corresponding to the activity distribution represented by the sinogram. Iterative algorithms that make use of ordered sets (OS-EM) can also be used in the 2D reconstruction process to reduce noise and provide high-quality images.[4] The use of iterative algorithms also simplifies the process of adding corrections for effects such as attenuation and scatter.

   The acquisition and reconstruction of 3D data sets are more complicated than that for 2D applications. First, it is not possible to perform the axial averaging of events recorded from two detectors in different detector rings. The origins of these data must be preserved in the acquisition process, and this results in a significant increase in the size of the acquired data set since $n^2$ sinograms are now required to accurately acquire the data. In addition, the reconstruction process is complicated by the fact that it is necessary to use a true 3D volume algorithm to accurately locate detected events in axial as well as transverse directions. Iterative reconstruction algorithms, although very time consuming and labor intensive, are well designed for this application. Currently, available systems offer this technique as an option, and it has proven useful in brain imaging because the imaging volume is relatively small and count rates are relatively low. Because of the added sensitivity provided by 3D imaging, a great deal of effort has been applied to develop accurate and efficient 3D algorithms and techniques to correct for scatter in order to improve contrast. These improvements have resulted in the 3D technique becoming the most prevalent choice for clinical PET imaging.

## Time-of-Flight PET

In conventional PET, the localization of a positron decay and the resultant production of annihilation radiation are represented by a LOR between the two detectors that detect the two annihilation photons. There is no way of identifying the precise position along the LOR where the decay process occurred. For many years, investigators have worked to solve this problem by using time-of-flight (TOF) techniques, but they have been limited by the response time of the detectors and the technology of timing measurements that have been available. The availability of fast LSO crystals and improvements in timing measurement capability now make the application a reality. Instead of using conventional timing circuitry to identify coincidence events within a timing window, TOF PET uses more sophisticated timing circuitry to measure the time difference between the detection of the two photons from an annihilation event. Since the photons travel at a known velocity, the speed of light ($c$), this time difference can be used to calculate the difference in distance of travel of the two photons between the two detectors involved in the measurement. Using this measurement and the known distance between the two detectors, the actual distance of travel of the two photons can be calculated (and therefore the location of the annihilation event). Current timing resolutions on the order of 0.6 ns yield an uncertainty on the order of 9 cm in the measurement of the location of the annihilation event. Thus, the conventional LOR between the two detectors is replaced with a LOR of approximately 9 cm whose center is the estimate of the location of the annihilation event.

The use of TOF PET technology results in improved contrast and spatial resolution by significantly reducing the uncertainty in the actual location of the annihilation event. Although signal processing is more intensive with this technology, improvements in lesion detection and image quality have been demonstrated in a commercial system using TOF technology, especially in large patients where random and scatter events are more prevalent.

## Quantitative Techniques

Because of the block detector technology used with PET systems, there is a dead time associated with measurements of activity distributions, and corrections for this effect must be implemented in order that the measurements are quantitatively accurate. When an interaction occurs in a crystal, a finite length of time is required to collect the light produced and process the resulting signal. If another event occurs in the same block while the first interaction is being processed, the light from the two events will be summed together by the photomultiplier tubes in that block, and the resulting signal will probably fall outside of the pulse height window. This effect will result in an erroneous measurement of count rate. Modern systems have dead time correction capability utilizing correction factors determined for the system as a function of count rate. These correction factors adjust for errors in count rate but cannot add the lost events back into the acquired image.

A state-of-the-art PET scanner may have several thousand discrete crystals coupled to hundreds of photomultiplier tubes. Thus, there are inherent differences in sensitivity between detector pairs in the measurement process, and it is necessary to correct for these differences in order for measurements of coincidence events to correspond to the activity distribution being imaged. This correction is generally accomplished by exposing each detector pair to a uniform source distribution, typically created by a rotating rod source of $^{68}$Ge and measuring the response of each detector pair. This data set is called a blank scan. The blank scan can be used to create normalization factors that are stored away and used to correct data subsequently acquired in image acquisition. Blank scans must be acquired frequently (at least weekly) in order to monitor system parameters and adequately correct for small changes in detector responses.

A second factor to be considered is the exponential attenuation of photons within the body. Photons are either absorbed or scattered by tissues based on the attenuation coefficients of these tissues and the distance of travel through the body. The attenuation effects are much more significant in coincidence imaging than in single photon imaging since both photons from a single annihilation process must pass through the body without interaction in order to be detected and counted as a coincidence event. The probability of this occurrence is much less than that for a single photon emitted from the same location to escape the body without interaction. These effects result in non-uniformities, distortions of intense structures, and edge effects. Therefore, it is necessary to correct for attenuation to eliminate these effects, especially in the thorax and abdomen where attenuation is non-uniform due to the presence of different tissue types. Since the brain is relatively uniform, it is possible to perform a calculated attenuation correction. This is accomplished by outlining the outer contour of the head, assuming uniform attenuation within this volume, and calculating correction factors to be applied to the raw projection data.

In the thorax and abdomen, because of the non-uniform attenuation, it is necessary to perform a measured attenuation correction. This approach is very accurate because attenuation of two annihilation photons from an annihilation event is independent of the location of the event. The total distance traveled through the patient is constant as shown in Fig. I.1.12A–C. It is therefore possible to measure the attenuation using an external source as shown in Fig. I.1.12D. In the past, this was typically accomplished by transmission scanning using a rotating rod source of $^{68}$Ge as in the acquisition of a blank scan for detector normalization, but with the patient present in the scan field. The transmission data can then be used to correct the raw projection data during the reconstruction process. Iterative reconstruction algorithms can be easily adapted to handle the attenuation correction process. Transmission scans with high counting statistics are required in order to prevent the addition of statistical noise in the corrected images. In the past, it was necessary to perform the transmission scan prior to administration of the radiopharmaceutical into the patient. This resulted in lengthened studies and the need for careful repositioning of the patient before acquiring the emission scan. More recent improvements in count rate capabilities have made it possible to acquire transmission scans after the patient has been injected with a radiopharmaceutical by increasing the activity in the transmission source. It

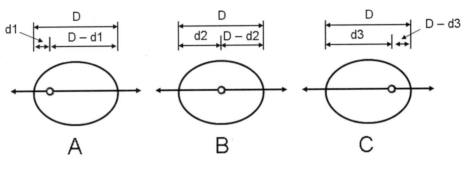

$$I = I_o \, e^{-\mu d1} \, e^{-\mu(D-d1)} = I_o \, e^{-\mu d2} \, e^{-\mu(D-d2)} = I_o \, e^{-\mu d3} \, e^{-\mu(D-d3)} = I_o \, e^{-\mu D}$$

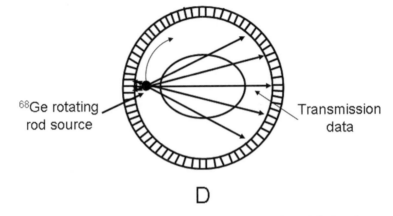

**Fig. I.1.12** The attenuation of two annihilation photons is independent of the location at which the two photons were produced, since the photon pair must always travel the same distance within the patient and escape without interaction in order to be detected as a true event (**A–C**). Thus, attenuation can be measured using a rotating rod source of a positron emitter such as $^{68}$Ge (**D**) (Reprinted with permission of Springer Science + Business Media from Vitola J, Delbeke D, eds. *Nuclear Cardiology and Correlative Imaging: A Teaching File*. New York: Springer-Verlag, 2004.)

has also been shown that it is possible to shorten the length of the transmission scan by using a process called segmented attenuation correction. In this process, attenuation coefficients are predetermined (based on certain tissue types) and limited in number. The measured attenuation coefficients from the transmission scan are then modified to match the closest allowed coefficients from the predetermined options. Figure I.1.13 shows a single coronal view reconstructed from a set of transmission scans, the corresponding view reconstructed from emission data using filtered backprojection, and the same view reconstructed using an OS-EM algorithm with attenuation correction.

The addition of transmission scanning permits accurate delineation of body contours. This fact makes it possible to limit image reconstruction to the areas defined by the contours. In addition, accurately knowing these contours permits the development of mathematical models for determining the contribution to the images of random and scatter events, and subsequently the implementation of correction methods to eliminate their effect. Work is currently ongoing in this area.

In order to make absolute measurements of activity in a region of the body, one additional calibration is necessary. A cylindrical phantom containing a very accurately

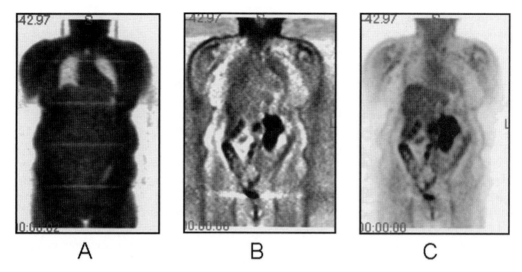

**Fig. I.1.13 (A)** A coronal view of a transmission data set acquired from a multi-ring PET scanner. **(B)** A coronal view of a patient with gastric cancer imaged with [18]F-FDG. The image was reconstructed without attenuation correction using filtered back projection. **(C)** The same coronal view of the [18]F-FDG distribution reconstructed with attenuation correction from the transmission data set shown in **(A)** using an iterative reconstruction algorithm (OS-EM) (Reprinted with permission of Springer Science + Business Media from Vitola J, Delbeke D, eds. *Nuclear Cardiology and Correlative Imaging: A Teaching File.* New York: Springer-Verlag, 2004.)

known distribution of activity is scanned and total counts (after attenuation correction) are determined. A quantitative calibration factor is then determined by dividing the measured counts per unit time by the concentration of activity in the phantom. This results in a calibration factor of counts/s per µCi/cc. To determine activity in a specific area, a region of interest is identified and the counts in the region are determined and converted to a count rate using the scan time, and the calibration factor is then used to calculate µCi/cc in the region. Current systems have the capability of measuring absolute activity to within 5%. In practice, it should be noted that the same acquisition and reconstruction algorithms (and filters) should be used in acquiring and processing the phantom data and the patient data in order to obtain accurate quantitative data. A quantitative measurement that has proven to be of use in some clinical applications is the standard uptake value (SUV). This factor is determined by normalizing the measured activity in a region to the administered activity per unit of patient weight. Using the SUV, regions of abnormal uptake can be compared to that of normal regions, and lesion uptake in serial scans can be compared.

## X-Ray Computed Tomography

As described in the Introduction, SPECT and PET imaging technologies often suffer from insufficient anatomical detail. These deficiencies can be resolved by incorporating the techniques of x-ray CT into the image acquisition and reconstruction process. This technology was introduced to the medical community in the early 1970s when Hounsfield and Ambrose[23] introduced a computerized x-ray tube-based tomographic scanner using reconstruction algorithms developed by McCormack[24] to provide images of tissue densities from acquired projections. CT scanning provides high quality and high spatial resolution ($\sim$ 1 mm) images of cross-sectional anatomy and therefore provides a significant portion of the anatomical images acquired in oncological applications, not only for diagnosis and staging of disease but also for simulations used for radiation treatment planning. CT images generally have a high sensitivity for lesion detection, but may have limited specificity in some applications. CT images are acquired as transmission maps with a high photon flux and are actually high-quality representations of tissue attenuation and thus can provide the basis for attenuation correction.

CT images are acquired by using a high-output x-ray tube and an arc of detectors in a fixed geometry to acquire cross-sectional transmission images of the patient as the x-ray tube and detectors configuration rapidly rotates around the patient as shown in Fig. I.1.14A, B. Current technology using multi-detector arrays and helical (spiral) scanning permits the simultaneous acquisition of as many as 64 thin slices (0.625 mm) in as little as 0.35 s. [If the rotation is 0.35 s, only a little more than half of the rotation is actually required to produce images.] The geometry of these third generation CT scanners results in the acquisition of transmission data in a fan beam geometry. However, each ray in a fan beam geometry can be represented by an equivalent ray in a parallel beam geometry.

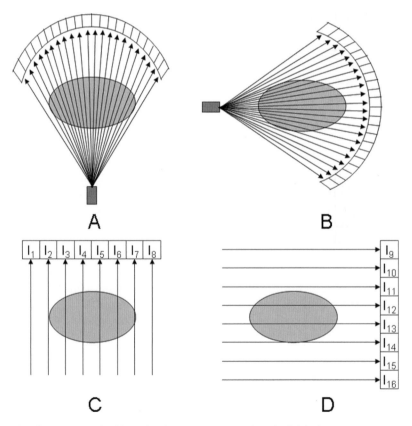

**Fig. I.1.14** CT data are acquired in a fan beam geometry where individual rays represent transmitted photon intensities from multiple projections around the patient (**A, B**). These data can be reformatted into an orthogonal geometry similar to that used for SPECT (**C, D**) (Reprinted by permission of the Society of Nuclear Medicine from: James A. Patton and Timothy G. Turkington. SPECT/CT Physical Principles and Attenuation Correction. *J Nucl Med Technol* 2008 36(1):1–10. Fig. 4.)

Therefore, a common approach is to convert the fan beam data to parallel beam geometry as illustrated diagrammatically in Fig. I.1.14C, D, in order to simplify the reconstruction process. This redistribution of data results in orthogonal data sets similar to that obtained from PET and SPECT. As many as 600 projection arrays are acquired in this manner in order to produce a high-quality transmission measurement of each slice of tissue.

Each measured ray ($I$) is the initial ray intensity ($I_0$) attenuated by a factor

$$I = I_0 e^{\sum_i -x_i\mu_i}$$

where the index $i$ represents all the different tissue type regions along the trajectory, $\mu_i$ are the effective attenuation coefficients for the different tissue regions, and $x_i$ are the corresponding thicknesses of the tissue regions, so that the sum represents the total attenuation through all regions. With filtered backprojection (or another tomographic reconstruction technique), these attenuation measurements obtained, along all rays at all angles, are used to produce cross-sectional arrays of tissue attenuation coefficients as shown in Fig. I.1.15A. The resulting arrays are high-quality images of body attenuation and therefore representative of body anatomy. In order to standardize the data and provide sufficient gray scale for display, the data are typically converted to CT numbers (Hounsfield units) as shown in Fig. I.1.15B by normalizing to the attenuation coefficient of water using the following equation:

$$\text{CT number} = [(\mu_{\text{tissue}} - \mu_{\text{water}})/\mu_{\text{water}}] \times 1000.$$

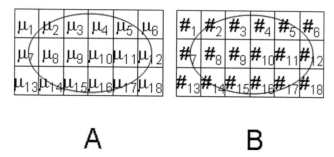

A                                    B

Fig. I.1.15  The transmitted intensities can be used to solve for attenuation coefficients ($\mu$) by using the un-attenuated intensity ($I_o$) by the attenuation equation ($I = I_o\, e^{-\mu x}$). Using filtered backprojection, an array of attenuation coefficients for each anatomical slice can be determined (A) and converted to an array of CT numbers for display purposes (B) (Reprinted by permission of the Society of Nuclear Medicine from: James A. Patton and Timothy G. Turkington. SPECT/CT Physical Principles and Attenuation Correction. *J Nucl Med Technol* 2008 36(1):1–10. Fig. 5.)

Based on this convention, the CT numbers of air and water are –1000 and 0, respectively. These images are typically displayed as $256 \times 256$ or $512 \times 512$ arrays, with pixels representing 0.5–2 mm of tissue, because of the high spatial resolution inherent in the measurements.[25,26]

## SPECT/CT and PET/CT

The integration of an emission tomography system (SPECT or PET) with a transmission tomography system (CT) into a single imaging unit sharing a common imaging table provides a significant advance in technology. Lang, Hasegawa, and colleagues[27] developed a prototype SPECT/CT imaging system using an array of solid-state detectors to acquire both the emission and transmission data. They subsequently integrated a commercial CT scanner and single-head SPECT camera to acquire sequential SPECT and CT scans using a common imaging table.[28] This work led to the introduction of the first commercially available SPECT/CT system.[29] At the same time, Townsend and colleagues integrated a commercially available PET scanner and CT scanner to provide sequential PET and CT scans using a common imaging table.[30,31] These works introduced a new era in nuclear medicine imaging. These combinations permit the acquisition of emission and transmission data sequentially in a single study with the patient in an ideally fixed position. Thus, the two data sets can be acquired in a registered format by appropriate calibrations, permitting the acquisition of corresponding slices from the two modalities. The CT data can then be used to correct for tissue attenuation in the emission scans on a slice-by-slice basis. Since the CT data are acquired in a higher resolution matrix than the emission data, it is necessary to decrease the resolution of the CT data to match that of the emission data. In other words, the CT data are blurred to match the emission data for attenuation correction.

One additional topic must be addressed in order to ensure the accuracy of the attenuation correction. The output of the x-ray tube used in CT provides a spectrum of photon energies from 0 keV up to the maximum photon energy (kVp = peak energy in keV) setting used for the acquisition as shown in Fig. I.1.16. Because low-energy photons are preferentially absorbed in tissue, the beam spectrum shifts toward the higher energy end as it passes through more tissue, thereby changing its effective $\mu$ and producing a variety of artifacts (beam-hardening effects) in images, and filtering of the beam to remove low-energy photons is required. The spectrum after filtering shown in Fig. I.1.16 has been "hardened" to reduce these effects. The resulting spectrum has an effective energy (mean) of approximately 70 keV in the example in Fig. I.1.16. Since attenuation effects vary with energy, it is necessary to convert the attenuation data acquired with CT to match the energy of the radionuclide used in the SPECT or PET acquisitions. For example in Fig. I.1.16, it is necessary to convert the attenuation data measured at an effective energy of 70–140 keV for $^{99m}$Tc. This is typically accomplished by using a bilinear model[32–34] relating attenuation coefficients at the desired energy to CT numbers measured at the effective energy of the CT beam of x-rays as shown in Fig. I.1.17. For CT numbers < 0, the measured tissue is assumed to be a combination of air and water, and the attenuation coefficient at the desired energy (140 keV) can be calculated from the CT number by the equation.

$$\mu_{tissue,140\,keV} = \frac{CT\# \ * \ (\mu_{water,140\,keV} - \mu_{air,140\,keV})}{1000}$$

This equation describes the first component of the bilinear curve in Fig. I.1.17. For CT numbers >0, the conversion is more complicated due to the measured tissue being a

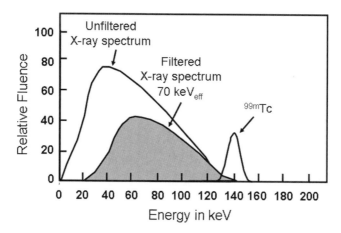

**Fig. I.1.16** Typical energy spectrum of x-rays from an x-ray tube. The shaded area shows the effects of filtration (beam hardening), which is used for CT scanning. These data can be used for attenuation correction of single photon emitters such as $^{99m}$Tc using the bilinear model shown in Fig. I.1.17 (Reprinted by permission of the Society of Nuclear Medicine from: James A. Patton and Timothy G. Turkington. SPECT/CT Physical Principles and Attenuation Correction. *J Nucl Med Technol* 2008 36(1):1–10. Fig. 7.)

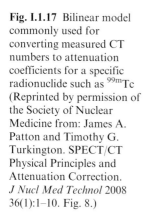

**Fig. I.1.17** Bilinear model commonly used for converting measured CT numbers to attenuation coefficients for a specific radionuclide such as $^{99m}$Tc (Reprinted by permission of the Society of Nuclear Medicine from: James A. Patton and Timothy G. Turkington. SPECT/CT Physical Principles and Attenuation Correction. *J Nucl Med Technol* 2008 36(1):1–10. Fig. 8.)

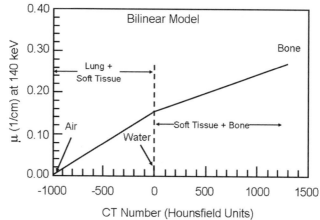

combination of water and bone. In this case, the attenuation coefficient at the desired energy (140 keV) can be calculated from the CT number by the equation

$$\mu_{tissue,\,140\,keV} = \mu_{water,\,140\,keV} + \frac{CT\# \, * \, \mu_{water,\,keVeff} * \left(\mu_{bone,\,140\,keV} - \mu_{water,\,140\,keV}\right)}{1000 * \left(\mu_{bone,\,keVeff} - \mu_{water,\,keVeff}\right)}$$

This equation describes the second component of the bilinear curve in Fig. I.1.17. In practice, the various attenuation coefficients for specific photon energy used in the SPECT or PET acquisition and the effective photon energy used in the CT acquisition can be found in a stored look-up table in the reconstruction algorithm. The conversion can then be performed using two simple linear relationships relating the attenuation coefficient at the desired energy and the measured CT numbers for specific measured tissues. From the attenuation coefficient data acquired with CT, correction factors can then be determined as shown in Fig. I.1.16, which can then be used to correct the SPECT or PET data (Fig. I.1.18) for attenuation, yielding the attenuation-corrected SPECT or PET images.[35,36]

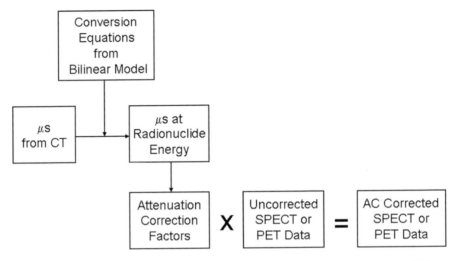

**Fig. I.1.18** Conversion equations from the bilinear model are used to convert attenuation coefficient values (ms) measured with CT to values corresponding to the energy of the radionuclide being imaged in order to determine factors for attenuation correction of SPECT or PET data

There are numerous advantages in the use of CT data for attenuation correction of emission data. First, the CT scan provides a very high photon flux which significantly reduces the statistical noise associated with the correction in comparison to other techniques (i.e., radionuclides used as transmission sources). Also, due to the fast acquisition speed of CT scanners, the total imaging time is significantly reduced by using this technology. Another advantage related to the high photon flux of CT scanners is that attenuation measurements can be made in the presence of radionuclide distributions with negligible contributions from photons emitted by the radionuclides (i.e., post-injection CT measurements can be performed). The use of CT also eliminates the need for additional hardware and transmission sources that often must be replaced on a routine basis. And, of course, the anatomical images acquired with CT can be fused with the emission images to provide functional anatomical maps for accurate localization of radiopharmaceutical uptake.

## Clinical SPECT/CT Systems

Clinical SPECT/CT systems currently available from manufacturers typically have dual-head scintillation cameras positioned in front of the CT scanner and sharing a common imaging table. There are two approaches to clinical SPECT/CT applications. The first approach is the use of a low-output, slow-acquisition CT scanner, the Hawkeye® with dual-head Infinia™ manufactured by General Electric Healthcare Systems. The CT scanner consists of a low-output x-ray tube (2.5 mA) and four linear arrays of detectors and can acquire four 5-mm anatomical slices in 13.6 s with a high contrast spatial resolution > 3 lp/cm. The images acquired with this system are not of sufficient quality to be used for billable procedures, but are sufficient to be used for attenuation correction and anatomical correlation with emission scans. The slow scan speed is actually an advantage in regions where there is physiological motion since the CT image blurring from the motion is comparable to that of the emission scans resulting in a good match in fused images. Radiation dose from this system is typically < 5 mGy (500 mrads) compared to values of 10–100 μGy (1–10 mrads) for applications using radioisotope transmission sources.

The second approach is to integrate commercially available CT scanners with dual-head scintillation cameras. The Symbia® with dual-head E-Cam manufactured by Siemens Medical Systems is available at present in one, two, and six slice versions with variable tube currents (20–345 mA), slice thicknesses of 0.6–10 mm, and rotational speeds of 0.6–1.5 s. The Precedence with dual-head Skylight manufactured by Philips Medical Systems is available in 16 and 64 slice versions with variable tube currents (20–500 mA), slice thicknesses of 0.6–12 mm, and rotational speeds as fast as 0.5 s. These systems exhibit high contrast spatial resolutions of 13–15 lp/cm with approximately 4–5 times the patient radiation dose of that from the Hawkeye® system. Since the CT scanners in the systems are commercially available diagnostic systems, the images produced are of sufficient quality to be used for billable procedures, in addition to the obvious attenuation correction and anatomical correlation applications. Radiation doses from these systems are on the order of 20 mGy (2 rads) when diagnostic quality images are produced. It should be noted that these systems can also be operated in a lower radiation dose mode by reducing the x-ray tube current. Although the images provided by this mode of operation typically are not of sufficient quality to be used for billable procedures, they are acceptable for attenuation correction and anatomical correlation applications.

## Clinical PET/CT Systems

Clinical PET/CT systems are only available with diagnostic CT scanners, and systems are generally acquired with 4, 8, 16, or 64 slice capability providing images of sufficient diagnostic quality to be used for billable procedures. As with SPECT/CT systems, the CT scanners can be operated at reduced tube current if the scans are only to be used for attenuation correction.

## Contrast Agents

Many diagnostic applications of CT scanning require the use of contrast agents administered either orally or intravenously to improve the visualization of soft tissue structures in the body. However, the use of a contrast CT scan for attenuation correction is a source of some concern. The introduction of a dense, high atomic number agent such as iodine increases the attenuation coefficients of the regions of tissue in which the contrast agent is located. This presence visually enhances the region in CT images by increasing the attenuation of the radiation beam in that region. However, when using the contrast CT scan for attenuation correction, the measured attenuation coefficients will be artificially increased potentially resulting in an artificial enhancement of the radionuclide distribution in the regions containing the contrast agent. In other words, the potential exists for the creation of artifacts of increased radionuclide uptake in those regions. For this reason, caution is indicated in the use of contrast CT scans for attenuation correction, and it is advised that the uncorrected SPECT or PET scan be carefully reviewed to insure that no artifacts have been created in the corrected images.

## *Beam-Hardening Artifacts*

It is not uncommon to see streak artifacts in CT scans in regions of the body containing dense bony structures. These artifacts are due to the preferential absorption of low-energy photons by the structures resulting in streaks of decreased photon flux in the final images. This phenomenon, known as beam hardening, is more severe in regions where metal objects such as surgical clips and prosthetic devices are present. In many instances, the presence of these artifacts will invalidate the use of the CT scan for attenuation correction in those regions.

## *Physiological Motion*

The accurate registration of a SPECT or PET scan with a CT scan depends on careful calibrations of the sequential data acquisition processes and assumes that there is no patient movement during the acquisitions. However, the natural physiological motion of the lungs and heart poses potential problems. These problems exist due to the fact that CT acquisitions are fast, i.e., images of multiple slices are acquired in less than a second, and SPECT and PET acquisitions are slow, i.e., several minutes per view. The relatively fast motion of the heart results in the motion being smoothed out in both data sets so that a reasonable registration is usually obtained. However, the slower motion of the lungs often results in a misregistration at the base of the lungs that can cause difficulty in the accurate localization of lesions in this area. PET/CT systems are now available with respiratory gating capability so that both the CT and the PET scan of the chest can accurately be registered by eliminating the effects of lung motion.

## *Radiation Dosimetry Considerations*

The replacement of conventional transmission sources with CT increases the concern regarding radiation dose to the patient. In the past, the radiation dose from transmission sources such as $^{153}$Gd used in SPECT and $^{68}$Ge used in PET was generally ignored due to the small values associated with their use in comparison to the dose from the radionuclides used in these studies. For example, the effective dose equivalent (EDE) for a PET transmission scan with $^{68}$Ge is on the order of 0.12 milli-Sieverts (mSv). However, when CT is used, the associated dose with this procedure is of such magnitude that it must be taken into consideration. The EDE for a diagnostic CT of the chest/abdomen/pelvis is on the order of 13 mSv assuming 140 kVp, 340 mA, 0.5 s rotation time, 5 mm slice, and 17.5 cm/s table feed. For comparison purposes, the EDE from a PET scan with 10 mCi of $^{18}$FDG is 11 mSv[37] and from a SPECT scan with 25 mCi of $^{99m}$Tc labeled white cells is 18.5 mSv.[37] Thus, the addition of the diagnostic CT increases the dose by 118% and 70%, respectively, in these two examples. If the CT scan is only to be used for attenuation correction, the tube current (mA) can be reduced by a factor of 4 or more, reducing the EDE to no more than 3.3 mSv. The attenuation measurement with CT would then increase the total EDE by only 30% and 18%, respectively, in the two examples. Every patient's study should be reviewed carefully prior to beginning the study in order that the CT acquisition parameters can be adjusted to achieve the desired data while minimizing radiation dose.

## Quality Assurance

In addition to the routine quality assurance procedures that are routinely performed with CT scanners and scintillation cameras with SPECT capability, it is important to routinely verify the accuracy of the registration techniques that are used with these combined systems. Errors in registration will cause inaccuracies in attenuation correction procedures and improper correlations of anatomy and function. All manufacturers recommend the scanning of an image registration phantom, such as the one shown in Fig. I.1.19, with recommended weekly or monthly frequencies. The phantom shown in Fig. I.1.19 has six radioactivity-filled syringes that are positioned along the three imaging axes. The phantom is scanned sequentially with the CT scanner, and scintillation camera and errors are calculated between the measured center locations of the syringes. These measurements are then compared with the acceptable errors for the system, typically 3–5 mm, in order to verify that the registration accuracy is sufficient for clinical applications. It may be important to do these measurements with substantial weight on the table to mimic the clinical situation.

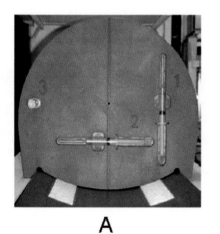
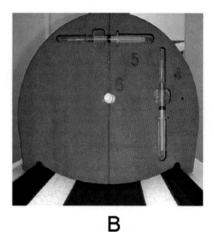

A                                                                    B

## CT – NM registration absolute values:

|  | X (mm) | Y (mm) | Z (mm) |
|---|---|---|---|
| Results | 0.39 | 0.61 | 1.36 |
| Acceptable Limits | 3.0 | 3.0 | 5.0 |

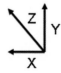

C

**Fig. I.1.19 (A–C)** Phantom used for quality assurance of the registration of images acquired with CT and SPECT in an integrated system (Reprinted by permission of the Society of Nuclear Medicine from: James A. Patton and Timothy G. Turkington. SPECT/CT Physical Principles and Attenuation Correction. *J Nucl Med Technol* 2008 36(1):1–10. Fig. 15.)

Currently, the most common application of attenuation correction techniques in nuclear medicine is cardiac perfusion imaging.[38] The use of an accurate attenuation correction can provide valuable information in making the correct diagnostic interpretation. However, slight misalignments of the transmission and emission scans, often due to patient motion, can result in artifacts in the attenuation-corrected images. Because of this potential problem, manufacturers typically provide correction software to adjust the alignment of the two data sets. An example of currently available attenuation correction quality control (ACQC) software provided by General Electric Healthcare Systems is shown in Fig. I.1.20. In Fig. I.1.20B, CT images of the myocardium in the standard three orthogonal views format are shown with the perfusion images fused to this data set and presented as contours typically set at 30% of maximum counts. In these images, there is an obvious misalignment that results in attenuation-corrected images with artifacts of decreased perfusion as shown in Fig. I.1.20A. Under cursor control, the data sets can be re-aligned in the three views resulting in correct alignment as shown in Fig. I.1.20D. This results in the production of accurate attenuation-corrected perfusion images (Fig. I.1.20C). This is a valuable quality assurance technique that should be used regularly to validate registration prior to final image reconstruction and display in order to increase the level of confidence of the inter-preting physician.[39]

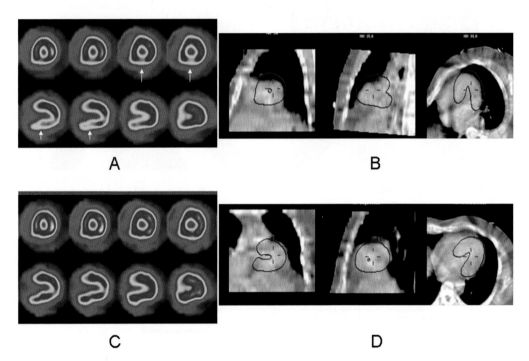

**Fig. I.1.20** Demonstration of the attenuation correction artifacts in a perfusion study (**A**) resulting from a misalignment of the CT and SPECT data sets (**B**) and the removal of these artifacts (**C**) after a re-alignment of the data sets (**D**) using registration quality assurance software (Reprinted by permission of the Society of Nuclear Medicine from: James A. Patton and Timothy G. Turkington. SPECT/CT Physical Principles and Attenuation Correction. *J Nucl Med Technol* 2008 36(1):1–10. Fig. 16.)

## Conclusions

The impact of the availability of hybrid imaging systems has been significant to diagnostic imaging. This impact is emphasized by the fact that during the past 2 years many scintillation cameras and most PET scanners have been purchased in combination with CT scanners in hybrid configurations. Clinicians now have the ability to image radiopharmaceutical distributions in registered format with anatomical images to accurately correlate function with anatomy and to improve image quality using the anatomical data for attenuation correction. This technology significantly improves the overall quality of the diagnostic information obtained and also provides data to improve therapeutic decisions thus enhancing patient care. The hybrid technology is now being extended to PET/MRI systems, and further advances are foreseen with this new capability.

# References

1. Anger HO, Rosenthal DJ. Scintillation camera and positron camera. In *Medical Radioisotope Scanning*. Vienna: International Atomic Energy Agency, 1959:59–75.
2. Kuhl DE, Edwards RQ. Image separation radioisotope scanning. *Radiology* 1963;80:653–662.
3. Kuhl DE, Edwards RQ. Cylindrical and section radioisotope scanning of the liver and brain. *Radiology* 1964;83:926–936.
4. Kuhl DE. A clinical radioisotope scanner for cylindrical and section scanning. In *Medical Radioisotope Scanning*, Vol. 1. Vienna: International Atomic Energy Agency, 1964:273–289.
5. Muehllehner G. A tomographic scintillation camera. *Phy Med Biol* 1971;16:87–96.
6. Keyes JW, Oleandea N, Heetderks WJ, Leonard PF, Rogers, WL. The humongotron: A scintillation camera transaxial tomography. *J Nucl Med* 1977;18:381–387.
7. Jaszczak RJ, Huard D, Murphy P, Burdine J. Radionuclide emission tomography with a scintillation camera. *J Nucl Med* 1976;17:551.
8. Galt JR, Germano G. Advances in instrumentation for cardiac SPECT. In DePuey EG, Berman DS, Garcia EV (eds): *Cardiac SPECT Imaging*. New York: Raven Press, 1995:91–102.
9. Garcia EV (ed). Imaging guidelines for nuclear cardiology procedures, part I. *J Nucl Cardiol* 1996;3:G3–45.
10. Shepp LA, Vardi Y. Maximum likelihood reconstruction for emission tomography. *IEEE Trans Med Imaging* 1982;MI-1:113–122.
11. Hudson HM, Larkin RS. Accelerated image reconstruction using ordered subsets of projection data. *J Nucl Med* 1994;13:601–609.
12. Muehllehner G, Buchin M, Dudek J. Performance parameters of a positron imaging camera. *IEEE Trans Nucl Sci* 1976;NS-23:528–537.
13. Patton JA. Instrumentation for coincidence imaging with multihead cameras. *Semin Nucl Med* 2000;30:239–254.
14. Robertson J, Marr R, Roseblurn B. Thirty-two crystal positron transverse section detector. In Freedman G (ed): *Tomographic Imaging in Nuclear Medicine*. New York: Society of Nuclear Medicine, 1973:151–153.
15. Burnham C, Brownell G. A multi-crystal positron camera. *IEEE Trans Nucl Sci* 1972;19:201–205.
16. Brownell G, Burnham C. MGH positron camera. In Freedman G (ed): *Tomographic Imaging in Nuclear Medicine*. New York: Society of Nuclear Medicine, 1973:154–164.
17. Ter-Pogossian MM, Phelps ME, Hoffman EJ, Mullani N. A positron-emission transaxial tomography for nuclear imaging (PETT). *Radiology* 1975;114:89–98.
18. Phelps ME, Hoffman E, Mullani N, Ter-Pogossian MM. Application of annihilation coincidence detection to transaxial reconstruction tomography. *J Nucl Med* 1975;16:210–224.
19. Phelps ME, Hoffman E, Mullani N, Higgins CS, Ter-Pogossian MM. Design considerations for a positron emission transaxial tomography (PETT III). *IEEE Trans Nucl Sci* 1976;NS-23:516–522.
20. Hoffman E, Phelps ME, Mullani N, Higgins CS, Ter-Pogossian MM. Design and performance characteristics of a whole body transaxial tomography. *J Nucl Med* 1976;17:493–503.
21. Phelps ME, Hoffman E, Huang S, Kuhl D. ECAT: A new computerized tomographic imaging system for positron emitting radiopharmaceuticals. *J Nucl Med* 1978;19:635–647.
22. Hoffman E, Ricci A, van der Stee LMAM, Phelps ME. ECATIII – Basic design considerations. *IEEE Trans Nucl Sci* 1983;NS-30:729–733.
23. Hounsfield G, Ambrose J. Computerized transverse axial scanning (tomography). Part I: Description of system. Part II: Clinical applications. *Br J Radiol* 1973;46:1016–1047.
24. McCormack A. Reconstruction of densities from their projections, with applications to radiological physics. *Phys Med Biol* 1973;18:195–207.
25. X-Ray Computed Tomography. In Bushberg JT, Seibert JA, Leidholdt, Jr. EM, Boone JM (eds): *The Essential Physics of Medical Imaging, Second Edition*. Philadelphia: Lippincott Williams & Wilkins, 2002:327–369.
26. Bruyant PP. Analytic and iterative reconstruction algorithms in SPECT. *J Nucl Med* 2002;43:1343–1358.
27. Lang TF, Hasegawa BH, Liew SC, Brown JK, Blankespoor S, Reilly SM, Gingold EL, Cann CE. A prototype emission-transmission imaging system. *IEEE Nucl Sci Symp Conf Rec* 1991;3:1902–1906.
28. Lang TF, Hasegawa BH, Liew SC, Brown JK, Blankespoor CS, Reilly SM, Gingold EL, Cann CE. Description of a prototype emission-transmission computed tomography imaging system. *J Nucl Med* 1992;33:1881–1887.

29. Patton JA, Delbeke D, Sandler MP. Image fusion using an integrated, dual-head coincidence camera with X-ray tube-based attenuation maps. *J Nucl Med* 2000;41:1364–1368.
30. Townsend DW, Beyer T, Kinahan PE, Brun T, Roddy R, Nutt R, Byars LG. The SMART scanner: A combined PET/CT tomography for clinical oncology. *IEEE Nucl Sci Symp Conf Rec*1998;2:170–1174, paper M5-1.
31. Beyer T, Townsend DW, Brun T, Kinahan PE, Charron M, Roddy R, Jerin J, Young J, Byars L, Nutt R. A combined PET/CT scanner for clinical oncology. *J Nucl Med* 2000;41:1369–1379.
32. Kinahan PE, Hasegawa BH, Beyer T. X-ray-based attenuation correction for positron mission tomography/computed tomography scanners. *Semin Nuc Med* 2003;33:166–179.
33. LaCroix KJ, Tsui BMW, Hasegawa BH, Brown JK. Investigation of the use of X-ray CT images for attenuation compensation in SPECT. *IEEE Trans Nucl Sci* 1994; NS-41:2793–2799.
34. Blankespoor SC, Xu X, Kalki CK, Brown JK, Tang HR, Cann CE, Hasegawa BH.Attenuation correction of SPECT using X-ray CT on an emission-transmission CT system: Myocardial perfusion assessment. *IEEE Trans Nucl Sci* 1996; NS-43:2263–2274.
35. Zaidi H, Hasegawa BH. Determination of the attenuation map in emission tomography. *J Nucl Med* 2003;44:291–315.
36. King MA, Glick SJ, Pretorius PH, Wells RG, Gifford HC, Narayanan MV, Farncombe T. Attenuation, scatter, and spatial resolution compensation in SPECT. In Wernick MN, Aarsvold JN (eds): *Emission Tomography: The Fundamentals of PET and SPECT*. London: Elsevier Academic Press, 2004:473–494.
37. Stabin, M, Stubbs JB, Toohey RE. *Radiation Dose Extimates for Radiopharmaceuticals*. Oak Ridge, TN: Radiation Internal Dose Information Center, ORNL, 1996.
38. Shaw LJ, Berman DS, Bax JJ, Brown KA, Cohen MC, Hendel RC, Mahmarian JJ, Williams KA, Ziffer JA. Computed tomographic imaging within nuclear cardiology, ASNC information statement – approved November 2004. *J Nucl Cardiol* 2005;12:131–142.
39. Tonge CM, Ellul G, Pandit M, Lawson RS, Shields RA, Arumugam P, Prescott MC. The value of registration correction in the attenuation correction of myocardial SPECT studies using low resolution computed tomography images. *Nucl Med Commun* 2006;27:843–852.

# Chapter I.2
# Normal Distribution, Variants, Pitfalls, and Artifacts

Ora Israel and Dominique Delbeke

## PET/CT Imaging with [18]F-Fluorodeoxyglucose

[18]F-fluorodeoxyglucose ([18]F-FDG) is an analog of glucose and therefore has a similar biodistribution. [18]F-FDG enters the cells by the same transport mechanism as glucose and is intracellularly phosphorylated by a hexokinase into [18]F-FDG-6-phosphate ([18]F-FDG-6-P). As an indicator of glucose metabolism, [18]F-FDG is not taken up only by malignant cells. In tissues with a low concentration of glucose-6-phosphatase, such as the brain, the myocardium, and most malignant cells, [18]F-FDG-6-P does not follow further enzymatic pathways and accumulates proportionally to the glycolytic cellular rate. Other tissues such as liver, kidney, intestine, muscle, and some malignant cells that exhibit variable degrees of glucose-6-phosphatase activity demonstrate lower levels of [18]F-FDG-6-P. Knowledge of the physiologic radiotracer biodistribution, normal patterns and variants, as well as benign conditions that accumulate [18]F-FDG are important for correct interpretation of clinical studies, mainly in cancer patients, as well as for other applications such as cardiology or infectious diseases.[1-3]

## *Normal [18]F-FDG Distribution and Physiologic Variants*

The cortex of the normal brain uses glucose as its substrate and cerebral [18]F-FDG activity is therefore physiologically high. In the region of the head and neck, normal [18]F-FDG uptake is identified in salivary glands including the submandibular and sublingual glands, the genioglossus and crico-arytenoid muscles, the lymphoid tissue of the Waldeyer's ring, and the vocal cords. Not infrequently, an [18]F-FDG positron emission tomography (PET) study will be the first test to demonstrate the presence of vocal cord paralysis, although the degree of hoarseness can often be quite modest. A paralyzed vocal cord typically has low uptake of [18]F-FDG, while intense uptake is seen in the remaining functional vocal cord and the controlling crico-arytenoid muscles.

The normal thyroid demonstrates only minimal [18]F-FDG uptake. Diffuse increased thyroid activity is seen mainly in thyroiditis, but also in Graves' disease, in patients with hypothyroidism receiving substitution treatment, or as a normal variant. Focal abnormal uptake in the thyroid is seen in ~1.5% of patients, is associated with malignancy in approximately one-third of cases, and therefore warrants further evaluation[4] (see Case II.4.4).

O. Israel (✉)
Department of Nuclear Medicine, Rambam Health Care Campus, Haifa, Israel; B. and R. Rappaport School of Medicine, Technion, Israel Institute of Technology, Haifa, Israel
e-mail: o_israel@rambam.health.gov.il

In the thorax, [18]F-FDG activity in the anterior upper mediastinum, mainly in young children during their first decade of life, represents physiologic thymic uptake. Increased [18]F-FDG activity can be also found along the esophagus, more common in its distal portion, best identified on sagittal views. Focal tracer uptake is more frequently seen at the gastro-esophageal junction and is difficult to differentiate from metastatic adenopathy, which is done mainly by the absence of lymph nodes corresponding to the sites of increased tracer uptake.

Myocardial [18]FDG uptake in normal subjects is variable and heterogeneous, related to serum glucose and free fatty acid (FFA) levels and the presence of associated conditions such as diabetes, or increased physical activity prior to administration of the radiotracer.[5] In cancer patients, intense cardiac [18]F-FDG uptake can obscure para-cardiac pathological foci. Prolonged fasting leads to a shift of cardiac substrate utilization from glucose to FFAs and thus reduces [18]F-FDG uptake in the heart. On the other hand, for evaluation of coronary artery disease, a glucose load is usually given to increase cardiac uptake of [18]F-FDG.

Abdominal uptake of [18]F-FDG related to the normal tracer biodistribution includes physiologic tracer activity within the gastrointestinal tract (GIT) of variable intensity and localization patterns. It is attributed to uptake by smooth muscles (mainly in the bowel), swallowed secretion, or excretion and intraluminal tracer concentration.[6,7] Moderate [18]F-FDG accumulation in the stomach, which involves as a rule the entire gastric wall, is more difficult to determine in a contracted stomach but relatively easy to identify following administration of oral contrast or water (negative contrast agent) for the computed tomography (CT) portion of the PET/CT study. Low intensity [18]F-FDG activity with a focal or diffuse pattern may be seen in the small bowel and the colon, potentially more prominent in the cecum, and is also related to abundant lymphoid tissue in the intestinal wall.[1] Uptake along the recto-sigmoid colon may appear focal on coronal images because of the antero-posterior organ orientation, but transaxial and sagittal images can identify the tubular pattern and avoid misinterpretation. Atypically located physiologic [18]F-FDG uptake in the GIT can be correctly localized by PET/CT to herniated bowel loops. However, precise PET/CT localization of [18]F-FDG foci to the GIT cannot differentiate between a physiologic or disease process.[8]

[18]F-FDG is excreted into the urine via the kidneys. Tracer accumulation in the renal collecting system, mainly when dilated, may obscure adjacent malignant sites or mimic suspicious lesions. Physiologic activity in the renal pelvis or ureter may be misinterpreted as nodal uptake on axial images because of its focal pattern. Viewing the sequence and continuity of uptake in cine mode and evaluation of coronal slices provide clarification in most cases. Placement of Foley catheters in the urinary bladder with irrigation, procedures recommended in the early days of [18]F-FDG imaging for optimized visualization of the pelvis, is rarely used since the introduction of hybrid PET/CT devices.

In the pelvis of female patients, unforeseen [18]F-FDG-avid sites located by the CT component to the uterus and ovaries should be assessed with knowledge of the age and mainly the menarchal status, specifically the phase of the menstrual cycle at the time of imaging. Premenopausal women can show physiologically increased endometrial [18]F-FDG uptake at mid-cycle, during the ovulatory phase, and at the menstrual flow phase, and physiologic ovarian uptake during the follicular, ovulatory, and the early luteal phase of the menstrual cycle (see Case II.12.1). After menopause, the probability of a malignant etiology of increased uterine or ovarian FDG uptake increases.[9,10]

In the resting state, there is only a low degree of [18]F-FDG uptake in the muscular system. In the region of the head and neck, uptake in laryngeal or masticatory muscles may mimic malignant foci. It is therefore important to keep the patient in a relaxed resting state, with no eating or talking during the uptake phase following injection of $^{18}$F-FDG. The linear pattern of the tracer uptake corresponding to muscles on PET/CT images excludes malignancy in the head and neck in most cases. In the torso, hyperventilation may increase uptake in the diaphragm, and anxiety-induced muscle tension increases uptake in the trapezius and paraspinal muscles.

Physiologic $^{18}$F-FDG uptake in brown adipose tissue (BAT) occurs predominantly in the younger age group and in females (see Case II.15.1). It is found more often in the head and neck region and less frequently in the thorax and infra-diaphragmatic in the pararenal and paracolic space. When the pattern of $^{18}$F-FDG uptake in BAT is asymmetric and focal, it can pose a diagnostic challenge. Localization of $^{18}$F-FDG activity to fatty tissue by PET/CT helps in understanding the etiology of the suspicious increased tracer focus.[8]

In the extremities, slightly increased $^{18}$F-FDG uptake that can be seen in the medial aspect of both thighs has been localized by PET/CT to blood vessels, either in vascular wall calcifications or due to some tracer retention within the blood pool. $^{18}$F-FDG uptake in the wall of large arteries increases in frequency with advancing age and has been observed in up to 60% of patients 50 years and older (see Case II.2.2). Significant accumulation of $^{18}$F-FDG can occur in selected muscular groups in the arms or legs following their recent increased use, and refraining from strenuous physical exercise during the 24 h prior to FDG imaging is therefore recommended.

## *Pitfalls and Artifacts on $^{18}$F-FDG Imaging*

If metal is detected on CT, attenuation-corrected PET images should be reviewed with caution and compared to the non-corrected data set. In areas adjacent to metal implants, attenuation-corrected PET images can show artifactual increased $^{18}$F-FDG activity. Disappearance or faint visualization of the $^{18}$F-FDG focus in the non-corrected images defines the artifactual nature of these findings. This occurs mostly in areas surrounding a metal hip or knee prosthetic implant, in the vicinity of metallic dental devices, and in the presence of a cardiac pacemaker implanted in the anterior upper chest wall. With improved attenuation correction algorithms, this pitfall has been partly solved. Increased $^{18}$F-FDG uptake adjacent to devices or implants unchanged between attenuation-corrected and uncorrected images may be related to the presence of a regional reactive inflammatory process adjacent to, for example, an intracholedocal stent or a thoracic port-a-cat. Detailed patient history and evaluation of CT images provide the differential diagnosis.

Misregistration can cause pitfalls in assessing the $^{18}$F-FDG avidity of pulmonary nodules or in defining precise localization of foci of increased tracer uptake in the region of the chest wall, due to motion and breathing artifacts. PET and CT acquisition can be performed with different breathing patterns, and imaging of the same anatomic region can occur during different parts of the breathing cycle for PET and CT. This pitfall is more significant for small lesions or those located at the base of the thorax where respiratory artifacts are more prominent and can be overcome by acquisition protocols using respiratory gating.

Misregistration due to even slight movements of the head (or foot) in various directions between the PET and CT acquisition can affect precise localization of $^{18}$F-FDG-avid foci. The same position on both sets of images is sometimes achieved by fixation of the organ during imaging using a hardware accessory.

Misregistration between PET and CT images in the abdomino-pelvic region can potentially result in superimposition of [18]F-FDG foci on faulty anatomic structures. It is caused mainly by changes in content with subsequent variations in distention of organs such as the stomach, bowel, or urinary bladder, or to a lesser extent due to shifting following bowel peristalsis and movement.

If difficulties are encountered at the time of tracer administration, extravasation into the soft tissues at the site of injection leads to radioisotope accumulation in draining healthy lymph nodes due to lymphatic reabsorption. [18]F-FDG should be injected through an intravenous catheter, and, when the study is performed for staging malignancies such as melanoma or breast cancer, in the arm opposite the primary lesion. Regional nodal uptake ipsilateral to the injection site should be interpreted with caution. The axillae are better evaluated with the arms positioned above the head.

## *Benign Processes Accumulating [18]F-FDG*

Any acute injury to soft tissues results in an inflammatory response associated with high uptake of [18]F-FDG by activated macrophages. A careful medical history and physical examination can avoid misinterpretation of [18]F-FDG related to inflammation such as acute arthritis in synovial joints or granulomatous processes such as tuberculosis[11] or sarcoidosis[12] among others.

New nodal [18]F-FDG-avid foci may represent a reactive process to a concurrent infection and is more common in the head and neck, axillary, and inguinal regions. On the other hand, recurrent uptake in nodes that were involved by cancer at presentation is more suspicious for relapse.

Recent rib fractures have intense tracer uptake, which tends to fade as the fracture heals. With complete healing, [18]F-FDG uptake disappears in most non-pathological rib fractures. Benign bone lesions such as fibrous dysplasia or osteomyelitis may also appear hypermetabolic. Degenerative changes and osteophytes can show mild to moderately increased tracer uptake in 15–20% of cases (see Case II.6.3). The CT component evaluated with bone and soft tissue windows can identify non-malignant skeletal lesions.[13]

In the thorax, post-obstructive pneumonitis may be confusing but should not be interpreted as tumor extension (see Case II.3.10). In the abdomino-pelvic region, benign [18]F-FDG-avid processes in the bowel include diverticulitis or adenoma of the rectum and sigmoid colon[1] (see Case II.3.7). Up to 18% of benign fibroid uterine tumors and leiomyoma, as well as benign ovarian lesions such as follicular ovarian cysts and hemorrhagic corpus luteus, are [18]F-FDG-avid.[14] Pelvic abscesses can be a major source for diagnostic errors with PET/CT because of their high [18]F-FDG avidity and the mass effect on CT. Foreign body reactions associated with an intra-uterine device also show increased [18]F-FDG uptake.

## *Treatment-Related Processes Accumulating [18]F-FDG*

Various treatment-related processes demonstrate increased [18]F-FDG activity, more common after surgery or radiation therapy. In the region of the head and neck, surgery can be complex and include partial removal of organs, often followed by radiotherapy to the same region. Knowledge of the surgical procedure and of the radiation port can help in understanding asymmetrical increased [18]F-FDG uptake.

In the chest, in patients receiving radiation treatment, a linear increased [18]F-FDG uptake located on CT along the esophagus may be consistent with radiation esophagitis. Paramediastinal geographically shaped [18]F-FDG uptake of mild intensity in the radiation port is very common in the weeks and months immediately following treatment due to radiation-induced inflammation and should not be misinterpreted as residual cancer (see Cases II.3.8 and II.3.9).

Pleurodesis is a procedure that generates an intense inflammatory process in the pleural space in order to minimize the accumulation of pleural effusions. Talc is also radiodense. PET/CT findings after pleurodesis are characterized by increased [18]F-FDG uptake and high density foci on CT located in the pleural space, representing the inflammatory reaction to talc. This procedure can mimic asbestos-induced calcified pleural plaques or mesothelioma, differentiated only by an individual patient's clinical history.

Mild to moderate [18]F-FDG activity may be seen at biopsy sites and along recent or infected surgical incisions for at least 6–8 weeks after the procedure and may disappear within a few months (see Case II.13.2). Increased tracer uptake in sites of colostomy has a diffuse, low-intensity pattern. Focal sites of higher intensity should raise the suspicion of cancer if, for example, they are located in nodules detected on the CT component and need to be further assessed.[15–18]

Increased [18]F-FDG activity may persist at tumor sites for several weeks following successful chemotherapy and for several months following radiation therapy, including radioimmunotherapy.

Thymic uptake can appear as a result of rebound thymic hyperplasia after chemotherapy, more common in older children and young adults. It needs to be differentiated from [18]F-FDG-avid mediastinal site of malignancy. The classic "inverted Y" shape of the thymus and comparison to the pre-treatment study can assist in differentiating between the two causes of uptake.[19,20]

Following granulocyte colony-stimulating factor (G-CSF) treatment, diffuse [18]F-FDG uptake of varying intensity occurs in the skeleton and in an enlarged spleen and decreases at approximately 1 month after completion of therapy. G-CSF-related intramedullary uptake should not be misinterpreted as malignant bone marrow involvement.[21]

## Summary

In order to avoid misinterpretation of [18]F-FDG-avid foci, it is very important to standardize the patient preparation prior to the study and the environment during the uptake period. The patients should be questioned and examined for post-operative findings or implants. Imaging at an appropriate timing after invasive procedures and therapeutic interventions is imperative. A 4-h fasting period is recommended including no consumption of beverages with sugar and no intravenous dextrose. Drinking water should be encouraged to keep the patient hydrated and promote diuresis that will limit artifacts from the renal collecting system and radiation exposure to the bladder. During the distribution phase, the patient should be relaxed and avoid talking, chewing, and any muscular activity.

## Physiologic Distribution of Other PET Tracers

### *[18]F-Fluoride*

[18]F-fluoride is a PET imaging tracer of the skeleton. Following rapid clearance from the blood and diffusion into the extracellular bone, fluid [18]F-fluoride is absorbed on the bone surface, forming fluoroapatite compounds. It was introduced as a bone-seeking imaging agent almost 50 years ago. Skeletal uptake of [18]F-fluoride is proportional to regional blood flow and bone turnover and is similar to that of [99m]Tc-diphosphonates agents. The normal pattern of [18]F-fluoride includes, therefore, uniform and homogenous uptake throughout the axial and appendicular skeleton. The kidneys and urinary bladder are visualized because of the urinary excretion of the radiotracer. Tracer uptake is increased in benign and malignant skeletal lesions, characterized by increased regional blood flow, high capillary permeability, and increased bone turnover. Whereas the mechanism of uptake for [18]F-fluoride is similar to that for other bone-imaging radiopharmaceuticals,[22] images are of higher quality due to the superior spatial resolution of the PET technology as compared to both planar and single photon emission computed tomography (SPECT) imaging using the [99m]Tc-radiopharmaceuticals.

   [18]F-fluoride is further addressed in Chapter III.2 (see Case III.2.4).[23,24]

### *[18]F-Fluorothymidine*

Malignant tumors are characterized by increased cell proliferation, which is responsible for their accelerated growth. DNA synthesis is a measure of proliferation, and thymidine is one of the main nucleotides required for this process. 3'-Deoxy-3'-fluoro thymidine ([18]F-FLT) is a derivative of thymidine used as a PET imaging tracer of DNA synthesis and, thus, an indicator of tumor grade and aggressiveness. Following its intracellular incorporation, [18]F-FLT is phosphorylated to [18]F-FLT-monophosphate and further to [18]F-FLT-triphosphate, which is metabolically trapped inside the cell. Uptake and retention of [18]F-FLT are dependent on phosphorylation by thymidine kinase but not on incorporation into DNA. [18]F-FLT is a preferential substrate for cytosolic thymidine kinase 1 (TK1) rather than the mitochondrial isozyme (TK2), which is important, since TK2 is maintained at low basal levels in all cells, while TK1 is increased up to tenfold in proliferating cells compared to those in a resting state.

   In the early 1990s, Higashi and colleagues[25] demonstrated in vitro that uptake of [18]F-FLT correlates with the tumor proliferative rate. Uptake of [18]F-FLT is lower compared to [18]F-FDG, but with a significant linear correlation.[26]

   [18]F-FLT does not cross the blood–brain barrier, and, therefore, uptake in the normal brain is only minimal, allowing easy imaging of high-grade cerebral tumors.[27] Whereas thymidine is retained in the myocardium due to the presence of TK2, this is not the case for [18]F-FLT because of the specificity of [18]F-FLT for TK1.[28] There is little uptake in normal organs in the chest including the myocardium. [18]F-FLT is therefore an useful agent for evaluation of malignancies of the chest.[26,29]

   [18]F-FLT uptake in the liver and bone marrow is higher as compared to [18]F-FDG. In the liver, there is retention of [18]F-FLT during glucuronidation. The marrow takes up [18]F-FLT because of its normal proliferative activity. [18]F-FLT is excreted by the kidneys, and therefore its use for evaluation of malignancies of the kidneys and bladder is limited.[30]

[18]F-FLT may be more specific than [18]F-FDG for detection of malignancy because of less retention in inflammatory cells. A study in mice with a sterile inflammatory lesion caused by turpentine demonstrated inflamed muscle-to-normal muscle uptake ratio of 4.8 with [18]F-FDG and 1.3 with FLT.[31] However, this was not confirmed in a study of patients with head and neck cancers in which both [18]F-FDG and [18]F-FLT gave comparable results for detection of malignancies and inflammatory lesions.[32]

## [18]F-Fluorocholine and [11]C-Choline

Radiolabeled choline tracers are PET imaging agents of membrane lipid synthesis.[33,34] Choline is a precursor for phospholipid biosynthesis, mainly lecithin, a principal component of cell membranes. Malignant cells characterized by a high proliferation rate need large amounts of phospholipids and will therefore demonstrate high uptake of choline. Inflammatory, infectious, and benign proliferative processes accumulate radiolabeled choline.

[11]C-choline has a very rapid blood clearance of approximately 7 min. Most of the tracer remains trapped within the cells, providing images of good diagnostic quality. There is minimal physiologic tracer uptake in organs, such as the brain and the myocardium, and moderate hepatic and pancreatic retentions. As [11]C-choline has minimal urinary excretion, it is a better tool in evaluation of bladder and prostate malignancies. PET images are, however, acquired, starting from the pelvis 3–5 min post-injection of [11]C-choline before even minimal excretion into the ureters and bladder occurs. [11]C-choline PET/CT has a higher accuracy as compared to PET stand-alone.

[18]F-Fluorocholine derivatives have also been synthesized. In addition to high liver, pancreas, and bowel activity, fluorocholine undergoes urinary excretion. However, the rapid blood clearance allows early imaging of the prostate before the tracer arrives to the bladder. The toxicity of fluorocholine may limit its use in humans.

These tracers have been suggested for imaging of malignant brain and prostate tumors. [11]C-choline is hampered by the short physical half-life of the radioisotope and by its rapid in vivo oxidation. [11]C-choline, including normal distribution, is further addressed in the evaluation of malignancies of the urinary tract, prostate, and testicular cancer in Chapter II.9 (see Cases II.9.3 through II.9.6).[35,36]

## [11]C-Acetate

[11]C-acetate has been first used to assess the oxidative metabolism of the myocardium. Possible biochemical pathways that lead to accumulation of [11]C-acetate in tumors include its entry into the Krebs cycle from acetyl coenzyme A (acetyl CoA) or as an intermediate metabolite; esterification to form acetyl CoA as a major precursor in β-oxidation for fatty acid synthesis; combining with glycine in heme synthesis; and through the use of citrate for cholesterol synthesis. Among these possible metabolic pathways, participation in FFA (lipid) synthesis is believed to be the dominant method of incorporation into tumors.

Radiolabeled acetate accumulates in tissues with high levels of anabolic metabolism such as the pancreas. Blood pool tracer activity clears within 2 min after administration, and tumor visualization nears maximal levels within about 5 min post-tracer injection, with very slow clearance of retained tracer thereafter. The pancreas is the only abdominal organ with consistently high uptake, with only variable uptake of moderate intensity in the liver and portions of the bowel. Activity clears from the renal parenchyma within 10 min after injection due to oxidation to carbon dioxide, and there is little appreciable urinary excretion.[37] Acetate can therefore be useful for imaging of renal, bladder, and prostate malignancies.[38] It has also been shown helpful for evaluation of hepatocellular carcinoma. [11]C-acetate is further addressed in Chapter II.7 (see Case II.7.1) and Chapter II.9 (see Case II.9.4).

## [11]C-Methionine

Assessment of amino-acid transport and protein metabolism is possible with [11]C-methionine. Methionine is taken up proportional to the amino-acid transport and is primarily metabolized in the liver and pancreas with no significant renal excretion. [11]C-methionine is used more commonly in Europe than in the United States. It has some advantages over [18]F-FDG for evaluation of cerebral tumors, for example, because of the low physiologic background uptake in the cortex. It has also been investigated for evaluation of prostate cancer.[39]

[11]C-methionine is further addressed in Chapter II.1 (see Case II.1.9) and in Chapter II.9.

## [18]F-Fluorodopamine

[18]F-Fluorodopamine ([18]F-FDOPA) is a PET imaging tracer of amino-acid transport and protein synthesis. Development of malignant tumors requires an increase in protein synthesis, which requires an increased amount of amino-acids. Their intracellular transport can therefore be a measure of the degree of protein synthesis. Tyrosine, among other amino-acids, is retained in tumor cells, which have a higher metabolic activity than that of normal tissues. Dopamine is synthesized from tyrosine. [18]F-FDOPA has been initially developed to assess dopamine precursors from the blood and their distribution in the brain. It is also taken up by malignancies such as melanoma and neuroendocrine tumors such as medullary thyroid cancer (MTC) and pheochromocytoma.[40] The pancreas demonstrates high [18]F-FDOPA uptake, and moderate activity is seen in the liver and spleen. In normal extrachromaffin organs, such as the pancreas, liver, and spleen, there is a decrease in uptake of approximately 50% between 10–20 min and 60–90 min post-administration.[41] [18]F-FDOPA is excreted by the kidneys. There is no bone marrow uptake of this tracer.[42]

## [18]F-Fluoromisonidazole

[18]F-fluoromisonidazole ([18]F-FMISO) is a PET tracer for imaging of hypoxia in malignant tumors. Hypoxia develops in large tumors because of the inability of tumor vessels to supply the oxygen demands of growing number of tumor cells. While hypoxia inhibits further cell division and can lead to cell death, it can also induce the appearance of adaptive processes for cell survival, with subsequent development of tumor progression and resistance to treatment. Well-oxygenated tumor cells are more sensitive to radiation as compared to hypoxic cells. [18]F-FMISO is metabolized by the liver and excreted by the kidneys and bladder, thus with high physiologic tracer uptake in these

organs, as well as in the bowel, most probably due to the presence of intraluminal anaerobic bacteria. Lung, myocardium, brain, and bone show a low degree of uptake. Because [18]F-FMISO binds selectively to hypoxic cells, it has been used for determining their presence and quantifying their amount in malignancies such as lung, brain, and head and neck tumors.[43,44]

## [68]Ga-Somatostatin Receptors

The conventional SPECT radiopharmaceutical for detection of somatostatin receptors, [111]In-diethylenetriaminepentaacetic acid (DTPA)-octreotide ([111]In-pentetreotide), binds preferentially to subtypes II and V receptors. DOTA-Tyr3-octreotide (DOTATOC) has improved binding affinity, internalization rate, and selectivity for somatostatin receptor II, and DOTA-1-NaI-octreotide (DOTANOC) has a broader somatostatin receptor subtype profile. These DOTA compounds have been labeled with [111]In, [68]Ga, and [90]Y for diagnostic and therapeutic applications.

The normal biodistribution of [68]Ga-Somatostatin receptors is similar to that of [111]In-DTPA-octreotide. These newer somatostatin analogs, DOTATOC and DOTANOC, have improved pharmacokinetics, faster tumor uptake, and more rapid clearance, resulting in an increased tumor-to-background contrast and improved tumor visualization. Labeling with the [68]Ga positron-emitting radioisotope adds the advantages of high-resolution imaging with enhanced lesion detectability and the ability to quantitate tracer uptake for planning and monitoring peptide receptor (see Case II.11.8).

## Physiologic Distribution of SPECT/CT Imaging Tracers

### [131]I- and [123]I-Iodine ([131]I and [123]I)

Although radioactive iodine is only poorly concentrated by most extrathyroidal tissues, physiologic uptake can be encountered in the salivary glands, the genitourinary system (mainly in the urinary bladder), the GIT (most commonly in the stomach and bowel), and the liver. Because no clear reference landmarks can be recognized on planar [131]I-scintigraphy, differentiating cancer-related uptake from sites of physiologic tracer activity or contamination requires accurate localization of radioiodine-avid sites. Localization of these foci may constitute a particular problem when surgical removal of metastases is indicated, especially when they are small or occur in regions exhibiting distorted anatomy due to previous surgery, and can be in most cases readily differentiated by SPECT/CT.[45]

Although radioiodine uptake is highly specific for thyroid tissue, a variety of false positive findings have been reported. These can rarely represent malignant foci of non-thyroid origin, such as small-cell lung cancer. Thymus can take up radioiodine in children and young adults. Pitfalls related to focal [131]I uptake have been related to physiologic activity in normal organs with distorted anatomy, in inflammatory processes, and in artifactual contamination of the skin (see Chapter II.10. and Cases II.10.1 and II.10.3).[46]

## $^{131}I$- and $^{123}I$-MIBG

Radioiodinated meta-iodo-benzylguanidine ($^{131}I$- and $^{123}I$-MIBG) is a SPECT imaging tracer for tumors that arise from adrenergic tissue, such as pheochromocytoma, neuroblastoma, and paraganglioma. Radioiodinated MIBG is taken up by chromaffin catecholamine storage granules because of its structural similarity to norepinephrine and transported into storage vesicles that are found in all organs with adrenergic innervation, as well as in the above-mentioned specific tumor types. Intravesicular $^{123}I$-MIBG is not subject to further metabolism, and this is the basis for performing scintigraphy of the tracer taken up by disease processes.

Physiologic uptake of radioiodinated MIBG is demonstrated in the normal salivary glands, thyroid, lungs, heart, liver, bowel, uterus, and prostate.[47] The excretory pathways of the tracer include the kidneys and urinary bladder. Faint physiologic uptake may also be observed in normal functioning adrenal glands. Despite recent optimization in acquisition and processing protocols, interpretation of radioiodinated MIBG scintigraphy is challenging. Foci of increased tracer uptake in locations other than the normal biodistribution are suspicious for the presence of disease. False positive studies are mainly due to artifactual findings.

SPECT/CT may be of value both in defining the pathological nature of a suspicious focus as well as to exclude the presence of disease. Physiological tracer uptake in sites of the normal tracer biodistribution may be of low intensity but nevertheless difficult to differentiate from pathology related to early, small tumor-load stages of disease, or to residual viable tumor after treatment. Precise SPECT/CT localization of a low-intensity uptake focus in areas with congruent structural disease-related changes may be of help for the final characterization of equivocal scintigraphic radioiodinated MIBG findings.[48,49]

MIBG is further addressed in the evaluation of endocrine tumors (see Cases II.11.4 and II.11.5) and pediatric malignancies (see Case II.15.5) in Chapters II.11 and II.15, respectively.

## $^{111}In$-DTPA-Octreotide

$^{111}In$-DTPA-octreotide ($^{111}In$-pentetreotide) is a SPECT tracer to image somatostatin receptor positive neuroendocrine tumors. It binds preferentially to somatostatin receptor subtypes II and V. Detection of all tumor sites is critical for referring patients to surgery and for its optimal planning.

$^{111}In$-DTPA-octreotide uptake has been demonstrated in physiological sites as well as benign conditions unrelated to neuroendocrine tumors. This is due to the high receptor status of normal organs, such as the pituitary gland, thyroid, liver, and spleen, or to the physiological excretion of the tracer via the kidneys or the bowel. Hepatobiliary excretion, accounting for 2% clearance of the administered dose, may lead to occasional visualization of the gallbladder, which can be misinterpreted as hepatic metastases.[50]

Imaging protocols recommend performing delayed studies that may demonstrate changes in tracer kinetics and provide the differential diagnosis between benign/physiologic and malignant sites of radiotracer uptake. Neuroendocrine tumors often arise in the abdomen and it is often difficult to precisely localize a suspicious lesion to organs such as the pancreas, small bowel, liver, or bone, without anatomic correlation. In the region of the liver, it is difficult to distinguish physiologic gallbladder accumulation from a lesion in the head of the pancreas, the right adrenal, or the small bowel. Foci of increased [111]In-DTPA-octreotide activity have been described in benign processes such as scar after recent surgery or colostomy, increased thyroid uptake in Graves' disease, accessory spleen, renal parapelvic cysts, and granulomatous lung processes need also to be differentiated from disease-related lesions. [1,51]

[111]In-DTPA-octreotide is further addressed in the evaluation of thyroid cancer (see Case II.10.5) and endocrine tumors (see Cases II.11.1, II.11.2, and II.11.3) in Chapters II.10 and II.11, respectively.

## [99m]Tc-Sestamibi

[99m]Tc-hexa-2-methoxyisobutylisonitrile ([99m]Tc-Sestamibi) is a lipophilic cation used for both myocardial and tumor imaging. The distribution of [99m]Tc-Sestamibi is proportional to blood flow, and, once intracellular, it is sequestrated primarily within the mitochondria in response to the electrical potential generated across the membranes. There is no tracer uptake in the normal brain. In the head and neck, there is physiological uptake in the salivary glands and normal thyroid gland. The uptake in the thyroid gland washes out over time, whereas there is retention in parathyroid adenoma. Therefore, dual phase imaging allows detection of parathyroid adenoma. There is homogenous uptake in the normal myocardium. Physiological uptake in the GIT, liver, and gallbladder can make interpretation of myocardial perfusion studies difficult.

[99m]Tc-Sestamibi is further addressed in the evaluation of endocrine tumors (see Cases II.11.6 and II.11.7) in Chapter II.11.

## [111]In- and [99m]Tc-HMPAO-Leucocytes (WBC)

Radiolabeled WBCs using either [99m]Tc-hexamethyl-propyleneamine oxime (HMPAO) or [111]In are SPECT tracers for imaging of acute and chronic infections. [111]In forms a lipophilic complex with oxine, a chelating agent that allows penetration of the WBC membranes. [111]In oxine does not preferentially seek out neutrophils, and therefore labels all types of cells. For this reason, leukocytes must be separated from the plasma prior to labeling. Intracellular [111]In oxine disassociates, [111]In binds to nuclear and cytoplasmic proteins, and the oxine then diffuses out of the cell. [99m]Tc-HMPAO is a lipophilic complex that easily penetrates cell membranes. After entering the WBC, this complex becomes hydrophilic, which, in turn, traps it within the cell. The labeling process is similar to [111]In labeling. Labeled WBCs subsequently localize in regions of inflammation/infection via the expected pathophysiologic mechanisms.

The biodistribution of radiolabeled WBCs is similar when using any of the radioisotopes, with activity concentrating mostly in the spleen, followed by uptake in the liver, bone marrow, and lungs. In addition, [99m]Tc-HMPAO-WBC will also commonly have nonspecific bowel, urinary, and gallbladder activity, which may be the result of excretion of secondary hydrophilic complexes of [99m]Tc-HMPAO. Bowel activity may be due to biliary excretion and appears in all patients at 24 h. Gallbladder activity is seen in less than 10% of patients. The time to image [99m]Tc-HMPAO-WBC is, in part, dependent on the type and location of a suspected infection.

Clinical indications for labeled WBC scintigraphy include osteomyelitis, especially in patients with complicated bones, when an infected joint prosthesis or following fracture is suspected. Labeled WBC scintigraphy has been also used in suspected vascular graft infections, diabetic foot, and abdominal infections.

[111]In-WBC is further addressed in the evaluation of infectious processes (see Cases III.3.1, III.3.2, and III.3.3) in Chapter III.3.

## [67]Ga-Citrate

[67]Ga is a SPECT tracer used at present mainly for imaging of infectious and inflammatory processes. Several shortcomings have led to the continuous decrease in the use of this agent, such as the spatial resolution capabilities of current technology for detection of small lesions, the physiologic biodistribution of this radiotracer, and nonspecific increased [67]Ga uptake in various processes. In addition, uncertainty in the anatomic localization of foci of increased tracer activity due to the lack of clear anatomic details hampers their characterization as normal or abnormal findings.

After intravenous administration of carrier-free [67]Ga, it is bound to the iron-binding plasma protein, transferrin. It is postulated that the high metabolic activity of malignant cells demands a high iron supply and therefore an increased density of transferrin receptors, thus explaining the increased [67]Ga accumulation in malignant versus benign tumors. Unfortunately, this binding of [67]Ga to plasma transferrin and lactoferrin, another plasma protein, also leads to delayed plasma clearance and to physiologic uptake in liver, spleen, bone marrow, breasts, nasal mucosa, and lacrimal and salivary glands. Physiologic lacrimal and salivary gland [67]Ga activity may become asymmetric and increase in intensity in inflammatory or obstructive processes, after unilateral resection or radiation therapy. While the mediastinum is a common site of involvement by various disease processes, hilar [67]Ga uptake of benign etiology has been described in up to one-third of mainly elderly patients and in the thymus in young children or in rebound hyperplasia after chemotherapy. In the abdomen and pelvis, physiologic [67]Ga activity in organs such as the liver and spleen, and its excretion via the urinary and more prominently the GIT, make this area especially difficult for interpretation. [67]Ga is also a bone-seeking agent, taken up by various skeletal lesions, not necessarily of malignant origin, such as bone fractures or degenerative changes. The benign pattern of increased radiotracer uptake in metabolically active brown fat has been recognized by PET/CT with [18]F-FDG, followed by SPECT/CT identifying its occurrence with [67]Ga as well.

[67]Ga-citrate is further addressed in the evaluation of soft tissue and skeletal infectious processes (see Cases III.3.1, III.3.2, and III.3.4) in Chapter III.3.

## [111]In-ProstaScint®

Capromab pendetide (ProstaScint®) is an Food and Drug Administration-approved [111]In-labeled murine IgG antibody to an intracellular component of the prostatic specific membrane antigen (PSMA). Although scintigraphy is difficult to interpret, preliminary results indicate that the sensitivity for the detection of pelvic nodal metastases either prior to surgery or after prostatectomy is much higher than with CT. ProstaScint® scintigraphy, including both planar and SPECT, has not gained wide acceptance for imaging of prostate cancer. A considerable amount of expertise is required to interpret these studies because of significant nonspecific binding and high blood pool and marrow activity, leading to a low target-to-background ratio. ProstaScint® uptake has been demonstrated in the GIT and bladder. Concurrent $^{99m}$Tc-RBC imaging is often utilized to differentiate retained vascular activity from pathological nodal activity. Fused SPECT/CT images are more useful and should be performed routinely.

## Case Presentations

### Case I.2.1 (DICOM Images on DVD)

**History**

This 20-year-old male with a history of Hodgkin's disease stage III who has completed chemotherapy 6 months earlier was referred to $^{18}$F-FDG PET/CT to assess response to therapy (Fig. I.2.1A–E).

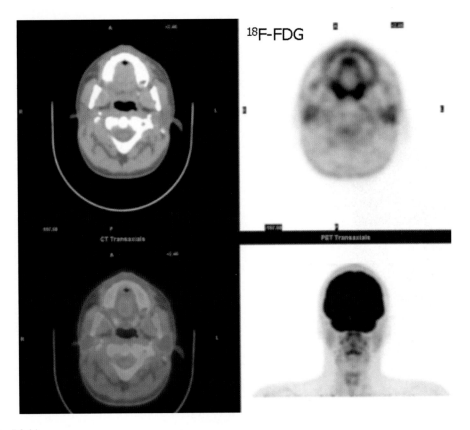

**Fig. I.2.1A**

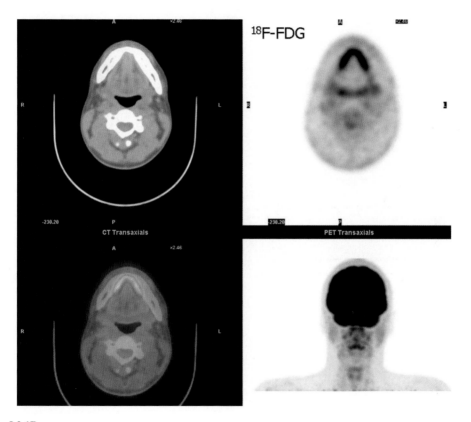

**Fig. I.2.1B**

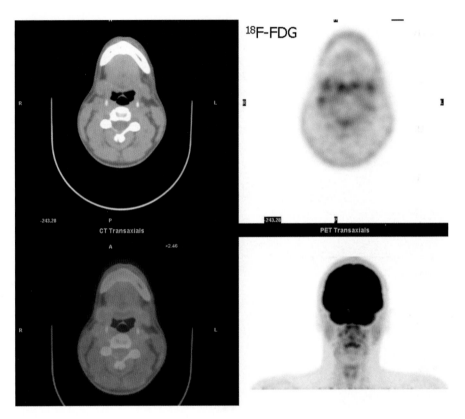

**Fig. I.2.1C**

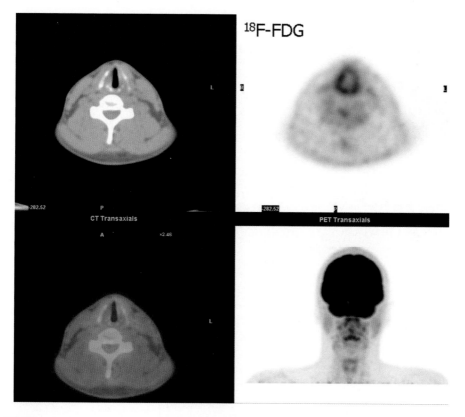

**Fig. I.2.1D**

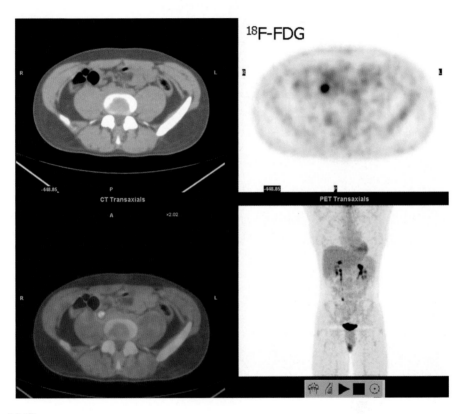

**Fig. I.2.1E**

**Findings**

There is normal distribution of [18]F-FDG in the lymphoid and glandular tissue of the head and neck. Radiotracer uptake is identified in the parotid glands (Fig. I.2.1A), lingular tonsils (Fig. I.2.1A and B), sublingual (Fig. I.2.1B) and submandibular glands (Fig. I.2.1C), and laryngeal muscles (Fig. I.2.1D). In addition, there is moderate uptake in a subcentimeter right level II lymph node (Fig. I.2.1C), most consistent with an inflammatory process.

On images of the torso, there is mild uptake in the myocardium as expected in a fasting patient and in the GIT. There is physiological tracer uptake in the kidneys, renal collecting system, and bladder as a result of renal [18]F-FDG excretion. Fusion images at the level of the upper pelvis (Fig. I.2.1E) demonstrate that the focal uptake in the mid-right abdomen corresponds to the location of the right ureter and is due to focal pooling of urine, with no lesion on CT.

**Discussion**

It is important to be familiar with the physiological distribution of [18]F-FDG and its variations. The lymphoid and glandular tissues of the neck demonstrate, as a rule, higher activity in young individuals. There is uptake in muscles in the neck, more prominent when activated, such as the laryngeal muscles of this patient, who was probably talking during the uptake phase. Fusion images help differentiate physiological versus pathological uptake, especially when unilateral or in patients with distorted anatomy who underwent surgery. For example, Fig. I.2.1F shows images of a different patient referred for initial staging of

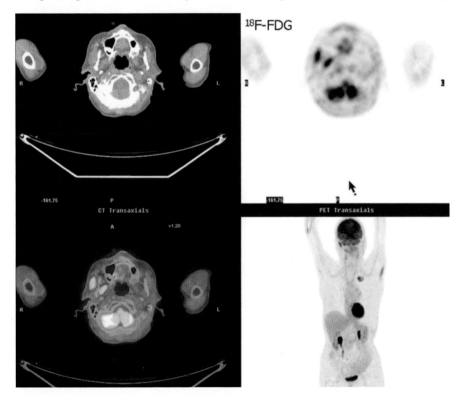

**Fig. I.2.1F**

non-small-cell lung carcinoma who has unilateral uptake in the right masseter and pterygoid muscles probably due to chewing during the uptake phase. Focal radiotracer uptake in the left upper lobe: primary lung cancer is seen on the maximum intensity projection (MIP) image.

### Diagnosis

1. Normal $^{18}$F-FDG distribution.
2. No evidence of residual Hodgkin's disease.

### Clinical Report: Body $^{18}$F-FDG PET/CT Imaging (for DVD cases only)

Indication

Restaging of lymphoma

History

This 20-year-old male with a history of Hodgkin's disease stage III has completed chemotherapy 6 months earlier and is referred to $^{18}$F-FDG PET/CT to assess response to therapy.

Procedure

The fasting blood glucose level was 90 mg/dl. A dose of 370 MBq (10 mCi) of $^{18}$F-FDG was administered intravenously in the right antecubital fossa. After a 60-min distribution time, PET/CT was performed in two separate acquisitions, one over the head and neck with the arms along the side and one over the torso with the arms elevated. For each acquisition, low-dose CT scan without contrast was performed, first for attenuation correction followed by tomographic PET images acquired over the brain, neck, thorax, abdomen, and pelvis.

Findings

*Quality of the study*: Good
*Head and neck*: There is physiological distribution of $^{18}$F-FDG in the gray matter and in the glandular and lymphoid tissue of the neck. Moderate uptake is noted in a subcentimeter lymph node in the level II right neck, most likely of inflammatory etiology.
*Chest*: There is mild physiological uptake in the myocardium.
*Abdomen and pelvis*: Physiological uptake is seen in the gastrointestinal and genitourinary tract.
*Musculoskeletal*: Unremarkable.

Disclaimers

Lesions less than 5 mm are likely below the resolution of PET. Lesions between 5 and 10 mm are detected with less sensitivity (50–80% range) than lesions greater than 10 mm.

Some inflammatory processes, such as infection (especially granulomatous), and post-traumatic or post-operative sites may show $^{18}$F-FDG uptake and be false positive for malignant lesions.

Impression

No evidence of residual or recurrent Hodgkin's disease.

## Case I.2.2

### History

A 67-year-old female with a history of medullary thyroid carcinoma and thyroidectomy presented with rising calcitonin levels at 40 pg/ml and was referred to $^{18}$F-FDG PET/CT with suspicion of recurrence (Fig. I.2.2).

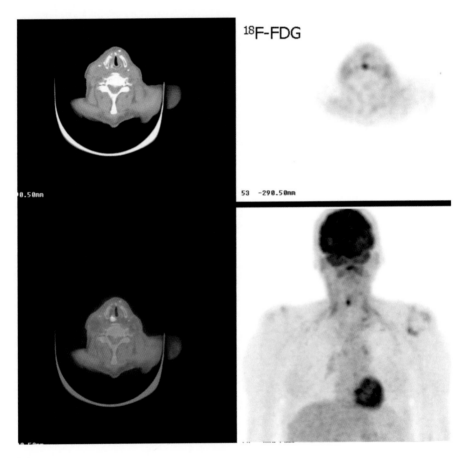

Fig. I.2.2

### Findings

There is asymmetrical tracer activity in the vocal cords, with less uptake on the left side, consistent with left vocal cord paralysis (Fig. I.2.2). There is no abnormal uptake in the neck to suggest recurrent MTC, but low-volume disease may be below PET resolution.

### Discussion

This patient shows the typical PET pattern of vocal cord paralysis that can be seen, among other settings, in patients after thyroidectomy and injury to the laryngeal nerve. These findings are also commonly seen in patients with tumor of lung apex and compression of the laryngeal nerve.[52]

Uptake of [18]F-FDG within the laryngeal muscles occurs commonly and is related to speech during the uptake phase. Subtle visualization of the laryngeal muscles may be seen even with limited vocalization. If the study is performed to evaluate head and neck carcinomas or lymphoma, this can constitute a problem for interpretation. Kostakoglu and colleagues[53] found a direct correlation between the intensity of speech during the uptake phase and the degree of [18]F-FDG activity in these muscles. Therefore, it is important to explain to patients that they should not speak after the tracer injection, and this is mandatory for patients who are being evaluated for head and neck tumors.

[18]F-FDG PET/CT in the evaluation of medullary thyroid carcinoma is discussed in Chapter II.10. and Cases II.10.5 and II.10.6.

## Diagnosis

1. Physiological [18]F-FDG uptake in asymmetrical vocal cords.
2. No evidence of [18]F-FDG-avid medullary thyroid carcinoma.

## *Case I.2.3*

### History

A 9-year-old female diagnosed with Hodgkin's disease, stage IIA, was treated with chemotherapy and achieved a complete remission. Nine months after completion of treatment, $^{18}$F-FDG PET/CT was performed during routine follow-up (Fig. I.2.3A, B).

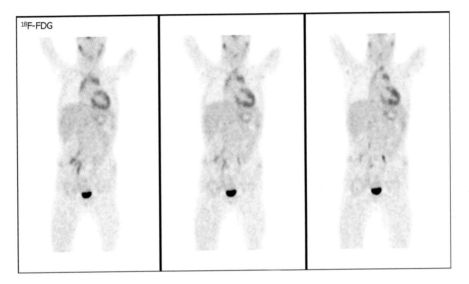

**Fig. I.2.3A**

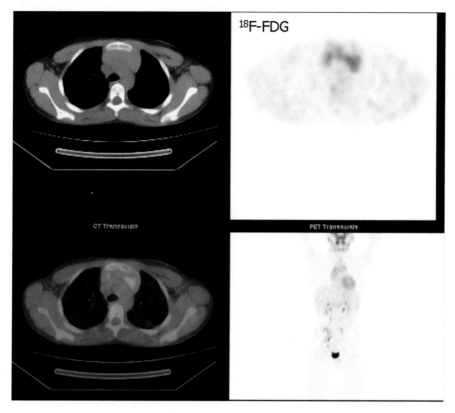

**Fig. I.2.3B**

## Findings

Selected coronal $^{18}$F-FDG PET slices (Fig. I.2.3A) show increased mediastinal tracer activity of moderate intensity with an "inverted Y" configuration. Fused PET/CT images (Fig. I.2.3B) localize the area of increased uptake to an enlarged thymus in the anterior mediastinum.

## Discussion

The findings are consistent with thymic hyperplasia in a child with Hodgkin's disease following chemotherapy. The thymus is an active organ during the first years of life, with subsequent involution and progression to fatty infiltration around puberty. In young children, the thymus demonstrates variable uptake of $^{18}$F-FDG. Thymic hyperplasia following chemotherapy is associated with increased $^{18}$F-FDG uptake and occurs in a relatively high number of children and adolescents and may be seen in young adults as well. The incidence of tracer uptake in a hyperplasic thymus is rather low during treatment but increases over the 12–24 months after completion of therapy and may persist even beyond this period of time. Duration of increased activity can reach a few years. Thymic $^{18}$F-FDG uptake is of mild to moderate intensity. This physiologic variant has to be differentiated from $^{18}$F-FDG-avid mediastinal malignant masses. The classic "inverted Y" pattern and the localization of the increased tracer activity to an enlarged thymus on fused images help in making the correct diagnosis.[19,20]

**Diagnosis**

1. Rebound thymic hyperplasia.
2. No evidence for residual active Hodgkin's disease.

## Case I.2.4

### History

This 23-year-old male with Hodgkin's disease was referred to $^{18}$F-FDG imaging for restaging (Fig. I.2.4).

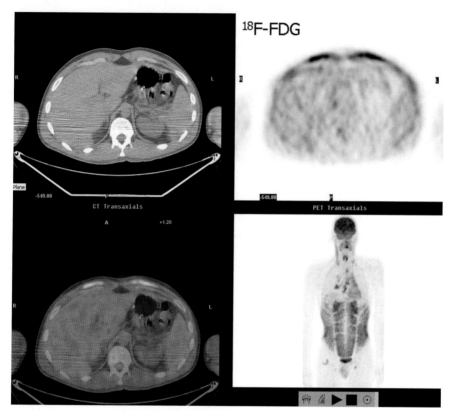

**Fig. I.2.4**

### Findings

The MIP image demonstrates diffuse $^{18}$F-FDG uptake in a pattern consistent with muscular uptake. PET/CT images confirm that the uptake is located in the musculature of the abdominal wall. Further history revealed that the patient had nausea and vomited during the uptake phase.

In addition, there are multiple foci of severely increased radiopharmaceutical uptake within in the chest, abdomen, and pelvis seen on the MIP image. Systematic review of the PET/CT images (not shown) demonstrated locations of these foci in the sternum, right rib, right sacroiliac joints, right femoral head, bilateral ischium, mediastinal lymph nodes, bilateral hilar lymph nodes, and periportal lymph nodes consistent with recurrent Hodgkin's disease.

**Discussion**

Increased [18]F-FDG uptake into muscle during activation or exercise has been previously described. The mechanism for the increased uptake is not entirely clear but appears to be distinct from the one involved with the regulation of glucose metabolism by insulin.[54] One possible explanation is increased blood flow and translocation and activation of protein carriers in response to calcium release from the sarcoplasmic reticulum during exercise.[55] At rest, skeletal muscles do not show significant accumulation of [18]F-FDG, but after exercise (as in this case) or if contraction takes place during the uptake period, in particular the first 30 min after injection of the radiopharmaceutical, there can be marked tracer accumulation in the musculature. This uptake can usually be distinguished from malignant disease because it is often symmetric and matches the anatomy of muscular groups. Occasionally, skeletal [18]F-FDG muscular uptake may be focal and asymmetric, a pattern that makes the differential diagnosis from malignant lesions difficult. This is of most concern when evaluating the neck region of patients with head and neck cancer and lymphoma. Therefore, it is very important to make the patient as comfortable as possible and avoid muscular contraction, including flexion of the neck, prior to and after the injection of the tracer. Diazepam has anxiolytic and muscle-relaxant effects and may offer a simple solution to differentiate between enhanced physiologic muscle uptake and malignant uptake.

**Diagnosis**

1. Recurrent Hodgkin's disease in the mediastinal, hilar, and periportal lymph nodes and skeleton.
2. Abdominal wall muscular uptake in a patient with nausea and vomiting.

## Case I.2.5

### History

This is a 49-year-old patient with a history of Hodgkin's disease diagnosed 10 years earlier. He had multiple episodes of recurrence, most recently in a right flank mass, in the right iliac wing, and right acetabulum, that were highly $^{18}$F-FDG-avid on an outside PET study. The patient was referred for bone marrow transplantation a few months later, and $^{18}$F-FDG PET/CT was performed for restaging (Fig. I.2.5A, B).

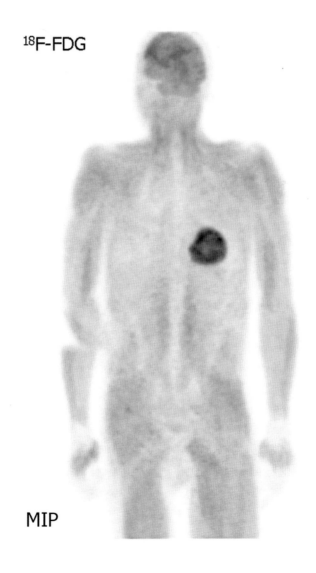

**Fig. I.2.5A**

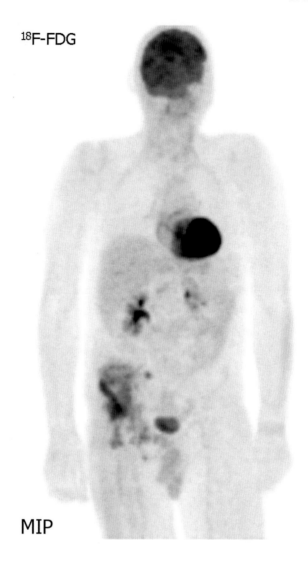

**Fig. I.2.5B**

**Findings**

There is diffuse muscular and myocardial $^{18}$F-FDG uptake, which markedly compromises detection of lymphoma (Fig. I.2.5A). Further history revealed that the patient had not complied with fasting instructions.

**Discussion**

The key to successful $^{18}$F-FDG imaging is appropriate patient preparation to minimize the appearance of artifactual uptake patterns. All patients are instructed to fast for at least 4 h and preferably 12 h and to drink plenty of acaloric clear fluids. The serum glucose level should be measured just before $^{18}$F-FDG administration to document euglycemia. Post-prandial insulin secretion promotes $^{18}$F-FDG uptake by skeletal muscle and myocardium, making [18]F-FDG less available for tumoral uptake.[56] Therefore, the sensitivity for detection of metastatic disease is decreased. The same considerations apply to diabetic patients who require delay of [18]F-FDG administration for 2 or 3 h after insulin injection. In this patient, blood glucose level was 129 mg/dl, but presumably the insulin level may still have been elevated. [18]F-FDG PET/CT was repeated 2 months later, with no interval treatment and after counseling the patient regarding the importance of fasting (Fig. I.2.5B). [18]F-FDG distribution is normal, and intense uptake is seen in the known recurrence in the right hemipelvis.

Hyperglycemia represents a limitation for the sensitivity of [18]F-FDG imaging. The excess of plasma glucose competes with [18]F-FDG and consequently reduces tracer uptake in tumors by up to 50%. Control of glycemia in diabetic patients and overnight fasting in normal patients are thus essential for high quality [18]F-FDG images. Not uncommonly, patients with diabetes present with hyperglycemia because they have been instructed to fast overnight and have not appropriately adjusted their medications. Furthermore, unrecognized diabetes is not uncommon in elderly patients with malignancies.

### Diagnosis

Suboptimal [18]F-FDG PET/CT study due to diffuse muscular uptake in a non-fasting patient.

## Case I.2.6

### History

This 79-year-old male with fever of unknown origin was referred to $^{18}$F-FDG PET/CT in search for the source of the prolonged febrile state (Fig. I.2.6A–C).

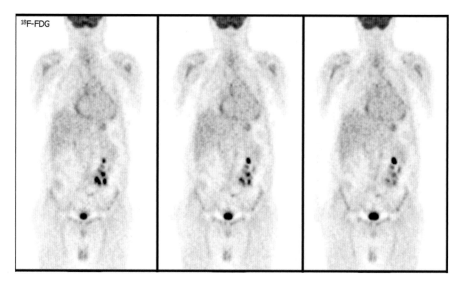

Fig. I.2.6A

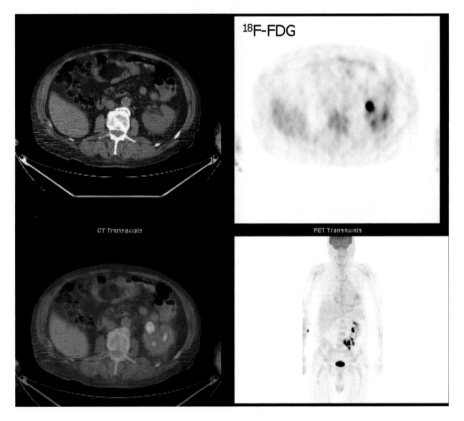

**Fig. I.2.6B**

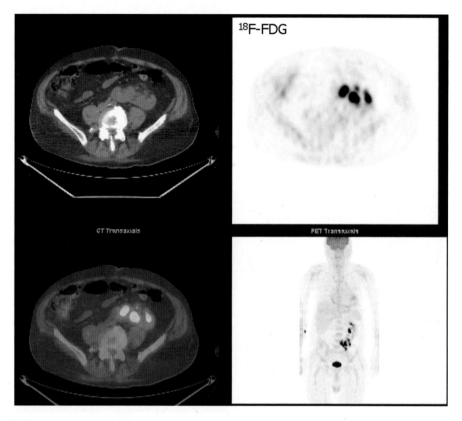

**Fig. I.2.6C**

### Findings

Selected coronal $^{18}$F-FDG-PET slices (Fig. I.2.6A) demonstrate a linear uptake around the contour of the heart. There are additional foci of high-intensity $^{18}$F-FDG uptake localized by fused PET/CT images to the right kidney (Fig. I.2.6B) and to the crossed ectopic left kidney situated below the right kidney in a horizontal position (Fig. I.2.6C).

### Discussion

The patient was diagnosed as idiopathic pericarditis and treated with non-steroidal inflammatory drugs with good response. Abdominal ultrasound confirmed the renal malformation. Increased $^{18}$F-FDG activity in the abdomen or pelvis can be identified by PET/CT as related to the mid-portion of a horseshoe kidney and, when located in the pelvis, to ectopic or transplanted kidneys and thus can be characterized as an anatomic variant and not to a clinically significant lesion. Urinary stasis occurs often in a hydronephrotic renal pelvis, in dilated ureters, or in bladder diverticula with focal accumulation of $^{18}$F-FDG. These anatomic variants can be defined on the CT component of the study. Instructing the patient to be well hydrated may be helpful to promote diuresis. Frequent voiding minimizes urinary collection and, at the same time, decreases radiation exposure to the genitourinary tract.

**Diagnosis**

1. Pericarditis.
2. Crossed ectopic transposition of the left kidney.

## Case I.2.7

### History

A 21-year-old female with Hodgkin's disease, stage IIB, completed chemotherapy and achieved complete remission. Routine follow-up $^{18}$F-FDG PET/CT imaging were performed over the next 3 years (Fig. I.2.7A-C).

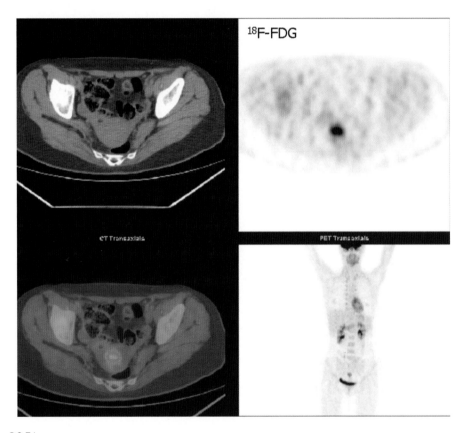

**Fig. I.2.7A**

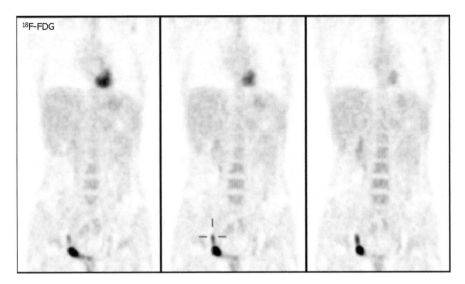

**Fig. I.2.7B**

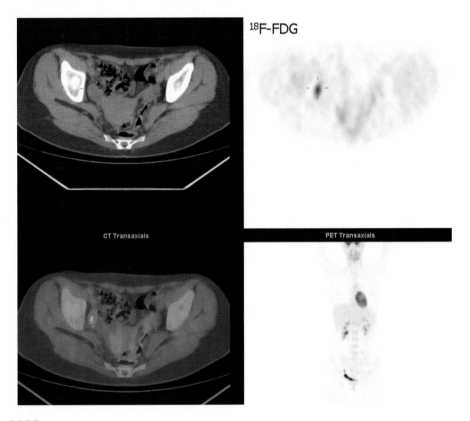

**Fig. I.2.7C**

**Findings**

PET/CT images of a study performed at 12 months after completion of chemotherapy demonstrate the presence of a focal region of moderately intense increased tracer activity in the mid-pelvis above the urinary bladder, as demonstrated on the MIP and transaxial PET images (Fig. I.2.7A) localized by PET/CT to the uterus. Selected coronal $^{18}$F-FDG slices of a repeat study performed 3 years after completion of treatment (Fig. I.2.7B, C marker), demonstrate the presence of an $^{18}$F-FDG-avid focus of mild intensity in the right lower pelvis, superior to a bladder diverticulum localized by fused PET/CT images to the right ovary.

**Discussion**

Detailed patient history indicated that the first study (Fig. I.2.7A) was performed during menstruation, and the increased uptake was therefore considered to represent physiologic tracer activity in the uterus, with no evidence for residual or recurrent Hodgkin. The second study (Fig. I.2.7B, C) was performed at mid-menstrual cycle and uptake in the right ovary was therefore defined as physiologic. The patient continues to remain in complete remission.

   Pelvic $^{18}$F-FDG uptake in female patients located by PET/CT to the uterus and ovaries should be interpreted in view of age, menarchal status, and phase of the menstrual cycle at the time the study was performed. In premenopausal women, physiologic endometrial $^{18}$F-FDG uptake can be seen at mid-cycle and during the menstrual flow phase. This physiologic activity can also be seen over the first few years after menopause, while the uterus is still functional, although the potential malignant etiology of increased uterine $^{18}$F-FDG uptake is higher. Focal increased physiologic $^{18}$F-FDG uptake in the ovaries in premenopausal women has been reported during the late follicular, the ovulatory, and the early luteal phase of the menstrual cycle and is an expression of increased ovarian function. In a post-menopausal patient, these same findings should raise concerns of malignancy.

**Diagnosis**

1. Physiologic $^{18}$F-FDG activity in uterus during menstruation and in right ovary at mid-menstrual cycle.
2. Hodgkin's disease during continuous complete remission.

## Case I.2.8

### History

This 25-year-old female was diagnosed with Hodgkin's disease during her pregnancy. She was referred for $^{18}$F-FDG PET/CT after delivery (Fig. I.2.8).

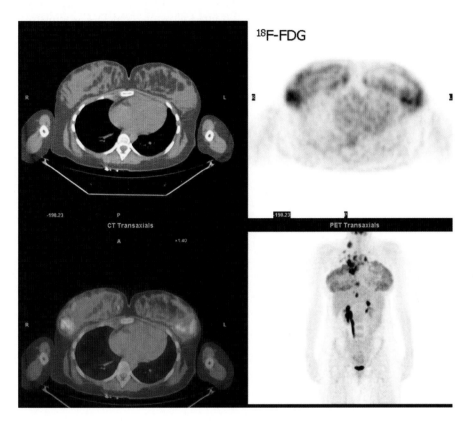

**Fig. I.2.8**

### Findings

There are multiple foci of abnormal $^{18}$F-FDG uptake in the chest and abdomen on the MIP image. Systematic review of the PET/CT images (not shown) demonstrated their localization to lymph nodes consistent with involvement with Hodgkin's disease. In addition, there is heterogeneous $^{18}$F-FDG uptake in the breasts because the patient was lactating and breastfeeding (Fig. I.2.8).

### Discussion

$^{18}$F-FDG uptake within breast tissue can be variable, related to the density of breast tissue and other factors such as lactation. Average standardized uptake values (SUVs) are 0.84 for dense breasts and 0.66 for nondense breasts.[58] Breast uptake SUV in this patient was above

5.0. Although not common, Hodgkin's disease may involve the breast. In the absence of the history of lactating breast, lymphomatous involvement would be a concern. While uptake in the breast is significantly increased during lactation, there is very little excretion of $^{18}$F-FDG in breast milk.[59] This is most probably due to intracellular trapping of $^{18}$F-FDG within the glandular tissue. Although the risk of radiation exposure to infants from ingesting breast milk is low, there is a higher risk of radiation exposure from being in close contact with the breast tissue during feeding. Current recommendations are that mothers discontinue breastfeeding for several hours following $^{18}$F-FDG administration.

**Diagnosis**

1. Lactating breasts.
2. Hodgkin's disease.

## Case I.2.9

### History

A 35-year-old female with uterine cervical cancer was evaluated 3 months after total hysterectomy and completion of radiotherapy. Follow-up CT showed an equivocal mass in the region of the surgical stump. The patient was referred for $^{18}$F-FDG PET/CT with the suspicion of recurrence (Fig. I.2.9A–D).

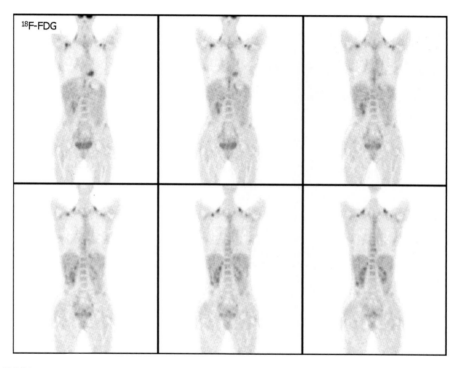

Fig. I.2.9A

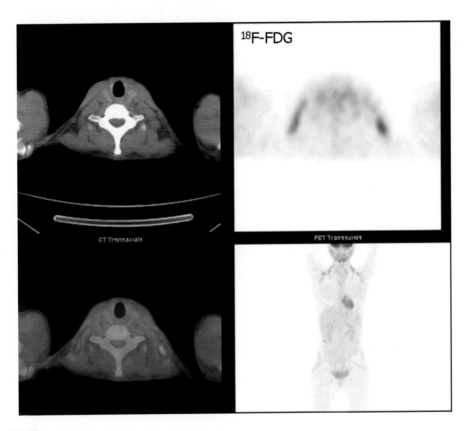

**Fig. I.2.9B**

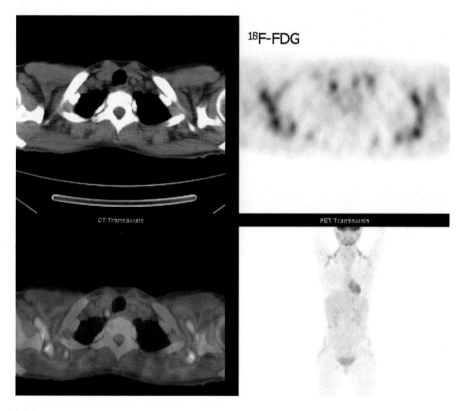

**Fig. I.2.9C**

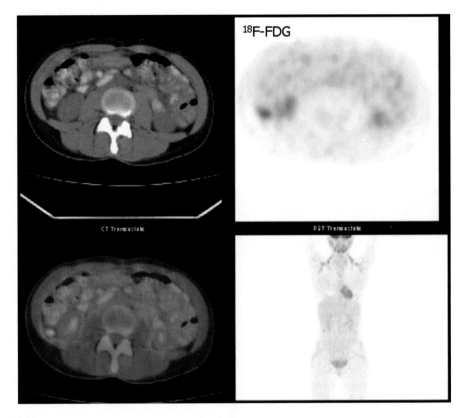

**Fig. I.2.9D**

**Findings**

Selected coronal [18]F-FDG PET slices (Fig. I.2.9A) demonstrate multiple areas of focal increased tracer activity in the lower neck, the shoulder girdle, and in the right pararenal region, adjacent to the lower pole of the right kidney. Fused PET/CT images localize these findings to adipose tissue in the neck (Fig. I.2.9B), shoulder girdle (Fig. I.2.9C), and the right pararenal space (Fig. I.2.9D). There is no focal abnormal tracer uptake in the pelvis.

**Discussion**

Physiologic [18]F-FDG uptake in BAT occurs predominantly in the younger age group and in females, unrelated to their body mass index.[8,60] It occurs mainly in the head and neck region and is less frequent in the thorax and infra-diaphragmatic in the pararenal and paracolic spaces. However, mainly these latter findings can be confounding, especially when they have an atypical, asymmetric focal pattern, or in the presence of additional abnormal cancer-related [18]F-FDG uptake. Increasing the patient's environmental temperature, administration of beta blockers or reserpine, or a change in diet prior to tracer injection and during the uptake phase reduces [18]F-FDG uptake in brown fat but has no significant effect on cancer-related sites.[61,62] Localization of [18]F-FDG foci to fatty tissue on the CT component of the study provides the final diagnosis.

**Diagnosis**

1. Physiologic$^{18}$F-FDG uptake in activated BAT in the neck and shoulder girdle, and asymmetric in the right pararenal space.
2. No evidence for recurrent cervical cancer.

## Case I.2.10

### History

This 50-year-old male with Menetrier's disease was referred to $^{18}$F-FLT PET/CT imaging to evaluate baseline uptake in that disease process (Fig. I.2.10).

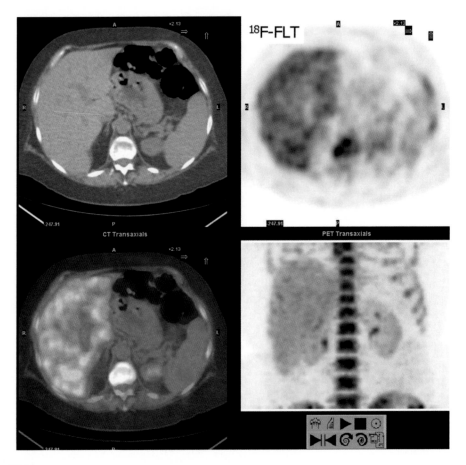

**Fig. I.2.10**

### Findings

This limited study over the abdomen illustrates the normal distribution of $^{18}$F-FLT in the liver and bone marrow. $^{18}$F-FLT is excreted by the kidneys. No abnormal uptake is seen in the thickened wall of the stomach.

### Discussion

As discussed earlier, $^{18}$F-FLT is a tracer of cell proliferation. Tracer uptake in normal hepatic parenchyma and bone marrow is higher than for $^{18}$F-FDG and can mask lesions with increased uptake in or adjacent to these organs. $^{18}$F-FLT is a promising radiotracer to monitor therapy when there is baseline uptake in the primary disease process. In this case, no abnormal uptake is seen in the wall of the stomach, and, therefore, $^{18}$F-FLT is unlikely to be helpful to monitor therapy of Menetrier's disease.

**Diagnosis**

Normal distribution of $^{18}$F-FLT in the abdomen.

## Case I.2.11

### History

This 50-year-old male with multicentric papillary thyroid cancer and lymph node metastases found at surgery was referred for post-ablative whole body scintigraphy 7 days after administration of 3,700 MBq (100 mCi) of $^{131}$I-iodine (Fig. I.2.11).

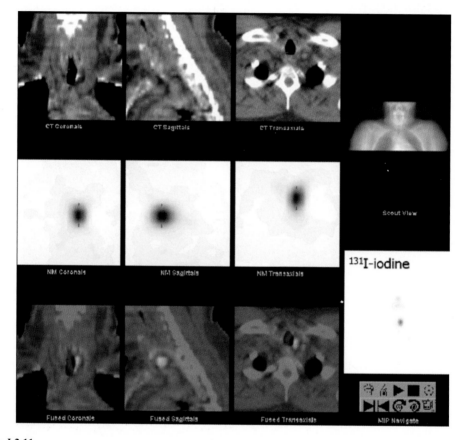

**Fig. I.2.11**

### Findings

SPECT/CT of the neck area was performed. As demonstrated on the MIP image (lower right corner), there is a single focus of intense tracer uptake in the left paramedian mid-cervical region, localized by SPECT/CT to left paratracheal remnant thyroid tissue.

### Discussion

Despite attempts for thyroidectomy to provide total removal of the gland, a variable amount of normal thyroid parenchyma persists and an ablative dose of $^{131}$I is administered. On post-therapeutic radioiodine whole body scintigraphy, the high activity contained in the parenchymal residue may hamper cervical N-staging, a limitation overcome by SPECT/CT.

**Diagnosis**

Papillary thyroid cancer with lymph node metastases at surgery, status post subtotal thyroidectomy and neck dissection, and $^{131}$I-iodine ablation, with evidence of remnant of the left lobe of the thyroid.

## Case I.2.12

### History

This 28-year-old female, status post subtotal thyroidectomy for papillary thyroid cancer, underwent whole body $^{131}$I-iodine scintigraphy at 7 days after the administration of 3,700 MBq (100 mCi) for ablation of thyroid remnant (Fig. I.2.12A, B).

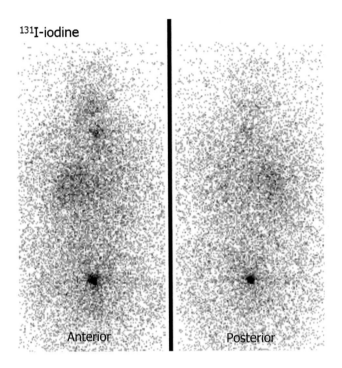

**Fig. I.2.12A**

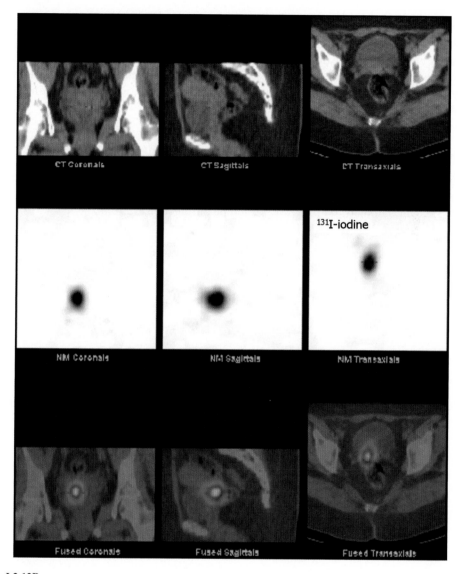

**Fig. I.2.12B**

## Findings

Planar whole body scintigraphy in the anterior and posterior view shows a focus of intense
[131]I-iodine uptake in the pelvis (Fig. I.2.12A). This focus is localized by SPECT/CT of the
pelvis to the uterus. Detailed patient interview indicated that the study was done during
menstruation, and a malignant etiology of this area of increased uptake was therefore
excluded (Fig. I.2.12B). An additional focus of mild increased activity in the lower neck,
seen only on the anterior view of the planar scintigraphy, was consistent with residual
[131]I-iodine uptake in remnant thyroid tissue (Fig. I.2.12A).

## Discussion

[131]I-iodine uptake in benign, non-malignant processes, often of inflammatory etiology, can represent clinically significant pitfalls in patients in whom metastatic well-differentiated thyroid cancer is suspected. Due to the lack of anatomic landmarks on [131]I-iodine whole body scintigraphy, these potential sources of false positive results have become more evident, mainly over recent years, with the use of hybrid SPECT/CT imaging.

## Diagnosis

1. Papillary thyroid cancer, status post surgery and [131]I-iodine ablation, no evidence of active malignancy.
2. Physiologic endometrial uptake of [131]I-iodine during menstruation.

## Case I.2.13

### History

This 49-year-old male was referred for $^{123}$I-MIBG scintigraphy with the clinical suspicion of a pheochromocytoma (Fig. I.2.13A–C).

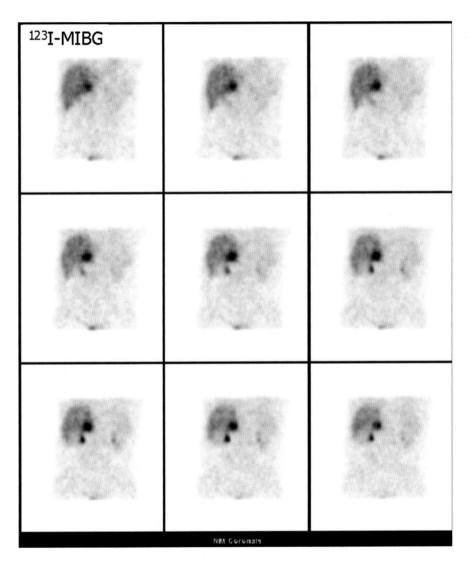

**Fig. I.2.13A**

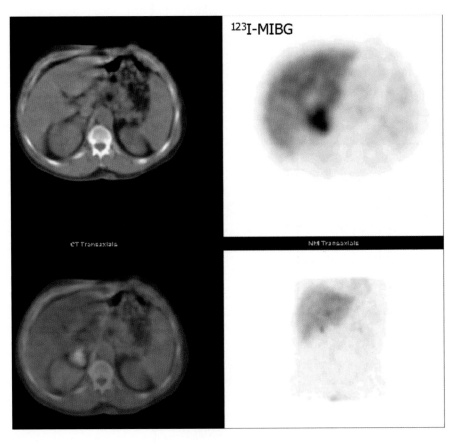

**Fig. I.2.13B**

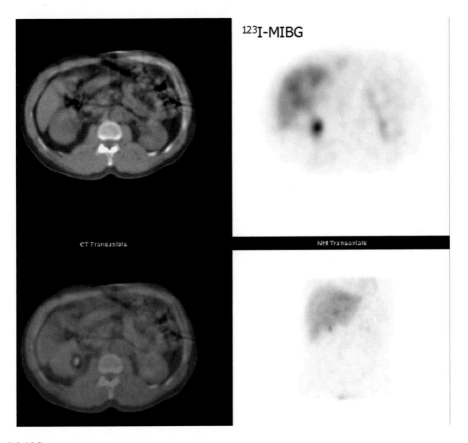

**Fig. I.2.13C**

**Findings**

Coronal SPECT slices of the abdomen–pelvic region demonstrate the presence of two foci of $^{123}$I-MIBG uptake in the right abdomen (Fig. I.2.13A). SPECT/CT localizes the upper focus to a slightly enlarged right adrenal gland (Fig. I.2.13B), consistent with a pheochromocytoma. The lower focus is localized by SPECT/CT to a somewhat dilated right renal pelvis (Fig. I.2.13C) thus representing physiologic urinary excretion of the tracer.

**Discussion**

Faint physiologic uptake of $^{123}$I-MIBG may be observed in normal functioning adrenal glands. $^{123}$I-MIBG is excreted via the urinary system, and stasis in the renal pelvis or ureters can lead to increased focal tracer uptake in these regions. Physiological tracer uptake in sites of the normal $^{123}$I-MIBG biodistribution may be of low intensity but nevertheless difficult to differentiate from pathology related to early stages of disease with small tumor-load, or to residual viable tumor after treatment. False positive $^{123}$I-MIBG studies are due mainly to artifactual findings. SPECT/CT may be of value in separating foci of disease with increased $^{123}$I-MIBG uptake from sites of physiologic tracer activity located in their close proximity.

**Diagnosis**

1. Right adrenal pheochromocytoma.
2. Slightly dilated right renal pelvis.

## Case I.2.14

### History

This 58-year-old female patient with clinically and laboratory-suspected hyperparathyroidism was referred for $^{99m}$Tc-Sestamibi scintigraphy for final diagnosis and localization of a parathyroid adenoma prior to the planned minimally invasive surgery (Fig. I.2.14A, B).

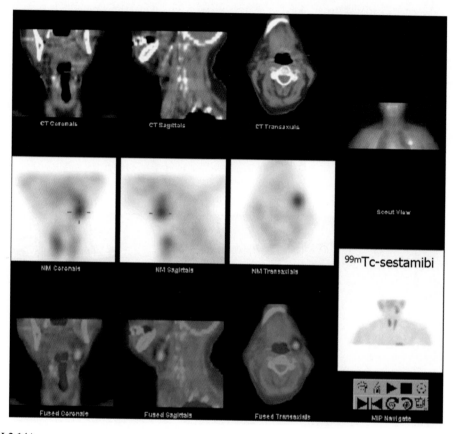

**Fig. I.2.14A**

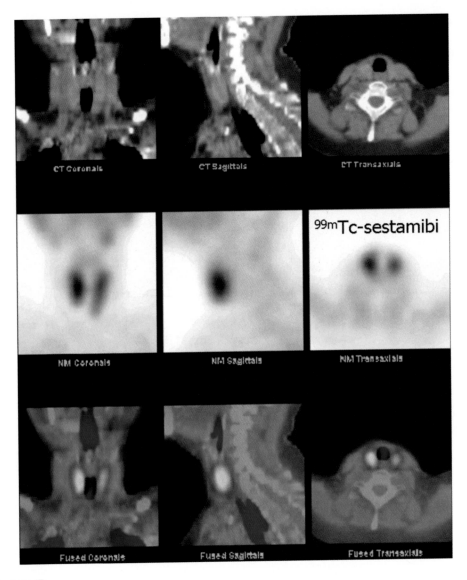

**Fig. I.2.14B**

**Findings**

As demonstrated on the MIP image (right lower corner, Fig. I.2.14A), a parathyroid adenoma was identified and localized by SPECT/CT (not shown) to the left lower pole of the thyroid. In addition, there is asymmetric focal increased $^{99m}$Tc-Sestamibi in the left submandibular region. SPECT/CT (Fig. I.2.14A) defines the physiologic nature of this focus of uptake localized to a normal left salivary gland. In contrast, there is atrophy of the right submandibular salivary gland as shown on the CT component, responsible for the asymmetric and suspicious appearance on MIP and SPECT images stand-alone. In addition, SPECT/CT at the level of the thyroid (Fig. I.2.14B) shows the presence of mild enlargement of the right lobe of the gland.

**Discussion**

Physiological $^{99m}$Tc-Sestamibi uptake in the salivary glands and normal thyroid can be misinterpreted as thyroid- or parathyroid-related pathology in the presence of anatomic variability due to previous surgery, goiter, or congenital anomalies. These entities can be readily identified by SPECT/CT, thus avoiding pitfalls and false positive results of $^{99m}$Tc-Sestamibi scintigraphy in the region of the head and neck.

**Diagnosis**

1. Left parathyroid adenoma.
2. Atrophy of right submandibular salivary gland.
3. Mildly enlarged right lobe of thyroid.

# References

1. Cook GJR, Fogelman I, Maisey MN. Normal physiological and benign pathological variants of 18-fluoro-2-deoxyglucose positron emission tomography scanning: Potential for error in interpretation. *Semin Nucl Med* 1996;26:308–314.
2. Engel H, Steinert H, Buck A, Berthold T, Boni RAH, von Schulthess GK. Whole body PET: Physiological and artifactual fluorodeoxyglucose accumulations. *J Nucl Med* 1996;37:441–446.
3. Bakheet SM, Powe J. Benign causes of 18-FDG uptake on whole body imaging. *Semin Nucl Med* 1998;28:352–358.
4. Kang KW, Kim SK, Kang HS, Lee ES, Sim JS, Lee IG, Jeong S-Y, Kim SW. Prevalence and risk of cancer of focal thyroid incidentaloma identified by 18F-fluorodeoxyglucose positron emission tomography for metastasis evaluation and cancer screening in healthy subjects. *Clin Endocrinol Metab* 2003;88:4100–4104.
5. Israel O, Weiler-Sagie M, Rispler S, Bar-Shalom R, Frenkel A, Keidar Z, Bar-Shalev A, Strauss HW. PET/CT quantitation of the effect of patient-related factors on cardiac $^{18}$F-Fluoro-deoxyglucose uptake. *J Nucl Med* 2007;48:234–239.
6. Shreve PD, Anzai Y, Wahl RL. Pitfalls in oncologic diagnosis with FDG PET imaging: physiologic and benign variants. *Radiographics* 1999;19:61–77.
7. Kim S, Chung JK, Kim BT, Kim SJ, Jeong JM, Lee DS, Lee MC. Relationship between gastrointestinal F-18- fluorodeoxyglucose accumulation of gastrointestinal symptoms in whole-body PET. *Clin Posit Imaging* 1999;2:273–280.
8. Bar-Shalom R, Gaitini D, Keidar Z, Israel O. Non-malignant FDG uptake in infradiaphragmatic adipose tissue – A new site of physiologic tracer biodistribution characterized by PET/CT. *Eur J Nucl Med* 2004;31:1105–1113.
9. Noci I, Borri P, Scarselli G, Chieffi O, Bucciantini S, Biagiotti R, Paglierani M, Moncini D, Taddei G. Morphological and functional aspects of the endometrium of asymptomatic post-menopausal women: does the endometrium really age? *Hum Reprod* 1996;11:2246–2250.
10. Kim SK, Kang KW, Roh JW, Sim JS, Lee ES, Park SY. Incidental ovarian F-18 FDG accumulation on PET: correlation with the menstrual cycle. *Eur J Nucl Med Mol Imaging* 2005;32:757–763.
11. Bakheet SMB, Powe J, Ezzat A, Rostom Al. F-18-FDG uptake in tuberculosis. *Clin Nucl Med* 1998;23:739–742.
12. Lewis PJ, Salama A. Uptake of fluorine-18-fluorodeoxyglucose in sarcoidosis. *J Nucl Med* 1994;35:1647–1649.
13. Love C, Tomas MB, Tronco GG, Palestro CJ. FDG PET of infection and inflammation. *Radiographics* 2005;25:1357–1368.
14. Saksena MA, Blake MA, Brachtel E, Harisinghani MG, Mueller PR. Uterine fibroid 18F-fluorodeoxyglucose (FDG) uptake on combined PET-CT: genitourinary- imaging the male and female pelvis with CT, MRI, and ultrasound. *AJR Am J Roentgenol* 2006;186 (suppl 4): A20–A24.
15. Agress H, Cooper BZ. Detection of clinically unexpected malignant and premalignant tumors with whole-body FDG PET: Histopathologic comparison. *Radiology* 2004;230:417–422.
16. Kamel EM, Thumshirn M, Truninger K, Schiesser M, Fried M, Padberg B, Schneiter D, Stoeckli SJ, von Schulthess GK, Stumpe KDM. Significance of incidental 18F-FDG accumulations in the gastrointestinal tract in PET/CT: Correlation with endoscopic and histopathological results. *J Nucl Med* 2004;45:1804–1810.
17. Gutman F, Alberini JL, Wartski M, Vilain D, Stanc EL, Sarandi F, Corone C, Tainturier C, Pecking AP. Incidental colonic focal lesions detected by FDG PET/CT. *Am J Roentgenol* 2005;185:495–500.
18. Israel O, Yefremov N, Bar-Shalom R, Kagana O, Frenkel A, Keidar Z, Fischer D. PET/CT detection of unexpected gastrointestinal foci of 18F-FDG uptake: Incidence, localization patterns, and clinical significance. *J Nucl Med* 2005;46:758–762.
19. Ferdinand B, Gupta P, Kramer EL. Spectrum of thymic uptake at 18F-FDG PET. *Radiographics* 2004;24:1611–1616.
20. Kawano T, Suzuki A, Ishida A, Takahashi N, Lee J, Tayama Y, Oka T, Yokota S, Inoue T. The clinical relevance of thymic fluorodeoxyglucose uptake in pediatric patients after chemotherapy. *Eur J Nucl Med Mol Imaging* 2004;31:831–836.
21. Sugawara Y, Fisher SJ, Zasadny KR, Kison PV, Baker LH, Wahl RL. Preclinical and clinical studies of bone marrow uptake of fluorine-1-fluorodeoxyglucose with or without granulocyte colony-stimulating factor during chemotherapy. *J Clin Oncol* 1998;16:173–180.

22. Bang S, Baug CA. Topographical distribution of fluoride in iliac bone of a fluoride-treated osteoporotic patient. *J Bone Miner Res* 1990;5:S87–S89.
23. Blake GM, Park-Holohan SJ, Cook GJ, Fogelman I. Quantitative studies of bone with the use of 18F-fluoride and 99mTc-methylene diphosphonate. *Semin Nucl Med* 2001;31:28–49.
24. Even-Sapir E, Mester U, Flusser G, Zuriel L, Kollender Y, Lerman H, Lievshitz G, Ron I, Mishani E. Assessment of malignant skeletal disease with 18F-fluoride PET/CT. *J Nucl Med* 2004;45:272–278.
25. Higashi K, Clavo AC , Wahl RL. In vitro assessment of 2-fluoro-2-deoxy-D-glucose, L-methionine, and thymidine as agents to monitor early response of a human adenocarcinoma cell line to radio-therapy. *J Nucl Med* 1993;34:773–780.
26. Dittmann H, Dohmen BM, Paulsen F, Eichhorn K, Eschmann SM, Horger M, Wehrmann M, Machulla HJ, Bares R. [(18)F]FLT PET for diagnosis and staging of thoracic tumors. *Eur J Nucl Med Mol Imaging* 2003;30:1407–1417.
27. Bendaly E, Sloan A, Dohmen B, Mangner TJ, Machulla HJ, Bares R, Muzik O, Shields AF. Use of 18F-FLT-PET to assess the metabolic activity of primary and metastatic brain disease. *J Nucl Med* 2002;43:111P–112P.
28. Munch-Petersen B, Cloos L, Tyrsted G, Eriksson S. Diverging substrate specificity of pure human thymidine kinases 1 and 2 against antiviral dideoxynucleosides. *J Biol Chem* 1991;266:9032–9038.
29. Dohmen BM, Shields AF, Dittman H, Fersis N, Eschmann SM, Philip P, Reimold M, Machulla HJ, Bares R. Use of [18F]FLT for breast cancer imaging. *J Nucl Med* 2001;42:29P.
30. Buchmann I, Neumaier B, Schreckenberger M, Reske S. [18F]3'-deoxy-3'-fluorothymidine-PET in NHL patients: whole-body biodistribution and imaging of lymphoma manifestations – A pilot study. *Cancer Biother Radiopharm* 2004;19:436–442.
31. van Waarde A, Cobben DC, Suurmeijer AJ, Maas B, Vaalburg W, de Vries EF, Jager PL, Hoekstra HJ, Elsinga PH. Selectivity of 18F-FLT and 18F-FDG for differentiating tumor from inflammation in a rodent model. *J Nucl Med* 2004;45:695–700.
32. Troost EG, Vogel WV, Merkx MA, Slootweg PJ, Marres HA, Peeters WJ, Bussink J, van der Kogel AJ, Oyen WJ, Kaanders JH.18F-FLT PET does not discriminate between reactive and metastatic lymph nodes in primary head and neck cancer patients. *J Nucl Med* 2007;48:726–735.
33. DeGrado TR, Baldwin SW, Wang S, Orr MD, Liao RP, Friedman HS, Reiman R, Price DT, Coleman RE. Synthesis and evaluation of (18)F-labeled choline analogs as oncologic PET tracers. *J Nucl Med* 2001;42:1805–1814.
34. DeGrado TR, Reiman RE, Price DT, Wang S, Coleman RE. Pharmacokinetics and radiation dosi-metry of 18F-fluorocholine. *J Nucl Med* 2002;43:92–96.
35. Martorana G, Schiavina R, Corti B, Farsad M, Salizzoni E, Brunocilla E, Bertaccini A, Manferrari F, Castellucci P, Fanti S. 11C-choline positron emission tomography/computed tomography for tumor localization of primary prostate cancer in comparison with 12-core biopsy. *J Urol* 2006;176:954–960.
36. Price DT, Coleman RE, Liao RP, Robertson C, Polascik T, Degrado T. Comparison of 18Fluorocho-line and 18Fluorodeoxyglucose for positron emission tomography of androgen dependent and andro-gen independent prostate cancer. *J Urol* 2002;168:273–280.
37. Shreve PD, Gross MD. Imaging of the pancreas and related diseases with PET carbon-11 acetate. *J Nucl Med* 1997;38:1305–1310.
38. Fricke E, Machtens S, Hofmann M, Van Den Hoff J, Bergh S, Brunkhorst T, Meyer GJ, Karstens JH, Knapp WH, Boerner AR. Positron emission tomography with 11C-acetate and 18F-FDG in prostate cancer patients. *Eur J Nucl Med Mol Imaging* 2003;30:607–611.
39. Toth G, Lengyel Z, Balkay L, Salah MA, Tron L, Toth C. Detection of prostate cancer with 11C-methionine positron emission tomography. *J Urol* 2005;173:66–69.
40. Vallabhajosula S. (18)F-labeled positron emission tomographic radiopharmaceuticals in oncology: an overview of radiochemistry and mechanisms of tumor localization. *Semin Nucl Med* 2007;37:400–419.
41. Taïeb D, Tessonnier L, Sebag F, Niccoli-Sire P, Morange I, Colavolpe C, De Micco C, Barlier A, Palazzo FF, Henry JF, Mundler O. The role of (18)F-FDOPA and (18)F-FDG-PET in the manage-ment of malignant and multifocal pheochromocytomas. *Clin Endocrinol* (Oxf) 2008;69:580–586.
42. Montravers F, Grahek D, Kerrou K, Ruszniewski P, de Beco V, Aide N, Gutman F, Grangé J-D, Lotz J-P, Talbot J-N. Can fluorodihydroxyphenylalanine PET replace somatostatin receptor scintigraphy in patients with digestive endocrine tumors? *J Nucl Med* 2006;47:1455–1462.
43. Graham MM, Peterson LM, Link JM, Evans ML, Rasey JS, Koh W-J, Caldwell JH, Krohn KA. Fluorine-18-fluoromisonidazole radiation dosimetry in imaging studies. *J Nucl Med* 1997;38:1631–1636.
44. Lee ST, Scott AM. Hypoxia positron emission tomography imaging with 18F-fluoromisonidazole. *Semin Nucl Med* 2007;37:4151–4161.

45. Tharp K, Israel O, Hausmann J, Bettman L, Martin LH, Daitzchman M, Sandler MP, Delbeke D. Impact of I-131 SPECT/CT images obtained with an integrated system in the follow up of patients with thyroid carcinoma. *Eur J Nucl Med* 2004, 31:1435–1442.
46. Shapiro B, Rufini V, Jarwan A, Geatti O, Kearfott KJ, Fig LM, Kirkwood ID, Gross MD. Artifacts, anatomical and physiological variants, and unrelated diseases that might cause false-positive whole-body 131-I scans in patients with thyroid cancer. *Semin Nucl Med* 2000;30:115–132.
47. Bonnin F, Lumbroso J, Tenenbaum F, Harymann O, Parmentier C. Refining interpretation of MIBG scans in children. *J Nucl Med* 1994;35:803–810.
48. Even-Sapir E, Keidar Z, Sachs J, Engel A, Bettman L, Gaitini D, Guralnik L, Werbin N, Iosilevsky G, Israel O. The new technology of combined transmission and emission tomography in evaluation of endocrine neoplasms. *J Nucl Med* 2001;42:998–1004.
49. Rozovsky K, Koplewitz BZ, Krausz Y, Revel-Vilk S, Weintraub M, Chisin R, Klein M. Added value of SPECT/CT for correlation of MIBG scintigraphy and diagnostic CT in neuroblastoma and pheochromocytoma. AJR *Am J Roentgenol* 2008;190:1085–1090.
50. Krausz Y, Shibley N, de Jong RBJ, Jaffe S, Glaser B. Gallbladder visualization with [111]In-labeled Octreotide. *Clin Nucl Med* 1994;19:133–135.
51. Krausz Y, Keidar Z, Kogan, Even-Sapir E, Bar-Shalom R, Engel A, Rubinstein R, Sachs J, Bocher M, Agranovicz S, Chisin R, Israel O. SPECT/CT hybrid imaging with In111-Pentetreotide in assessment of neuroendocrine tumors. *Clin Endocrinol* 2003;59:565–573.
52. Kamel EM, Goerres GW, Burger C, von Schulthess GK, Steinert HC. Recurrent laryngeal nerve palsy in patients with lung cancer: detection with PET-CT image fusion – report of six cases. *Radiology* 2002;224:153–156.
53. Kostakoglu L, Wong JCH, Barrington SF, Cronin BF, Dynes AM, Maisey MN. Speech-related visualization of laryngeal muscles with Fluorine-18-FDG. *J Nucl Med* 1996;37:1711–1713.
54. Barrington SF, Maisey MN. Skeletal muscle uptake of Fluorine-18-FDG: Effect of oral Diazepam. *J Nucl Med* 1996;37:1127–1129.
55. Barnard RJ, Youngren JF. Regulation of glucose transport in skeletal muscle. *FASEB J* 1992;6:3238–3244.
56. Huitink JM, Visser FC, van Leeuwen GR, van Lingen A, Bax JJ, Heine RJ, Teule GJJ, Visser CA. Influence of high and low plasma insulin levels on the uptake of fluorine-18 fluorodeoxyglucose in myocardium and femoral muscle, assessed by planar imaging. *Eur J Nucl Med* 1995;22:1141–1148.
57. Lindholm P, Minn H, Leskinen-Kallio S, Bergman J, Ruotsalainen U, Joensuu H. Influence of the blood glucose concentration on FDG uptake in cancer – a PET study. *J Nucl Med* 1993;34:1–6
58. Kumar R, Chauhan A, Zhuang H, Chandra P, Schnall M, Alavi A. Standardized uptake values of normal breast tissue with 2-deoxy-2-[F-18]fluoro-D-glucose positron emission tomography: variations with age, breast density, and menopausal status. *Mol Imaging Biol* 2006;8:355–362.
59. Hicks RJ, Binns D, Stabin MG. Pattern of uptake and excretion of 18F-FDG in the lactating breast. *J Nucl Med* 2001;42:1238–1242.
60. Yeung HW, Grewal RK, Gonen M, Schöder H, Larson SM. Patterns of (18)F-FDG uptake in adipose tissue and muscle: a potential source of false-positives for PET. *J Nucl Med* 2003;44:1789–1796.
61. Gelfand MJ, O'Hara SM, Curtwright LA, Maclean JR. Pre-medication to block [(18)F]FDG uptake in the brown adipose tissue of pediatric and adolescent patients. *Pediatr Radiol* 2005;35:984–990.
62. Williams G, Kolodny GM. Method for decreasing uptake of 18F-FDG by hypermetabolic brown adipose tissue on PET. *AJR Am J Roentgenol* 2008;190:1406–1409

# Part II
# Clinical Applications in Oncology

# Chapter II.1
# Tumors of the Central Nervous System

**Aaron C. Jessop, Ronald C. Walker, and Dominique Delbeke**

## Introduction

Malignant cerebral tumors represent a small percentage (approximately 2%) of all malignancies, but have poor prognosis due to high morbidity and mortality. According to the American Cancer Society, in 2007 there were 23,300 new benign cerebral tumors and 20,500 new malignant cerebral tumors diagnosed in the United States, with an estimated number of resulting deaths of 12,760. Malignancies of the central nervous system (CNS) are the second most common malignancy in patients under the age of 20 (after hematologic malignancies) and are the leading cause of death from solid tumors in children and the third leading cause of death from cancer in the 15- to 34-year-old age group.[1]

Metastatic disease is the most common intracranial tumor in adults with a 10 times higher incidence than primary tumors. Primary cerebral tumors are a diverse group of neoplasms and can be classified as gliomas and non-gliomas. The later group includes 27% of primary cerebral tumors,[2] such as meningiomas, malignant tumors such as primary CNS lymphoma (representing 1–2%), medulloblastoma, rare CNS germ cell tumors, as well as pituitary adenomas that are typically benign. Gliomas are the most common primary cerebral tumors, representing 40–50% of cases. They arise from glial cells such as astrocytes, ependymal cells, and oligodendrocytes. Low-grade gliomas (WHO grades I and II) include oligodendrogliomas and astrocytomas. High-grade gliomas (WHO grades III and IV) include anaplastic astrocytomas and glioblastoma multiforme. Glioblastoma multiforme is the most common type and represents 51% of primary gliomas; it is also the most aggressive and most resistant to treatment (WHO grade IV).[3,4]

Intracranial tumors are also classified as intra- and extra-axial. Intra-axial tumors such as gliomas arise from the cerebral parenchyma. Extra-axial tumors arise from structures outside of the brain, such as the meninges.

Diagnosis and staging of cerebral tumors are routinely performed by anatomical imaging modalities such as magnetic resonance imaging (MRI) and computed tomography (CT). MRI is considered the gold standard modality because it gives excellent anatomical information regarding the location and extent of disease.[5] [18]F-fluorodeoxyglucose ([18]F-FDG) imaging is a useful adjunct to anatomical assessment because it adds metabolic information. [18]F-FDG imaging can provide useful data in the initial evaluation of cerebral tumors since poorly differentiated tumors typically demonstrate higher metabolic rates. Further into the course of disease, [18]F-FDG

A.C. Jessop (✉)
Department of Radiology and Radiological Sciences, Vanderbilt University Medical Center,
Nashville, TN, USA
e-mail: a.jessop@vanderbilt.edu

imaging can also help in the differential diagnosis of radiation necrosis from recurrent tumor, which is very difficult to make by contrast-enhanced CT or MRI. With the use of positron emission tomography (PET)/CT, there is improved anatomical localization of focal metabolic abnormalities. The sensitivity for detection of cerebral lesions increases by the addition of CT. Due to the relatively intense physiologic $^{18}$F-FDG uptake in the gray matter in the brain, some lesions may not be discernable by $^{18}$F-FDG PET alone. PET also has inferior spatial resolution compared to CT and thus may not detect small lesions in the brain that are visible on the accompanying CT images.

## Physiologic Distribution of $^{18}$F-FDG in the CNS

$^{18}$F-FDG crosses the blood–brain barrier similar to glucose and is transported intracellularly by the membrane-bound glucose uptake and transporter proteins (Glut – predominantly Glut-1 through Glut-5). Inside the cell, $^{18}$F-FDG is phosphorylated by hexokinase, producing $^{19}$F-FDG-6-phosphate, effectively trapping the $^{18}$F-FDG within the cell. Due to the low concentration of glucose-6-phosphatase in the brain, very little of the $^{18}$F-FDG-6-phosphate is dephosphorylated, and, therefore, there is insignificant diffusion back across the cell membrane into the extracellular space. Unlike glucose-6-phosphate, $^{18}$F-FDG-6-phosphate does not serve as a substrate for the enzymes of the glycolytic pathway, and $^{18}$F-FDG-6-phosphate is accumulated in the cytosol, proportional to the activity and level of expression of the Glut proteins and of the enzymes hexokinase and glucose-6-phosphatase.

Since the brain is metabolically active and only uses glucose as a substrate, $^{18}$F-FDG accumulation is high compared to other tissues of the body. $^{18}$F-FDG uptake in white matter is about one-third to one-fourth that of gray matter. $^{18}$F-FDG uptake is therefore predominant in the cerebral cortex, cerebellum, basal ganglia, and thalamus. High physiologic $^{18}$F-FDG uptake is also found in the extraocular muscles.

Many factors can alter the distribution of $^{18}$F-FDG in the CNS. Insulin stimulates $^{19}$F-FDG uptake in somatic cells, and, therefore, injection of insulin or the presence of postprandial, endogenous insulin often results in relatively diminished $^{18}$F-FDG uptake in the brain, with alternatively increased uptake within skeletal muscle and other soft tissues. Medications, such as sedatives, general anesthetics, and corticosteroids, can also result in a decrease in cortical $^{18}$F-FDG uptake. Benzodiazepines, sometimes used to reduce the uptake within brown adipose tissue, can also cause decreased $^{18}$F-FDG uptake within the brain.

While the adult pattern of $^{18}$F-FDG uptake in the brain is established by the age of 2, there are subtle differences between the normal adult distribution of $^{18}$F-FDG and that in the brain of younger patients. In the newborn, there is decreased perfusion and metabolism of the frontal and parieto-temporal cortical regions, while that of basal ganglia, visual cortex, and sensory-motor cortex are similar to that of an adult, thus resulting in an immature pattern of $^{18}$F-FDG uptake in the brain.[6] Aging can also alter the distribution of $^{18}$F-FDG. Dementia can alter the normal distribution of $^{18}$F-FDG in the brain and, by the resulting pattern of distribution, can help characterize the particular type of dementia sometimes years before clinical signs or symptoms occur.

For proper interpretation of PET/CT images of the brain, images must, when necessary, be re-oriented along the anterior–posterior commissure (AC–PC) line and be examined along each of the three classic projections (axial, coronal, and sagittal). If other studies are available for comparison (e.g., MRI or CT), processing the PET/CT images to provide similar orientation, slice thickness, and windowing to the comparison studies is essential. Comparison with current MRI or CT can be critical to answer specific questions, such as in evaluation of a previously described structural abnormality.


## Initial Evaluation and Staging of Primary Cerebral Tumors

MRI is the current gold standard for the initial imaging evaluation of cerebral tumors. T1-weighted, pre- and post-contrast, and T2-weighted MRI images, sometimes with additional less common sequences, provide excellent anatomical detail necessary for determining the size and anatomical location of cerebral tumors. Cerebral tumors typically demonstrate increased signal (bright) on T2-weighted images and decreased signal (dark) on T1-weighted images. Enhancement with IV gadolinium occurs with breakdown of the blood–brain barrier, commonly seen with high-grade gliomas or metastases. Low-grade gliomas do not always enhance. Other clinically relevant imaging findings associated with cerebral tumors that are common on MRI include edema, mass effect, herniation, hemorrhage, degree of vascularity, and signs of increased intracranial pressure, such as hydrocephalus.

[18]F-FDG PET/CT can serve as a valuable adjunct to MRI in the evaluation of primary cerebral tumors by providing a noninvasive means of evaluating the metabolic status of tumors. In gliomas, the degree of uptake correlates directly with the histological grade of the tumor. Low uptake (equal or less than that of white matter) is seen in low-grade gliomas, while high-grade gliomas generally demonstrate uptake that is twice that of white matter or higher. The degree of uptake also correlates with overall prognosis. Patients with low uptake have been shown to have a longer median survival than patients with cerebral tumors that are more metabolically active. If uptake is equal or higher than 1.4 times that of gray matter, the prognosis is very poor, with a median survival of less than 6 months.[7]

[18]F-FDG PET/CT can be useful in the initial evaluation of cerebral tumors by providing guidance for stereotactic biopsy. Some cerebral gliomas may be well differentiated in some regions and yet contain less-differentiated cells in others. Using [18]F-FDG PET/CT to target to the site of maximum activity increases the accuracy of the procedure by decreasing the biopsy sampling error. [18]F-FDG PET/CT guidance for biopsy is particularly helpful when access to the lesion is difficult. The use of PET/CT to guide stereotactic cerebral biopsy has increased the diagnostic yield and accuracy for both [18]F-FDG and [11]C-methionine.[8] One of the advantages of imaging with [11]C-methionine is the absence of background uptake in the normal cerebral cortex. Therefore, both low-grade and high-grade gliomas are better delineated on [11]C-methionine than on [18]F-FDG studies. However, [11]C-methionine accumulates in all tumor types and therefore does not allow for a good differentiation between low- and high-grade gliomas. Despite this limitation, a correlation between areas of highest [11]C-methionine uptake and those with highest [18]F-FDG uptake has been found.[9] Where available, [11]C-methionine, in combination with MRI, has gained a place in defining neurosurgical strategies that aim at delineating the entire tumor volume for resection under neuronavigation or for radiosurgery.[10]

[18]F-FDG PET/CT is also useful in the evaluation of primary CNS lymphoma, particularly in patients with acquired immune deficiency syndrome (AIDS) who are at greater risk than the general population. Patients with AIDS are also at an increased risk for opportunistic infections, including toxoplasmosis of the brain. Accurate differentiation between these two entities is paramount, since prompt and appropriate treatment for either of these

diagnoses differs and is essential for a favorable outcome. CNS lymphoma and cerebral toxoplasmosis can show similar patterns on CT or MRI. On [18]F-FDG PET/CT imaging, CNS lymphoma is typically intensely [18]F-FDG avid relative to normal cerebral uptake, whereas infection from toxoplasmosis usually is not.

## Evaluation of Treated Primary Cerebral Tumors

MRI evaluation of a previously treated cerebral tumor can be limited by the inability to distinguish between tumor recurrence and treatment-related changes, specifically post-surgical gliosis and radiation-induced injury. Radiation therapy causes damage to the vascular endothelial cells and oligodendrocytes, resulting in edema, necrosis, and reactive gliosis. On MRI, this entity appears as increased signal intensity on T2-weighted images. There is often contrast enhancement on both MRI and CT, due to disruption of the blood–brain barrier, and, therefore, these treatment-related changes can be indistinguishable from recurrent tumor.

[18]F-FDG PET/CT can be particularly useful in this clinical setting, distinguishing radiation injury from recurrent tumor. As a rule, lesions that are equivocal or suspicious on MRI and demonstrate high uptake on [18]F-FDG PET/CT represent tumor recurrence.[11] False positive [18]F-FDG results can occur early after treatment due to the normal surgically induced inflammatory response or to focal subclinical seizure activity related to the surgical or radiation injury as well, which can all show increased [18]F-FDG uptake.

In patients with low-grade glioma, [18]F-FDG PET/CT can provide a noninvasive means of evaluation for malignant transformation. New high [18]F-FDG uptake in a previously diagnosed low-grade glioma can be diagnostic of tumor transformation to an aggressive state and worsening of prognosis. A limitation of [18]F-FDG imaging is the fact that this tracer does not accumulate significantly in low-grade glioma and therefore does not allow detection of recurrent disease, which can be, however, done with [11]C-methionine.[12]

## Evaluation of Cerebral Metastases

Cerebral metastases are the most common intracranial tumors in adults, 10 times more common than primary cerebral tumors. With advances in systemic chemotherapy leading to an increase in survival of patients with malignancies, the incidence of cerebral metastases is rising, and they occur in 20–40% of adult cancer patients. Cancers of the lung and breast, and melanoma are the most common malignancies to metastasize to the brain.

Cerebral metastases result from hematogenous tumor spread and are most often found at the gray/white junction due to changes in the caliber of blood vessels in this region. Detection of these cerebral lesions is of great importance since they can be life-threatening. Gadolinium-enhanced MRI is the diagnostic test of choice when cerebral metastases are suspected. The detection rate of cerebral metastases on [18]F-FDG imaging is low compared to contrast-enhanced CT or MRI. However, cerebral metastases can be detected prior to the onset of neurological symptoms on whole-body [18]F-FDG PET/CT examinations when the brain is included in the field of view.

$^{18}$F-FDG PET/CT is suboptimal for detection of cerebral metastases because of the normally high tracer uptake in the brain, reducing the tumor-to-background ratio of subtle cerebral lesions. The heterogeneity of $^{18}$F-FDG accumulation among cerebral lesions (even of the same histological type and in the same patient), the often small size of the lesions, and their frequent proximity to metabolically active gray matter are all factors that contribute to the relatively low sensitivity of 68% of $^{18}$F-FDG imaging for detection of cerebral metastases. These lesions can appear hyper-, iso-, or hypometabolic relative to surrounding cerebral activity.[13,14]

It is essential that the interpreting physician examines the PET and PET/CT fusion images of the brain as well as the CT. Important clinical information can also be gained by viewing the cerebral images of the CT component of the PET/CT at appropriate window-width and window-level settings. Without careful inspection of the CT images of the brain where intense $^{18}$F-FDG uptake is seen in a physiologic state, small metastatic lesions, below the resolution of PET or demonstrating $^{18}$F-FDG uptake of similar intensity to the surrounding cortex, are easily missed. Also, many lesions in the brain may be visible only on the anatomic localization CT images, with the PET and PET/CT fusion images appearing normal.

## Evaluation of Meningiomas

Meningiomas are the most common non-glial intracranial tumor, accounting for 13–19% of surgical interventions for intracranial lesions. The incidence of meningiomas is estimated to be 1.4%, with most remaining asymptomatic, often diagnosed as incidental findings. Nonetheless, the high prevalence in the population, the focal signs and symptoms that can occur from these tumors, and the sometimes associated skeletal changes all combine to create the large number of surgical procedures related to this tumor.

Meningiomas occur twice as often in women than in men, with two peak ages: between 15 and 19 years and between 70 and 79 years. In men, the prevalence increases throughout life until the 7th decade. Below the age of 16, meningiomas are reported more commonly in males.

Meningiomas are non-glial tumors arising from the arachnoidal layer of the meninges and are usually benign (WHO grade 1). The WHO 2000 classification for meningiomas includes three groups: typical meningioma (with variants including several pathologic types), atypical meningiomas, and anaplastic (malignant) meningiomas. Atypical and anaplastic mengiomas are more aggressive and can invade the cerebral cortex. They occur with a higher prevalence in children than in adults, with 28% of these childhood tumors being malignant meningiomas or meningeal sarcomas. Meningiomas can metastasize, though only rarely.

While meningiomas can occur in any location where there are arachnoid cap cells, including the vertebral column, they are more frequent in areas with arachnoid granulations. About 50% of meningiomas occur along the convexities or near the superior sagittal sinus. Other common locations include the Sylvian fissure, near the sella turcica, the sphenoid wings, and the olfactory grooves, as well as the posterior fossa in the region of the tentorium or the petrous bone, especially involving the cerebellopontine angle. Rarely, meningiomas can arise from an intraventricular location in the choroid plexus. Meningiomas are typically broad-based, attached to the dura, and seen as extra-axial masses, with a less clear-cut pattern in certain locations, such as in the Sylvian fissure or along the basal cisterns.

While multiplanar MRI, with and without gadolinium, is the mainstay for cerebral lesions, many of the characteristics of meningiomas are identifiable on PET/CT, especially on the CT portion. The typical pattern is a well-defined, extra-axial tumor with displacement of the cortex. Calcifications are commonly present and may make the mass appear slightly hyperdense relative to the brain. The mass is usually hypometabolic relative to gray matter. If this is not the case, an atypical metastasis or another, more aggressive process, including an atypical or malignant meningioma, should be strongly considered. Reactive hyperostosis of the adjacent cranium is an indicator of tumor invasion of the bone, highly specific for meningiomas. If IV contrast is given, the "dural tail sign" may be visible, representing a region of the dura adjacent to the tumor that is thickened and enhanced. This phenomenon represents areas of reactive change in the meningeal tissues near the meningioma, but not tumor involvement if located at more than 1 cm from the mass.[15,16]

## Summary

$^{18}$F-FDG imaging is a valuable adjunct to MRI or contrast-enhanced multidetector CT in the evaluation of intracranial lesions. It can provide a noninvasive means to evaluate the metabolic rate of primary cerebral tumors, with a powerful correlation with both tumor grade and prognosis. PET/CT, by providing anatomic localization of the regions with greatest metabolic activity, can aid in selection of high-yield biopsy sites. $^{18}$F-FDG imaging is of value in the differential diagnosis between primary CNS lymphoma and toxoplasmosis in patients with AIDS. In patients with meningioma, the degree of $^{18}$F-FDG uptake correlates with the proliferation rate and is a predictor of the likelihood of recurrence after surgical resection. In previously treated cerebral tumor patients, $^{18}$F-FDG PET or PET/CT is useful for distinguishing treatment-induced changes and/or radiation necrosis from recurrent/residual tumor.

Although contrast-enhanced CT and MRI are the standard of care for evaluation of cerebral metastases, $^{18}$F-FDG PET/CT can also demonstrate metastatic brain lesions. Interpreting physicians should independently examine the PET, CT, and fusion PET/CT images carefully, at appropriate window-width and window-level settings, for evidence of clinically significant lesions in the visualized portions of the brain.

In addition to $^{18}$F-FDG, $^{11}$C-methionine has the advantage of accumulating in both low- and high-grade gliomas, resulting in good delineation of these tumors as compared to $^{19}$FDG, also due to low background uptake of this tracer in normal cortex. $^{11}$C-methionine offers the potential to detect recurrent low-grade gliomas and to better delineate the entire tumor volume for resection under neuronavigation or for radiosurgery.

## *Guidelines and Recommendations for the use of $^{18}$F-FDG PET and PET/CT*

The National Comprehensive Cancer Network (NCCN) has incorporated $^{18}$F-FDG PET and PET/CT in the practice guidelines and management algorithm of a variety of malignancies including brain cancer. The use of $^{18}$F-FDG PET (PET/CT where available) is recommended in the following clinical scenarios: 1) Identification of low-grade gliomas undergoing malignant conversion; 2) Differentiation of radiation effect from tumor recurrence; 3) Guidance of biopsy to site of maximum uptake; 4) Planning radiation therapy.[17]

## Case Presentations

## *Case II.1.1*

### History

This 40-year-old female presented with new-onset neurological symptoms affecting the left side of her body. MRI of the brain revealed abnormally increased signal on T2-weighted images involving the cortex and subcortical white matter in the anterior part of the right frontal lobe with no abnormal enhancement. The patient was referred to $^{18}$F-FDG PET/CT of the brain for further characterizing the lesion seen on MRI (Fig. II.1.1A, B).

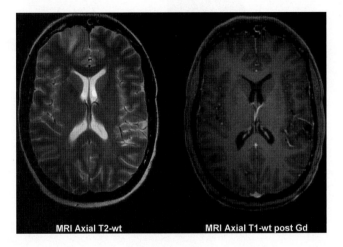

**Fig. II.1.1A**

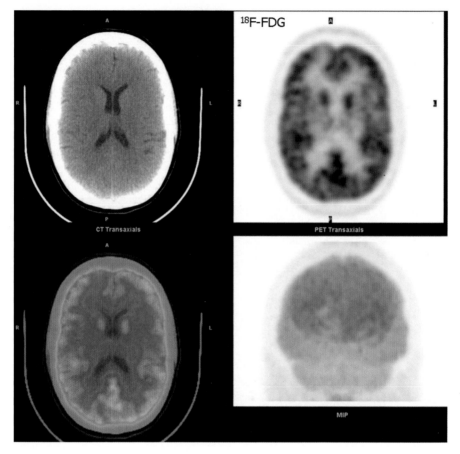

**Fig. II.1.1B**

**Findings**

There is moderately decreased uptake in the gray matter and the subcortical white matter in the anterior part of the right frontal lobe (Fig. II.1.1B), corresponding to an area of decreased density on CT and to the area of the lesion demonstrated on MRI (Fig. II.1.1A). There are no foci of abnormally increased [18]F-FDG uptake (Fig. II.1.1B).

**Discussion**

The focal region of decreased uptake corresponding to the abnormality visualized on MRI is most consistent with a low-grade cerebral tumor. The patient was referred for biopsy, which revealed a well-differentiated WHO grade II oligodendroglioma.

This case demonstrates the usefulness of [18]F-FDG PET/CT for noninvasive characterization of cerebral tumors by evaluating their metabolic activity. The degree of [18]F-FDG uptake correlates significantly with the histological grade of a glioma.[18] Low-grade gliomas, as seen in this case, typically have uptake similar to or less than that of white matter. If, on the other hand, uptake in a primary cerebral tumor is equal to or greater than that of normal gray matter, the tumor is most likely a high-grade glioma. If uptake is greater than that of white matter, but less than that of gray matter, evaluation can be more difficult. While semiquantification can be performed, measurement of standardized uptake values (SUV) is of limited significance in the evaluation of cerebral tumors.[19]

[18]F-FDG PET/CT findings may be subtle if the metabolic activity of the tumor is similar to that of the normal surrounding cortex. It is thus essential to directly compare the [19]F-FDG PET/CT to a recent MRI to verify the correct anatomic location of the lesion in question.

The relationship between [18]F-FDG uptake and the histological grade of a glioma was first described by Di Chiro and colleagues in 1982.[20] A more recent retrospective study was performed by Padma and colleagues[21] and evaluated the ability of [18]F-FDG imaging to predict the pathologic grade of glioma and duration of survival. It reported that 86% of patients with low uptake (equal to or less than white matter) on [18]F-FDG PET had low-grade gliomas on histology as compared to 94% of patients with high uptake (more than white matter) who had high-grade gliomas. The degree of uptake also correlated significantly with patient survival with a median of 29 months for patients with low uptake as compared to 11 months for those with high uptake.

**Diagnosis**

Low-grade glioma (oligodendroglioma, WHO grade II).

## Case II.1.2

### History

This 40-year-old male presented with a history of a right frontal lobe low-grade glioma (grade II, oligodendroglioma) and had received radiation therapy 7 years previously. He has been followed by annual MRI for evidence of tumor recurrence and was referred to $^{19}$F-FDG PET/CT for further evaluation after his most recent MRI demonstrated a slight increase in tumor volume (Fig. II.1.2A, B).

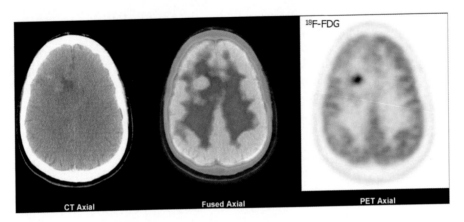

**Fig. II.1.2A**

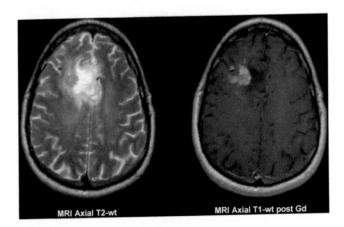

**Fig. II.1.2B**

### Findings

On $^{18}$F-FDG PET/CT, there is a focus of intense uptake located in the white matter of the right frontal lobe, of higher intensity as compared to that of gray matter, corresponding on CT to a lesion with heterogeneous density with associated surrounding edema (Fig. II.1.2A). This correlates with the high signal lesion on the T2-weighted (left) and region of enhancement on the post-gadolinium T1-weighted (right) axial MRI images (Fig. II.1.2B).

**Discussion**

The intense $^{18}$F-FDG uptake in the right frontal lobe lesion is most consistent with a high-grade tumor. Although no baseline PET/CT was performed to establish the presence and degree of $^{18}$F-FDG avidity of the original lesion, the high degree of uptake is suggestive of a region of focal transformation to a high-grade primary cerebral tumor in a patient with a previously treated low-grade entity. The patient was asymptomatic at the time of $^{18}$F-FDG PET/CT, but deteriorated rapidly over the next year despite aggressive treatment.

This case demonstrates the usefulness of $^{18}$F-FDG PET/CT in evaluating primary cerebral tumors and for detecting malignant transformation of low-grade gliomas. The degree of $^{18}$F-FDG uptake is inversely correlated with prognosis. In a study of 28 patients with known low-grade gliomas, De Witte and colleagues[22] performed F-FDG PET imaging at baseline. After a mean follow-up interval of 27 months, 67% of patients with high uptake died or developed recurrence after treatment, whereas all patients with low uptake at baseline were alive.

Although the visual assessment of the degree of uptake is often sufficient for differentiation of low-grade (same or less than white matter) from high-grade (more than gray matter) primary cerebral tumors, semiquantization can be performed when visual assessment of the level of uptake is equivocal.[23,24] A tumor-to-white matter ratio of 1.5 or more has been suggested as an appropriate cutoff level for discrimination between low- and high-grade cerebral tumors.[25]

**Diagnosis**

Recurrent glioma with transformation from low grade to high grade tumor.

## *Case II.1.3*

### History

This 27-year-old male was diagnosed with primary CNS diffuse large B-cell lymphoma. He underwent six cycles of high-dose methotrexate and was referred for restaging with $^{19}$F-FDG PET/CT and MRI (Fig. II.1.3 A, B).

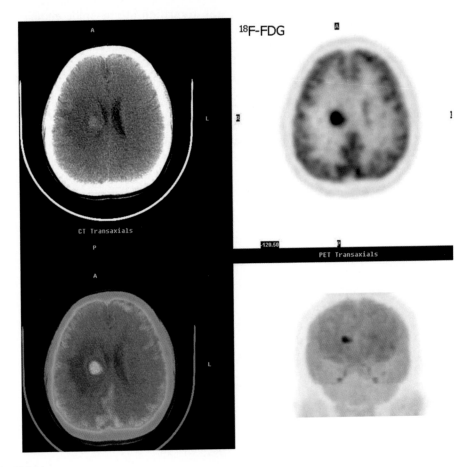

Fig. II.1.3A

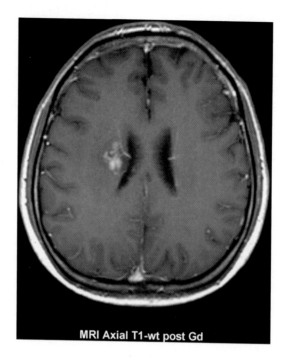

**MRI Axial T1-wt post Gd**

**Fig. II.1.3B**

## Findings

There is a focus of $^{18}$F-FDG uptake of significantly higher intensity than that of the gray matter, within the right centrum semiovale corresponding to an $18 \times 11$ mm hyperdense lesion visualized on CT (Fig. II.1.3A).

The gadolinium-enhanced T1-weighted MRI image (Fig. II.1.3B), which was performed a few weeks prior to the $^{18}$F-FDG PET/CT, reveals an enhancing mass in the right centrum semiovale corresponding to the location of the hypermetabolic focus visualized on the $^{19}$F-FDG PET/CT images.

## Discussion

The enhancing lesion visualized on MRI demonstrates $^{18}$F-FDG uptake on PET/CT that is significantly greater than that of normal gray matter. This is consistent with persistent high-grade tumor in this region. The patient has completed a course of treatment for the known lymphoma, and, therefore, this focus of persistent uptake represents residual viable tumor.

Primary lymphoma of the CNS is rare, representing 1–3% of all primary cerebral tumors. Most are diffuse large B-cell lymphomas and intensely $^{18}$F-FDG avid. They occur more commonly in immunosuppressed patients, such as those with AIDS. Common sites of occurrence are the cerebral hemispheres, basal ganglia, and corpus callosum.[26]

The appearance on MRI can be very similar to other entities, such as a toxoplasmosis abscess. AIDS patients are at an increased risk for both CNS lymphoma and opportunistic toxoplasmosis infections. Rapid distinction between these two entities is necessary, as prompt initiation of appropriate treatment is essential. When diagnosis is uncertain on MRI, $^{18}$F-FDG PET/CT can help in the differential diagnosis between these two entities.

Primary CNS lymphoma is typically intensely FDG avid relative to gray matter, while toxoplasmosis is not.

Whole-body [18]F-FDG PET/CT is also useful in the initial staging of CNS lymphoma, with occult sites of systemic disease found in up to 15% of patients who are otherwise believed to have localized disease only.[27] Restaging can also be performed with [18]F-FDG PET/CT to evaluate for persistent or recurrent metabolically active disease.

**Diagnosis**

Primary residual active lymphoma of the CNS.

## Case II.1.4 (DICOM Images on DVD)

### History

This 41-year-old human immunodeficiency virus (HIV)-positive patient presented to the emergency department with neurological symptoms and fever. MRI of the brain revealed an 18 mm thin-walled ring-enhancing lesion in the left basal ganglia, with significant associated edema exerting a moderate mass effect upon the adjacent lateral ventricle. The patient was referred to [18]F-FDG PET/CT for further characterization of the lesion (Fig. II.1.4 A, B).

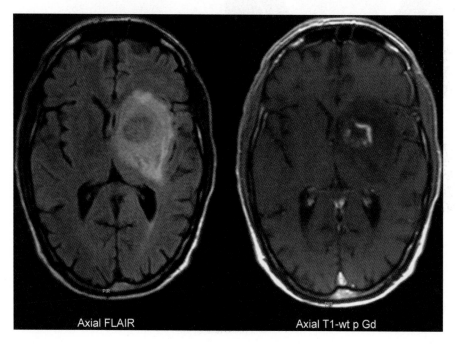

Fig. II.1.4A

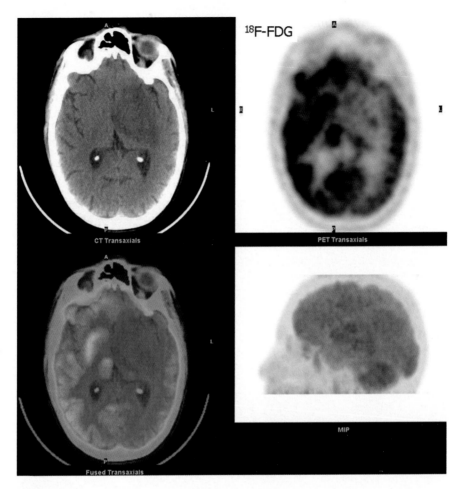

**Fig. II.1.4B**

**Findings**

There is low metabolism in the region of the left basal ganglia (Fig. II.1.4B) corresponding to the anatomic location of the lesion identified on the MRI (Fig. II.1.4A). There is also a relative diffuse decrease in [18]F-FDG uptake throughout the left cerebral hemisphere as compared to the right (Fig. II.1.4B).

**Discussion**

Decreased [18]F-FDG uptake in the region of the ring-enhancing lesion visualized on MRI is most consistent with a toxoplasmosis abscess of the brain. Based on the [18]F-FDG PET/CT findings, the patient was started on anti-toxoplasmosis therapy and improved clinically over the next several days. An MRI performed several weeks later demonstrated marked improvement.

This case demonstrates the utility of [18]F-FDG PET/CT in distinguishing AIDS-related lymphoma from toxoplasmosis of the brain in HIV-positive patients. Due to immuno-suppression, HIV-infected patients are prone to develop both opportunistic infections and malignancies such as lymphoma, with 50% of cerebral lesions in these patients representing toxoplasmosis and 30% CNS lymphoma, while 20% have other pathological processes such as progressive multifocal leukoencephalopathy (PML) or fungal infection.[28]

Infection by the intracellular protozoan parasite, *Toxoplasma gondii*, may cause focal cerebral lesions or diffuse meningoencephalitis. On MRI and CT, these lesions appear as single or multifocal ring-enhancing lesions, most common in the basal ganglia, thalamus, and gray/white matter junction. It is not always possible to distinguish primary CNS lymphoma from toxoplasmosis on the basis of CT or MRI alone.[29] F-FDG PET/CT can be a useful modality for distinguishing the various etiologies by revealing the metabolic activity of the lesions. Primary CNS lymphoma usually demonstrates intense [18]F-FDG avidity. Toxoplasmosis, as seen in this case, is not [18]F-FDG avid relative to the cerebral cortex and allows for accurate diagnosis.[30,31]

PML must also be considered in the differential diagnosis of hypometabolic lesions in HIV-positive patients, although they can be occasionally hypermetabolic. Fungal infections are commonly hypermetabolic, but not frequent in the HIV-positive population.

## Diagnosis

Toxoplasmosis abscess of the brain.

## Clinical Report: Brain [18]F-FDG PET/CT (for DVD cases only)

Indication

Evaluation of a left cerebral lesion in an HIV-positive patient.

History

This 41-year-old male with a history of HIV infection presented with a large lesion in the left basal ganglia on CT and MRI. [18]F-FDG PET/CT is performed in order to differentiate between toxoplasmosis and lymphoma.

Procedure

The fasting blood glucose level was 132 mg/dl. [18]F-FDG (9.7 millicuries, 359 MBq) was administered intravenously in a right antecubital vein. Following a 45 min distribution time, CT without contrast was acquired to correct for attenuation, followed by PET of the brain.

Findings

   *Quality of the study*: The quality of the study is good.

   *Brain*: There is relative decreased uptake within the region of the left basal ganglia relative to the brain, corresponding to the anatomic location of the 18 mm lesion identified on the above-mentioned MRI of the brain performed the same day. There is diffuse decreased $^{18}$F-FDG uptake throughout the left cerebral hemisphere in comparison to the right.

Impression

There is relatively decreased $^{18}$F-FDG metabolism within the left basal ganglia mass, most consistent with a toxoplasmosis abscess of the brain.

## Case II.1.5

### History

This 63-year-old male was recently diagnosed with non-small-cell lung cancer with a large right hilar and paratracheal mass. He also had extensive adenopathy throughout the mediastinum visualized on a chest CT. The patient was referred to $^{18}$F-FDG PET/CT for initial staging prior to radiation therapy (Fig. II.1.5).

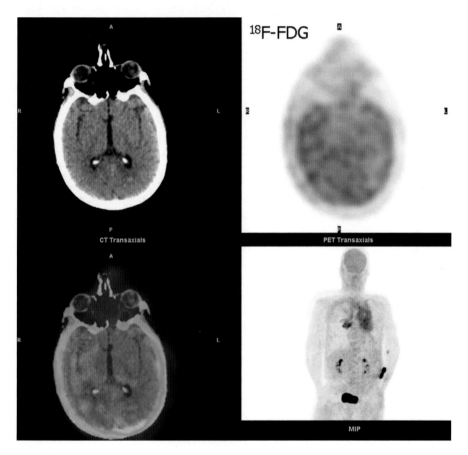

**Fig. II.1.5**

### Findings

The quality of the study is limited due to diffusely diminished uptake within the cerebral cortex, which may be due to a non-fasting or hyperglycemic state. There is also misregistration of the PET and CT images due to patient motion. While there are no focal abnormalities visualized on the limited-quality PET images, on CT images there are two small subcentimeter hyperattenuating lesions in the left parieto-occipital white matter (Fig. II.1.5).

The MIP image demonstrates intense $^{18}$F-FDG uptake within a right hilar mass and mediastinal adenopathy. There is moderately increased $^{18}$F-FDG uptake within the left upper lobe corresponding ground glass opacification on CT (not shown).

## Discussion

The hyperattenuating lesions in the left parieto-occipital white matter visualized on the CT images are most consistent with cerebral metastases. The patient had advanced stage disease and developed pulmonary decompensation. He declined radiation therapy and died within a few days.

Cerebral metastases are the most common intracranial tumors in adults and occur in 20–40% of cancer patients, most commonly in cancers of the lung, breast, and melanoma. Cerebral metastases result from hematogenous spread.[3]

Despite the limited quality of the study, valuable clinical information was gained by viewing the CT images of the brain. Without their careful inspection, it can be easy to miss small metastatic lesions that may be below the resolution of PET or that may demonstrate iso-intense [18]F-FDG uptake compared to surrounding cortex.

Gadolinium-enhanced MRI of the brain is the diagnostic test of choice when metastases are suspected, but asymptomatic lesion can be found prior to the onset of neurological symptoms on whole-body [18]F-FDG PET/CT examinations when the brain is included in the field of view. Metastases to the brain typically appear on non-contrast CT scans as focal regions of hypodense or isodense mass lesion(s) near the gray–white junction, with associated vasogenic edema, possibly also with a mass effect.[32] Some lesions may appear hyperdense on non-contrast CT because of acute intra-tumoral hemorrhage or from increased tissue density of the tumor itself.[33]

The diffusely diminished [18]F-FDG uptake within the brain in this case is most likely due to hyperglycemia. The fasting blood glucose was measured at 170 mg/dl prior to [18]F-FDG administration. High levels of plasma glucose causes competitive inhibition of [18]F-FDG transport into cells, including neurons. Sedating medications can also result in decreased [18]F-FDG uptake within the brain.

## Diagnosis

1.  Stage IV non-small-cell lung cancer with cerebral metastases.
2.  Poor [18]F-FDG uptake within the brain due to hyperglycemia.

## Case II.1.6

### History

This 61-year-old male has a history of non-small-cell lung cancer treated with resection 3 years previously. A recent CT of the chest revealed a small pulmonary nodule in the left lower lobe, suspicious of recurrence. The patient was referred to whole-body $^{19}$F-FDG PET/CT imaging for restaging. Images of the brain are shown (Fig. II.1.6A, B, C).

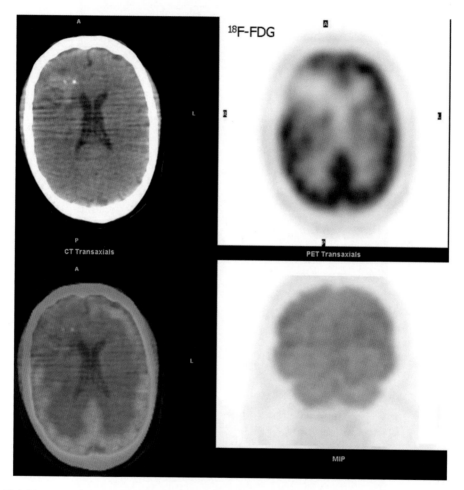

**Fig. II.1.6A**

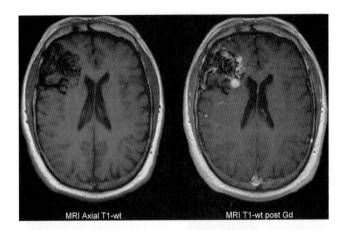

**Fig. II.1.6B**

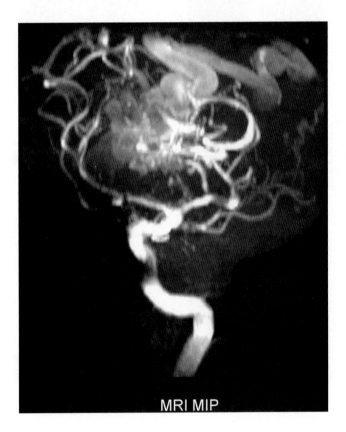

**Fig. II.1.6C**

## Findings

$^{18}$F-FDG PET/CT images of the brain reveal a large focus of decreased $^{18}$F-FDG uptake in the right frontal lobe (Fig. II.1.6A). On CT, this corresponds to a large, intra-axial hyperdense mass, with small, punctate calcifications. There is a subtle mass effect on the right frontal lobe with mildly decreased attenuation. There is no midline shift. Of note, the small left lower lobe pulmonary nodule (not shown) did not demonstrate [18]F-FDG avidity.

## Discussion

Due to the patient's history of lung cancer, metastasis must be considered in the differential diagnosis of the cerebral lesion. Given the CT appearance, a primary cerebral tumor (specifically a high-grade glioma) should be considered, although the diminished [18]F-FDG uptake would favor a low-grade tumor or a benign process.

MRI of the brain was performed for further evaluation (Fig. II.1.6B, C), revealing multiple serpiginous flow void regions in a large corresponding region measuring 51 × 46 mm, with large varicose draining cortical veins extending to the sagittal sinus. This appearance was most consistent with a large cerebral arterio-venous malformation (AVM).

AVMs are abnormal conglomerations of arteries and veins in which a loss of normal vascular organization and the lack of a capillary bed lead to arterio-venous shunting.[34] Approximately half of patients with symptomatic cerebral AVMs first present with intra-cerebral hemorrhage. Other presentations include seizure, headache, and focal neurological deficits. Many cerebral AVMs are asymptomatic and incidentally discovered on CT or MRI. The annual risk of hemorrhage is estimated to be in the range of 2–4%, with a 5–10% chance of death and a greater chance of permanent neurological deficit. Treatment options include surgical resection, radiosurgery, endovascular embolization, or some combination of these options.[35]

It is not uncommon to encounter unexpected but potentially significant findings when interpreting PET/CT examinations.[36] Some of these unexpected findings are only seen on the CT portion of the examination since they are not [18]F-FDG-avid. Nonetheless, they may be clinically significant and should be reported according to guidelines for appropriate training of nuclear medicine physicians and diagnostic radiologists for interpretation and reporting of PET/CT examinations.[37,38]

## Diagnosis

Right frontal cerebral arterio-venous malformation (AVM).

## Case II.1.7 (DICOM Images on DVD)

### History

This is a 60-year-old male with a history of a right frontotemporal glioblastoma multiforme diagnosed 10 months previously, treated with surgical resection followed by radiation and chemotherapy. A recent MRI revealed heterogeneous enhancement of the right temporal lobe with posterior and medial extension toward the region of prior treatment. He was referred to [18]F-FDG PET/CT to help differentiate recurrent tumor from late, delayed radiation injury (LDRI) (Fig. II.1.7A, B).

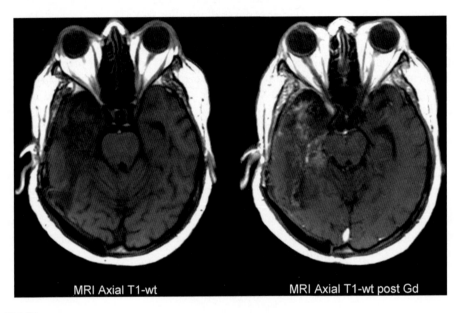

MRI Axial T1-wt                          MRI Axial T1-wt post Gd

Fig. II.1.7A

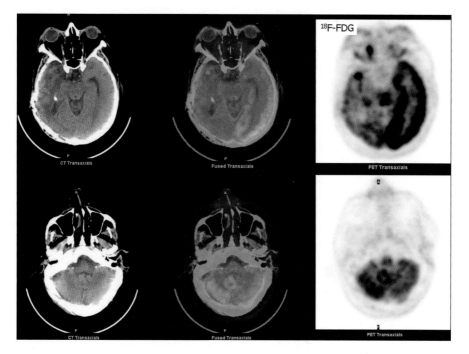

**Fig. II.1.7B**

## Findings

There is diffusely decreased uptake throughout the residual right temporal and parieto-temporal regions consistent with therapy-induced changes as well as a small focus of intensely increased uptake in the anterior tip of the right temporal lobe measuring $10 \times 9$ mm (Fig. II.1.7B, upper row) corresponding to a focus of abnormal enhancement on the recent MRI (Fig. II.1.7A). There is also intense $^{18}$F-FDG uptake corresponding to the region of abnormal enhancement seen on the MRI extending from anterior to posterior along the temporal horn of the right lateral ventricle (best seen on the PET-only image). There is asymmetrically decreased activity in the left cerebellum (Fig. II.1.7B, bottom row).

## Discussion

The diffusely diminished uptake throughout the right temporal and parieto-temporal regions is most likely due to therapy-induced changes. The focal areas of intense $^{19}$F-FDG uptake in the right temporal lobe are most consistent with recurrent glioblastoma multiforme. The asymmetrically decreased activity in the left cerebellum represents crossed cerebellar diaschisis.

Glioblastoma multiforme is the most malignant cerebral tumor, with a median survival of 1 year. Despite aggressive multimodality therapy including surgery, radiation therapy, and chemotherapy, prognosis remains poor.[39]

Following treatment of high-grade gliomas, evaluation for tumor recurrence can be a clinical challenge. Neurological symptoms that develop after treatment may be attributable to either recurrent tumor or to necrosis of the tumor and surrounding cortex. Areas of necrosis appear as edematous masses on MRI and CT that enhance due to increased permeability of the blood–brain barrier. These changes can occur from several weeks to several months or even years following therapy. Changes associated with radiation necrosis – LDRI – can be indistinguishable from recurrent high-grade tumor.

Metabolic [18]F-FDG imaging can be helpful in differentiating between recurrent cerebral tumors and radiation injury, with sensitivity in the 80–90% range and a specificity of 50–90%.[40] Most recurrent high-grade tumors demonstrate marked [19]F-FDG uptake. Conversely, radiation injury results in tissue necrosis that does not accumulate [18]F-FDG.

Crossed cerebellar diaschisis occurs when a cerebral hemispheric abnormality results in under-stimulation of the contralateral cerebellar hemisphere, resulting in decreased metabolic activity with resultant decrease in [18]F-FDG uptake relative to the other hemisphere. These findings reflect the functional relationship between the cerebral cortex and the cerebellum.[41]

## Diagnosis

1. Recurrent glioblastoma multiforme.
2. Diminished uptake in the right temporal region due to previous treatment.
3. Crossed cerebellar diaschisis.

## Clinical Report: Brain [18]F-FDG PET/CT (for DVD cases only)

Indication

Restaging of glioblastoma multiforme.

History

This 60-year-old male with a right frontotemporal glioblastoma multiforme diagnosed 10 months ago and treated with surgical resection, radiation, and chemotherapy experienced progressive lower extremity weakness for the last 3 months. Recent MRI revealed heterogeneous enhancement of the right temporal lobe extending in a posterior and medial direction from the location of the original tumor. The patient is referred for [18]F-FDG PET/CT to differentiate between suspected recurrence and treatment-related changes.

Procedure

The fasting blood glucose level was 91 mg/dl. [18]F-FDG (11.7 millicuries, 433 MBq) was administered via a right antecubital vein. Following a 70 min distribution time, CT of the brain without contrast was acquired to correct for attenuation followed by acquisition of PET images.

Findings

*Quality of the study*: The quality of the study is good.

*Brain*: There is physiologic distribution of $^{18}$F-FDG throughout the gray matter. There is diffusely decreased uptake throughout the right temporal and parieto-temporal regions, consistent with therapy-induced changes. There is a small focus of intensely increased $^{18}$F-FDG uptake in the anterior tip of the residual right temporal lobe, $10 \times 9$ mm in size, corresponding to a focus of abnormal enhancement on the recent MRI. There is also intense $^{18}$F-FDG uptake, corresponding to the region of abnormal enhancement seen on the MRI, extending in the anterior to posterior direction along the temporal horn of the right lateral ventricle. Asymmetrically decreased $^{18}$F-FDG activity is seen in the left cerebellum.

Impression

1. Recurrent glioblastoma multiforme of the right temporal lobe.
2. Therapy-related changes of the right temporal and parieto-temporal regions.
3. Crossed cerebellar diaschisis.

## *Case II.1.8*

### History

This 41-year-old female with a right below-the-elbow amputation for a clear-cell sarcoma of the wrist 4 years previously was referred for a whole-body [18]F-FDG PET/CT for periodic surveillance with no clinical evidence of disease (Fig. II.1.8A).

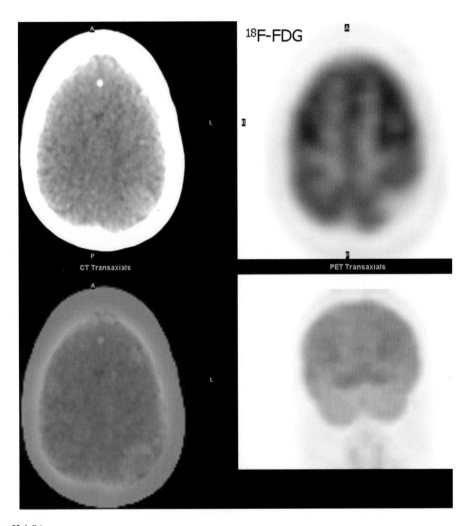

**Fig. II.1.8A**

**Findings**

There is a non-[18]F-FDG avid mass just to the left of, and below the vertex corresponding to an intracranial, extra-axial mass that appears to be dural-based, with an extrinsic mass effect on the brain (Fig. II.1.8A). The mass is slightly hyperdense relative to the cerebral parenchyma on CT and has a maximum axial dimension of 21 mm. Uptake is clearly less than gray matter and very close to white matter. The mass was not visible until the window-width and window-level settings were optimized for visualization of the intracranial regions. MRI was recommended to better characterize the mass.

There are no [18]F-FDG avid foci on the whole-body examination to suggest recurrent malignancy.

**Discussion**

The presence of an extra-axial, well-defined intracranial mass in an asymptomatic patient with no other evidence of residual tumor is most suggestive of a benign meningioma, the most common non-glial intracranial tumor. However, [18]F-FDG uptake in sarcomas can be variable, and uptake is difficult to judge due to the nearby normal uptake in gray matter.

Sagittal MRI (Fig. II.1.8B, upper row, T1-weighted, pre- and post-gadolinium, upper left and right, respectively) with sagittal PET (Fig. II.1.8B, lower left) and fused PET/CT (Fig. II.1.8B, lower right) demonstrate findings that are most consistent with a meningioma based on the anatomic and signal characteristics of the mass on the MRI, including the uniform and intense enhancement pattern, the [18]F-FDG uptake pattern, and the CT appearance. The post-gadolinium MRI images also demonstrate a "dural tail sign" (small arrow, Fig. II.1.8B upper right) of enhancement trailing from the mass into the adjacent meninges. Despite these strong characteristics favoring a benign meningioma, the patient elected to have the mass resected. Diagnosis of a well-differentiated meningioma was confirmed at pathologic examination of the surgical specimen.

Most meningiomas seen on [18]F-FDG PET/CT will appear similar to this example: an incidental mass with minimal uptake and mild (if any) mass effect on the brain. Edema, sometimes severe, can be seen in the underlying brain, but is not specific for the type or aggressiveness of the meningioma. The differential diagnosis includes metastatic disease, lymphoma, and inflammatory processes such as sarcoidosis or tuberculosis, Wegener's granulomatosis, rheumatoid nodules, fungal disease, and leutic gummas. Other conditions that can mimic a meningioma, with or without associated calcifications, include a cranial osteoma, chronic subdural or epidural hematoma, or an old abscess or empyema. Granulomatous disease processes more commonly involve the basilar meninges than the convexities.

Just as [18]F-FDG uptake is directly related to aggressiveness of gliomas, investigators have shown the same relationship between uptake and tumor grade of meningiomas. In a report of 62 patients, the degree of [18]F-FDG uptake was directly and significantly correlated with the proliferation rate ($p < 0.025$) and cellularity ($p < 0.01$) of the tumor.[42]

In a similar report of 75 patients, the meningioma-to-contralateral gray matter ratio (TGR) of [18]F-FDG uptake was found to reliably discriminate between typical WHO grade I and WHO grade II or III meningiomas, especially in a fasting patient. SUV measurements were inferior to the TGR for tumor grade discrimination. Increased blood glucose levels in

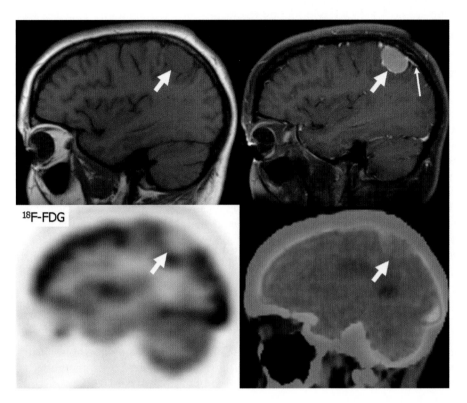

**Fig. II.1.8B**

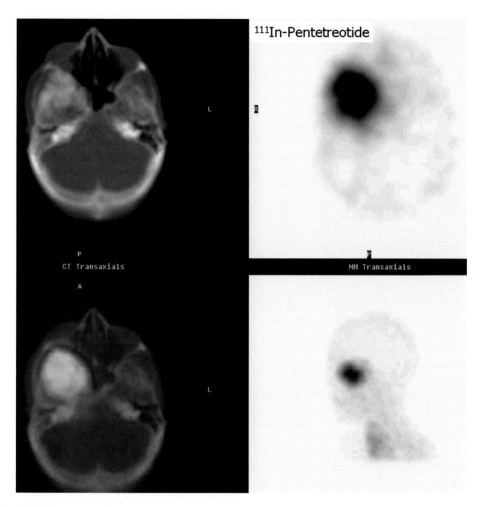

**Fig. II.1.8C**

either diabetic or non-fasting patients caused false positive results with an apparent relative increase in the tumor uptake.[43]

While there is extensive literature concerning the role of $^{18}$F-FDG imaging in evaluation of meningiomas, there is also a role for the use of $^{111}$In-pentetreotide SPECT/CT. The majority of meningiomas are somatostatin-receptor expressing and, especially if over 25 mm in size, are well demonstrated with $^{111}$In-pentetreotide. A particular advantage of $^{111}$In-pentetreotide SPECT/CT over $^{18}$F-FDG PET/CT in this clinical setting is the lack of physiologic cerebral uptake of $^{111}$In-pentetreotide, thus improving the tumor-to-background ratio compared to $^{18}$F-FDG. In the example of $^{111}$In-pentetreotide imaging with SPECT/CT demonstrated in Fig. II.1.8C the tumor is easily visible against the low background, and the accompanying CT demonstrates the hyperostosis induced by bone involvement with the meningioma. Because of the resolution limitations of medium energy collimators, 25 mm is the lower size range for $^{111}$In-pentetreotide detectability rate of suspected meningiomas. Early experimental work with $^{68}$Ga-DOTATOC[44] and $^{19}$F-FLT,[45] both PET agents providing superior resolution relative to $^{111}$In and minimal normal cerebral uptake, suggests that these PET imaging agents will demonstrate meningiomas to good advantage.

**Diagnosis**

Incidental extra-axial, intracranial mass, surgically proven to be a benign or typical meningioma.

# Case II.1.9*

## History

A 55-year-old male patient was referred to brain $^{11}$C-methionine PET imaging 6 years after resection of a WHO grade II (low-grade) oligodendroglioma of the right temporal lobe because of indeterminate CT and MRI evaluations for recurrent tumor (Fig. II.1.9A, B, C).

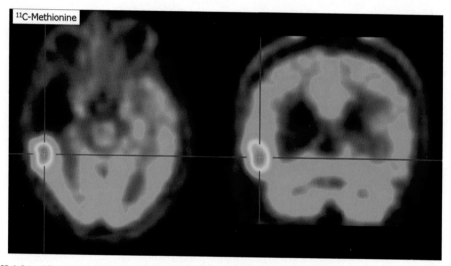

**Fig. II.1.9A**  (Courtesy of K. Van Laere and L. Mortelmans, University Hospital Leuven, Belgium.)

*  This case is courtesy of K. Van Laere and L. Mortelmans, University Hospital Leuven, Belgium.

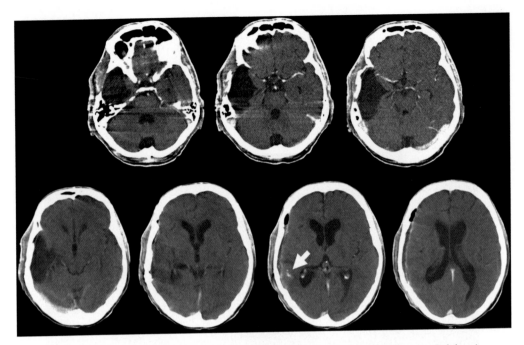

**Fig. II.1.9B** (Courtesy of K. Van Laere and L. Mortelmans, University Hospital Leuven, Belgium.)

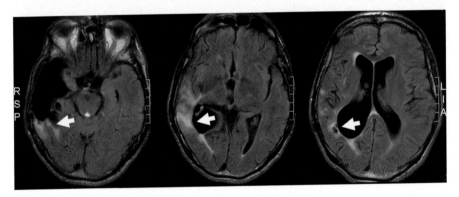

**Fig. II.1.9C** (Courtesy of K. Van Laere and L. Mortelmans, University Hospital Leuven, Belgium.)

## Findings

The axial (left) and coronal (right) $^{11}$C-methionine PET images of the brain (Fig. II.1.9A) demonstrate a focal area of intense uptake corresponding to the region of subtle enhancement on post-IV contrast axial CT (Fig. II.1.9B, arrow) and the region of increased signal on the axial FLAIR MRI images (Fig. II.1.9C, arrows) in the posterior margin of the surgical bed. There are obvious surgical changes due to prior resection in the right temporal and parieto-temporal region, and, therefore, the findings on CT and MRI could be due to post-surgical gliosis or recurrent tumor. The $^{11}$C-methionine-to-background ratio uptake (SUVmax/SUVbackground) yields a metabolic index of 2.95.

## Discussion

$^{18}$F-FDG PET/CT is of limited value in evaluation of low-grade gliomas due to the relatively low metabolic rate of these tumors compared to normal cortex.

A common feature of cerebral tumors, including low-grade gliomas, is active protein synthesis, which is above that of normal cortex and is supported by active transport of amino-acids, including methionine, occurring even with an intact blood–brain barrier. Thus, in cerebral tumors with low metabolic rates (e.g., low-grade gliomas), $^{11}$C-methionine (a radiolabeled amino-acid) PET imaging can demonstrate increased uptake in the tumor compared to the surrounding cortex, unlike $^{18}$F-FDG. In this patient, there is a clear-cut focal region of intense uptake in the posterior margin of the patient's surgical bed (Fig. II.1.9A), corresponding to the abnormalities seen on the CT and MRI mentioned earlier, with a ratio of abnormal to normal cerebral tissue of 2.95. While the reported significant ratio of tumor to normal cerebral tissue differs between reported series, a ratio of ≥1.6 usually indicates tumor physiology.[12]

Increased amino-acid active transport is not specific for primary brain glioma and has been reported for gliomas of all grades, metastatic disease, and meningiomas. Radiation or surgically induced gliosis and normal cerebral tissue all have a very low level of protein synthesis. Both $^{18}$F-FDG and $^{11}$C-methionine PET are useful for demonstrating the location of high-grade cerebral tumors when uptake of either PET tracer will be above that of normal gray matter.[5,8–10,46]

$^{11}$C-methionine PET, especially co-registered with corresponding MRI images, can also provide a valuable tool to confirm low-grade glioma presence and/or recurrence, as well as provide biopsy or surgical guidance for tumor resection. $^{11}$C-methionine is the most evaluated PET imaging agent for these indications, but other amino-acids, labeled with either $^{11}$C or $^{19}$F have been evaluated and show promising results as well.[5,8–10,46]

## Diagnosis

Recurrent low-grade oligodendroglioma of the residual right parieto-temporal lobe.

## Follow-Up

Repeat resection of the recurrent grade II oligodendroglioma was performed. The patient was alive and clinically free of disease 2 years after repeat surgical resection, 8 years after initial surgery, and 10 years after initial diagnosis.

# References

1. Jemal A, Siegel R, Ward E, Murray T, Xu J, Thun MJ. Cancer statistics, 2007. *CA Cancer J Clin* 2007;57:43–66.
2. http://www.cancer.gov/cancertopics/pdq/treatment/adultbrain/healthprofessional.
3. Buckner JC, Brown PD, O'Neill BP, Meyer FB, Wetmore CJ, Uhm JH. Central nervous system tumors. *Mayo Clin Proc* 2007;82:1271–1286.
4. Norden AD, Wen PY. Glioma therapy in adults. *Neurologist* 2006;12:279–292.
5. Chen W. Clinical applications of PET in brain tumors. *J Nucl Med* 2007;48:1468–1481.
6. Chugani HT, Phelps ME, Mazziotta JC. Positron emission tomography study of human brain functional development. *Ann Neurol* 1987;22:487–497.
7. Di Chiro G. Positron emission tomography using [18F] fluorodeoxyglucose in brain tumors. A powerful diagnostic and prognostic tool. *Invest Radiol* 1987;22:360–371.
8. Pirotte BJ, Lubansu A, Massager N, Wikler D, Goldman S, Levivier M. Results of positron emission tomography guidance and reassessment of the utility of and indications for stereotactic biopsy in children with infiltrative brainstem tumors. *J Neurosurg* 2007;107:392–399.
9. Pirotte B, Goldman S, Massager N, David P, Wikler D, Vandesteene A, Salmon I, Brotchi J, Levivier M. Comparison of 18F-FDG and 11C-methionine for PET-guided stereotactic brain biopsy of gliomas. *J Nucl* 2004;45:1293–1298.
10. Pirotte B, Goldman S, Van Bogaert P, David P, Wikler D, Rorive S, Brotchi J, Levivier M. Integration of [11C]methionine-positron emission tomographic and magnetic resonance imaging for image-guided surgical resection of infiltrative low-grade brain tumors in children. *Neurosurgery* 2005;57(1 Suppl):128–139.
11. Hustinx R, Pourdehnad M, Kaschten B, Alavi A. PET imaging for differentiating recurrent brain tumor from radiation necrosis. *Radiol Clin North Am* 2005;43:35–47.
12. Terakawa Y, Tsuyuguchi N, Iwai Y, Yamanaka K, Higashiyama S, Takami T, Ohata K. Diagnostic accuracy of ¹¹C-Methionine PET for differentiation of recurrent brain tumors from radiation necrosis after radiotherapy. *J Nucl Med* 2008; 49:694–699.
13. Griffeth LK, Rich KM, Dehdashti F, Simpson JR, Fusselman MJ, McGuire AH, Siegel BA. Brain metastases from non-central nervous system tumors: evaluation with PET. *Radiology* 1993;186:37–44.
14. Rohren EM, Provenzale JM, Barboriak DP, Coleman RE. Screening for cerebral metastases with FDG PET in patients undergoing whole-body staging of non-central nervous system malignancy. *Radiology* 2003;226:181–187.
15. Shaman MA, Zak IT, Kupsky WJ. Best cases from the AFIP: Involuted sclerotic meningioma. *Radiographics* 2003;23:785–789.
16. Smirniotopoulos JG, Murphy FM, Rushing EJ, Rees JH, Schroeder JW. From the archives of the AFIP patterns of contrast enhancement in the brain and meninges. *Radiographics* 2007;27:525–551.
17. Podoloff DA, Ball DW, Ben-Josef E, Benson AB, Cohen SJ, Coleman RE, Delbeke D, Ho M, Ilson DH, Kalemkerian GP, Lee RJ, Loeffler JS, Macapinlac HA, Morgan RJ, Siegel BA, Singhal S, Tyler DS, Wong RJ. NCCN Task Force: Clinical Utility of PET in a Variety of Tumor Types Task Force. *J Natl Compr Canc Netw* 2009;7 Suppl 2:S1–S23. www.nccn.org/professionals/physician_gls/f_guidelines.asp
18. Bénard F, Romsa J, Hustinx R. Imaging gliomas with positron emission tomography and single-photon emission computed tomography. *Semin Nucl Med* 2003;33:148–162.
19. Hustinx R, Smith RJ, Benard F, Bhatnagar A, Alavi A. Can the standardized uptake value characterize primary brain tumors on FDG-PET? *Eur J Nucl Med* 1999;26:1501–1509.
20. Di Chiro G, DeLaPaz RL, Brooks RA, Sokoloff L, Kornblith PL, Smith BH, Patronas NJ, Kufta CV, Kessler RM, Johnston GS, Manning RG, Wolf AP. Glucose utilization of cerebral gliomas measured by [18F] fluorodeoxyglucose and positron emission tomography. *Neurology* 1982;32:1323–1329.
21. Padma MV, Said S, Jacobs M, Hwang DR, Dunigan K, Satter M, Christian B, Ruppert J, Bernstein T, Kraus G, Mantil JC. Prediction of pathology and survival by FDG PET in gliomas. *J Neurooncol* 2003;64:227–237.
22. De Witte O, Levivier M, Violon P, Salmon I, Damhaut P, Wikler Jr D, Hildebrand J, Brotchi J, Goldman S. Prognostic value positron emission tomography with [18F]fluoro-2-deoxy-D-glucose in the low-grade glioma. *Neurosurgery* 1996;39:470–476; discussion 476–477.
23. Meyer PT, Schreckenberger M, Spetzger U, Meyer GF, Sabri O, Setani KS, Zeggel T, Buell U. Comparison of visual and ROI-based brain tumour grading using 18F-FDG PET: ROC analyses. *Eur J Nucl Med* 2001;28:165–174.

24. Borbély K, Nyáry I, Tóth M, Ericson K, Gulyás B. Optimization of semi-quantification in metabolic PET studies with 18F-fluorodeoxyglucose and 11C-methionine in the determination of malignancy of gliomas. *J Neurol Sci* 2006; 246:85–94.

25. Delbeke D, Meyerowitz C, Lapidus RL, Maciunas RJ, Jennings MT, Moots PL, Kessler RM. Optimal cutoff levels of F-18 fluorodeoxyglucose uptake in the differentiation of low-grade from high-grade brain tumors with PET. *Radiology* 1995;195:47–52.

26. Mohile NA, Abrey LE. Primary central nervous system lymphoma. *Neurol Clin* 2007; 25:1193–1207.

27. Mohile NA, Deangelis LM, Abrey LE. The utility of body FDG PET in staging primary central nervous system lymphoma. *Neuro Oncol* 2008;10:223–228.

28. Ciricillo SF, Rosenblum ML. Use of CT and MR imaging to distinguish intracranial lesions and to define the need for biopsy in AIDS patients. *J Neurosurg* 1990;73:720–724.

29. Offiah CE, Turnbull IW. The imaging appearances of intracranial CNS infections in adult HIV and AIDS patients. *Clin Radiol* 2006;61:393–401.

30. Hoffman JM, Waskin HA, Schifter T, Hanson MW, Gray L, Rosenfeld S, Coleman RW. FDG-PET in differentiating lymphoma from nonmalignant central nervous system lesions in patients with AIDS. *J Nucl Med* 1993; 34:567–575.

31. O'Doherty MJ, Barrington SF, Campbell M, Lowe J, Bradbeer CS. PET scanning and the human immunodeficiency virus-positive patient. *J Nucl Med* 1997;38:1575–1583.

32. Young RJ, Sills AK, Brem S, Knopp EA. Neuroimaging of metastatic brain disease. *Neurosurgery* 2005;57(5 Suppl):S10–23; discussion S1–4.

33. Nguyen TD, DeAngelis LM. Brain metastases. *Neurol Clin* 2007;25:1173–1192.

34. Friedlander RM. Clinical practice. Arteriovenous malformations of the brain. *N Engl J Med* 2007; 356:2704–2712.

35. Choi JH, Mohr JP. Brain arteriovenous malformations in adults. *Lancet Neurol* 2005;4:299–308.

36. Bruzzi JF, Truong MT, Marom EM, Mawlawi O, Podoloff DA, Macapinlac HA, Munden RF. Incidental findings on integrated PET/CT that do not accumulate 18F-FDG. *AJR Am J Roentgenol* 2006;187:1116–1123.

37. Coleman RE, Delbeke D, Guiberteau MJ, Conti PS, Royal DD, Weinreb JC, Siegel BA, Federle MF, Townsend DW, Berland LL. Concurrent PET/CT with an integrated imaging system: Intersociety dialogue from the joint working group of the American College of Radiology, the Society of Nuclear Medicine, and the Society of Computed Body Tomography and Magnetic Resonance. *J Nucl Med* 2005;46:1225–1239.

38. Delbeke D, Coleman RE, Guiberteau MJ, Brown ML, Royal HD, Siegel BA, Townsend DW, Berland LL, Parker JA, Hubner K, Stabin MG, Zubal G, Kachelriess M, Cronin V, Holbrook S. Procedure guideline for tumor imaging with 18F-FDG PET/CT. *J Nucl Med* 2006;47:885–895.

39. Krex D, Klink B, Hartmann C, von Deimling A, Pietsch T, Simon M, Sabel M, Steinbach JP, Heese O, Reifenberger G, Weller M, Schackert G, for the German Glioma Network. Long-term survival with glioblastoma multiforme. *Brain* 2007;130 (Pt 10):2596–2606.

40. Langleben DD, Segall GM. PET in differentiation of recurrent brain tumor from radiation injury. *J Nucl Med* 2000;41:1861–1867.

41. Otte A, Roelcke U, von Ammon K, Hausmann O, Maguire RP, Missimer J, Müller-Brand J, Radü EW, Leenders KL. Crossed cerebellar diaschisis and brain tumor biochemistry studied with positron emission tomography, [18F]fluorodeoxyglucose and [11C]methionine. *J Neurol Sci* 1998;156:73–77.

42. Lippitz B, Cremerius U, Mayfrank L, Bertalanffy H, Raoofi R, Weis J, Böcking A, Büll U, Gilsbach JM. PET-study of intracranial meningiomas: Correlation with histopathology, cellularity and proliferation rate. *Acta Neurochirurgica* 1996;65:108–111.

43. Cremerius U, Bares R, Weis J, Sabri O, Mull M, Schröder JM, Gilsbach JM, Buell U. Fasting improves discrimination of grade 1 and atypical or malignant meningioma in FDG-PET. *J Nucl Med* 1997;38:26–30.

44. Henze M, Schuhmacher J, Hipp P, Kowalski J, Becker DW, Doll J, Mäcke HR, Hofmann M, Debus J, Haberkorn U. PET imaging of somatostatin receptors using [$^{68}$GA]DOTA-D-Phe$^{1}$-Try$^{3}$-Octreotide: first results in patients with meningiomas. *J Nucl Med* 2001;42:1053–1056.

45. Rutten I, Cabay JE, Withoffs N, Lemaire C, Aerts J, Baart V, Hustinx R. PET/CT of skull base meningiomas using 2-$^{18}$F-Fluoro-L-Tyrosine: Initial report. *J Nucl Med* 2007; 48:720–725.

46. Coope D, Cizek J, Eggers C, Vollmar S, Heiss W-D, Herholz K. Evaluation of primary brain tumors using $^{11}$C-Methionine PET with reference to a normal methionine uptake map. *J Nucl Med* 2007;48:1971–1980.

# Chapter II.2
# Hybrid Imaging of Head and Neck Malignancies

Arie Gordin, Marcelo Daitzchman, and Ora Israel

## Introduction

Head and neck cancer represents approximately 2–4% of all malignancies in the United States, with an annual incidence of 38,000 new cases.[1] The majority of these malignancies (over 90%) are squamous cell carcinoma (SCC) of the larynx, oropharynx, and oral cavity. Early detection and accurate staging of head and neck tumors are critical for selecting the appropriate treatment and therefore are of prognostic significance. After therapy, early detection of recurrence has been shown to improve patient outcome.[2]

Computed tomography (CT) and magnetic resonance imaging (MRI) are the standard imaging modalities for assessing head and neck cancer. These tests are, however, based on morphological diagnostic criteria, such as nodal size and contrast enhancement patterns, which do not always accurately reflect the presence of malignancy.[3] In particular, distinction between treatment-related changes and recurrent or residual tumor using imaging modalities that rely on morphologic criteria is challenging and has a limited accuracy due to the distorted regional anatomy caused by previous surgery and/or radiation therapy.[4]

Fluorine-18 fluorodeoxyglucose ($^{18}$F-FDG) positron emission tomography (PET) plays an increasing role in the assessment of head and neck cancer, both for initial staging[5] and for monitoring patients after treatment.[6,7] PET is a functional diagnostic test that reflects metabolism and biology of the tumor, has been proven to be superior to both CT and MRI in the assessment of cancer of the head and neck,[6–9] but is limited by the lack of anatomical landmarks. Precise localization of suspicious foci of increased tracer uptake is difficult in the presence of low background activity. The region of the head and neck has a complex anatomy with a variety of extremely important but also delicate structures. Additionally, variable degrees of uptake of $^{18}$F-FDG are encountered in the region of the head and neck due to sites of physiologic biodistribution of the tracer and to $^{18}$F-FDG avidity of benign, mainly inflammatory, processes, unrelated to cancer. Regional physiologic $^{18}$F-FDG uptake seen in the lymphoid tissue of the Waldeyer ring, in the salivary glands, in active or strained skeletal muscles (mainly the vocal cords and neck muscles), and in activated brown fat tissue in the neck and shoulder girdle has to be differentiated from cancer.[10] Paralysis of one of the vocal cords can cause an increased uptake in the other cord due to excessive use. Asymmetric physiologic $^{18}$F-FDG uptake is frequently seen in the mastication muscles, sternocleidomastoid muscle, and various other neck muscles due to strain or

A. Gordin (✉)
Department of Otolaryngology, Head and Neck Surgery, The Hospital for Sick Children, Toronto, ON, Canada
e-mail: a_gordin@rambam.health.gov.il

D. Delbeke, O. Israel (eds.), *Hybrid PET/CT and SPECT/CT Imaging*,
DOI 10.1007/978-0-387-92820-3_4, © Springer Science+Business Media, LLC 2010

excessive use. Warthin's tumor and pleomorphic adenoma, benign lesions of the salivary gland, have been described to accumulate $^{18}$F-FDG and can be erroneously interpreted as malignancy.[11]

PET/CT allows for sequentially acquiring PET and CT studies in a single session and provides fused imaging data of clinically significant anatomic and metabolic information. It improves the anatomic localization of $^{18}$F-FDG-avid abnormalities and reduces the number of equivocal interpretations, while also defining the functional significance of structural abnormalities seen on CT or MRI.[12,13]

## Staging of Head and Neck Carcinoma

Accurate assessment of the stage of disease at presentation is essential for planning the appropriate therapeutic strategies in patients with head and neck cancer. Head and neck cancer is staged by the tumor, nodes, metastases (TNM) classification (Table II.2.1).

**Table II.2.1** Head and neck cancer staged by the TNM (tumor, nodes, metastases) classification (reprinted with permission from Greene FL, Page DL, Fleming, ID, Fritz AG, Balch CM, Haller DG, Morrow M. (eds): *The AJCC Cancer Staging Manual, Sixth Edition.* New York: Springer-Verlag, 2002.)

| Stage | Grouping | | |
|-------|----------|------|------|
| 0     | Tis      | N0   | M0   |
| I     | T1       | N0   | M0   |
| II    | T2       | N0   | M0   |
| III   | T3       | N0   | M0   |
|       | T1       | N1   | M0   |
|       | T2       | N1   | M0   |
|       | T3       | N1   | M0   |
| IVA   | T4a      | N0   | M0   |
|       | T4a      | N1   | M0   |
|       | T1       | N2   | M0   |
|       | T2       | N2   | M0   |
|       | T3       | N2   | M0   |
|       | T4a      | N2   | M0   |
| IVB   | T4b      | Any N | M0  |
|       | Any T    | N3   | M0   |
| IVC   | Any T    | Any N | M1  |

The T stage is defined by the size of the tumor and the number of involved subsites. While accurate T-staging of head and neck tumors varies to some degree stage T1–T3 indicates, as a rule, an increasing size of the primary malignancy, and T4 defines tumor invasion of surrounding structures.

N-staging of head and neck tumors relates to size, number of nodal metastases and their relation to the primary tumor (contra- or ipsilateral). Cervical lymph nodes are classified and identified by their location in relationship to other anatomical structures in the neck including the sternocleidomastoid muscle, jugular vein, carotid artery, submandibular gland, digastric muscle, hyoid bone, cricoid cartilage, as well as the clavicle and manubrium (Diagram II.2.1).

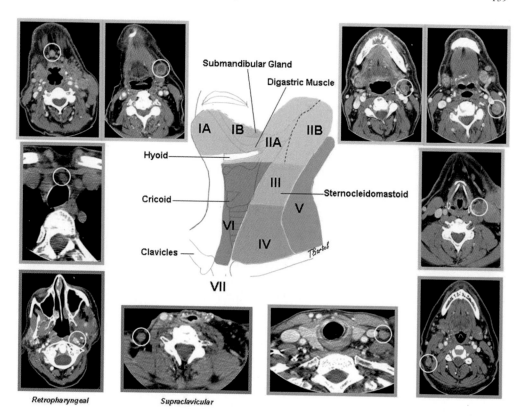

**Diagram II.2.1** Cervical lymph nodes are classified and identified by their location in relationship to other anatomical structures in the neck including the sternocleidomastoid muscle, jugular vein, carotid artery, submandibular gland, digastric muscle, hyoid bone, cricoid cartilage, as well as the clavicle and manubrium (reproduced with permission from the Society of Nuclear Medicine. From Twyla Bartel, Ronald Walker, Laurie Jones-Jackson, Victoria Major, Hemendra Shah, Dominique Delbeke. *Module Oncology CT/Head and Neck. Lifelong Learning and Assessment Program; 2008.* www.snm.org/llsap.)

*Level I* nodes are located above the hyoid and anterior to the submandibular gland, including level IA, submental, and IB nodes, located laterally to IA nodes. They drain the face, tongue, lip, mouth mucosa, floor of the mouth, and nasal cavity. *Level II* upper jugular nodes extend between the base of the skull and the inferior margin of the hyoid and from the posterior aspect of the sternocleidomastoid muscle to the submandibular gland, including IIA jugulo-digastric nodes, located anterior, lateral, and medial to the internal jugular vein and IIB nodes in a more posterior location. They drain the oral and nasal cavity, tonsils, ear, retropharyngeal region, and parotid glands. *Level III* middle jugular nodes drain the naso-, oro-, and hypopharynx, the oral cavity, and larynx. They are located between the hyoid bone and the cricoid cartilage, behind the margin of the sternocleidomastoid muscle and lateral to the carotid. *Level IV* inferior jugular nodes drain the hypopharynx, subglottic larynx, thyroid, and esophagus and lie between the cricoid cartilage and the clavicle, lateral to the carotid. *Level V* posterior triangle nodes drain the posterior scalp and neck, the naso- and oropharynx, and lie posteriorly along the sternocleidomastoid muscle, subdivided into VA nodes located from the base of the skull to the cricoid and VB between the cricoid and the clavicle. *Level VI* anterior compartment nodes draining the thyroid, glottic and subglottic larynx, piriform sinus, and esophagus are located between the hyoid bone and the manubrium and axially between the carotid arteries. *Level VII* upper mediastinal nodes drain the thyroid, parathyroids, and esophagus and lie medial to the carotid arteries from the superior aspect of the manubrium to the innominate veins.

Although [18]F-FDG PET/CT shows similar or even higher detection rates of primary head and neck tumors as compared to conventional imaging modalities,[5,14] its use for T-staging is limited mainly because it does not provide anatomical details comparable to MRI required for planning of surgery and radiotherapy. Performance of PET/CT can be improved by administration of intravenous (IV) contrast and changes in CT acquisition parameters.[15]

The presence of lymph node metastases is an important prognostic factor. The cure rate declines by almost 50% in the presence of regional lymph node involvement.[16] PET/CT is reported to have a higher sensitivity (90–100%) and specificity (85–100%) as compared to contrast CT or MRI (60–90% and 33–90%, respectively) for detecting metastatic cervical lymph nodes.[13,17,18] However, it is not clear whether more accurate N-staging affects patient management. The real challenge in management is in patients with a negative (N0) neck. The probability of a patient with primary head and neck cancer and a N0 neck (defined as such by clinical examination and conventional imaging modalities) to have pathological (N+) neck disease at surgery is between 10 and 45%.[16] Elective neck dissection is recommended whenever the risk for occult neck metastases of a specific head and neck SCC is above 20% (for example, base of tongue and supraglottic SCC). If an imaging test has the potential to improve and correctly identify or exclude neck metastases, patients could be spared unnecessary neck dissection. [18]F-FDG PET, as a stand-alone modality, missed most occult neck metastases in group of patients with oral and oropharyngeal SCC, and this failure has been attributed to the small size of these lesions.[19] Recently, Schoder and colleagues[20] reported a sensitivity of 67% and specificity of 95% for PET/CT in detecting cervical node metastases in a group of patients with clinically defined N0 cancer. However, despite the relatively high accuracy, the authors concluded that surgical management of the N0 neck should not based only on PET/CT findings.

Patients with advanced stage head and neck cancer have a 25% chance of developing distant metastases and 10% chance of having a synchronous malignancy.[21] This group of patients may especially benefit from a pretreatment PET/CT study since detection of distant metastases or a synchronous tumor will change the treatment plan dramatically. [18]F-FDG PET scans the whole body and therefore has the advantage of disclosing unexpected tumor foci outside the head and neck region with a high sensitivity. The superiority of [18]F-FDG imaging over anatomic modalities for diagnosis of distant metastases in patients with head and neck tumors has been demonstrated by several studies.[19,21] Fleming and colleagues reported a 15% detection rate of distant metastases in a group of pretreated head and neck cancer patients, with 70% of the cases having stage III and IV disease.[22] The addition of CT to PET improved the anatomic characterization of distant hypermetabolic foci and made additional imaging tests obsolete, especially in advanced disease.

## Cervical Lymph Node Metastases of Unknown Tumors

Management of patients with metastatic SCC in cervical lymph nodes and no clear evidence of the site of the primary head and neck tumors are a diagnostic as well as a therapeutic challenge. In 2–9% of patients that present with a neck mass that proves to be a metastatic node at biopsy, the primary tumor cannot be identified by the routine diagnostic work-up, which includes physical examination, conventional imaging tests, and panendo-scopy with guided biopsies.[23,24] Detection of the primary tumor improves the patient's prognosis as it allows targeted therapy.[25] The detection rate of the primary tumor in patients with metastatic cervical lymph nodes using PET stand-alone [18]F-FDG imaging varies in reported studies between 8 and 50%,[26,27] the high variability being related at least in part to different inclusion criteria, with an average detection rate (reported in a meta-analysis of nine studies) of 30%.[25] This relatively low overall detection rate has been attributed to the resolution limit of PET (approximately 5 mm) and the high physiological uptake of [18]F-FDG in the region of the head and neck.[24] The detection rate of [18]F-FDG PET/CT for primary tumors in patients with metastatic neck nodes ranges between 40 and 65%.[28,29] PET/CT has been shown to provide data with further clinical impact in up to 60% of patients in this category mainly by improving the localization of tracer uptake foci.[28] Hybrid imaging decreases the false-positive rate attributed to [18]F-FDG PET, thus leading to an increase in sensitivity. However, at present, the cost effectiveness of PET/CT and the impact of this imaging procedure on the outcome of patients with metastatic neck cancer of unknown origin are still unclear and require further investigation.[29]

## Monitoring Response to Therapy

Treatment options in patients with cancer of the head and neck include surgery, radiation therapy, chemo-radiation, and combinations of the above, depending on the stage of disease. Early assessment of treatment response to chemo-radiation or radiotherapy is highly significant since salvage surgery performed after completion of these initial treat-ments improves local disease control. Assessing treatment response is facilitated if pre- and post-treatment [18]F-FDG PET/CT studies are available for comparison. Timing of the post-treatment study should consider a delay of 8–12 weeks after completion of radiotherapy in order to decrease the potential for false-positive results caused by an inflammatory radiation-related reaction.[29] A delay of 4–8 weeks is recommended if the patient received only chemotherapy. The sensitivity of [18]F-FDG imaging for detecting responders to treatment ranges between 70 and 90%.[2,30] Measurement of [18]F-FDG activity in tumors before and during therapy using the standard uptake value (SUV) has demonstrated that responding tumors show a decrease in tracer uptake, while in non-responding tumors the uptake persists.[29] PET/CT represents a good modality for identi-fying patients who show only partial response with residual active disease and is superior to CT or MRI in detecting post-chemo-radiation residual disease with a sensitivity of 90%.[4,30] A relatively high false-positive rate in [18]F-FDG PET assessment of patients after treatment is related to the frequency of inflammatory changes in the region of the head and neck, persisting for longer periods of time after completion of treatment. PET/CT performed at 12 weeks after the end of radiotherapy has been reported to have sensitivity of 93–100% for detection of residual tumors.[2] A negative PET/CT study after treatment is highly reliable, while a positive scan may indicate the presence of residual disease unless there are clinical or other imaging signs suggestive of an inflam-matory or infectious process that may explain the presence of abnormally increased [18]F-FDG uptake.

## Diagnosis and Restaging of Recurrence

Early detection of recurrent head and neck cancer is important since, if salvage surgery is performed, it can improve patient's outcome and prognosis. The regional head and neck anatomy is distorted by post-surgical and/or radiation therapy changes. The distinction between post-therapeutic changes and residual or recurrent tumor using imaging tests that rely on morphologic criteria is difficult, and, therefore, in this particular setting, CT and/or MRI have a limited accuracy.[4] Furthermore, biopsy of irradiated tissue is associated with high morbidity and may lead to radionecrosis or failure to heal. [18]F-FDG imaging has a high sensitivity for detection of recurrent disease in patients with head and neck cancer, regardless of the primary treatment modality, ranging between 78 and 96%, as compared to 38–80% for CT or MRI.[6–9,13,31,32] [18]F-FDG accumulates in metabolically active tissue, including inflammation and infection, which are known post-irradiation sequels.[13,33] PET/CT is therefore of particular value in this group of patients. Landmarks provided by CT are essential in the presence of the complicated head and neck anatomy and the known potential pitfalls of increased [18]F-FDG uptake in this region. PET/CT improved the confidence of interpretation, reduced the number of equivocal foci of [18]F-FDG uptake, and thus led to a decrease in the number of further non-invasive imaging, as well as invasive biopsy procedures performed for diagnostic purposes, associated also with a reduction in morbidity, costs, and emotional stress.[13]

Laryngeal cancer is an excellent example for the value of PET/CT. Laryngeal edema that persists after radiation treatment confronts the surgeon with a diagnostic dilemma, with recurrence being diagnosed in 50% of patients. Laryngeal biopsy under general anesthesia is the gold standard for diagnosis of recurrence but can cause additional edema, chondro-radionecrosis, and impairment of airways leading to tracheotomy. Direct laryngoscopy with biopsy has a low specificity and negative predictive value (NPV), with an up to 30% false-negative rate.[34] PET/CT was reported to have a sensitivity 92% and specificity of 96% in a group of patients with a suspected recurrent laryngeal carcinoma.[35] A positive PET/CT study can accurately guide biopsy to the hypermetabolic foci in an edematous larynx and thus achieve two goals: decrease sampling errors and avoid damage to normal but edematous laryngeal structures. In patients with a negative PET/CT study, unnecessary biopsy can be at least temporarily prevented, unless there is a high clinical suspicion for recurrent disease. PET/CT was also shown to have a significant impact on patient care. PET/CT altered further clinical management in 31–50% of the patients with head and neck cancer, mainly by eliminating the need for previously planned diagnostic procedures, guiding biopsy to a specific metabolically active area inside an edematous region, and by inducing a change in the planned therapeutic approach.[13,22]

## Planning of Radiotherapy

Radiotherapy is frequently used as a treatment method in head and neck cancer. Three-dimensional radiotherapy and intensity-modulated radiation therapy (IMRT) are the principal modalities because they allow accurate delivery of high doses of radiation, leading to improved local control and reduced morbidity. CT and MRI are the current modalities widely used for target volume selection and delineation. [18]F-FDG PET can define tumor volumes in a different way than anatomic imaging. [18]F-FDG-based radiation treatment planning has led to a significant reduction in size of radiotherapy fields, thus sparing more normal tissues.[36] The use of [18]F-FDG imaging for radiation treatment planning has been recommended but is still under evaluation. Large prospective studies, currently being performed, will establish the protocol for the routine clinical use of PET/CT for this specific important indication.

## Summary

[18]F-FDG PET/CT has become a widely used imaging modality in patients with head and neck cancer. At presentation, PET/CT has a proven value in staging, especially in patients with advanced disease. It can identify unknown and synchronous primary tumors with higher performance indices when compared to conventional imaging modalities. In assessment of loco-regional disease, PET/CT provides better anatomical localization of foci with abnormal [18]F-FDG uptake and reduces significantly the number of false-positive or equivocal results. It also detects distant metastases with a high sensitivity. PET/CT is highly reliable for monitoring response to treatment of head and neck cancer and can be used to select patients for salvage surgery. When an [18]F-FDG PET/CT study of a head and neck cancer patient is negative, additional clinical and radiological follow-up can be postponed, at least temporarily. A positive study should encourage and guide the surgeon to obtain tissue diagnosis.

## Guidelines and Recommendations for the Use of [18]F-FDG PET and PET/CT

The National Comprehensive Cancer Network (NCCN) has incorporated FDG PET and PET/CT in the evaluation and management algorithm of a variety of malignancies including head and neck cancer.[37] The use of [18]F-FDG PET (PET/CT where available) is recommended: (1) for occult malignancies when other tests do not identify a primary tumor; (2) for the initial staging of nasopharyngeal carcinoma for detection of distant metastases and (3) for the initial staging and restaging of head and neck carcinoma.

A multidisciplinary panel of experts reviewed meta-analyses and systematic reviews published in the FDG PET literature before March 2006 and made recommendations for the use of FDG PET in oncology.[38] The panel concluded

1) that [18]F-FDG PET should be added to the imaging tests routinely used to identify unknown primary head and neck tumors;
2) that [18]F-FDG PET should not be routinely added to CT or MRI in the diagnostic work-up of primary tumor head and neck malignancies;
3) that [18]F-FDG PET should routinely be added to CT or MRI to improve nodal or distant-disease staging of head and neck cancer; and
4) that [18]F-FDG PET should routinely be added to conventional imaging in the diagnostic work-up of patients with a potential recurrence of head and neck cancer.

# Case Presentations

## *Case II.2.1*

### History

This 49-year-old man was diagnosed with metastatic SCC in a cervical lymph node with no known primary tumor. [18]F-FDG PET/CT was performed in order to identify the primary tumor and to exclude additional metastases (Fig. II.2.1).

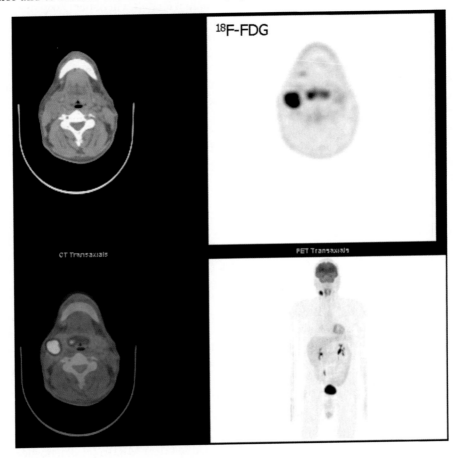

**Fig. II.2.1**

### Findings

Intense [18]F-FDG uptake is seen in a level 2 enlarged necrotic right submandibular lymph node, 28 mm in diameter. An additional focus of lower intensity uptake was localized by CT to the lingual tonsil at the level of the base of tongue, more prominent on the right (Fig. II.2.1).

### Discussion

Biopsy from the base of tongue revealed the primary SCC. The patient received chemo-radiation with boost of radiation to the primary tumor and to the right neck, following an organ-sparing protocol of the upper left neck. Follow-up PET/CT performed 6 months after completion of treatment showed complete regression of the primary tumor and the nodal metastasis.

Patients with SCC metastatic to cervical lymph nodes without an identified primary tumor pose a diagnostic and therapeutic challenge. Head and neck carcinomas are characterized by loco-regional progression, and therefore treatment consists of wide-field irradiation and neck dissection. Identification of the primary tumor improves prognosis as it allows targeted therapy and may thus reduce the toxicity associated with wide-field irradiation. The detection rate of $^{18}$F-FDG PET/CT of primary tumors of the head and neck ranges between 40 and 65%[28,29] and is superior to that of PET stand-alone, CT, or MRI. The limiting factor for the performance of $^{18}$F-FDG PET/CT is probably related to its resolution. Many primary tumors encountered in this clinical scenario are very small or superficially located and thus more difficult to detect by PET/CT. The management of this patient was changed by the results of the $^{18}$F-FDG PET/CT study. The initial plan of delivering full-dose wide-field irradiation was modified, and the patient received a boost to the primary tumor and the metastatic site, avoiding irradiation to the left upper neck.

**Diagnosis**

SCC of the base of tongue, metastatic to a right submandibular lymph node.

## Case II.2.2

### History

This 68-year-old man with a recently diagnosed laryngeal tumor showed multiple small pulmonary nodules on chest CT and was referred to $^{18}$F-FDG PET/CT for staging. The presence of distant lung metastases would obviously lead to a change in treatment (Fig. II.2.2A-C).

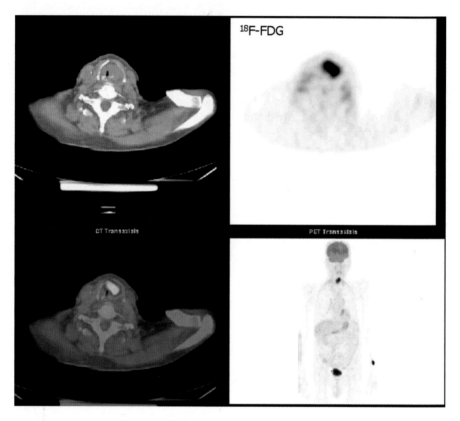

Fig. II.2.2A

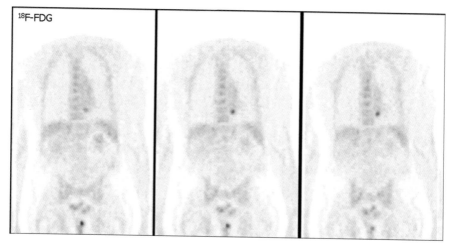

Fig. II.2.2B

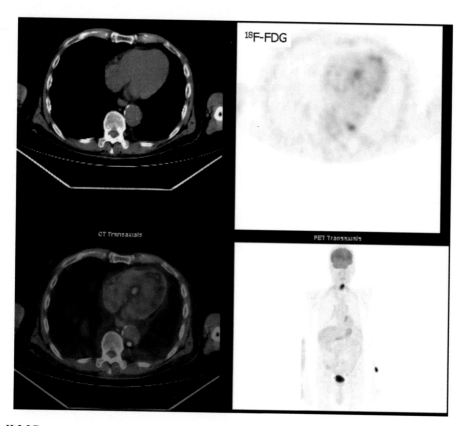

Fig. II.2.2C

## Findings

An area of intense $^{18}$F-FDG uptake is seen in anterior neck localized by CT to a large paraglottic mass originating from the left vocal cord, 33 × 20 mm in size, invading the left thyroid cartilage and crico-aritenoid joint, and crossing the midline through the anterior commissure, representing the primary laryngeal tumor (Fig. II.2.2A). An additional focus of moderate intensity $^{18}$F-FDG uptake is seen in the left posterior mediastinum (Fig. II.2.2B) localized by CT to a low-density lesion to the posterior wall of the descending thoracic aorta, 8 × 16 mm in size, consistent with an $^{18}$F-FDG -avid soft atheroma with an eccentric thrombus (Fig. II.2.2C). The pulmonary nodules on CT did not accumulate $^{18}$F-FDG (not shown).

## Discussion

This is a case of advanced laryngeal cancer with no distant metastases. The patient underwent curative treatment by a larynx preservation protocol. There was no evidence of pulmonary metastases on clinical and imaging follow-up.

The lungs are the most common site of distant metastases in head and neck tumors. The significance of small pulmonary nodules in patients with extrathoracic malignancy was recently reviewed by Jeong and colleagues.[39] Between 4 and 18% of subcentimeter lesions are malignant. PET/CT is suboptimal for detection of such nodules due to the current resolution limitation of PET. Hyun and colleagues[40] reported a malignancy rate of 20% in subcentimeter pulmonary nodes negative by PET/CT. $^{18}$F-FDG avidity in single small pulmonary nodule suggests metastasis, while a negative study requires close follow-up. In the present case, the pulmonary nodules disappeared on a follow-up CT.

The increased uptake in the aortic thrombus was an incidental finding. PET images showed a focus of increased $^{18}$F-FDG uptake localized by CT to the aortic wall. It was impossible to localize and determinate the etiology of the uptake by stand-alone PET. $^{18}$F-FDG has been shown to accumulate in vulnerable plaques due to the high metabolic activity of the inflamed cap.

## Diagnosis

1. Locally advanced laryngeal carcinoma.
2. No evidence of pulmonary metastasis.
3. $^{18}$F-FDG -avid soft atheroma in the wall of the thoracic aorta.

## Case II.2.3 (DICOM Images on DVD)

### History

This 46-year-old man has a history of undifferentiated nasopharyngeal carcinoma, treated by induction chemotherapy and full-dose radiotherapy 4 years prior to current examination. He presented with a new mass in the right neck, and MRI demonstrated edema and widening of the nasopharynx and a 1 cm lymph node in the right neck. The patient was referred for [18]F-FDG PET/CT with suspected loco-regional recurrence, to define the whole extent of disease (Fig. II.2.3A, B).

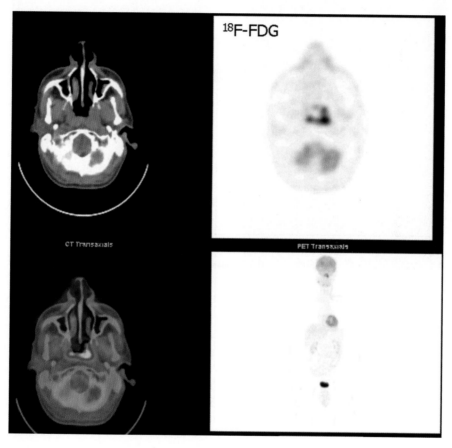

**Fig. II.2.3A**

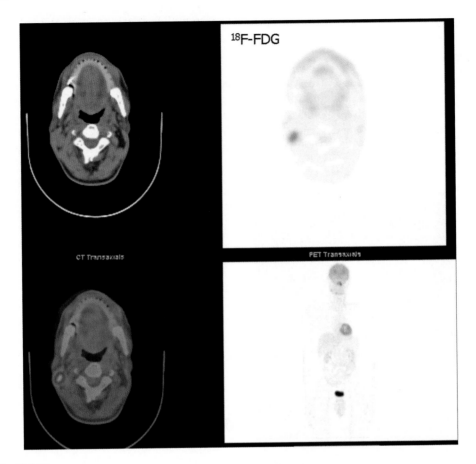

**Fig. II.2.3B**

### Findings

There is a focus of intense [18]F-FDG uptake in the left nasopharynx. CT shows diffuse thickening of the nasopharyngeal wall. PET/CT localizes the abnormal [18]F-FDG uptake to the posterior and left lateral aspect of the nasopharyngeal wall, with no increased tracer uptake demonstrated in the right nasopharynx (Fig. II.2.3A). In addition, there is a focus of increased [18]F-FDG uptake, in an enlarged, 19 mm retro-jugular level 5 lymph node in the right upper neck (Fig. II.2.3B).

### Discussion

The findings are consistent with local (nasopharynx) and regional (cervical lymph node) recurrence. Biopsy from the nasopharynx and fine needle aspiration (FNA) from the suspicious node confirmed this diagnosis.

Post-irradiation edema poses a challenge for conventional imaging in head and neck tumors. The value of CT and MRI in these cases is very limited due to inability to differentiate between post-radiation sequel and recurrence.[4,35] PET will show the suspicious pathologic [18]F-FDG uptake without the anatomic details necessary in order to perform an accurate biopsy or surgical procedure. Combined morphologic and metabolic PET/CT images guide interventions to a specific metabolically active area inside an edematous region. This increases the probability of correct tissue sampling while also reducing the damage to the surrounding areas.

### Diagnosis

1. Recurrent nasopharyngeal carcinoma and associated post-radiotherapy edema.
2. Right cervical lymph node metastasis.

### Clinical Report Case II.2.3: Body $^{18}$F-FDG PET/CT (for DVD cases only)

Indication

Restaging nasopharyngeal carcinoma.

History

This 46 year-old man has a history of undifferentiated nasopharyngeal carcinoma, treated by induction chemotherapy and full dose radiotherapy four years prior to current examination. He presented with a new mass in the right neck and MRI demonstrated edema and widening of the nasopharynx and a 1 cm lymph node in the right neck.

Procedure

The fasting blood glucose was 129 mg/dL at time of injection of 481 MBq (13.0 mCi) of $^{18}$F-FDG via the right antecubital vein. After a 60 min distribution time, a whole-body low-dose CT was acquired for anatomic localization and to correct for attenuation, without contrast, from the vertex to the upper thighs. PET images were then acquired over the same anatomic regions. The arms were positioned along the sides of the torso.

Findings

*Quality of the study*: The quality of this study is good.

*Neck*: There is a focus of intense $^{18}$F-FDG uptake in the left nasopharynx. CT shows diffuse thickening of the nasopharyngeal wall. PET/CT localizes the abnormal $^{18}$F-FDG uptake to the posterior and left lateral aspect of the nasopharyngeal wall, with no increased tracer uptake demonstrated in the right nasopharynx. There is a focus of increased $^{18}$F-FDG uptake in an enlarged, 19 mm retro-jugular level 5 lymph node in the right upper neck.

In addition, on the PET component there is physiologic $^{18}$F-FDG uptake in lymphoid and glandular tissues of the neck and in both vocal cords. On CT, there are normal size submental level 1 lymph nodes. A hypodense, predominantly fatty round mass is demonstrated at the base of the left neck, consistent with a small lipoma.

*Chest*: No sites of abnormal increased $^{18}$F-FDG activity are seen on the PET component. On CT, there are multiple high-density lesions in the region of the heart, consistent with multiple coronary calcifications.

*Abdomen and pelvis*: No sites of abnormal increased $^{18}$F-FDG activity are seen on the PET component. On CT low-density round lesions are demonstrated in the cortex of the right kidney, consistent with renal cysts. Multiple small retroperitoneal lymph nodes are seen in the left mid-abdomen. Hyperdense pelvic lesions are seen in calcifications in the iliac arteries.

*Musculoskeletal*: Multiple degenerative changes and osteophytes are seen in thoracic and lumbar vertebrae, with no significant $^{18}$F-FDG uptake.

Impression

1. Recurrent nasopharyngeal carcinoma and associated post-radiotherapy edema.
2. Right cervical lymph node metastasis.
3. Additional CT findings as described above.

## Case II.2.4

**History**

This 46-year-old man with a history of heavy smoking and alcohol abuse was diagnosed with SCC of the right true vocal cord (T1N0M0) and was treated by radiotherapy. Eighteen months after completion of treatment, he complained of new onset of hoarseness. Flexible laryngoscopy revealed decreased mobility of the right vocal cord and mild laryngeal edema with no obvious glottic mass. CT of the region of the head and neck showed swelling of the right vocal cord. The patient was referred for $^{18}$F-FDG PET/CT for a suspected loco-regional recurrence (Fig. II.2.4A, B).

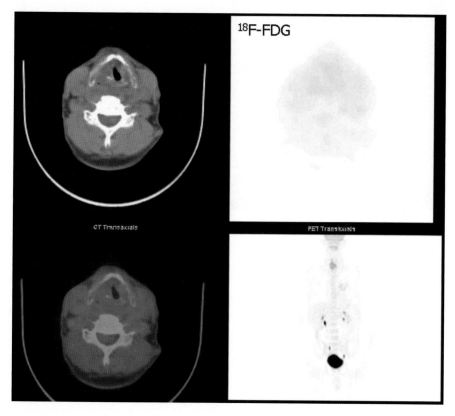

**Fig. II.2.4A**

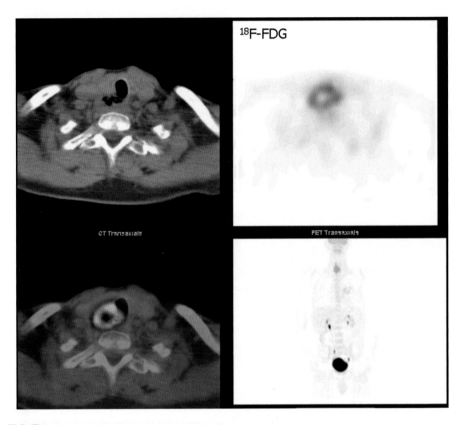

**Fig. II.2.4B**

**Findings**

CT at the level of the true vocal cords demonstrates rotation of the larynx to the left and marked thickening of the right vocal cord and the paraglottic space, with no corresponding abnormal [18]F-FDG uptake (Fig. II.2.4A). An area of increased abnormal circular [18]F-FDG uptake is demonstrated in the anterior neck region, at the level of the upper trachea and esophagus, localized by fused PET/CT images to the upper esophagus, with extension to the paraesophageal and paratracheal region (Fig. II.2.4B). An additional focus of abnormal [18]F-FDG uptake was found corresponding to a right lower lobe (RLL) lung nodule (not shown).

**Discussion**

PET/CT findings are suspicious for a second primary tumor in the upper esophagus with lung metastasis. Esophagoscopy and FNA from the RLL lesion confirmed the diagnosis. Although the patient had hoarseness and laryngeal swelling demonstrated by endoscopy and CT, there was no evidence of local recurrence. The clinical symptoms were related to recurrent laryngeal invasion by the esophageal tumor.

Second primary tumors are relatively prevalent in the head and neck region, especially in smokers and alcohol abusers. Lin and colleagues[41] reported an incidence of 8–10% second aero-digestive malignancies in a large group of patients with oral cavity and laryngeal carcinoma, with a fivefold increased risk in smokers and twofold associated with alcohol use. Stokkel and colleagues[42] found a synchronous primary in 12 out of 68 patients with head and neck SCC using $^{18}$F-FDG PET, while conventional imaging modalities detected only 5 of those 12 patients. Whole-body $^{18}$F-FDG PET imaging has the advantage of detecting unexpected tumor foci inside and outside the head and neck region with a high sensitivity. Distant metastases and synchronous or second primary tumors in the aero-digestive tract have a high likelihood of being hypermetabolic and therefore $^{18}$F-FDG avid. In this patient, PET/CT allowed accurate diagnosis of a second malignancy and thus significantly changed further clinical management. The patient underwent esophagoscopy, instead of the previously planned laryngeal biopsy, with confirmation of the esophageal tumor. In addition, diagnosis of a pulmonary metastasis defined the treatment strategy in this patient.

**Diagnosis**

1. Esophageal carcinoma (second primary malignancy).
2. Pulmonary metastasis.
3. Laryngeal edema with no evidence of recurrent laryngeal tumor.

## *Case II.2.5*

### History

This 51-year-old man has a history of glottic (laryngeal) tumor (T2N0M0) treated by radiotherapy. The patient returned 24 months later with new onset of dyspnea. Flexible laryngoscopy reveled paralysis of the right vocal cord but no evidence of recurrent tumor. CT of the region of the head and neck showed mild supraglottic and glottic thickening. The patient was referred for $^{18}$F-FDG PET/CT prior to performing a laryngeal biopsy (Fig. II.2.5).

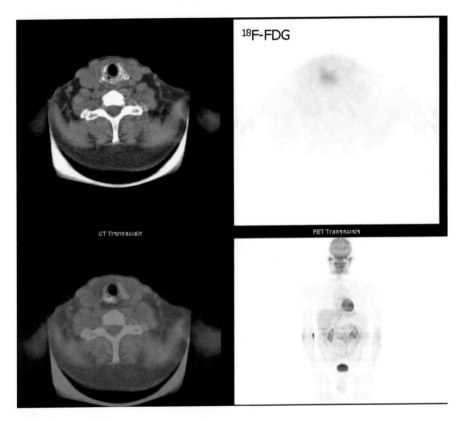

**Fig. II.2.5**

### Findings

There is an area of increased $^{18}$F-FDG uptake in the anterior neck. CT at the same level demonstrates mild thickening and erosive changes of the posterior larynx, with a differential diagnosis of recurrence versus post-radiation changes. PET/CT images localize the $^{18}$F-FDG-avid lesion to the cricoid cartilage in the posterior subglottic area (Fig. II.2.5).

### Discussion

Biopsy diagnosed recurrent tumor. Surgery and radiation therapy alter the normal laryngeal anatomy. Treatment-related edema, fibrosis, inflammation, and scarring are the limiting factors that hamper the role of physical examination and anatomic imaging with CT or MRI for diagnosis of recurrent laryngeal cancer.[6] Direct laryngoscopy with biopsy has a low reported specificity and NPV, with a false-negative rate of up to 30% in patients with suspected recurrent laryngeal cancer.[34] In a study by Ward and colleagues,[43] four laryngoscopies were needed to diagnose local recurrent tumor growth in patients with edema of the larynx after radiotherapy.

[18]F-FDG imaging has clear advantages in identifying local laryngeal recurrence,[8,9,13] and PET/CT improves the anatomic localization of [18]F-FDG-avid abnormalities in laryngeal tumors.[13] A recent study showed that a positive PET/CT study can accurately guide biopsy to hypermetabolic foci in an edematous larynx and achieve two goals: decrease previously described sampling errors and avoid damage to normal but edematous laryngeal structures. In this patient, stand-alone PET images cannot be used for planning of biopsy or surgery.[35] Hybrid PET/CT images localize the abnormal [18]F-FDG uptake to a specific anatomic region, the posterior right crycoid cartilage, and therefore precisely guided biopsy to a site that probably would not have been included in the initial planning.

**Diagnosis**

Recurrent laryngeal cancer.

## *Case II.2.6*

### History

This 54-year-old woman was diagnosed with supraglottic (laryngeal) carcinoma (T3N1M0) and treated by chemo-radiation. She developed post-radiation radiochondronecrosis of the larynx, which required urgent tracheotomy and hyperbaric chamber treatment. The upper airway obstruction improved gradually and allowed decanulation, but the patient continued to suffer from severe laryngeal edema persisting for more than 12 months. The patient underwent laryngeal biopsy which was negative for recurrence but led to worsening of the edema and airway obstruction.

CT of the region of the head and neck showed mark supraglottic and glottic edema (mainly on the right). The patient was referred for [18]F-FDG PET/CT to define the precise localization or exclude local recurrence, knowing that an additional laryngeal biopsy will lead to tracheotomy (Fig. II.2.6).

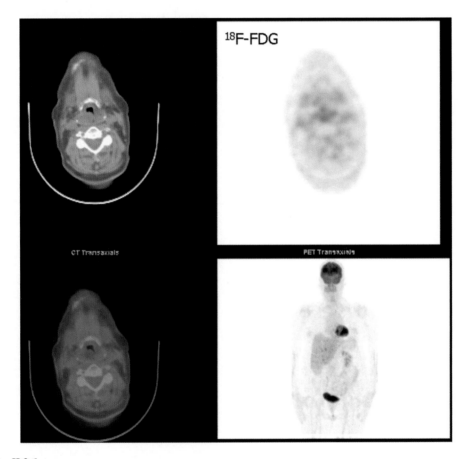

**Fig. II.2.6**

**Findings**

Whole-body imaging showed no foci of increased $^{18}$F-FDG uptake, including the region of the supraglottic thickening, more prominent of the right, which is demonstrated on CT (Fig. II.2.6).

**Discussion**

Laryngeal biopsy was avoided because of the lack of $^{18}$F-FDG uptake in the suspicious anatomic lesion as seen on PET/CT. A follow-up study performed 12 months later showed no significant change with persistent thickening on CT and no abnormal $^{18}$F-FDG uptake. The patient was free of recurrent disease for an additional 2 years follow-up.

After treatment, imaging is of particular clinical value in monitoring response, as well as for early diagnosis of recurrence. CT and MRI that rely on structural changes are unreliable in making the differential diagnosis between post-treatment changes and residual or recurrent tumor.[4] Biopsy of irradiated tissue is associated with high morbidity and may lead to failure to heal. $^{18}$F-FDG imaging has been reported to have a higher sensitivity and specificity for detection of recurrent disease in patients with head and neck cancer as compared to conventional imaging modalities.[6–9]

Laryngeal edema that persists after radiation treatment confronts the surgeon with a diagnostic dilemma. Recurrence is diagnosed in 50% of this patient group. Laryngeal biopsy under general anesthesia is the gold standard for diagnosis of recurrence but can cause additional edema, chondro-radionecrosis, and impairment of airways leading to tracheotomy. Post-radiation laryngeal edema is a relatively common finding, and performing a biopsy on every patient will be associated with a low yield of positive biopsy. $^{18}$F-FDG PET/CT is very beneficial in this scenario. As discussed above, CT and MRI are unreliable with a very low specificity (14% in a recent study[13]). $^{18}$F-FDG PET had a high sensitivity (90%) but was also associated with a high false-positive rate (25%) in a group of patients with laryngeal cancer,[35] mainly due to $^{18}$F-FDG accumulation in nonmalignant metabolically active tissue, including inflammation and infection, known post-irradiation sequels. In contrast, PET/CT has been reported to have a sensitivity of 92% and specificity of 96%.[35]

Therefore, in patients with a negative $^{18}$F-FDG PET/CT study, biopsy can be at least temporarily postponed, unless there is a high clinical suspicion for recurrent disease.

**Diagnosis**

Post-radiation laryngeal edema, no evidence of recurrence.

## Case II.2.7

### History

This 42-year-old woman was diagnosed with SCC of the base of tongue (T2N0M0) and was treated by primary surgical resection and post-operative radiotherapy. Follow-up CT performed at 2 years after completion of treatment demonstrated asymmetry of the base of tongue. Differential diagnosis included post-radiation changes and a low probability suspicion of local recurrence. The patient was referred for [18]F-FDG PET/CT to exclude or confirm the presence of local recurrence (Fig. II.2.7).

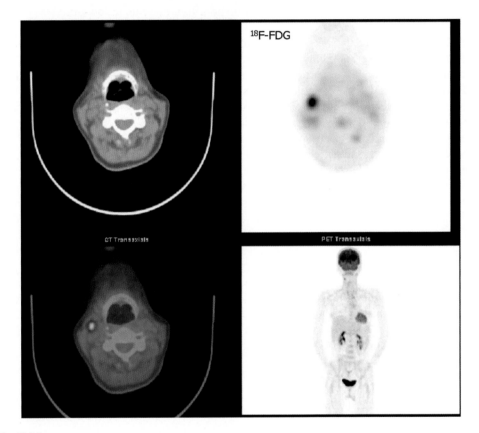

**Fig. II.2.7**

### Findings

On the CT component, there was mild thickening in the region of the base of tongue with no congruent abnormal [18]F-FDG activity (not shown). There is, however, a focus of abnormal [18]F-FDG uptake in the right upper neck, localized by fused images to a normal size, 11 mm diameter, right jugulodigastric level 2 lymph node. Reevaluation of the pre-referral CT study demonstrated the presence of this same lymph node, which was not considered as suspicious due to its small diameter (Fig. II.2.7). Additional findings on PET/CT include more normal size or slightly enlarged retro-jugular lymph nodes showing no [18]F-FDG uptake.

**Discussion**

PET/CT findings were consistent with a single metastasis in a right, normal size cervical lymph node. FNA was negative, but right neck dissection was performed and detected a 11 mm lymph node, positive for SCC.

Conventional imaging modalities rely on morphological criteria for malignancy, including nodal size and contrast enhancement patterns, which do not always accurately reflect the presence of active tumor. The reported sensitivity, specificity, and accuracy of CT for diagnosis of cervical nodal metastases are 88, 86, and 87%, respectively.[17] Specificity was even lower when using the 10 mm size criterion, 39% for CT and 48% for MRI.[3] Vermeersch and colleagues[44] reported a significantly higher sensitivity and specificity for $^{18}$F-FDG PET as compared to CT/MRI for detection of cervical lymph node metastases, with additional studies supporting these results.[13,17,18] Furthermore, PET/CT improves the specificity for detecting small lymph node metastases for a similar sensitivity (due to PET resolution limitations).[20] In this patient, neck dissection was performed because of the positive results of the PET/CT study, in spite of the negative FNA.

**Diagnosis**

1. Right cervical lymph node metastasis.
2. No evidence of local recurrence.

## *Case II.2.8*

### History

This 50-year-old man was diagnosed with laryngeal carcinoma (T3N0M0) and was treated by chemo-radiation. Two years after treatment, the patient developed severe laryngeal obstruction, and biopsy was positive for recurrence. CT of the chest demonstrated a suspicious nodule in the middle lobe of the right lung. The patient was referred to [18]F-FDG PET/CT for restaging prior to further treatment planning (Fig. II.2.8A-C).

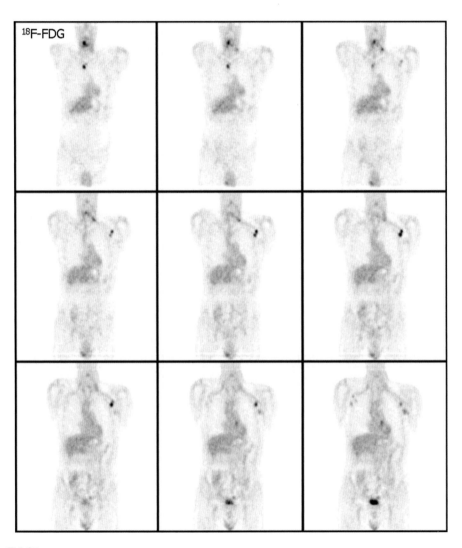

**Fig. II.2.8A**

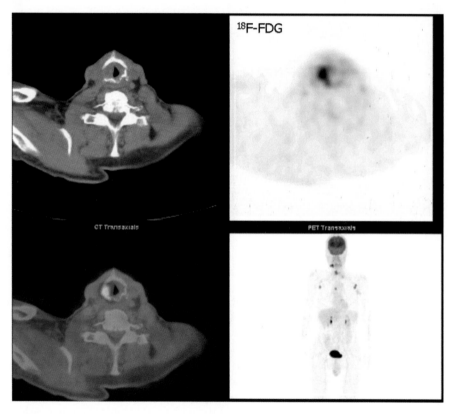

**Fig. II.2.8B**

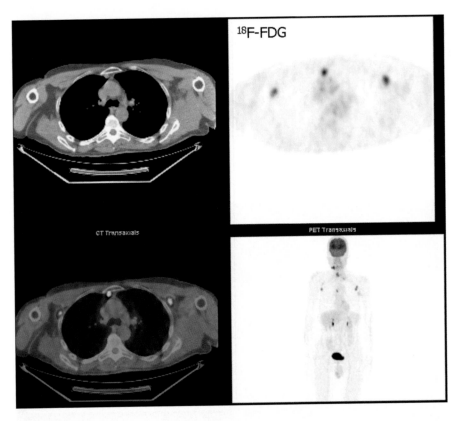

Fig. II.2.8C

## Findings

Coronal PET slices show multiple foci of abnormal $^{18}$F-FDG uptake (Fig. II.2.8A). Transaxial slices at the level of the larynx (Fig. II.2.8B) demonstrate an $^{18}$F-FDG-avid lesion in the anterior cervical region localized by fused images to a mass seen on CT in the right subglottic region, 25 × 16 mm in size, with erosion of the cricoid cartilage, representing the known local recurrence. Transaxial slices at the level of the upper mediastinum (Fig. II.2.8C) show increased $^{18}$F-FDG uptake in the anterior mediastinum and both axillary regions, localized by fused images to bilateral axillary lymphadenopathy (17 and 22 mm diameter) and a right anterior retrosternal lymph node, 11 mm diameter. Additional foci of abnormal $^{18}$F-FDG uptake were seen in right submandibular and left lower neck lymphadenopathy and a subpleural lung nodule in the right middle lobe (not shown).

## Discussion

Diagnosis of loco-regional recurrence and multiple distant metastases was confirmed by FNA from the axillary lymph nodes and the pulmonary nodule. The patient was not considered a surgical candidate due to massive metastatic spread.

Early detection of distant metastases is important for planning the therapeutic strategy and predicting patient outcome. Several studies have demonstrated the superiority of $^{18}$F-FDG PET and lower sensitivity of conventional imaging modalities for diagnosis of distant metastases in patients with head and neck tumors.[19,21] Performing a whole-body MRI survey is generally impractical for staging or restaging of malignant tumors. [18]F-FDG imaging, as true whole-body modality, has the advantage of detecting unexpected tumor foci outside the region of the head and neck with high sensitivity, further facilitated by the highly metabolic activity of distant metastases. A positive [18]F-FDG PET/CT is highly reliable, with low rates of false-positive results.[13]

**Diagnosis**

1. Local laryngeal recurrence.
2. Multiple cervical and axillary lymph node metastases.
3. Pulmonary metastasis.

## Case II.2.9

### History

This 62-year-old man was diagnosed with non-small-cell lung cancer 6 years prior to current examination and was treated by right upper lobe lobectomy followed by post-operative chemo- and radiotherapy. Follow-up CT of the chest detected a small, 6 mm nodule in the upper part of the right lung. The patient was referred for $^{18}$F-FDG PET/CT to exclude or confirm the presence of recurrence (Fig. II.2.9).

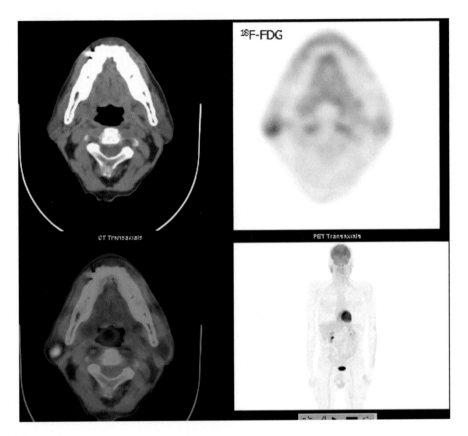

**Fig. II.2.9**

### Findings

On the CT component, there is a nodule with ill-defined borders, 6 mm in diameter in the upper part of the right lung with no congruent abnormal $^{18}$F-FDG activity (not shown). There is, however, a focus of abnormal $^{18}$F-FDG uptake in the right upper neck, localized by fused images to hyperdense lesion in the right parotid (Fig. II.2.9). There were no additional findings on PET/CT.

## Discussion

PET/CT findings were consistent with a hypermetabolic lesion in the right parotid gland, suspicious for metastasis. FNA diagnosed a right parotid Whartin's tumor.

Symmetrical uptake of [18]F-FDG by the salivary gland is relatively common and usually does not pose a diagnostic dilemma. Asymmetric [18]F-FDG parotid uptake could suggest a benign or malignant primary tumor or a metastatic lesion to parotid lymph nodes. Basu and colleagues[45] reported on the significance of incidental [18]F-FDG uptake in the parotid glands and its impact on patient management. All (18/25) patients with symmetrical or diffuse asymmetrical uptake were free of parotid tumors, while 5/7 focal asymmetric uptake patients had primary or metastatic parotid tumors.

Warthin's tumor is one of the benign parotid tumors (about 15% of all salivary gland tumors). It tends to accumulate [18]F-FDG intensively and could be mistaken for malignant lesion. Histologically, Warthin's tumor consists of epithelial parenchyma and lymphoid stroma. It is believed that the high [18]F-FDG uptake in this tumor could derive from a large number of mitochondria in the inner ductal layer or from activated lymphocytes in the lymphoid stroma. Ozawa and colleagues[46] tried to use different imaging modalities as a diagnostic tool to differentiate between benign and malignant parotid tumors. Warthin's tumors had the same SUV levels as malignant tumors and concluded that tumor characteristic cannot be determinate based on [18]F-FDG uptake. Salivary gland scintigraphy using [99m]Tc-pertechnetate can be used to differentiate between the last two. Warthin's tumor tends to accumulate [99m]Tc-pertechnetate, while malignant tumors do not.[11] Final diagnosis of the suspicious lesion should be made based on tissue sample.

## Diagnosis

1. Right parotid Warthin's tumor.
2. No evidence of recurrent lung cancer.

# References

1. Jemal A, Tiwari R, Murray T, Ghafoor A, Samuels A, Ward E, Feuer EJ, Thun MJ. Cancer statistics, 2004. *Cancer J Clin* 2004;54:8–29.
2. Quon A, Fischbein NJ, McDougall IR, Le Q-T, Loo Jr BW, Pinto H, Kaplan MJ. Clinical role of 18F-FDG PET/CT in the management of squamous cell carcinoma of the head and neck and thyroid carcinoma. *J Nuc Med* 2007;48(Supp 1):58–67.
3. Curtin H, Ishwararn H, Mancuso H, Dalley RW, Caudry DJ, McNeil BJ. Comparison of CT and MRI imaging in staging of neck metastases. *Radiology* 1998;207:123–130.
4. Lowe VJ, Dunphy FR, Varvares M, Kim H, Wittry M, Dunphy CH, Dunleavy T, McDonough E, Minster J, Fletcher JW, Boyd JH. Evaluation of chemotherapy response in patients with head and neck cancer using FDG PET. *Head Neck* 1997;19:666–674.
5. Adams S, Baum RP, Stuckensen T, Bitter K, Hör G. Prospective comparison of FDG PET with conventional imaging modalities (CT, MRI, US) in lymph node staging of head and neck cancer. *Eur J Nucl Med* 1998;25:1255–1260.
6. Anzai Y, Caroll WR, Quint DJ, Bradford CR, Minoshima S, Wolf GT, Wahl RL. Recurrence of head and neck cancer after surgery or irradiation: prospective comparison of FDG PET and MR imaging diagnoses. *Radiology* 1996;200:135–141.
7. McGuirt WF, Greven K, Williams Dr, Keyes JW, Watson N, Watson N, Cappellari JO, Geisinger KR. PET scanning in head and neck oncology: A review. *Head and Neck* 1998;20:208–215.
8. Kresnik K, Mikosch P, Gallowitsch HJ, Kogler D, Wieser A, Heinisch M, Unterweger O, Raunik W, Kumnig G, Gomez I, Grünbacher G, Lind P. Evaluation of head and neck cancer with $^{18}$F-FDG PET: a comparison with conventional methods. *Eur J Nucl Med* 2001;28:816–821.
9. Lowe VJ, Boyd JH, Dunphy FR, Kim H, Dunleavy T, Collins BT, Martin D, Stack Jr BC, Hollenbeak C, Fletcher JW. Surveillance for recurrent head and neck cancer using PET. *J Clin Oncol* 2000;18:651–658.
10. Blodgett TM, Fukui MB, Snyderman CH, Branstetter IV BF, McCook BM, Townsend D, Meltzer CC. Combined PET-CT in the head and neck: part 1. Physiologic, altered physiologic, and artefactual FDG uptake. *Radiographics* 2005;25:897–912.
11. Uchida Y, Minoshima S, Kawata T, Motoori K, Nakano K, Kazama T, Uno T, Okamoto Y, Ito H. Diagnostic value of FDG PET and salivary gland scintigraphy for parotid tumors. *Clin Nucl Med* 2005;30:170–176.
12. Fukui MB, Blodgett TD, Meltzer CC. PET/CT imaging in recurrent head and neck cancer. *Semin US, CT & MRI* 2003;24:157–163.
13. Gordin, A, Golz, A, Keidar Z, Daitzchman M, Bar-Shalom R, Israel O. The role of FDG-PET/CT imaging in head and neck malignancies -impact on diagnostic accuracy and patient care. *Otolaryngol Head Neck Surg* 2007;137:130–137.
14. Ha PK, Hdeib A, Goldenberg D, Jacene H, Patel P, Koch W, Califano J, Cummings CW, Flint PW, Wahl R, Tufano RP. The role of positron emission tomography and computed tomography fusion in the management of early-stage and advanced stage primary head and neck squamous cell carcinoma. *Arch Otolaryngol* 2006;132:11–16.
15. Alberico RA, Husain SH, Sirotkin I. Imaging in head and neck oncology. *Surg Oncol Clin N Am* 2004;13:13–35.
16. Shah J. Cervical lymph node metastases: diagnostic, therapeutic and prognostic implications. *Oncology* 1990;4:61–69.
17. Schwartz DL, Ford E, Rajendran J, Yueh B, Coltrera M, Virgin J, Anzai Y, Haynor D, Lewellyn B, Mattes D. FDG-PET/CT imaging for preradiotherapy staging of head and neck squamous cell carcinoma. *Int J Radiat Oncol* 2005;61:129–136.
18. Schoder H, Yeung HW. Positron emission imaging of head and neck cancer, including thyroid carcinoma. *Semin Nucl Med* 2004;34:180–197.
19. Stoeckli SJ, Steinert H, Pfaltz M, Schmid S. Is there a role for PET with FDG in the initial staging of nodal negative oral and oropharyngeal SCC. *Head Neck* 2002;24:345–349.
20. Schoder H, Carlson DL, Kraus DH, Stambuk HE, Gönen M, Erdi YE, Yeung HWD, Huvos AG, Shah JP, Larson SM, Wong RJ. FDG PET/CT for detecting nodal metastases in patients with oral cancer staged N0 by clinical examination and CT/MRI. *J Nucl Med* 2006;47:755–762.
21. Tenkos T, Rosenthal E, Lee D, Taylor R, Marn CS. Positron emission tomography in evaluation of stage III and IV head and neck cancer. *Head Neck* 2001;23:1056–1060.

22. Fleming AJ, Smith SP, Paul CM. Impact of PET/CT on previously untreated head and neck cancer patients. *Laryngoscope* 2007;117:1173–1179.
23. Muir C. Cancer of an unknown primary site. *Cancer* 1995;75:353–356.
24. Jereczek-Fossa BA, Jassem J, Orecchia R. Cervical lymph node metastases of squamous cell carcinoma from unknown primary. *Cancer Treat Rev* 2004;30:153–164.
25. Johansen J, Eigtved A, Buchwald C, Theilgaard SA. Implication of 18F-Fluoro-2-Deoxy-D-Glucose positron emission tomography on management of carcinoma of unknown primary in the head and neck: A Danish cohort study. *Laryngoscope* 2002;112:2009–2014.
26. Greven KM, Keyes Jr JW, Williams 3rd, McGuirt WF, Joyce MT. Occult primary tumors of the head and neck: lack of benefit from positron emission tomography imaging with FDG. *Cancer* 1999;86:114–118.
27. Assar OS, Fischbein NJ, Caputo GR, Kaplan MJ, Price DC, Singer MI, Dillon WP, Hawkins RA. Metastatic head and neck cancer: Role and usefulness of FDG PET in locating occult primary tumors. *Radiology* 1999;210:177–181.
28. Wartski M, Le Stanc E, Gontier E, Vilain D, Banal A, Tainturier C, Pecking A, Paul A, Alberini JL. In search of unknown primary tumor presenting with cervical metastases: performance of hybrid FDG-PET-CT. *Nucl Med Comm* 2007;28:365–371.
29. Zimmer LA, Branstetter BF, Nayak JV, Johnson JT. Current use of 18f-Fluorodeoxyglucose positron emission tomography and computed tomography in squamous cell carcinoma of the head and neck. *Laryngoscope* 2005;115:2029–2034.
30. Kitagawa Y, Nishizawa S, Sano K, Ogasawara T, Nakamura M, Sadato N, Yoshida M, Yonekura Y. Prospective comparison of 18F-FDG-PET with conventional imaging modalities (MRI, CT and 67 Ga scintigraphy) in assessment of combined intraarterial chemotherapy and radiotherapy for head and neck carcinoma. *J Nucl Med* 2003;44:198–206.
31. Wong VJ, Lin DT, Schoder H, Patel SG, Gonen M, Wolden S, Pfister DG, Shah GP, Larson SM, Kraus DH. Diagnostic and prognostic value of 18-FDG PET for recurrent head and neck squamous cell carcinoma. *J Clin Oncol* 2002;20:4199–4208.
32. Kunkel M, Forster GJ, Reichert TE, Jeong J-H, Benz P, Bartenstein P, Wagner W, Whiteside TL. Detection of oral squamous cell carcinoma by 18-FDG PET: implications for prognosis and patient management radiation treatment planning with an integrated positron emission and computer tomography: A feasibility study. *Cancer* 2003;98:2257–2265.
33. Schoder H, Yeung HWD, Gonen M, Kraus D, Larson SM. Head and neck cancer: clinical usefulness and accuracy of PET/CT image fusion. *Radiology* 2004;231:65–72.
34. Brouwer J, Bodar EJ, De Bree R, Lankendijk JA, Castelijns JA, Hoekstra OS, Leemans CR. Detecting recurrent laryngeal carcinoma after radiotherapy: room for improvement. *Eur Arch Otorhin* 2004;261:417–422.
35. Gordin A, Daitzchman M, Doweck I, Yefremov N, Golz A, Keidar Z, Bar-Shalom R, Kuten A, Israel O. FDG PET/CT imaging in patients with carcinoma of the larynx: diagnostic accuracy and impact on clinical management. *Laryngoscope* 2006;116:273–278.
36. Geets X, Daisne JF, Tomsej M, Duprez T, Lonneux M, Grégoire V. Impact of the type of imaging modality on target volumes delineation and dose distribution in pharyngo-laryngeal squamous cell carcinoma: Comparison between pre and per-treatment studies. *Radiother Oncol* 2006;78:291–297.
37. Podoloff DA, Advani RH, Allred C, Benson AB, Brown E, Burstein HJ, Carlson RW, Coleman RE, Czuczman MS, Delbeke D, Edge SB, Ettinger DS, Grannis FW, Hillner BE, Hoffman JM, Keil K, Komaki R, Larson SM, Mankoff DA, Rozenzweig KE, Skibber JM, Yahalom J, Yu JM, Zelenetz AD. NCCN task force report: Positron Emission Tomography (PET/Computed tomography (CT) scanning in cancer. *J Natl Compr Canc Netw* 2007;5(Suppl 1):S1–S22. www.nccn.org/professionals/physician_gls/f_guidelines.asp
38. Fletcher JW, Djulbegovic B, Soares HP, Siegel BA, Lowe VJ, Lyman GH, Coleman E, Wahl R, Paschold JC, Avril N , Einhorn LH, Suh WW, Samson D, Delbeke D, Gorman M, Shields AF. Recommendations for the use of FDG( fluorine-18, (2-[$^{18}$F] Fluoro-2-deoxy-D-glucose) positron emission tomography in oncology. *J Nucl Med* 2008;49:480–508.
39. Jeong YJ, Yi CA, Lee KS. Solitary pulmonary nodules: Detection, characterization, and guidance for further diagnostic workup and treatment. *AJR Am J Roentgenol* 2007;188:57–68.
40. Joo HY, Yoo IR, Kim SH. Clinical significance of small pulmonary nodules with little or no FDG uptake on PET/CT images of patients with nonthoracic malignancies. *J Nucl Med* 2007;48:15–21

41. Lin K, Patel SG, Chu PY, Matsuo JMS, Singh B, Wong RJ, Kraus DH, Shaha AR, Shah JP, Boyle JO. Second primary malignancy of the aerodigestive tract in patients treated for cancer of the oral cavity and larynx. *Head and Neck* 2005;27:1042–1048.
42. Stokkel MP, Moons KG, Ten Broek FW, van Rijk PP, Hordijk GJ. 18F-fluorodeoxyglucose dual-head positron emission tomography as procedure for detecting simultaneous primary tumors in cases of head and neck cancer. *Cancer* 1999;86:2370–2377.
43. Ward PH, Calcaterra TC, Kagan AR. The enigma of post-irradiation edema and recurrent or residual carcinoma of the larynx. *Laryngoscope* 1975;85:522–529.
44. Vermeersch H, Loose D, Ham H, Otte A, Van de Wiele C. Nuclear medicine imaging for the assessment of primary and recurrent head and neck carcinoma using routinely available traces. *Eur J Nucl Med Mol Imaging* 2003;30:1689–1700.
45. Basu S, Houseni M, Alavi A. Significance of incidental fluorodeoxyglucose uptake in the parotid glands and its impact on patient management. *Nucl Med Commun* 2008;29:367–373.
46. Ozawa N, Okamura T, Koyama K, Nakayama K, Kawabe JK, Shiomi S, Yamane H, Inoue Y. Retrospective review: Usefulness of a number of imaging modalities including CT, MRI, technetium-99m pertechnetate scintigraphy, gallium-67 scintigraphy and F-18-FDG PET in the differentiation of benign from malignant parotid masses. *Radiat Med* 2006;24:41–49.

# Chapter II.3
# Lung Cancer

Ronald C. Walker, Laurie B. Jones-Jackson, Aaron C. Jessop, and Dominique Delbeke

## Introduction

In 2004, an estimated 173,700 Americans were diagnosed with lung cancer; of these, about 164,440 (95%) will die of their disease. Despite decades of research, the prognosis for lung cancer remains dismal, with a 5-year survival rate of 14%. Nonetheless, benefits have been realized for most patients, mainly through improved quality of life and some prolonged survival. Importantly, lung cancer can be curable if detected in its early stages.[1]

Lung cancer is divided into two types, non-small cell and small cell. Non-small-cell lung cancer (NSCLC) is comprised of several subtypes, predominantly adenocarcinoma, squamous-cell, and large-cell carcinoma, all of which are treated similarly. Small-cell lung cancer (SCLC) is a highly aggressive neuroendocrine carcinoma treated primarily with chemotherapy and, sometimes, radiotherapy. Maximum benefit to the patient with lung cancer, both for treatment of the malignancy and for management of tumor- or treatment-related complications, occurs when patient care is delivered by a multidisciplinary team of physicians providing subspecialty expertise. Careful coordination of the treatment regimens is essential for optimal patient outcome.[1]

## Indeterminate Pulmonary Nodules

Indeterminate pulmonary nodules can be solitary or multiple. Multiple indeterminate nodules are usually metastatic or due to infectious or inflammatory etiologies. A solitary pulmonary nodule (SPN) is an approximately round lesion, less than 3 cm in diameter and completely surrounded by lung parenchyma. Lesions larger than 3 cm are called masses and have a higher frequency of malignancy. The reported incidence of cancer associated with SPNs varies from 10 to 70%. Of benign etiologies, about 80% are due to infectious granulomas and about 10% are pulmonary hamartomas. Biopsy is required for definitive diagnosis.

An SPN is found in about 0.1–0.2% of all chest radiographs. In the United States, an estimated 150,000 such nodules are identified each year. Since bronchogenic carcinoma as the underlying etiology of the SPN has been increasing in incidence, and because the 5-year survival in patients undergoing resection with curative intent decreases from 80 to 5% in

R.C. Walker (✉)
Department of Radiology and Radiological Sciences, Vanderbilt University Medical Center,
Nashville, TN, USA
e-mail: ronald.walker5@va.gov

D. Delbeke, O. Israel (eds.), *Hybrid PET/CT and SPECT/CT Imaging*,
DOI 10.1007/978-0-387-92820-3_5, © Springer Science+Business Media, LLC 2010

patients with advanced disease, preoperative evaluation of SPNs, at least for differentiation between benign and malignant entities, it a very important goal.

SPNs are typically discovered incidentally on a chest radiograph or a chest computed tomography (CT). Although the chest radiograph can provide information regarding the presence or absence of associated calcification, lesion margination (e.g., spiculated, smooth, lobulated), size, and growth rate, chest CT imaging is the standard of care for SPN evaluation.[2]

If a newly discovered SPN has spiculated margins, the nodule should be considered as malignant until proven otherwise. Scalloped or lobulated margins are associated with an intermediate probability of cancer. Smooth borders are more commonly seen with a benign diagnosis, though this is not a specific pattern and can be encountered in metastatic nodules as well.[2]

Calcifications within a nodule are suggestive but not diagnostic of a benign lesion. Accurate evaluation of the calcification pattern associated with a nodule is best done with CT. A laminated or central calcified pattern is typical for a granuloma. The classic "popcorn" pattern is most often seen with a lung hamartoma. In approximately 50% of SPNs due to hamartomas, high-resolution CT can show a definitive pattern of fat and cartilage. Stippled or eccentric calcification patterns have been associated with malignancy. Cancer can also occur adjacent to or engulf a benign calcification, resulting in an eccentric appearance. In patients with a history of sarcoma, dense calcified nodules should not be dismissed as benign.[2,3]

Comparison of current to prior imaging results is of great value in evaluation of SPNs. If previous studies are available, the growth rate of a nodule can be estimated. A 30% increase in diameter of a sphere represents a doubling of volume. Volume doubling time for lung cancer is rarely less than a month or more than a year. A nodule that was not present on a radiograph less than 2 months old is thus unlikely to be malignant. While stability of size for 2 years is widely accepted to indicate a benign etiology, this should only be determined by comparing state-of-the-art CT studies, including thin slices and breath-hold acquisition protocols. In the proper context, this can be done as a limited CT without IV contrast in order to reduce radiation to the patient, to decrease the chances for possible complications related to IV contrast, and to decrease costs. However, some malignancies, notably bronchoalveolar carcinoma (BAC) and lung carcinoid, can appear stable in size for 2 years, especially on chest radiograph. Stable size on chest radiograph of an SPN for 2 years has a positive predictive value (PPV) for a benign etiology of only 65%. Thus, the "2-year rule" should be used with caution, and, for high-risk patients, additional comparison imaging for more than 2 years should be considered.[4]

Although the appropriate interval for follow-up imaging is variable, depending on the specific context, standard follow-up imaging should be performed at 3-month intervals for the first year after the discovery of the SPN followed by 6-month intervals for the second year. Follow-up of nodules less than 5 mm diameter by CT may detect growth in as little as 1 month (modern CT accurately demonstrates changes in diameter as small as 0.3 mm), but the efficacy and appropriateness for such close interval follow-up for these very small nodules are still under investigation.[2]

## Non-surgical Evaluation of Pulmonary Nodules

Non-invasive diagnostic modalities used to determine the etiology of pulmonary nodules include CT densitometry, contrast-enhanced CT (CECT), bronchoscopy, transthoracic fine-needle aspiration biopsy (FNA-Bx), and $^{18}$F-fluorodeoxyglucose ($^{18}$F-FDG) imaging.

CT densitometry relies on measurement of attenuation values expressed in Hounsfield units (HU). Accurate calibration of the CT scanner is mandatory for meaningful HU measurements, using a CT reference phantom for comparison. Small nodules may not be accurately measured due to volume averaging. However, when sufficient calcium is present, nodules may demonstrate a HU number above a threshold value, suggesting a benign etiology (usually due to calcification in a granuloma). The CT is performed without IV contrast, during breath-hold. In one large multicenter trial using CT densitometry, only one of 66 nodules defined as benign was subsequently proven as malignant. CT densitometry can sometimes be helpful, but it is not definitive for characterization of SPNs.[5]

The degree of nodule enhancement on CT after the injection of IV contrast is useful to help differentiate benign from malignant lesions. In a multicenter trial, investigators reported a median enhancement for malignant nodules of 38.1 HU compared to 10.0 HU for benign lesions. While there was a certain degree of overlap in enhancement between benign and malignant nodules, a "cut-off" threshold of 15 HU resulted in a sensitivity, specificity, accuracy, PPV, and negative predictive value (NPV) for the diagnosis of malignancy of 98, 58, 77, 68, and 96%, respectively.[6]

The sensitivity of bronchoscopy for diagnosis of a malignant SPN ranges from 20 to 80%, depending on the nodule size, its accessibility via the bronchial tree, and the prevalence of cancer in a specific population. For nodules less than 1.5 cm in diameter, the sensitivity is 10%, increasing to 40–60% for lesions 2–3 cm in diameter. When CT demonstrates bronchial contact with a nodule, the sensitivity of bronchoscopic diagnosis increases to 70%.

Transthoracic FNA-Bx successfully identifies the etiology of a peripheral SPN as either malignant or benign in up to 95% of cases. For malignant nodules, the sensitivity ranges from 80 to 95%, with specificities ranging from 50 to about 90%. In one study of over 200 patients, the PPV was 98.6% and NPV 96.6%. For SPN less than 2 cm in diameter, the sensitivity of FNA-Bx for detection of malignancy is still greater than 60%, but with a false-negative rate of up to 30%. Complications for FNA-Bx occur more often than for bronchoscopic biopsy, with an incidence of pneumothorax of up to 30%.

In a large collaborative study of CT screening for lung cancer, Henschke and colleagues[8] reported the results of the International Early Lung Cancer Action Program in which 31,267 asymptomatic persons at risk were screened with low-dose CT between 1993 and 2005. During this period, 27,456 repeat screenings were performed with CT at intervals from the baseline examination varying between 7 and 18 months. Lung cancer was verified in 464 patients, of which 412 (85%) had stage I disease. The estimated 10-year survival was 88% in the patients with stage I disease who accepted treatment. Eight patients declined treatment, and all died within 5 years. These results are significantly better as compared to the 5-year survival of about 70% for stage I NSCLC, accidentally discovered during chest radiograph performed for other reasons.[9]

## [18]F-FDG PET/CT for Evaluation of Pulmonary Nodules

[18]F-FDG imaging is well established in the non-invasive evaluation of SPNs. In general, the degree of uptake of the [18]F-FDG is directly related to the likelihood of malignancy, though false-positive results occur, usually from infectious or inflammatory etiologies such as pneumonia, fungal or tuberculosis (TB) infection, sarcoidosis, and autoimmune processes, such as rheumatoid pulmonary disease.[10] Likewise, false-negative results occur, mainly in small nodules (under 1 cm in diameter, due to the point spread function and respiratory motion) or in malignancies with a low metabolic rate (pulmonary carcinoid, BAC, and less common adenocarcinomas and metastases).[11] [18]F-FDG positron emission tomography (PET)/computed tomography (CT) is becoming widely used for differentiating benign

from malignant nodules. According to a recent meta-analysis, its estimated sensitivity for identifying a malignant process is 97% and its specificity is 78%.[12]

Semi-quantitative indices have been used to separate benign from malignant lesions. The most common indices are the standardized uptake value (SUV) and the lesion to lung background ratio (L/B). While reliable SUV measurements require rigorous quality control for accuracy, visual estimate of the degree of uptake relative to that of the normal hepatic parenchyma is often adequate for clinical purposes. An SUV of 2.5 is accepted by most centers as the best threshold to help differentiate benign from malignant lesions in the lungs. If a lesion larger than 1 cm in diameter has an SUV lower than 2.5, malignancy is less likely but not excluded. Recent work has shown that there is an approximately 20% chance of malignancy in SPNs up to 1 cm in diameter with either no perceptible [18]F-FDG uptake or uptake that was just discernable above pulmonary background.[13]

Although non-diagnostic of etiology, the degree of [18]F-FDG uptake in an SPN can be helpful in clinical management, especially in combination with the morphological characteristics on the CT portion of the PET/CT, the degree of enhancement on a contrast-enhanced CT, patient risk factors, etc. Indeed, Gambhir and colleagues[14] reported a decision-analysis model using the information provided by the PET and CT components of the PET/CT examination to enhance cost-effectiveness of evaluation of SPNs, demonstrating a theoretical reduction in unnecessary surgery by 15% and estimated cost savings ranging from $91 to $2,200 per patient. In a cost-analysis of [18]F-FDG PET in evaluation of SPN, Gould and colleagues[15] demonstrated that [18]F-FDG imaging was cost-effective for patients with discordant pre-test probability of malignancy and CT findings, as well as for an intermediate pre-test probability for malignancy and high-risk surgical candidates.

Dual time point imaging of pulmonary nodules has also been suggested as a means to differentiate between malignant and benign etiologies. [18]F-FDG imaging of the SPN is performed twice, typically 1 and 2 h after tracer injection. As a rule, benign nodules demonstrate little or no change in uptake between the two studies, whereas most of the malignant nodules demonstrate an increase of 10% or more in intensity of uptake. This technique is still to be considered investigational.[16]

## Guidelines for Evaluation of Indeterminate Nodules

No evidence-based guidelines completely define the proper evaluation of SPNs. The American College of Radiology has published criteria for choosing the most appropriate tests in given circumstances, according to available evidence and expert opinion, incorporating nodule diameter, patient age, smoking history, and nodule margin characteristics.[17] Lesions are classified as low, moderate, or high-risk groups for malignancy based on these criteria. Unfortunately, these guidelines are qualitative rather than quantitative and do not suggest how to best assess probability in a specific nodule. In addition, these criteria do not address evaluation of a lesion relative to the surgical risk for a specific patient.[2]

The pre-test probability of cancer determines the most cost-effective means for evaluation of a SPN. In one analysis, greatest cost-effectiveness was achieved with radiographic (chest radiograph or CT) follow-up when the probability of cancer was below 12%, CT and [18]F-FDG imaging when the probability was intermediate (12–69%), CT followed by either biopsy or surgery when the probability was high (69–90%), and surgery when the probability for malignancy was very high (above >90%).[14] However, determining the probability of cancer in a given SPN is sometimes problematic. Indeed, a multivariate model incorporating age, cigarette-smoking status, the presence or absence of a prior history of cancer for the patient, the diameter of the nodule, the presence or absence of spiculation, and the location of the nodule (upper lobe versus lower lobe) had similar accuracy to expert physician judgment in predicting a malignant SPN.[2]

## Non-Small-Cell Lung Carcinoma (NSCLC)

### TNM Staging of NSCLC

The basis for staging of NSCLC is the International Staging TNM system (Chart II.3.1).[18] Management of patients with newly diagnosed NSCLC is based on establishing the

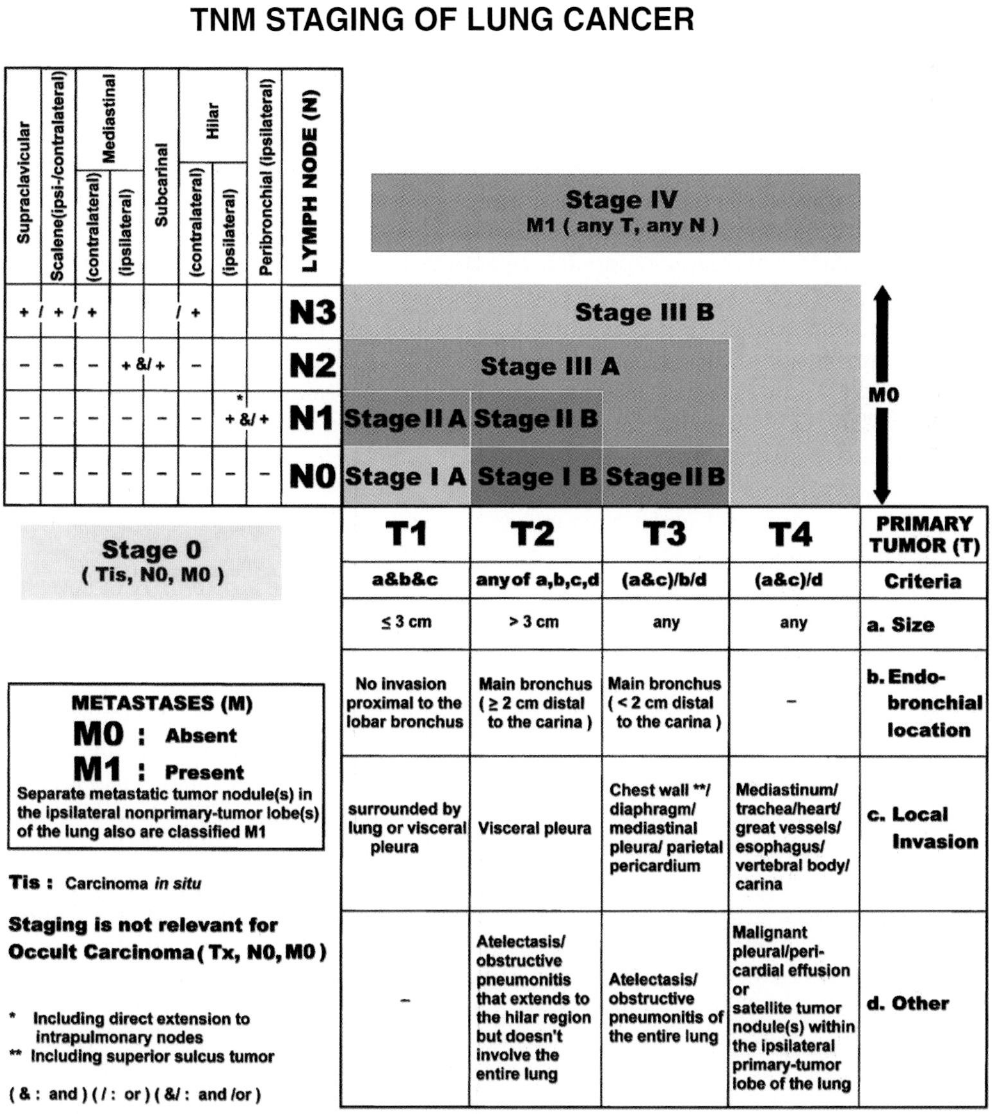

## TNM STAGING OF LUNG CANCER

| Supraclavicular | Scalene(ipsi-/contralateral) | Mediastinal (contralateral) | Mediastinal (ipsilateral) | Subcarinal | Hilar (contralateral) | Hilar (ipsilateral) | Peribronchial (ipsilateral) | LYMPH NODE (N) | | | |
|---|---|---|---|---|---|---|---|---|---|---|---|
| | | | | | | | | | Stage IV M1 ( any T, any N ) | | |
| + / + / + | | | | | / + | | | **N3** | Stage III B | | |
| – | – | – | + &/ + | – | | | | **N2** | Stage III A | | |
| – | – | – | – | – | – | +&/+ * | | **N1** | Stage II A | Stage II B | |
| – | – | – | – | – | – | – | – | **N0** | Stage I A | Stage I B | Stage II B |

| | T1 | T2 | T3 | T4 | PRIMARY TUMOR (T) |
|---|---|---|---|---|---|
| **Stage 0** ( Tis, N0, M0 ) | a&b&c | any of a,b,c,d | (a&c)/b/d | (a&c)/d | Criteria |
| | ≤ 3 cm | > 3 cm | any | any | a. Size |
| **METASTASES (M)** **M0** : Absent **M1** : Present | No invasion proximal to the lobar bronchus | Main bronchus (≥ 2 cm distal to the carina ) | Main bronchus (< 2 cm distal to the carina ) | – | b. Endo-bronchial location |
| Separate metastatic tumor nodule(s) in the ipsilateral nonprimary-tumor lobe(s) of the lung also are classified M1 | surrounded by lung or visceral pleura | Visceral pleura | Chest wall **/ diaphragm/ mediastinal pleura/ parietal pericardium | Mediastinum/ trachea/heart/ great vessels/ esophagus/ vertebral body/ carina | c. Local Invasion |
| **Tis :** Carcinoma *in situ* **Staging is not relevant for Occult Carcinoma( Tx, N0, M0)** | – | Atelectasis/ obstructive pneumonitis that extends to the hilar region but doesn't involve the entire lung | Atelectasis/ obstructive pneumonitis of the entire lung | Malignant pleural/peri-cardial effusion or satellite tumor nodule(s) within the ipsilateral primary-tumor lobe of the lung | d. Other |

\* Including direct extension to intrapulmonary nodes
\*\* Including superior sulcus tumor

( & : and ) ( / : or ) ( &/ : and /or )

Chart II.3.1  TNM staging of NSCLC (Reproduced with permission of American College of Chest Physicians from Silvestri et al.[20])

presence and/or extent of spread to the mediastinum or beyond (the N and M status). Accurate staging of NSCLC following diagnosis is very important because both the choice of treatment and the prognosis differ significantly by stage. This information will determine if the patient is a candidate for potentially curative treatment (surgery) or not. If resection for cure is not an option, accurate determination of the extent of disease is still of value for planning other therapeutic strategies such as chemotherapy associated with radiation, chemotherapy alone, or simple supportive care.[1]

## [18]F-FDG Imaging for Staging of NSCLC at Presentation: Comparison to CT

Chest CT remains the most commonly used initial staging modality for NSCLC, though there is strong evidence to support the use of [18]F-FDG imaging in many clinical settings.

Birin and coworkers[19] performed a systematic review of 17 studies comparing the accuracy of [18]F-FDG PET to CT in detection of mediastinal lymph node metastases in patients with NSCLC. The point on the receiver operating characteristic curve with equal sensitivity and specificity for [18]F-FDG PET was Q = 0.90 (95% CI, 86–95%), significantly superior to the corresponding value of 0.70 for CT (95% CI, 65–75%), p < 0.0001. All studies included in this review reported a superior accuracy of [18]F-FDG PET compared to CT in detection of mediastinal lymph node metastases.

The American College of Chest Physicians (ACCP) has published guidelines for non-invasive staging of NSCLC based on a meta-analysis of data from a variety of imaging modalities (CT, PET, PET/CT, bone scintigraphy, and magnetic resonance imaging [MRI]).[20] Using CT for staging of NSCLC 40% of mediastinal lymph nodes classified by size criteria (>1 cm short axis diameter) to be malignant were finally diagnosed as benign, whereas 20% of mediastinal lymph nodes thought to be benign were involved with metastatic disease. Clearly, CT alone is inappropriate for staging most patients with NSCLC.

Pooled data from studies that met acceptance criteria for the ACCP guidelines report that IV contrast-enhanced chest CT had a sensitivity of 51% and a specificity of 85% for identification of mediastinal lymph node metastases, thus establishing the limited ability of this imaging modality to either confirm or exclude mediastinal nodal involvement. [18]F-FDG imaging was clearly superior to CT in evaluation of metastatic mediastinal lymphadenopathy, with pooled estimates of sensitivity and specificity of 74 and 85%, respectively, and should be therefore considered for any patient in whom treatment with curative intent is contemplated (Chart II.3.2). Importantly, [18]F-FDG imaging could also detect occult extra-thoracic disease not seen by other imaging modalities in 1–8% of patients thought to have stage I disease and 7–18% of patients thought to have stage II disease. These relatively large numbers of unsuspected distant metastases discovered by [18]F-FDG imaging in patients classified as stage I by conventional imaging (CI) may explain, at least in part, the only 50% 5-year survival of patients with stage I disease.

Lardinois and colleagues[21] in a prospective study evaluated the accuracy for tumor, nodes, metastases (TNM) staging in 50 patients with proven or suspected NSCLC using CT alone, [18]F-FDG PET alone, visually correlated CT with [18]F-FDG PET, and truly integrated [18]F-FDG PET/CT. Tumor and nodal stages were verified histologically. Metastatic disease was confirmed either with histological examination or with complementary imaging. Integrated [18]F-FDG PET/CT provided additional information in 20 of 49 patients (41%) compared to side-by-side correlation of [18]F-FDG PET

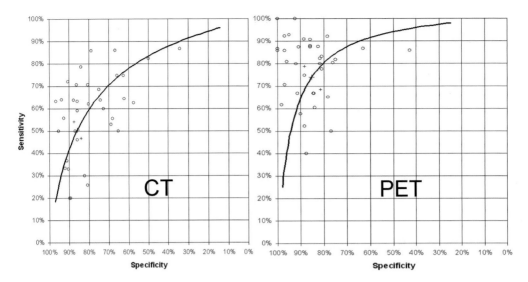

**Chart II.3.2** ROC curves from a meta-analysis assessing accuracy of mediastinal nodal staging by contrast-enhanced CT (left) and [18]F-FDG imaging (right) demonstrate the superior performance of metabolic data as compared to anatomic information alone (Reproduced with permission of American College of Chest Physcians from Silvestri et al.[20])

and CT. Integrated [18]F-FDG PET/CT had superior diagnostic accuracy compared to CT alone, PET alone, or CT and PET scans interpreted side-by-side.

Toloza and colleagues,[22] in a large meta-analysis and literature review, compared the accuracy of CT, [18]F-FDG PET, MRI, and endoscopic ultrasound (EUS) for mediastinal staging correlated with clinical evaluation (symptoms, physical findings, and laboratory results) in predicting metastatic disease in patients with either NSCLC or SCLC. Results were verified by long-term follow-up, histological confirmation and subsequent CI (brain and abdominal CT, and skeletal scintigraphy). [18]F-FDG imaging demonstrated superior accuracy compared to either CT or EUS for detection of mediastinal metastases. The NPV of clinical data for cerebral, abdominal, and skeletal metastases was greater or equal to 90%, suggesting that routinely imaging these regions in patients with lung cancer without evidence of advanced disease (present in 40% at diagnosis) may not be necessary.[22]

## Detection of Extra-Thoracic Metastases

Diagnosis of extra-thoracic metastatic disease at time of diagnosis of NSCLC prevents unnecessary attempts at curative surgery. Emphasis is placed on high-yield areas more commonly involved with metastatic spread, specifically the adrenal glands, liver, brain, and skeletal system. Detection of metastatic disease is limited to macroscopic lesions that are within the resolution of the used device. MRI is the modality of choice for evaluation of the superior sulcus of the lung and the brachial plexus. In many patients, the presence of extensive extra-thoracic disease is obvious on the initial chest CT, revealing involvement of the bone, liver, adrenal glands, etc. When this is indeed the case, further staging efforts to determine full extent of involvement (e.g., cerebral metastases) should be performed only when they can further impact clinical care.[23]

The use of whole-body [18]F-FDG imaging for extra-thoracic staging is evolving and may in future prove to be the diagnostic modality of choice. [18]F-FDG has limited sensitivity of approximately 60% for detection of cerebral metastases because of the high physiological tracer uptake in the gray matter. MRI remains the state of the art for detection of cerebral metastases, though CECT is acceptable. However, if the brain is in the field of view on the [18]F-FDG PET/CT study, careful examination will reveal unexpected metastases in about 0.5% of cases.[24] Adrenal glands are another common site for metastatic spread in NSCLC. In a series of 20 cancer patients with 24 incidental adrenal masses, [18]F-FDG PET was able to separate 10 benign from 14 malignant lesions in all cases.[25] Benign adrenal adenomas have as a rule [18]F-FDG uptake that is less than or similar to that of the normal hepatic parenchyma. For detection of skeletal metastases, [18]F-FDG imaging has a similar sensitivity to bone scintigraphy but with superior specificity.[26]

## Impact of [18]F-FDG Imaging on Management of NSCLC at Presentation

Up to 50% of thoracotomies performed with curative intent for NSCLC are "futile" due to the presence of unknown advanced local disease or metastatic spread. If discovered pre-operatively, these patients would have been upstaged and categorized as surgically incurable. Since these futile thoracotomies are associated with increased morbidity, mortality, and expense, decreasing the number of such ineffective procedures is in the interest of the patient and the health-care system.[27,28]

[18]F-FDG imaging used to stage patients with NSCLC changes patient management in 19–41% of cases. The multicenter PLUS trial[27] included 188 patients from 9 hospitals who were randomized to CI and CI+[18]F-FDG PET. The end point of evaluation was futile thoracotomy. The percentage of patients referred for "effective" thoracotomy was similar in each group (41% for the CI arm versus 44% for the CI + PET arm). However, the percentage of futile thoracotomies was significantly higher in the CI arm (41%) compared the CI + PET arm (21%). Despite adding the cost of the [18]F-FDG PET to the CI + PET scan group, the total cost of care after 1 year of follow-up on a per patient basis was less for the group performing the additional [18]F-FDG PET study due to the savings resulting from prevention of futile thoracotomies. This study demonstrated that the total cost of care was lower for patients who received CI + PET. It was difficult to quantify gains from decrease in patient morbidity/mortality and possible prolongation of survival from improved baseline staging.[27]

## [18]F-FDG Imaging for Monitoring Therapy of NSCLC

Only a few reports describe the role of [18]F-FDG imaging in evaluation of response to treatment, restaging, and detection of recurrence of NSCLC.

MacManus and colleagues[29] reported using [18]F-FDG PET and CT in 73 patients treated mostly with chemoradiation, followed by repeat imaging at a median interval of 70 days. PET demonstrated significantly more complete responders than CT, and both modalities were concurrent in only 40% of patients. Indeterminate responses on CT were related to atelectasis or pneumonitis, with none by PET. While both PET and CT responses were significantly related to duration of survival on univariate analysis, only PET response remained significant on multivariate analysis (p < 0.0001). Additionally, failure to achieve a complete response by PET (PET-CR) was significantly associated with shortened time to progression (p < 0.0009), whereas failure to achieve CT-CR was not (p < 0.089).

Pöttgen and colleagues[30] evaluated response to treatment via changes in the SUVmax between the pretreatment PET/CT and scans obtained during neoadjuvant chemoradiation therapy in a retrospective study of 50 patients, correlated with proven surgical histopathological response and with time to failure. A change in SUVmax of 55% had a sensitivity of 94% and specificity of 86% for major histopathological response, defined as 10% or less residual viable tumor cells. The degree of anatomic CT response was not significantly correlated with histopathological response.

Cerfolio and coworkers[31] performed a prospective trial of 93 patients with proven N2 (stage IIIA) NSCLC evaluated with PET/CT and CT before and after neoadjuvant chemo radiotherapy. While for evaluation of mediastinal lymph nodes PET/CT after treatment was false negative in 20% and false positive in 25% of patients, it had a higher accuracy than CT for all pathologic stages. When the pre- to post-treatment decrease in uptake was higher than 75%, the likelihood ratio that the patient was a complete responder was 6.1, as compared to 9.1 for only partial response with a decrease above 55%. Similarly, Eschmann and colleagues[32] found that patients with a decrease above 60% in SUVmax had better long-term survival compared to those showing a lower decrease in SUVmax (5-year survival 60 versus 15%, respectively, p < 0.0007). Patients with a decrease in SUVmax of 25% or less had a 5-year survival below 5% and were considered non-responders. Weber and colleagues,[33] in a prospective study of 57 patients with stage IIIB or IV NSCLC, showed that a decrease in SUVmax of more than 20% differentiated metabolic "responders" from "non-responders."

## Detection of Recurrence and Restaging with $^{18}$F-FDG PET or PET/CT

In a prospective evaluation of 30 consecutive stage IIIA-N2 NSCLC patients, restaging after induction chemotherapy $^{18}$F-FDG PET/CT had a better sensitivity and accuracy than reexamination by mediastinoscopy, 77 versus 29% (p < 0.0001) and 83 versus 60% (p = 0.012), respectively.[34] Repeat mediastinoscopy was hampered by the presence of adhesions and fibrosis related to the baseline staging procedure.

The performance of $^{18}$F-FDG imaging for detection of NSCLC recurrence and for its differential diagnosis from treatment-related tracer uptake resulted in a sensitivity of 93%, specificity 89%, accuracy 92%, PPV 96%, and NPV 80%.[35] The intensity of $^{18}$F-FDG uptake measured as average SUVmax was significantly higher in recurrent tumors as compared to treatment-related hypermetabolic changes. Patients with low-intensity $^{18}$F-FDG uptake in recurrent tumors had a better median survival as compared to high-uptake relapses. For patients with recurrent disease who underwent additional surgery, the SUV of the recurrent tumor was the only independent prognostic factor for long-term survival of 3 years or more. This prospective study demonstrates the accuracy of PET compared to CT alone in detection of lung cancer recurrence, differentiating recurrent tumor from treatment-related uptake and in identifying patients likely to benefit from a second surgery.

## Summary

The ACCP concluded that CT of the chest provides high-resolution anatomic images but has a poor accuracy for differentiating benign from malignant mediastinal lymphadenopathy relative to $^{18}$F-FDG imaging, which demonstrated superior sensitivity and specificity in both the mediastinum and in detection of extra-thoracic metastatic disease. Nonetheless, with either test, abnormal findings require confirmation by tissue biopsy.

Accurate initial staging can eliminate about half of futile thoracotomy procedures. Staging with[18]F-FDG imaging is recommended for all stage IB–IIIB patients who are candidates for potentially curative treatment and is also suggested for stage IA patients considered for surgery especially if at high risk due to co-morbid conditions. [18]F-FDG PET/CT detects extra-thoracic metastases missed on CI in up to 20% of patients. MRI with contrast is the modality of choice for detection of cerebral metastases and other selected areas such as the superior sulcus of the lung and brachial plexus.

Response to treatment is better assessed with [18]F-FDG PET/CT as compared to CT alone and, due to technical factors related to the presence of adhesions or fibrosis, compared to reexamination with mediastinoscopy as well. The superiority of [18]F-FDG PET/CT for post-treatment evaluation is less demonstrative than at baseline, primarily due to treatment-induced [18]F-FDG uptake. No study has yet demonstrated an improvement in ultimate outcome resulting from application of this information.

## Small-Cell Lung Carcinoma (SCLC)

### *[18]F-FDG PET and PET/CT for Staging, Restaging, and Assessment of Treatment Response of SCLC*

SCLC accounts for 13–20% of primary pulmonary malignancies. Untreated SCLC has an aggressive course with a median survival of 2–4 months after diagnosis. SCLC has a simple staging classification of limited versus extensive disease based on the Veterans Administration Lung Cancer Study Group.[36] Limited disease encountered in about 30% of patients at diagnosis involves ipsilateral thoracic, mediastinal, or supraclavicular lymph nodes. Extensive disease spreads beyond these confines. Except for rare cases of surgically treated limited SCLC, staging determines the choice between chemotherapy and radiation for limited versus chemotherapy alone for extensive disease. Classically, initial staging of patients with SCLC involves a CI regimen consisting of a diagnostic CT of the chest, abdomen, and pelvis, bone scintigraphy, and either CECT or MRI of the brain. [18]F-FDG imaging has been reported to have favorable detection rates for SCLC. However, the limited number of studies to date have not convincingly established an improvement in outcome for SCLC patients based on the results of these examinations.[37]

Schumaker and coworkers[38] compared the performance of [18]F-FDG PET scans for baseline staging of SCLC patients to CI and found that [18]F-FDG imaging resulted in either upstaging of patients or demonstrated a greater extent of disease than that appreciated by CT without any change in stage.

In a retrospective review of 46 patients with SCLC, Pandit and colleagues[39] found that [18]F-FDG PET imaging was positive in all tumors, it staged correctly all patients, intensity of uptake showed an inverse correlation with prognosis, and overall survival was significantly worse in patients showing residual [18]F-FDG after treatment. These authors concluded that [18]F-FDG imaging provides accurate staging information of powerful prognostic significance in treated and untreated SCLC.

In a study of 120 patients, [18]F-FDG PET had a sensitivity of 100% for detection of SCLC. CT and [18]F-FDG PET were congruent in staging 63% of patients.[40] Of the incongruent cases, [18]F-FDG PET was correct in 73% and incorrect in 15% and changed the stage in 12% of patients, mainly by upstaging to extensive disease. In only 1 of 120 patients did [18]F-FDG PET stage incorrectly by missing a cerebral metastasis. [18]F-FDG PET was significantly superior to CT for detection of extra-thoracic disease excluding cerebral metastases, where either MRI or CECT was superior with a sensitivity of 100 versus 46%, respectively.

## *Summary*

[18]F-FDG imaging demonstrates a uniformly high sensitivity for detection of SCLC, superior to CI at staging or restaging, excluding diagnosis of cerebral metastases. While the outcome of patients with SCLC may not benefit from the addition of [18]F-FDG PET/CT, the overall cost of care and patient morbidity might be lower if this modality substitutes for CT. As with NSCLC, [18]F-FDG can correctly demonstrate extensive disease in patients where CT suggests limited disease, thereby properly triaging the patient to chemotherapy versus chemoradiation. False-positive [18]F-FDG PET/CT may occur in patients with SCLC, thus imaging results must be proven by other means before potentially curative procedures are withheld in patients who are upstaged from limited to extensive disease on the basis of [18]F-FDG imaging.

## Malignant Pleural Mesothelioma

### *Introduction*

Malignant mesothelioma is an aggressive neoplasm of serosal surfaces such as the pleura, the pericardium, and the peritoneum. Once rare, the incidence of malignant pleural mesothelioma (MPM) is increasing worldwide as a result of widespread asbestos exposure, with a latency period from exposure to tumor of up to 30–40 years. This rising incidence is not expected to peak for another 10–20 years. The predicted total economic burden to both government and industry for compensation related to asbestos exposure in the next 40 years is estimated to be of up to $200 billion for the United States and $80 billion for Europe.[41]

Approximately 80% of patients with MPM are men. They typically present with pleural effusion associated with shortness of breath. Over 60% have chest wall or pleuritic pain, with weight loss and fatigue occurring in less than 30% at diagnosis. Due to chest wall fixation in areas of involvement, lung expansion is impaired and secondary pneumonia is common. Most cases are not diagnosed until 2–3 months after the onset of symptoms.[41] The median survival from time of diagnosis of MPM is 12 months. Prognosis is worse in patients with extensive disease, poor performance status, elevated white-cell counts, anemia, thrombocytosis, sarcomatoid histology, and high [18]F-FDG uptake.[41] Death is more commonly due to local invasion than distant metastases. Local progression can lead to mediastinal spread, which may result in obstruction of the superior vena cava or cardiac tamponade. Other complications include chest wall destruction with subcutaneous invasion and spinal cord compression. The contralateral lung and/or the peritoneal cavity are involved by MPM in 10–20% of cases.[41]

The International Mesothelioma Interest Group has published a modified TNM staging system for MPM to predict prognosis (Table II.3.1). CT, MRI, PET, thoracoscopy, and mediastinoscopy are used in the preoperative assessment of MPM. Laparoscopy is useful to evaluate for spread to the peritoneum. Final staging requires surgery.[42]

**Table II.3.1**  New international staging system for diffuse MPM

**T-Tumor status**

**T1**

T1a – tumor limited to ipsilateral parietal pleura

T1b – tumor in ipsilateral parietal pleura with scattered foci in ipsilateral visceral pleura

**T2**

Tumor involving each of the ipsilateral pleural surfaces (parietal, mediastinal, diaphragmatic, and visceral) with at least one of the following:
- involvement of the diaphragmatic muscle
- confluent visceral pleural spread (including into the fissures) *OR* extension of tumor from the visceral pleura into the lung parenchyma

**T3**

Locally advanced but potentially resectable involving all ipsilateral pleural surfaces with at least one of the following:
- involvement of the endothoracic fascia
- extension into the mediastinal fat
- solitary, completely resectable focus of tumor in the soft tissues of the chest wall
- non-transmural involvement of the pericardium

**T4**

Describes locally advanced technically non-resectable tumor involving all of the ipsilateral pleural surfaces with at least one of the following:
- diffuse or multi-focal extension into the chest wall with or without rib destruction
- direct extension of tumor
  o to the peritoneum *or*
  o to the contralateral pleura *or*
  o to one or more mediastinal organs *or*
  o to the spine *or*
  o to the internal surface of the pericardium with or without a pericardial effusion *or*
  o involvement of the myocardium *or*

**N – Lymph Node Status**

NX  Regional nodes cannot be assessed

N0  No regional node metastases

N1  Metastases to the ipsilateral bronchopulmonary or hilar nodes

N2  Metastases to the subcarinal or ipsilateral mediastinal nodes, including ipsilateral internal mammary nodes

N3  Metastases to the contralateral mediastinal, contralateral internal mammary, or supraclavicular nodes (either ipsilateral or contralateral)

**M – Metastases**

MX  Presence of metastases cannot be assesed

M0  No distant metastases

M1  Metastases present

**TNM Staging and Classification**

| Stage | Tumor | Node | Metastasis |
| --- | --- | --- | --- |
| IA | T1a | N0 | M0 |
| IB | T1b | N0 | M0 |
| II | T2 | N0 | M0 |
| III | Any T3 | Any N1 or N2 | M0 |
| IV | Any T4 | Any N3 | Any M1 |

(Reproduced with permission of Elsevier from Rusch[42]).

The most frequent diagnostic dilemma in MPM is the difficult differentiation from adenocarcinoma in cases with chest wall invasion. Cytological evidence of MPM in the pleural fluid is found in 30–85% of cases, though FNA-Bx is at times required, especially if there is no pleural effusion. Direct thoracoscopic biopsy is rarely needed.[41] At presentation, chest radiograph will demonstrate a pleural effusion and occasionally a pleural-based mass. Advanced MPM demonstrates an encasing "rind" of tumor in the involved hemithorax, often with lobulation, as well as pleural effusion and possibly rib destruction. Calcified pleural "plaques" indicate prior asbestos exposure but are not diagnostic of MPM. CT demonstrates pleural-based masses in 92% of cases, with or without thickening of the interlobular septa and/or pleural effusion. Invasion of the chest wall is seen in 18% of cases at diagnosis. It is not known why MPM will sometimes produce localized masses and at other times an encasing rind of tumor. MRI may be of value in determining the full extent of the mesothelioma, particularly when involvement of the ribs and/or the diaphragm is uncertain on CT, for planning of radiation therapy and for evaluation of spinal cord involvement.[41]

## [18]F-FDG Imaging of MPM

As with staging and restaging of other chest malignancies, [18]F-FDG imaging may distinguish benign from malignant pleural masses and detect extra-thoracic disease, thus its value in staging of MPM. Increasing SUV values are inversely correlated with prognosis. Early reports suggest that PET/CT imaging can differentiate tumor from fibrosis and necrosis more accurately and can determine the response to treatment better than either PET or CT alone.[41]

In an early report of 63 patients undergoing [18]F-FDG PET mainly for preoperative staging and also for assessment of recurrence after surgery, Flores and colleagues[43] showed that PET detected all but one stage 1A patient and improved detection of supraclavicular (N3) or extra-thoracic (M1) disease over conventional staging. However, overall T and N staging by PET was disappointingly poor, with sensitivities of only 19 and 11%, respectively, due to poor detection of tumor extent and of mediastinal lymph node involvement.

In a review of [18]F-FDG PET/CT in MPM, Truong and coworkers[44] reported overall sensitivity, specificity, PPV, NPV, and accuracy for T4 disease of 67, 93, 86, 82, and 83%, respectively. Due to respiratory or cardiac motion, both PET/CT and MRI are relatively poor compared to CT at demonstrating trans-diaphragmatic or trans-pericardial spread of tumor. Poor PET/CT results were reported for assessment of mediastinal nodes with false negatives due to the inability to demonstrate microscopic disease and false positives in [18]F-FDG-avid reactive nodes in patients with chronic pulmonary disease, with an overall sensitivity of 38%, specificity 78%, and accuracy 59%.[44] Mediastinoscopy-guided nodal biopsy must be performed for optimal mediastinal lymph node staging.

While CT is still the mainstay in imaging of MPM, MRI with and without gadolinium and [18]F-FDG PET/CT offer benefits over CT alone in demonstration of tumor extent, in the detection of extra-thoracic disease and in the identification of optimal sites for biopsy. Biopsy guidance is especially useful since MPM can occur in a focal, localized region in patients who often have antecedent diffuse pleural thickening.[45]

## Assessment of Metabolic Response to Treatment of MPM

Surgery is useful for palliation, such as local control of recurrent effusions. Debulking surgery has been also suggested. The consensus expert opinion is that surgery, whether tumor debulking or radical resection (extrapleural pneumonectomy), is best performed in combination with other treatments, such as adjuvant chemotherapy, radiotherapy, or immunotherapy. Until recently, chemotherapy demonstrated uniformly poor response rates, of less than 20%. However, a number of multicenter studies trials with new therapeutic regimens appear more encouraging. Experimental animal study have also been encouraging when an apoptosis-inducing agent is added to chemotherapy. Local radiotherapy directed to surgical sites decreases seeding of tumor and can provide palliation of chest wall pain.[41] Assessment of metabolic response to treatment in non-resectable MPM, defined as a decrease of at least 25% in [18]F-FDG uptake between the pretreatment study and a repeat test after two cycles of chemotherapy, correlated with improved time to progression and with borderline significance to overall survival, whereas CT did not.[46]

## Summary

The increasing incidence of MPM will result in future years in the need for improvements in diagnosis, treatment, and prevention of this aggressive malignancy which is associated with high mortality rates and high costs of patient management and economic compensations. Over the last decade, [18]F-FDG imaging has been incorporated in the evaluation algorithms of MPM at initial diagnosis and staging. [18]F-FDG PET/CT is of value to optimize sites for high-yield biopsy and to spare futile attempts at curative treatment. Early reports also suggest that [18]F-FDG PET/CT is superior to other imaging modalities in early assessment of MPM response to treatment. All imaging results must, of course, be verified by other means if potentially curative treatment would be withheld based on the imaging findings.

## Guidelines and Recommendations for the Use of F-FDG PET and PET/CT

The National Comprehensive Cancer Network (NCCN) has incorporated [18]F-FDG PET and PET/CT in the practice guidelines and management algorithm of a variety of malignancies including NSCLC.[47] The use of [18]F-FDG PET (PET/CT where available) is recommended in the following clinical scenarios:

1) Diagnosis of patients with one or two pulmonary nodules.
2) Initial staging except if multiple distant metastases.
3) Restaging stage III and IV after 2 to 3 months after treatment or before surgery.
4) Restaging in patients with symptoms suggestive of recurrence.

A multidisciplinary panel of experts reviewed meta-analyses and systematic reviews published in the [18]F-FDG PET literature before March 2006 and made recommendations for the use of FDG PET in oncology.[48] The panel concluded that

1) [18]F-FDG PET should routinely be obtained in the initial staging of patients with SPN.
2) [18]F-FDG PET should routinely be added to the conventional work-up of NSCLC patients.

3) $^{18}$F-FDG PET should be obtained in the diagnostic work-up of lung cancer patients for distant metastases.
4) The evidence is insufficient to support the use of $^{18}$F-FDG PET in the management of SCLC.

# Case Presentations

## *Case II.3.1*

### History

This 41-year-old female with cancer of the breast, being restaged after bilateral mastectomy and transverse rectus abdominis myocutaneous (TRAM) flap reconstruction 3 years prior to the current examination, was lost to follow-up until recently. Re-evaluation with CT demonstrated interval development of a pulmonary nodule of the right lower lobe (RLL). The patient was referred to [18]F-FDG PET/CT for restaging of her breast cancer and evaluation of the pulmonary nodule (Fig. II.3.1).

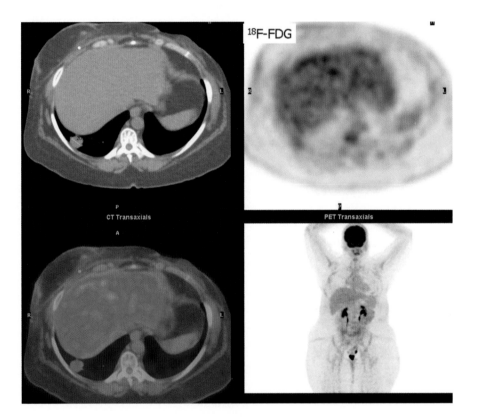

**Fig. II.3.1**

### Findings

The [18]F-FDG PET/CT study (Fig. II.3.1) demonstrates a relatively well-defined pulmonary nodule in the posterior aspect of the RLL, 20 mm in diameter, with moderate [18]F-FDG uptake, of similar intensity as the liver. Changes related to previous surgeries are noted on CT. There was no other evidence of tumor recurrence.

## Discussion

This pulmonary nodule is apparently new, though its true age since the surgery for breast cancer 3 years ago is uncertain as there have been no interval examinations. The major diagnostic considerations would include metastatic disease, primary pulmonary neoplasm or a non-calcified granuloma. Surgical changes are noted and appear well-healed. There is no apparent tumor recurrence otherwise on either the diagnostic CT examinations of the chest, abdomen, or pelvis (not shown) or the whole-body [18]F-FDG PET/CT. If the whole-body [18]F-FDG PET/CT would have demonstrated other tracer-avid foci suggestive of tumor recurrence, these may have been ideal biopsy targets for confirmation.[2,3,4,7]

The two major options for this patient relative to this indeterminate pulmonary nodule include biopsy at this time or continued radiographic surveillance. If the later option is elected, it is best performed with a limited, thin-cut CT without radiographic contrast, superior to plain films for detection of increase in size of a nodule, and cheaper than a full diagnostic CT of the chest. A minimum periodic follow-up of 2 years by CT from the time of discovery of the nodule should be performed before stability can be assumed. Since the nodule is shown to have only mild [18]F-FDG avidity, following this nodule with PET/CT is not cost-effective. Most patients with early stage breast cancer are not likely to benefit from routine restaging with [18]F-FDG PET/CT.[4]

## Diagnosis

Solitary pulmonary nodule with moderate uptake, likely a metastasis.

## Follow-up

The patient declined biopsy. A follow-up CT 3 months later revealed multiple additional non-calcified pulmonary nodules, consistent with breast cancer pulmonary metastases.

## Case II.3.2

### History

This 48-year-old man was referred for evaluation of a 30 mm RLL pulmonary mass. Seven years ago, a melanoma was removed from his left chest with negative margins. The patient recently complained of new right-sided chest pain, initially ascribed as possible cholecystitis. Ultrasound revealed a small right pleural effusion and a pulmonary mass abutting the right hemidiaphragm. A diagnostic CT of the chest confirmed the presence of the mass with minimal pleural thickening versus fluid. A CT-guided core biopsy demonstrated caseating granulomatous reaction with negative special staining for etiology. (Ziehl–Neelsen and Gomori's methenamine silver stains were negative for acid-fast and fungal organisms, respectively.) The patient denies fever, chills or sweats, hemoptysis, productive cough, or wheezing. He quit smoking 20 years ago.

Despite his prior history of melanoma, the patient had no imaging examinations until recently, so the actual age of the pulmonary findings is uncertain. He is referred to $^{18}$F-FDG PET/CT for a whole-body examination due to his somewhat confusing and inconclusive history as well as physical and laboratory findings (Fig. II.3.2).

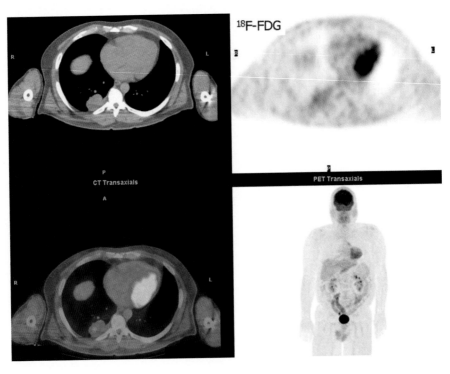

Fig. II.3.2

**Findings**

A 33 mm RLL pulmonary mass is identified, abutting the pleural surface and right hemi-diaphragm, demonstrating moderate [18]F-FDG uptake, similar to that of the liver (Fig. II.3.2). There is also a 13 mm lymph node in the aorto-pulmonary window with moderate [18]F-FDG uptake (not shown). No other enlarged or [18]F-FDG-avid lymph nodes are seen. The lung fields are otherwise clear, without nodules or infiltrates, and the previously described right pleural effusion has resolved. There is minimal pleural thickening in the region of the mass with the remainder of the pleura appearing normal.

**Discussion**

This examination demonstrates the non-specific nature of [18]F-FDG PET/CT. Given the patient's prior history of an aggressive malignancy (melanoma), the size of the abnormality (most pulmonary masses 30 mm in diameter or greater are malignant), and the prior smoking history, malignancy including either a primary or metastatic lesion was much more likely than a benign etiology. The [18]F-FDG PET/CT examination was performed for verification that other lesions were not present or in order to plan a repeat biopsy if discovered. The test confirmed that the findings were limited to the pulmonary mass and a presumably reactive mediastinal node.[2,4,10,11]

Despite the proven powerful clinical utility of [18]F-FDG PET/CT, the interpreting physician must remember that uptake of the radiopharmaceutical is related to the regional metabolic rate and that it does not replace a biopsy. Tissue verification must be obtained, particularly before a specific treatment strategy is contemplated.[13]

**Diagnosis**

Granulomatous infection presenting as a solitary, moderately [18]F-FDG-avid, pulmonary mass.

## *Case II.3.3*

### History

This 51-year-old female presented 1 month earlier with chest pain. CT of the chest obtained at that time revealed a lobulated 23 × 25 mm left upper lobe non-calcified pulmonary nodule. The patient was referred to $^{18}$F-FDG PET/CT for further evaluation of this pulmonary nodule (Fig. II.3.3A, B).

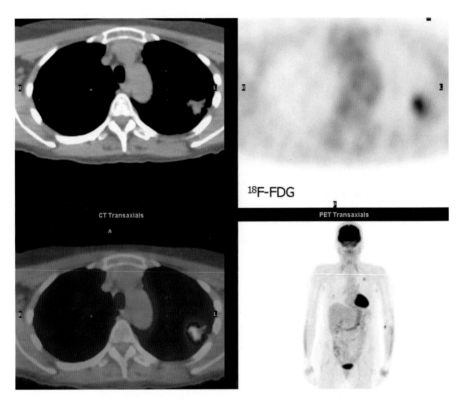

**Fig. II.3.3A**

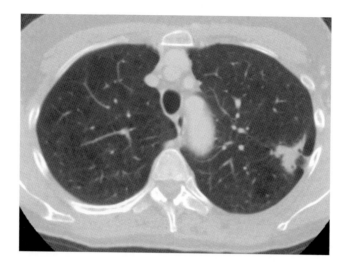

**Fig. II.3.3B**

## Findings

There is a spiculated non-calcified nodule at the periphery of the left upper lobe with intense uptake of [18]F-FDG. Both the PET/CT (Fig. II.3.3A) and the axial diagnostic CT (Fig. II.3.3B) demonstrate the "tethering" of the visceral pleural surface by the spiculated margins of this nodule. A needle biopsy at the time of the diagnostic CT (which also shows severe bullous emphysema) revealed NSCLC, for which the patient underwent a left upper lobe resection.

## Discussion

[18]F-FDG PET/CT demonstrated in a single examination not only the intense uptake in the spiculated nodule, but also provided a whole-body evaluation for staging the presumed malignancy. The appearance of the nodule alone, non-calcified and with spiculated margins, was sufficient to warrant biopsy. However, PET/CT provided the whole-body staging. The main value of PET/CT in this clinical setting is to exclude the presence of unsuspected metastases that would have rendered futile any attempts at a surgical cure. There was no evidence either clinically or on the basis of the PET/CT that the patient has disease beyond the left lung, and, therefore, surgery was performed, with resection of the left upper lobe revealing NSCLC.[27,28]

## Diagnosis

NSCLC of the left upper lobe with tumor involvement of the visceral pleura.

## Case II.3.4

### History

This 45-year-old woman with a history of bronchoalveolar cell (BAC) cancer in the left upper lobe diagnosed 4 years prior to current examination underwent lobectomy with sparing of the lingular region, including removal of an 80 mm tumor with clear surgical margins and negative lymph nodes. One year later, after six cycles of chemotherapy, three lingular nodules were resected, all revealing BAC with clear margins. Three years after her initial diagnosis, the patient presented with an ill-defined new, irregular right upper lobe pulmonary lesion, with needle biopsy indicating a well-differentiated BAC. She was referred to [18]F-FDG PET/CT for restaging prior to planned resection of this metastatic versus additional primary NSCLC (Fig. II.3.4).

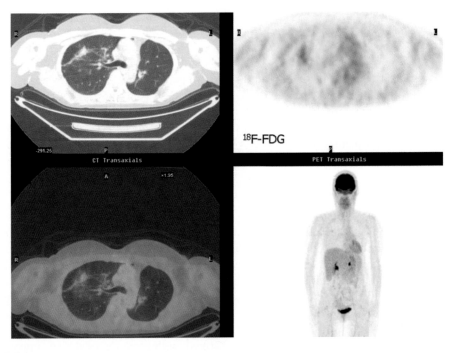

**Fig. II.3.4**

### Findings

Moderate [18]F-FDG uptake is seen in the irregular, ill-defined, approximately 30 mm right upper lobe pulmonary lesion. Spiculated margins are seen, some of which extend to the pleural surface (Fig. II.3.4). No other areas of abnormal uptake are seen.

Additional findings on CT include surgical changes from resection of the left upper lobe, with volume loss resulting in left shift of the mediastinum.

**Discussion**

In one whole-body examination, $^{18}$F-FDG PET/CT demonstrates the new pulmonary nodule to be solitary, favoring a new primary malignancy rather than metastatic disease. The spiculated characteristics of the margins are also strongly suggestive of new, multi-focal BAC rather than metastatic disease, which usually demonstrates relatively well defined, though sometimes lobulated margins. However, the PET/CT findings are not specific in this regard.

This new tumor demonstrates moderate $^{18}$F-FDG uptake, of similar intensity to activity in the liver. It is not uncommon, however, for BAC to demonstrate no, minimal, or only mild $^{18}$F-FDG uptake above background. Accordingly, any new pulmonary nodule, regardless of low uptake, should be followed for a minimum of 2 years from discovery at periodic intervals. In a high-risk setting, such as this patient, biopsy is indicated at time of discovery regardless of the results of PET/CT, unless the test would have demonstrated a better region to biopsy or the presence of widespread metastatic disease.[2,4,10,12,13,34]

**Diagnosis**

Bronchoalveolar cell lung cancer, presumed new primary, right upper lobe.

**Follow-up**

The patient elected to undergo resection of the right upper lobe and recovered well. Three years later, the patient developed several new pulmonary nodules in the residual left lung, found on biopsy to be adenocarcinoma of the lung, a malignancy of different histology.

## *Case II.3.5*

### History

This 58-year-old male, with a newly found right perihilar pulmonary nodule on CT, underwent surgical resection of a right perihilar NSCLC 2 years prior to current examination followed by radiation treatment. The patient was referred to $^{18}$F-FDG PET/CT for restaging (Fig. II.3.5A,B).

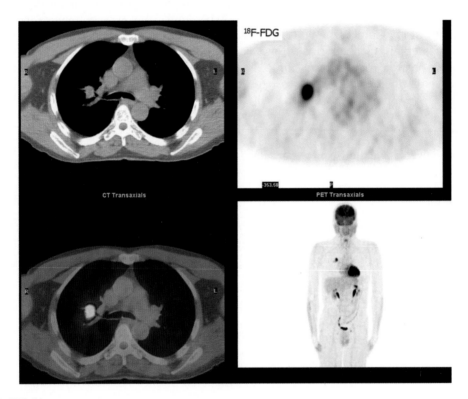

Fig. II.3.5A

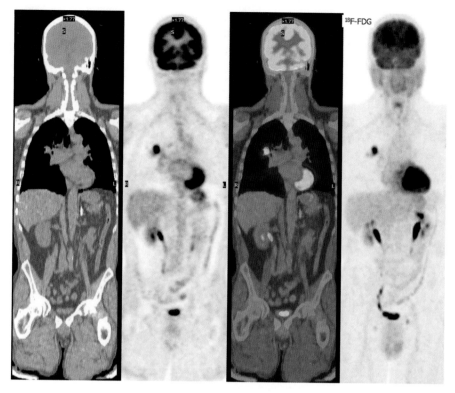

**Fig. II.3.5B**

## Findings

There is intense [18]F-FDG activity within a 30 mm right perihilar mass (Fig. II.3.5A, B), consistent with local tumor recurrence of the known NSCLC. Faint [18]F-FDG uptake in the rib located anterior to the old surgical site (not shown) most probably represents post-surgical changes, although neoplastic involvement could not be excluded.

## Discussion

Although cancers that recur after therapy may be staged with the same TNM criteria that are used in the pretreatment clinical staging, the significance of these criteria may not be the same. The restage classification of recurrent cancer (rTNM) is considered separately for therapeutic guidance, estimation of prognosis, and end-results reporting at that time in the patient's clinical course.

Since the primary tumor of the perihilar region has been resected and this region has been radiated, the new 30 mm mass with focal [18]F-FDG uptake is highly suggestive of local tumor recurrence, presumably in a lymph node, restaging the patients as rTNM stage IIA (with N1 disease, see Table II.3.1). The size of the recurrence is borderline at 30 mm, the upper range of diameter for stage IIA. (Had this perihilar nodal recurrence been >30 mm in greatest axial diameter, the patient would be restaged as stage IIB.)[20]

Treatment options for this patient would include additional radiation therapy (if prior dosages delivered to this region will permit), chemotherapy, or a second surgery to resect this area of localized recurrence. Hellwig and colleagues[35] have shown using $^{18}$F-FDG PET/CT guidance that lung cancer patients undergoing surgical resection for an area of localized recurrence have superior survival compared to those that did not undergo repeat surgery. $^{18}$F-FDG PET/CT whole-body restaging can help identify patients who are more likely to benefit from repeat surgery. If more widespread disease is found and the patient is upstaged, this may prevent unnecessary attempts at local surgical control.

## Diagnosis

Locally recurrent NSCLC, recurrent TNM stage IIA.

## Case II.3.6

### History

This 83-year-old male with a significant smoking history had a newly discovered left perihilar pulmonary lesion on a chest radiograph obtained during evaluation for an abdominal aortic aneurysm. Needle biopsy was suggestive for but not diagnostic of malignancy. The patient was referred to $^{18}$F-FDG PET/CT for further evaluation of this mass, staging of his presumed lung cancer, and selection of a high-yield location for biopsy (Fig. II.3.6A, B).

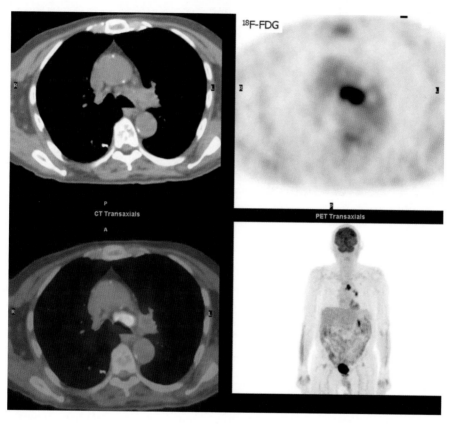

Fig. II.3.6A

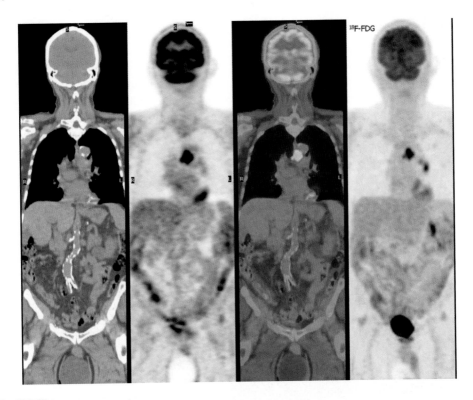

**Fig. II.3.6B**

## Findings

Images from the whole-body [18]F-FDG PET/CT study (Fig. II.3.6A, B) reveal a left
perihilar ill-defined 17 mm lesion with intense [18]F-FDG uptake, as well as a 24 mm left
hilar and ipsilateral mediastinal lymph nodes, including a 24 mm node in the aorto-pulmonary window, 10 mm pretracheal, and 24 mm subcarinal adenopathy.

The coronal images of the PET/CT scan (Fig. II.3.6B) also demonstrate the known
abdominal aortic aneurysm and a large scrotal hydrocele.

## Discussion

By PET/CT, the patient has stage IIIA disease and is still a candidate for potentially
curative surgery. Undetected disease in contralateral mediastinal lymph nodes would
upstage the patient to non-surgical stage IIIB tumor. Options for further preoperative
evaluation would include mediastinoscopy for sampling of contralateral lymph nodes. If
positive, this would prevent a futile thoracotomy in this elderly patient with advanced
atherosclerotic disease and severe emphysema. PET/CT identified several areas for "high-
yield" biopsy, and a directed diagnostic transbronchial biopsy of the pretracheal lymph
nodes indicated a NSCLC.[19–28]

## Diagnosis

NSCLC, stage IIIA.

## Case II.3.7

### History

This 73-year-old male with a 120 pack per year history of smoking, emphysema, and an aortic aneurysm had chest radiographs 6 months prior to current examination, which demonstrated a left upper pulmonary mass. Subsequent CT confirmed two lesions in the left upper lobe measuring 33 and 10 mm, respectively, and a moderate-sized left pleural effusion. The patient underwent mediastinoscopy with biopsy of a right paratracheal lymph node and demonstrated poorly differentiated NSCLC. The patient was referred for initial whole-body staging by [18]F-FDG PET/CT (Fig. II.3.7A, B).

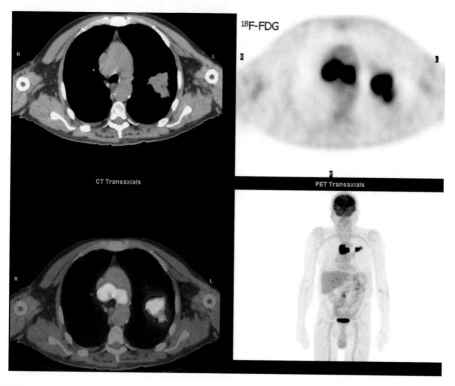

Fig. II.3.7A

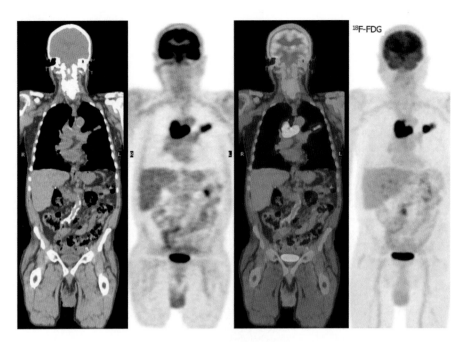

**Fig. II.3.7B**

### Findings

The transaxial (Fig. II.3.7A) and coronal (Fig. II.3.7B) images reveal intense [18]F-FDG uptake in a left upper lobe mass. There is similar intense [18]F-FDG uptake in mediastinal lymph nodes that reach the contralateral mediastinum, specifically the right paratracheal region. Additional findings include the patient's known severe atherosclerotic disease. There is slightly focal uptake in the region of the mid-transverse colon, best seen on the maximum intensity projection (MIP) images (Fig. II.3.7A, B). Colonoscopy was recommended.

### Discussion

The whole-body [18]F-FDG PET/CT scan demonstrates stage IIIB NSCLC with no evidence of stage IV disease with distant metastases. The single focal area of uptake in his mid-transverse colon was evaluated with colonoscopy to exclude the presence of an extra-thoracic malignancy, either primary or metastatic, and revealed a potentially pre-malignant adenomatous polyp.[23]

This patient is not a candidate for surgical cure. His initial staging mediastinoscopy and whole-body [18]F-FDG PET/CT imaging can be used for planning his medical and/or radiation treatment, as well as for assessment of response to treatment and for restaging.[19–28]

### Diagnosis

1. NSCLC, stage IIIB.
2. Adenomatous polyp in the transverse colon.

## Case II.3.8 (DICOM Images on DVD)

### History

This 48-year-old female with a recently diagnosed NSCLC of the right upper lobe was treated preoperatively with radiation, which was completed 2 weeks prior to current examination. The patient was considered at this time to be in stage IIIA based on prior mediastinal lymph node biopsies. She was referred to $^{18}$F-FDG PET/CT for restaging, to determine if the patient is a potential candidate for surgical cure (Fig. II.3.8A, B).

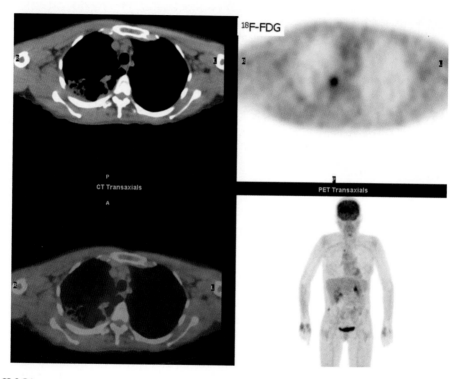

**Fig. II.3.8A**

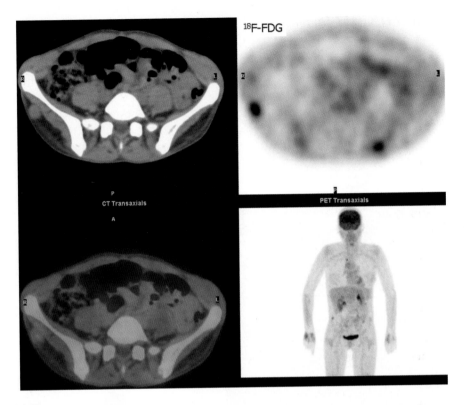

**Fig. II.3.8B**

## Findings

Figure II.3.8A demonstrates an intense [18]F-FDG-avid 26 × 19 mm right upper lobe lesion consistent with the primary tumor. On the CT there are presumed radiation therapy changes (versus less likely, post-obstructive pneumonitis) in the nearby lung. Minimal residual mediastinal [18]F-FDG uptake is seen in an 11 mm subcarinal node and an 8 mm right paratracheal node.

Figure II.3.8B demonstrates [18]F-FDG-avid lesions in a soft tissue nodule of the right gluteal region, 17 mm in diameter, and a subcentimeter lesion within the *longissimus thoracis* muscle on the left, adjacent to the posterior iliac wing. The MIP image demonstrates more extra-thoracic lesions.

## Discussion

Since the presence of extra-thoracic disease upstages the patient from IIIA to IV, at least one of these lesions should be biopsied for verification. Upstaging in this case changes treatment from potentially curative to palliative. PET/CT has also identified the locations that are most amenable to needle-core biopsy. By precise staging, the patient will benefit from correct treatment options and will not be undertreated. Both the patient and the healthcare system will benefit from avoiding the morbidity and expense of a futile thoracotomy.[19-28]

While recent radiation therapy can suppress uptake in areas of tumor and induce an inflammatory response that can mask subtle evidence of tumor, areas outside the radiation field are neither suppressed nor masked. $^{18}$F-FDG PET/CT can still be useful in restaging patients who have had recent radiation therapy by detection of tumor outside the radiation field.

**Diagnosis**

1. NSCLC, stage IV.
2. Radiation pneumonitis.

**Clinical Report: Body $^{18}$F-FDG PET/CT Imaging (for DVD cases only)**

Indication

Restaging of NSCLC.

History

This 48-year-old female with a recently diagnosed right upper lobe NSCLC completed radiation therapy to the right upper lobe and mediastinum 2 weeks prior to current examination and was staged as stage IIIA disease based on available information. The patient presents for verification of staging by $^{18}$F-FDG PET/CT prior to thoracotomy.

Procedure

The fasting blood glucose was 160 mg/dL at time of injection of 481 MBq (13.0 mCi) of $^{18}$F-FDG via the right antecubital vein. After a 60 min distribution time, a whole-body low-dose CT was acquired for anatomic localization and to correct for attenuation, without contrast from the vertex to the upper thighs. PET images were then acquired over the same anatomic regions. The arms were positioned along the sides of the torso.

Findings

 *Quality of the study*: The overall quality of the study is good.
 *Head and neck*: There is physiologic uptake of $^{18}$F-FDG within the gray matter of the brain and in the glandular and lymphoid tissues of the neck.
 *Chest*: Intense $^{18}$F-FDG uptake is seen within a 26 × 19 mm right upper lobe lesion, which likely represents the primary malignancy. On CT, there is an infiltrate in the right upper lobe, which represents either radiation pneumonitis and/or post-obstructive pneumonia. No significant $^{18}$F-FDG activity is otherwise seen in the lung or right hilus.
 Minimal $^{18}$F-FDG uptake is seen within an 11 mm subcarinal node and in an 8 mm right paratracheal node. There is an incidental 24 mm septal bleb within the RLL.
 *Abdomen and pelvis*: Physiologic uptake of $^{18}$F-FDG is seen within the gastro-intestinal and genito-urinary systems. Intense $^{18}$F-FDG uptake is seen within an 18 mm focal soft tissue mass posterior to the left kidney. Intense focal splenic $^{18}$F-FDG uptake is seen corresponding to a lesion measuring 20 mm in its greatest axial diameter. Focal lesions are most compatible with metastatic disease.
 *Musculoskeletal system*: Intense $^{18}$F-FDG uptake is seen within a 17 mm subcutaneous nodule in the right gluteal area, suspicious for metastasis. This gluteal lesion is very amenable to percutaneous needle-core biopsy for verification of disseminated metastatic disease. There is a sub-centimeter soft tissue focus of intense $^{18}$F-FDG uptake in

the left *longissimus thoracis* muscle adjacent to the posterior iliac wing, suspicious for a soft tissue metastasis. No skeletal metastases are identified.

Impression

1. Intense $^{18}$F-FDG activity within the 28 × 19 mm right upper lobe nodule, compatible with the known primary malignancy.
2. Radiation pneumonitis and/or post-obstructive pneumonia within the right upper lobe.
3. Intense $^{18}$F-FDG uptake within an 18 mm soft tissue nodule posterior to the left kidney and 20 mm splenic lesion most compatible with metastases.
4. Intense $^{18}$F-FDG uptake within a subcentimeter lesion within the left *longissimus thoracis* muscle adjacent to the posterior iliac wing, most likely a metastasis.
5. Intense $^{18}$F-FDG uptake in a 17 mm subcutaneous nodule in the right gluteal area suspicious for metastatic disease. This lesion is particularly amenable to needle-core biopsy for tissue confirmation.

## Case II.3.9

### History

This 45-year-old male with newly diagnosed SCLC presented with a 6-month history of increasing shortness of breath, weight loss, intermittent hemoptysis, and fever. He has a 30 pack per year history of smoking. A recent MRI of the brain is normal. A recent diagnostic CT of the chest, abdomen, and pelvis revealed no evidence of spread of tumor beyond the chest. Bone marrow aspiration/biopsy was negative for tumor. The patient was referred to [18]F-FDG PET/CT for initial staging to exclude occult disease not seen on the CI examinations (Fig. II.3.9).

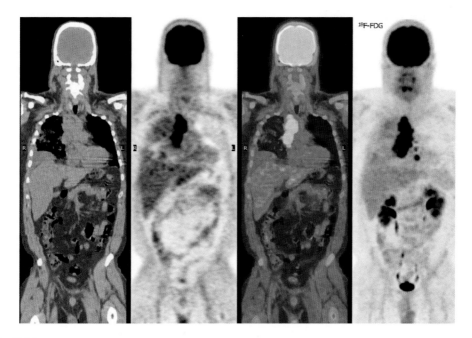

Fig. II.3.9

### Findings

There is intensely increased [18]F-FDG uptake within a bulky mediastinal mass, which begins at the thoracic inlet in the right paratracheal region, extending inferiorly to the subcarinal, right hilar, and right infrahilar regions and measures $78 \times 44 \times 130$ mm (Fig. II.3.9).

There is also intense [18]F-FDG uptake within contralateral mediastinal lymph nodes on the left, posterior to the aorta, at the costovertebral angle, extending from the level of the carina inferiorly to the level of the mid-heart. The largest lymph node measures $15 \times 30$ mm in the transaxial view.

In the right hemithorax, there is a diffuse fibronodular infiltrate with mildly increased [18]F-FDG uptake, most likely of inflammatory etiology. There is mildly increased [18]F-FDG uptake in a large right pleural effusion probably of malignant etiology.

**Discussion**

SCLC accounts for 13–20% of primary lung cancers. SCLC has a simple staging classification of limited-stage versus extensive disease. As with NSCLC, [18]F-FDG imaging reveals sites of disease missed on CI, especially extra thoracic metastases, excluding the brain, where MRI is superior, thus improving staging and restaging of patients. PET/CT in this case demonstrates the extent of disease to include the mediastinal nodes adjacent to the descending aorta. Since the extent of disease is limited to an area that is potentially treatable by radiation, the patient has limited-stage disease and received combined chemotherapy and radiation therapy.[39–40]

**Diagnosis**

SCLC, limited-stage disease.

## Case II.3.10 (DICOM Images on DVD)

### History

This 47-year-old woman with known left chest mesothelioma had Hodgkin's lymphoma 28 years ago and was treated with chemotherapy, splenectomy, and radiation to the mantle and periaortic lymph nodes. Two years prior to current examination, the patient developed shortness of breath. A chest radiograph showed a left pleural effusion, with subsequent chest CT suggesting pleural nodularity, subsequently found on biopsy to represent MPM. The patient was referred to $^{18}$F-FDG PET/CT for restaging following her most recent course of experimental chemotherapy (Fig. II.3.10A,B).

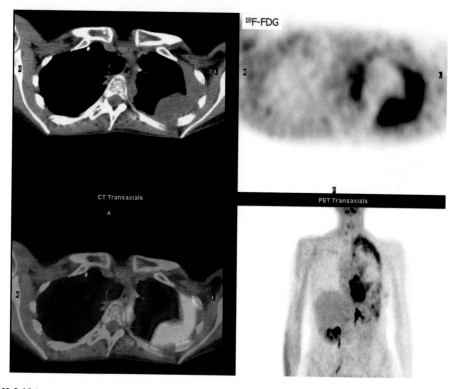

Fig. II.3.10A

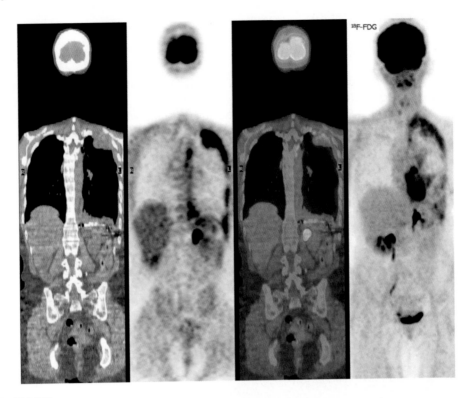

**Fig. II.3.10B**

## Findings

There is irregular pleural thickening in the left hemithorax measuring up to 30 mm, with [18]F-FDG uptake varying in intensity, with no evidence of involvement of the pulmonary parenchyma (Fig. II.3.10A, B). Old surgical changes from the prior pleurodesis are seen in the left lower hemithorax, including areas of presumed dystrophic calcifications and scarring (Fig. II.3.10B).

## Discussion

The diffuse pleural thickening on the left with variable areas of nodularity and uptake is classic for MPM. This tumor can spread by direct extension into the mediastinum, chest wall, pulmonary parenchyma, or peritoneal cavity. While there are areas of pleural thickening on the right, especially in the paravertebral region at the mid-thoracic level, they do not demonstrate uptake and are stable compared with prior examinations (not shown). In the present case, disease appears therefore confined to the left hemithorax. Pleurodesis is usually associated with a granulomatous inflammatory reaction. Therefore, [18]F-FDG avidity may be due to a combination of uptake in inflammatory and malignant cells.

Many, but not all, cases of MPM are associated with prior exposure to asbestos, smoking, or both. Some cases are sporadic, without an obvious etiology. However, patients with a history of prior radiation treatment for Hodgkin's lymphoma, especially 20 years or more previously, have an increased risk for a variety of secondary malignancies, especially solid tumors. The risk of secondary malignancies increases with the duration after initial treatment. The patients at greatest risk are those treated at a relatively young age, as with this patient who was treated at the age of 19, and with combined radiation and chemotherapy. Most secondary solid tumors occur in or at the edge of the radiation field, as in this case. The risk of secondary hematologic malignancies, especially non-Hodgkin's lymphoma, increases with time, but less than the risk for solid tumors. While it cannot be proven that this patient's MPM is associated with the prior administration of chemo- and radiation therapy for Hodgkin's lymphoma that she received 28 years previously at the age of 19, particularly since she has never smoked and has no asbestos exposure history.[41–46,49]

**Diagnosis**

MPM of the left hemithorax and/or reactive inflammation to former pleurodesis.

**Clinical Report (Body [18]F-FDG PET/CT for DVD cases only)**

Indication

Staging of MPM.

History

This 47-year-old woman with a known left chest mesothelioma had Hodgkin's lymphoma diagnosed 28 years previously and was treated with chemotherapy, splenectomy, and radiation to both mantle and periaortic lymph nodes. Two years ago, the patient developed shortness of breath, with a chest radiograph showing a left pleural effusion and chest CT suggesting pleural nodularity. The patient then underwent thoracoscopy and pleurodesis with biopsy obtained at that time demonstrating MPM.

Procedure

The fasting blood glucose level was 67 mg/dL at time of injection of the radioisotope. The patient was administered 362 MBq (9.8 mCi) of [18]F-FDG intravenously in the right antecubital fossa. After 55 min of distribution time, a whole-body low-dose CT scan without contrast was acquired for anatomic localization and to correct for attenuation with the patient's arms to the sides, from the vertex to the upper thighs. PET imaging was then acquired over the same anatomic regions.

Findings

   *Quality of the study*: The overall quality of the study is good.
   *Head and neck*: There is physiologic distribution of the radiopharmaceutical in the brain, excluding relatively decreased [18]F-FDG uptake within the right hemisphere with associated atrophy, consistent with the patient's history of stroke. The soft tissues of the remainder of the head and neck reveal a normal uptake pattern of the radiopharmaceutical with no abnormal adenopathy or other significant findings seen in this region.
   *Chest*: Intense [18]F-FDG uptake is identified, corresponding to irregular pleural thickening within the left hemithorax, with nodularity more pronounced in the superior half. Surgical scarring and clips are present within the posterior, inferior, and medial aspect

of the left chest, with intense $^{18}$F-FDG avidity, corresponding to an area of known prior pleurodesis and biopsy. A small non-$^{18}$F-FDG-avid pleural effusion is present at the base of the left lung. The tracer uptake in the pleural thickening on the left is heterogeneous, with some areas demonstrating moderate and other areas intense uptake. The pleural thickening is also seen to be irregular, with some areas being more nodular than others, with maximum thickness perpendicular to the chest wall of about 3 cm.

On the right, there are scattered areas of mild pleural thickening, though none of these regions demonstrate uptake above normal skeletal muscle. There are bilateral small fibronodular densities and sub-centimeter pulmonary nodules, too small to characterize by either PET or CT, with none of these demonstrating tracer uptake above background.

CT reveals a multi-nodular goiter, with one of the nodules in the superior pole on the right demonstrating mild $^{18}$F-FDG avidity.

*Abdomen and pelvis*: CT demonstrates the presence of surgical clips within the abdomen, a previous splenectomy, and a ptotic right kidney with horizontal orientation. No abnormal uptake, mass lesions, or other evidence of tumor spread to the abdomen or pelvis are seen.

*Musculoskeletal*: No skeletal metastases are seen. Excluding the soft tissue findings described above, no additional significant findings are noted for age.

Impression

1. $^{18}$F-FDG uptake corresponding to left pleural thickening which may be due to a combination of avidity of inflammatory and malignant cells. No evidence of extrathoracic disease.
2. Decreased $^{18}$F-FDG uptake within the right cerebral hemisphere consistent with the patient's known prior stroke.
3. Sequelae of prior splenectomy 28 years ago for Hodgkin's lymphoma.
4. Additional CT findings as described herewith.

## Case II.3.11

### History

This 69-year-old male with newly diagnosed NSCLC was referred to $^{18}$F-FDG PET/CT imaging for initial staging (Fig. II.3.11A, B).

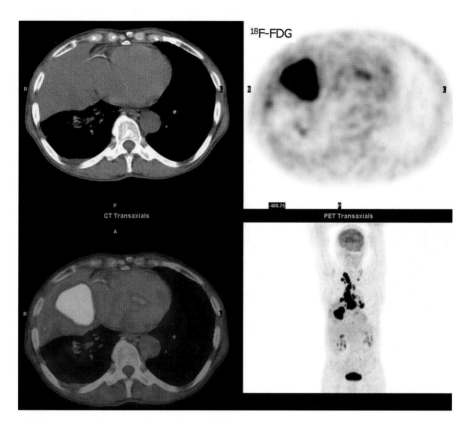

Fig. II.3.11A

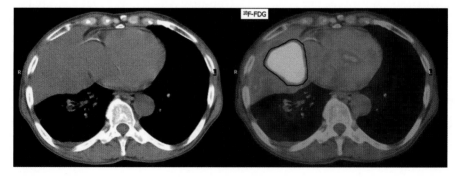

Fig. II.3.11B

## Findings

PET/CT demonstrates widespread disease bilateral in the chest and mediastinum, extending to the lower neck on both sides, clearly representing stage IV disease (Fig. II.3.11A). The patient also has severe chronic lung disease from smoking. He was symptomatic at the time of diagnosis with a productive cough and chest pain. The radiation therapist wished to maximize palliative treatment to the tumor while sparing as much lung function as possible.

Using the "metabolic margins" as defined by the $^{18}$F-FDG uptake (Fig. II.3.11B, right) on the fused PET/CT image, more accurate tumor contours were defined compared to the larger region of lung opacification on the corresponding CT image (Fig. II.3.11B, left). The PET/CT data were DICOM transferred to the radiation treatment planning workstation, where radiation ports were defined for treatment. In this specific patient, the change in the radiation field from using PET/CT data resulted in a decrease in gross tumor volume (GTV) of 43%. Following chemoradiation treatment, the patient's productive cough and chest pain were greatly improved. Preservation of as much lung function as possible was obtained for the remainder of the patient's life.

## Discussion

Several articles have reported on the use of $^{18}$F-FDG imaging in radiation treatment planning compared to CT alone. The use of PET/CT results in changes in GTV that range from 30 to 60%. In 16% of cases, PET/CT changed the intent of treatment from curative to palliative by demonstrating unsuspected stage IV disease. An important but as yet unanswered question relates to the use of the PET data to define tumor margins since change in intensity settings will result in apparent change in tumor margins. While various studies report using thresholds of 20–40% of SUVmax to define tumor margins, there is no validated threshold reported in the literature at this time. Indeed, the use of good judgment rather than an arbitrary threshold is of paramount importance in defining tumor contours because of many confounding factors that are often present, especially in the lungs, where apparent extent or intensity of uptake can be changed by respiratory motion, nearby infection/inflammation, and cardiac uptake, for example.[50]

Despite these limitations, the use of $^{18}$F-FDG PET/CT is being rapidly and widely accepted in radiation therapy planning. While inter observer variation in tumor margins exists, this averages less than with CT only. The most prominent changes in treatment planning have been reported in cases where the PET data allow discrimination of tumor from atelectasis, or with the inclusion of PET-positive lymph nodes that appeared normal on CT in the radiation field. While these results indicate that $^{18}$F-FDG PET/CT has an important role in radiation treatment planning, no large studies have yet proven a statistically significant improvement in long-term patient outcome.[51]

## Diagnosis

Stage IV NSCLC with extensive associated atelectasis and post-obstructive pneumonitis.

# References

1. Spira A, Ettinger D. Multidisciplinary management of lung cancer. *N Engl J Med* 2004;350:379–392.
2. Ost D, Fein A, Feinsilver S. The solitary pulmonary nodule. *New Engl J Med* 2003; 348:2535–2542.
3. Erasmus JJ, Connoly JE, McAdams HP, Roggli VL. Solitary pulmonary nodules: Part I. Morphologic evaluation for differentiation of benign and malignant lesions. *Radiographics* 2000;20:43–58.
4. Yankelevitz DF, Henschke CI. Does 2-year stability imply that pulmonary nodules are benign? *AJR Am J Roentgenol* 1997;168:325–328.
5. Zerhouni EA, Stitik FP, Siegelman SS, Naidich DP, Sagel SS, Proto AV, Muhm JR, Walsh JW, Martinez CR, Heelan RT. CT of the pulmonary nodule: a cooperative study. *Radiology* 1986;160: 319–327.
6. Swensen SJ, Viggiano RW, Midthun DE, Müller NL, Sherrick A, Yamashita K, Naidich DP, Patz EF, Hartman TH, Muhm JR, Weaver AL. Lung nodule enhancement at CT: Multicenter study. *Radiology* 2000;214:73–80.
7. Conces DJ Jr, Schwenk GR Jr, Doering PR, Glant MD. Thoracic needle biopsy: Improved results utilizing a team approach. *Chest* 1987;91:813–816.
8. Henschke CI, Yankelevitz DF, Libby DM, Pasmantier MW, Smith JP, Miettinen OS. The international early lung cancer action program investigators. Survival of patients with stage I lung cancer detected on CT screening. *New Engl J Med* 2006;255:1763–1771.
9. Unger M. A pause, progress and reassessment in lung cancer screening. *New Engl J Med* 2006;355: 1822–1824.
10. Winer-Muram H. The solitary pulmonary nodule. *Radiology* 2006;239:34–49.
11. Gupta NC, Frank AR, Dewan NA, Redepenning LS, Rothberg ML, Mailliard JA, Phalen JJ, Sunderland JJ, Frick MP. Solitary pulmonary nodules: detection of malignancy with PET with 2-[F-18]-fluoro-2-deoxy-D-glucose. *Radiology* 1992;184:441–444.
12. Gould MK, Maclean CC, Kuschner WG, Rydzak CE, Owens DK. Accuracy of positron emission tomography for diagnosis of pulmonary nodules and mass lesions: A meta-analysis. *JAMA* 2001;285: 914–924.
13. Joo Hyun O, Ie Ryung Y, Sung Hoon K, Sohn HS, Chung HK. Clinical significance of small pulmonary nodules with little or No 18 F-FDG uptake on PET/CT images of patients with nonthoracic malignancies. *J Nucl Med* 2007;48:15–21.
14. Gambhir SS, Shepherd JE, Shah BD, Hart E, Hoh CK, Valk PE, Emi T, Phelps ME. Analytical decision model for the cost-effective management of solitary pulmonary nodules. *J Clin Oncol* 1998;16: 2113–2125.
15. Gould MK, Sanders GD, Barnett PG, Rydzak CE, Maclean CC, McClellan MB, Owens DK. Cost-effectiveness of alternative management strategies for patients with solitary pulmonary nodules. *Ann Intern Med* 2003;138:724–735.
16. Matthies A, Hickeson M, Cuchiara A, Aliva A. Dual time point 18 F-FDG PET for the evaluation of pulmonary nodules. *J Nucl Med* 2002;43:871–875.
17. Henschke CI, Yankelevitz D, Westcott J, Davis SD, Fleishon H, Gefter WB, McLoud TC, Pugatch RD, Sostman HD, Tocino I, White CS, Bode FR, Swensen SJ. Work-up of the solitary pulmonary nodule. *Radiology* 2000;215:Suppl:607–609.
18. Mountain C. Revisions in the international system for staging lung cancer. *Chest* 1997;111:1710–1717.
19. Birim O, Kappetein AP, Stijnen T, Bogers AJJC. Meta-analysis of positron emission tomographic and computed tomographic imaging in detecting mediastinal lymph node metastases in non small cell lung cancer. *Ann Thorac Surg* 2005;79:375–381.
20. Silvestri GA, Gould MK, Margolis ML, Tanoue LT, McCrory D, Toloza C, Detterbeck F. Noninvasive staging of non-small cell lung cancer: ACCP evidenced-based clinical practice guidelines (2nd Edition). *Chest* 2007;132:178S–201S.
21. Lardinois D, Weder W, Hany TF, Kamel EM, Korom S, Seifert B, von Schulthess GK, Steinert HC. Staging of non-small-cell lung cancer with integrated positron-emission tomography and computed tomography. *New Engl J Med* 2003;348:2500–2507.
22. Toloza EM, Harpole L, McCrory DC. Noninvasive staging of non-small cell lung cancer: A review of the current evidence. *Chest* 2003;123:137S–146S.
23. MacManus, MP, Hicks, RJ, Matthews, JP, Hogg A, McKenzie AF, Wirth A, Ware RE, Ball DL. High rate of unsuspected distant metastases by PET in apparent stage III non-small-cell

lung cancer: Implications for radical radiation therapy. *Int J Radiat Oncol Biol Phys* 2001;50: 287–293.

24. Ludwig V, Komori T, Kolb DC, Martin WH, Sandler MP, Delbeke D. Cerebral lesions incidentally detected on FDG PET images of patients evaluated for body malignancies. *Mol Imaging Biol* 2002;4:359–362.

25. Boland GW, Goldberg MA, Lee MJ, Mayo-Smith WW, Dixon J, McNicholas MM, Mueller PR. Indeterminate adrenal masses in patients with cancer. Evaluation at PET with 2-(F-18)-fluoro-2-deoxy-D-glucose. *Radiology* 1995;194:131–134.

26. Bury T, Barreto A, Daenen F, Barthelemy N, Ghaye B, Rigo P. Fluorine-18 deoxyglucose positron emission tomography for the detection of bone metastases in patients with non-small cell lung cancer. *Eur J Nucl Med* 1998;25:1244–1247.

27. Verboom P, van Tinteren H, Hoekstra OS, Smit EF, van den Bergh J, Schreurs A, Stallaert R, Velthoven P, Comans E, Diepenhorst F, Mourik JC, Postmus PE, Boers M, Grijseels EWM, Teule GJJ, Uyl-de Groot CA, the PLUS study group. Cost-effectiveness of FDG-PET in staging non-small cell lung cancer: The PLUS study. *Eur J Nucl Med Mol Imaging* 2003;30:1444–1449.

28. van Tinteren H, Hoekstra OS, Smit EF,van den Bergh J, Schreurs A, Stallaert R, van Velthoven P, Comans E, Diepenhorst F, Verboom P. Effectiveness of positron emission tomography in the pre-operative assessment of patients with suspected non-small-cell lung cancer: the PLUS multicentre randomised trial. *Lancet* 2002;359:1388–1393.

29. MacManus MP, Hicks RJ, Matthews JP, McKenzie A, Rischin D, Salminen EK, Ball DL. Positron emission tomography is superior to computed tomography scanning for response-assessment after radical radiotherapy or chemoradiotherapy in patients with non-small-cell lung cancer. *J Clin Oncol* 2003;21:1285–1292.

30. Pöttgen C, Levegrün S, Theegarten D, Marnitz S, Grehl S, Pink R, Eberhardt W, Stamatis G, Gauler T, Antoch G, Bockisch A, Stuschke M. Value of 18F-fluoro-2-deoxy-D-glucose-positron emission tomography/computed tomography in nonsmall cell lung cancer for prediction of pathologic response and times to relapse after neoadjuvant chemoradiotherapy. *Clin Cancer Res* 2006;12: 97–106.

31. Cerfolio RJ, Bryant AS, Buddhiwardhan O. Restaging patients with N2 (stage IIIa) non-small cell lung cancer after neoadjuvant chemoradiotherapy: A prospective study. *J Thorac Cardiovasc Surg* 2006;131:1229–1235.

32. Eschmann SM, Friedel G, Paulsen F, Reimold M, Hehr T, Budach W, Dittmann H, Langen H, Bares R. Repeat 18 F-FDG PET for monitoring neoadjuvant chemotherapy in patients with stage III nonsmall cell lung cancer. *Lung Cancer* 2007;55:165–171.

33. Weber WA, Petersen V, Schmidt B, Tyndale-Hines L, Link T, Peschel C, Schwaiger M. Positron emission tomography in non-small-cell lung cancer: Prediction of response to chemotherapy by quantitative assessment of glucose use. *J Clin Oncol* 2003;21:2651–2657.

34. De Leyn P, Stoobants S, Dewever W, Lerut T, Coosemans W, Decker G, Nafteux P, Van Raemdonck D, Mortelmans L, Nackaerts K, Vansteenkiste J. Prospective comparative study of integrated positron emission tomography-computed tomography compared with remediastinoscopy in the assessment of residual mediastinal lymph node disease after induction chemotherapy for mediastinoscopy proven stage IIIA-N2 nonsmall cell lung cancer: A Leuven Lung Cancer Group study. *J Clin Oncol* 2006;24: 3333–3339.

35. Hellwig D, Groschel A, Graeter TP, Hellwig AP, Nestle U, Schäfers HJ, Sybrecht GW, Kirsch CM. Diagnostic performance and prognostic impact of FDG-PET in suspected recurrence of surgically treated nonsmall cell lung cancer. *Eur J Nucl Med Mol Imaging* 2006;33:13–21.

36. Green FL, Page DL, Fleming ID, Fritz AG, Balch CM, Haller DG, Morrow M. *AJCC Cancer Staging Handbook, sixth edition.* New York: Springer, 2004.

37. Samson DJ, Seidenfeld J. Simon GR, Turrisi AT 3rd, Bonnell C, Ziegler KM, Aronson N. Evidence for management of small cell lung cancer: ACCP evidence-based clinical practice guidelines (2nd edition). *Chest* 2007;132:314S–323S.

38. Schumacher T, Brink I, Mix M, Reinhardt M, Herget G, Digel W, Henke M, Moser E, Nitzsche E. FDG-PET imaging for the staging and follow-up of small cell lung cancer. *Eur J Nucl Med* 2001;28: 483–488.

39. Pandit N, Gonen M, Krug L, Larson SM. Prognostic value of [18 F]FDG-PET imaging in small cell lung cancer. *Eur J Nucl Med* 2003;30:78–84.

40. Brink I, Schumacher T, Mix M, Ruhland S, Stoelben E, Digel W, Henke M, Ghanem N, Moser E, Nitzsche EU. Impact of [18 F]FDG-PET on the primary staging of small-cell lung cancer. *Eur J Nucl Med Mol Imaging* 2004;31:1614–1620.

41. Robinson BWS, Lake RA. Advances in malignant mesothelioma. *N Engl J Med* 2005;353:1591–1603.

42. Rusch VW. A proposed new international TNM staging system for malignant pleural mesothelioma from the international mesothelioma interest group. *Lung Cancer* 1996;14:1–12.

43. Flores RM, Akhurst T, Gonen M, Larson S. Rusch V. Positron emission tomography defines metastatic disease but not locoregional disease in patients with malignant pleural mesothelioma. *J Thorac Cardiovasc Surg* 2003;126:11–15.

44. Truong MT, Marom EM, Erasmus JJ. Preoperative evaluation of patients with malignant pleural mesothelioma: Role of integrated CT-PET imaging. *J Thorac Imaging* 2006;21:146–153.

45. Wang ZJ, Reddy GP, Gotway MB, Higgins CB, Jablons DM, Ramaswamy M, Hawkins RA, Webb WR. Malignant pleural mesothelioma: Evaluation with CT, MR imaging, and PET. *Radio Graphics* 2004;24:105–119.

46. Ceresoli GL, Chiti A, Zucali PA, Rodari M, Lutman RF, Salamina S, Incarbone M, Alloisio M, Santoro A. Early response evaluation in malignant pleural mesothelioma by positron emission tomography with [18 F]Fluorodeoxyglucose. *J Clin Oncol* 2006;24:4587–4593.

47. Podoloff DA, Advani RH, Allred C, Benson AB, Brown E, Burstein HJ, Carlson RW, Coleman RE, Czuczman MS, Delbeke D, Edge SB, Ettinger DS, Grannis FW, Hillner BE, Hoffman JM, Keil K, Komaki R, Larson SM, Mankoff DA, Rozenzweig KE, Skibber JM, Yahalom J, Yu JM, Zelenetz AD. NCCN task force report: Positron emission tomography (PET/Computed tomography (CT) scanning in cancer. *J Natl Compr Canc Netw* 2007;5 (suppl 1): S1–S22. www/nccn.org/professionals/physician_gls/f_guidelines.asp.

48. Fletcher JW, Djulbegovic B, Soares HP, Siegel BA, Lowe VJ, Lyman GH, Coleman E, Wahl R, Paschold JC, Avril N, Einhorn LH, Suh WW, Samson D, Delbeke D, Gorman M, Shields AF. Recommendations for the Use of FDG(fluorine-18, (2-[18 F]Fluoro-2-deoxy-D-glucose) positron emission tomography in oncology. *J Nucl Med* 2008;49:480–508.

49. Abrahamsen A Foss, Andersen A, Nome O, Jacobsen AB, Holte H, Abrahamsen J Foss Kvaløy S. Long-term risk of second malignancy after treatment of Hodgkin's disease: the influence of treatment, age and follow-up time. *Ann Oncol* 2002;13:4786–4791.

50. Macapinlac H. Clinical applications of positron emission tomography/computed tomography treatment planning. *Semin Nucl Med* 2008;38:137–140.

51. Greco C, Rosenzweig K, Cascinic GL, Tamburrini O. Current status of PET/CT for tumour volume definition in radiotherapy treatment planning for non-small cell lung cancer (NSCLC). *Lung Cancer* 2007;57:125–134.

# Chapter II.4
# Breast Cancer

Simona Ben-Haim and Vineet Prakash

## Introduction

Breast cancer is the most common cancer in women in the Western world and the second leading cause of cancer-related death in women with an age-adjusted incidence of 117.7 women per year in 2004.[1] The National Cancer Institute estimates 178,480 women will be diagnosed with breast cancer and 40,640 will die of breast cancer in 2007 in the United States, most of them of progressive metastatic disease.

Staging of the tumor is based on the tumor, nodes, metastases (TNM) classification,[2] briefly summarized herewith. The primary tumor is classified as T0–T4, where T0 indicates in situ tumor with no associated invasion of normal breast tissue; T1–T3 indicate a tumor not larger than 2 cm, between 2 and 5 cm, or larger than 5 cm in the greatest dimension, respectively; and T4 indicates a tumor of any size with direct extension to chest wall or skin.

The status of the regional lymph nodes is defined by N, where Nx indicates nodes cannot be assessed (e.g., which have been previously removed); N0 indicates no regional lymph node metastasis; N1 indicates metastasis to movable ipsilateral axillary node(s); N2 indicates metastasis to ipsilateral fixed axillary or internal mammary node(s); and N3 indicates metastasis to ipsilateral infraclavicular or internal mammary and axillary or supraclavicular node(s). The pathological status of lymph nodes is defined by pN and further classified according to the number of lymph nodes as defined by immunohistochemical or molecular methods and by the size of the metastasis.

The status of distant metastasis (M) can be either M0 (no distant metastasis) or M1 (distant metastasis).

Accurate diagnosis and staging, efficient monitoring of response to therapy, and early diagnosis of disease recurrence are essential for the selection of the most appropriate therapeutic strategy and major determinants of patient's prognosis and survival.[3]

The role of fluorodeoxyglucose (FDG) positron emission tomography (PET)/computed tomography (CT) in evaluation of patients with primary and recurrent breast cancer has been recently reviewed.[3–5]

S. Ben-Haim (✉)
Institute of Nuclear Medicine, University College London Hospital NHS Trust, London, UK
e-mail: simona.ben-haim@uclh.nhs.uk

D. Delbeke, O. Israel (eds.), *Hybrid PET/CT and SPECT/CT Imaging*,
DOI 10.1007/978-0-387-92820-3_6, © Springer Science+Business Media, LLC 2010

# $^{18}$F-FDG PET and PET/CT for the Detection and Staging of Breast Cancer

At the time of initial diagnosis and staging of breast cancer, $^{18}$F-fluorodeoxyglucose ($^{18}$F-FDG) imaging is of controversial clinical value. Initially $^{18}$F-FDG PET was reported to have high sensitivity and specificity (ranging between 85–95% and 80–95%, respectively). It has been shown, however, of limited diagnostic value in detecting small noninvasive primary breast tumors, in staging the axillary region, and in the detection of osteoblastic metastases.[6,7] These discordant results can be explained, at least in part, by the different histopathology and size of the tumors. Lower sensitivity has been reported in better differentiated and slow-growing tumors and in noninvasive breast cancer, whereas better performance has been demonstrated for the detection of primary invasive breast cancer with an overall sensitivity, specificity, and accuracy of 90, 93, and 92%, respectively.[6] Among the invasive subtypes, infiltrating ductal carcinoma has higher $^{18}$F-FDG uptake and is therefore detected at higher sensitivity when compared with the infiltrating lobular subtype.[4] With respect to tumor size, detection of small tumors is limited by the resolution of the imaging systems. Sensitivity for the detection of subcentimeter tumors is 25%, compared with 84% for tumors 1–2 cm in size and 92% for tumors larger than 2 cm.[4]

There is only limited data on the use of $^{18}$F-FDG PET for the diagnosis of in situ carcinoma of the breast. PET was negative in all 12 patients with tumors smaller than 2 cm and was positive in 3 of 6 patients with larger in situ carcinomas.[4] Different locations of the primary tumors within the breast were also assessed. Patients with inner quadrant breast tumors had a six-fold greater frequency of extra-axillary $^{18}$F-FDG-avid metastases and are at a greater risk of progressive metastatic disease than patients with outer quadrant tumors. False-positive results have been reported in cases of inflammation, fibrous dysplasia, and fibroadenoma.[8]

Axillary lymph node involvement is the most important prognostic indicator in breast cancer patients, as well as an important factor for planning therapy. In a study of 360 patients, Wahl and colleagues[9] report a sensitivity of 61% and a specificity of 80% for axillary nodal staging, suggesting that $^{18}$F-FDG PET may fail to detect disease involvement in small nodes or micrometastatic disease. $^{18}$F-FDG PET is therefore not routinely recommended for axillary staging of patients with newly diagnosed breast cancer. Sentinel node identification and biopsy is the standard of care for staging the axilla in early breast cancer. There is strong evidence that the histopathology of the sentinel node predicts involvement of the other nodes in the region. The sentinel node(s) can be localized at minimally invasive surgery in 92–100% of patients using an intraoperative probe. False-negative sentinel nodes have been reported in <3% of patients, but many of these have occurred in patients with multicentric tumors. In fact, one investigator has reported a higher incidence (43%) of tumor when only the sentinel node was examined than when all the nodes within the axilla (29%) were examined, indicative of more accurate staging. The routine use of lymphoscintigraphy in patients with clinically negative axillary nodes results in the avoidance of axillary lymphadenectomy in patients who do not have lymphatic tumor and reduces morbidity and costs considerably. A good review of this topic is available.[10]

In contrast, $^{18}$F-FDG PET performs well and better than CT in detection of internal mammary and mediastinal metastases with sensitivity, specificity, and accuracy of 85, 90, and 88% for PET versus 54, 85, and 73% for CT, respectively.[6] Similar results were reported in studies assessing the performance of combined modality $^{18}$F-FDG PET/CT in patients with breast cancer.[7,11]

# $^{18}$F-FDG PET and PET/CT for the Detection of Metastatic Breast Cancer

$^{18}$F-FDG PET/CT has the ability to detect and further characterize distant metastatic disease sites in patients with breast cancer. Between 16 and 30% of patients with loco-regional recurrence are diagnosed using this modality as having distant metastases. Also, 24% of patients with breast cancer develop distant metastases within 18 months following diagnosis of disease recurrence.[12] $^{18}$F-FDG PET has been reported to have an overall sensitivity of 84–93% and a negative predictive value >90% for detection of distant metastases.[6]

$^{18}$F-FDG PET is more accurate than CT for the detection of nodal mediastinal involvement with sensitivity and specificity of 85 and 90% versus 50 and 83% for PET and CT, respectively. Furthermore, $^{18}$F-FDG PET accurately detects distant metastatic disease with a sensitivity of 80–97% and specificity of 75–94%.[13] In 6 of 21 patients that had dedicated breast magnetic resonance imaging (MRI) and $^{18}$F-FDG imaging, $^{18}$F-FDG PET/CT had a sensitivity of 100% for the detection of distant metastases, leading to a change in the therapeutic management of these patients.[10]

The skeleton is the most common site for distant metastases in breast cancer. Skeletal scintigraphy has a high overall sensitivity for the detection of skeletal metastases, which is, however, lower for detection of lytic lesions or foci confined to the bone marrow. $^{18}$F-fluoride PET has a higher sensitivity compared to $^{99m}$Tc-methylene diphosphonate bone scintigraphy, showing focally increased uptake in both osteolytic and osteoblastic skeletal metastases, but in benign lesions as well.[5] $^{18}$F-FDG PET has also been assessed for the detection of skeletal metastases and sensitivity ranges from 56 to 100%.[14,15] In 55 breast cancer patients with skeletal metastases, Nakai and colleagues[16] reported a sensitivity of 100% for the detection of lytic skeletal metastases with $^{18}$F-FDG PET versus 70% for bone scintigraphy. In sclerotic, osteoblastic metastases, the sensitivities were 56 and 100%, respectively. $^{18}$F-FDG PET/CT provides structural information of skeletal lesions on the CT component in addition to the assessment of their metabolic activity on PET. Du and colleagues[15] assessed sequentially 146 skeletal lesions in 25 patients with suspected recurrence of breast cancer with $^{18}$F-FDG PET/CT. Increased $^{18}$F-FDG uptake was present in 94% of osteolytic, 82% of mixed, and 61% of osteoblastic skeletal lesions. After treatment, 81% of the osteolytic $^{18}$F-FDG-avid lesions became osteoblastic and tracer-negative, with only the large lesions remaining $^{18}$F-FDG-avid. Of the $^{18}$F-FDG-avid osteoblastic lesions, 48% remained positive and increased in size on CT, consistent with disease progression.[15]

# $^{18}$F-FDG PET and PET/CT for the Detection and Staging of Recurrent Breast Cancer

Local or regional recurrence occurs in 7–35% of patients with breast cancer.[17] Early diagnosis of disease recurrence and exact localization and definition of its extent are of utmost importance for choosing the most appropriate therapeutic strategy.

In asymptomatic patients with rising serum tumor markers, $^{18}$F-FDG PET has an accuracy of 87–90% for the diagnosis of recurrent or metastatic breast cancer, compared with an accuracy of 50–78% for conventional imaging.[17,18] Weir and coworkers[19] have assessed the role of $^{18}$F-FDG PET/CT in the management of 165 patients with breast cancer. $^{18}$F-FDG PET/CT was of particular value in a subgroup of 27 patients with suspected recurrent disease. Recurrence was confirmed in 31% of patients, with [18]F-FDG PET having a 5% false-negative and a 20% false-positive rate. In 30% of patients with newly diagnosed recurrence, [18]F-FDG PET identified additional distant metastases, thus providing important information for further management decisions.[19] In a comprehensive meta-analysis, Isasi and colleagues[20] reported a mean sensitivity of 93% and a mean specificity of 82% in the diagnosis of recurrent breast cancer using [18]F-FDG PET.

[18]F-FDG PET performs better than conventional imaging modalities in the assessment of disease recurrence. Furthermore, [18]F-FDG PET findings also guide changes in the management of these patients. In 45 asymptomatic breast cancer patients with elevated serum tumor markers, [18]F-FDG PET detected recurrence in 24 patients and was superior to the combination of several conventional imaging modalities (CT, MRI, ultrasound (US), and X-rays) that detected recurrent tumor in 21 patients.[21] Eubank and colleagues[22] retrospectively assessed 125 patients with suspected recurrent breast cancer. [18]F-FDG PET was more accurate in defining the extent of disease in 67% and indicated a change of management in 32% of patients.

The specificity of [18]F-FDG imaging improves significantly by using combined molecular-anatomical PET/CT imaging.[18,23,24] Fueger and coworkers[23] assessed the specific role of [18]F-FDG PET/CT in breast cancer patients with suspected tumor recurrence and reported an accuracy of 90% for PET/CT as compared with 79% for PET. The specificity of [18]F-FDG PET was only partially improved by using PET/CT. False-positive results were related to the [18]F-FDG avidity of inflammatory lesions. Similar findings with sensitivity, specificity, and accuracy values of 90, 71, and 83%, respectively, were reported by Radan and colleagues.[24] False-negative findings included subcentimeter lesions, and false-positive findings were caused by inflammation. A change in management of breast cancer is most frequently noted in patients suspected of loco-regional disease recurrence who are considered for aggressive local therapy, in whom [18]F-FDG PET/CT detects disseminated disease having an impact on further management of up to 50% of these patients.[24]

Dedicated breast MRI is gaining a major role in the diagnosis and management of breast cancer, and specifically after treatment. In 40 women with suspected recurrence of breast cancer who were assessed after conservative therapy, Belli and colleagues[25] have demonstrated that MRI can differentiate post-therapy changes from recurrent breast cancer with a sensitivity, specificity, and accuracy of 100, 89, and 95%, respectively, and a negative predictive value of 100%. Goerres and coworkers[26] have shown better sensitivity for MRI (79 versus 100%), better specificity for [18]F-FDG PET (94 versus 72%), and comparable accuracy of both methods (88% for MRI and 84% for [18]F-FDG PET) in 32 patients with suspected recurrent breast cancer.

Based on preliminary data indicating that whole-body [18]F-FDG PET/CT may be more useful than other imaging modalities in the detection of recurrent breast cancer, it has been suggested that [18]F-FDG PET/CT could be used as the first diagnostic procedure in this group of patients, provided that prospective data from larger patient cohorts will confirm initial results.

## [18]F-FDG Imaging to Monitor Therapy of Breast Cancer

[18]F-FDG PET has been used to assess the response to treatment in patients with breast cancer. Only little clinical data are available on assessment of response to radiation therapy alone. Radiotherapy-induced inflammatory changes may cause increased [18]F-FDG

activity both in the region of the tumor and in radiosensitive normal tissues, such as bone marrow, gonads, salivary glands, gastrointestinal tract, and larynx that demonstrate toxicity within a few days, or in lung, liver, kidney, spinal cord, and brain that may demonstrate radiation damage in weeks or months. In patients with breast cancer studied with [18]F-FDG PET before and after radiation therapy alone, increased [18]F-FDG uptake may indicate tumor progression.[27]

More data are available in breast cancer patients treated with chemotherapy.[27,28] In 61 patients that completed therapy for breast cancer, [18]F-FDG PET was more accurate than other imaging modalities for predicting outcome with a positive and negative predictive values of 93 and 84% versus 85 and 59% for other imaging modalities, respectively, and a prognostic accuracy of 90%.[29] Early response to therapy has been assessed as well. [18]F-FDG PET results after a single course of chemotherapy are highly accurate in the prediction of treatment response. [18]F-FDG PET has been reported to detect a metabolic response with decreasing tracer uptake as early as 8 days after initiation of therapy, also significantly preceding anatomic changes.

Standard uptake value (SUV) measurements were used for serial follow-up studies. In patients receiving hormonal therapy, metabolic flare occurs 7–10 days after initiating the administration of tamoxifen with an increase in tumor SUV of $1.4 \pm 0.7$.[27,28,30] A significant decrease in SUV after the first and second cycles of chemotherapy compared to baseline was shown in patients who responded to chemotherapy, whereas nonresponders showed no significant change.[30] Berriolo-Riedinger and colleagues[31] have evaluated the predictive value of reduced [18]F-FDG uptake following the first course of neoadjuvant therapy in breast cancer patients. The relative decrease in SUV was significantly greater in those patients who achieved as compared to those who did not achieve a complete response (85% versus 22%). Moreover, in multivariate analysis the change in SUV was the only predicting factor of complete response.[31]

## [18]F-FDG PET/CT for Radiation Therapy Planning in Breast Cancer

PET/CT images may be more useful than CT alone for radiation therapy planning. Following surgery of breast cancer, there are several appropriate radiation therapy protocols. When there is no evidence of macroscopic disease, [18]F-FDG PET/CT is not helpful for radiation planning. While studies using [18]F-FDG PET/CT for radiation treatment planning in malignancies such as head and neck, lung, colon, and gynecological tumors report promising results, no clinical data are yet available in breast cancer. [18]F-FDG PET/CT can nevertheless contribute significantly for radiation therapy planning in patients with suspected recurrent breast cancer, allowing for a better delineation of the tumor volume and for an increased precision for radiation therapy delivery in these patients.[32]

## Summary

[18]F-FDG PET/CT appears to be of limited value in the diagnosis and early staging of breast cancer, mainly in small-sized, noninvasive, slow-growing tumors. It is, therefore, not routinely used for preoperative staging of patients with breast cancer. Sentinel lymph node identification and biopsy is the standard of care for staging early breast cancer.

However, [18]F-FDG PET/CT is useful as part of the preoperative staging of high-risk patients, in the assessment of distant metastatic spread, in some patients with primary tumors larger than 2 cm, and in patients with dense breasts or fibrocystic changes. [18]F-FDG PET/CT is superior to conventional imaging modalities in identifying distant disease sites and in the assessment of recurrent breast tumors, and is also a useful prognostic indicator, with a significant impact on patient management decisions. Preliminary studies indicate a potential role for [18]F-FDG PET/CT as a first diagnostic modality in the assessment of patients with suspected recurrent breast cancer and in more precise planning of radiation therapy.

# Guidelines and Recommendations for the Use of [18]F-FDG PET and PET/CT

The National Comprehensive Cancer Network (NCCN) has incorporated [18]F-FDG PET and PET/CT in the evaluation and management algorithm of a variety of malignancies.[33] At the present time, [18]F-FDG PET and PET/CT have not been incorporated in the NCCN management algorithms for breast cancer. The NCCN recommends the use of [18]F-FDG PET and PET/CT:

(1) As adjunct to other imaging for initial evaluation for recurrent or metastatic disease
(2) As clinically indicated when other imaging is equivocal

Promising data but more research are needed for the use of [18]F-FDG PET and PET/CT in

(1) loco-regional staging for locally advanced disease;
(2) early response indicator for systemic therapy;
(3) treatment response in metastatic disease, particularly in the skeleton.

[18]F-FDG PET and PET/CT is not indicated for

(1) screening or detecting for primary tumors;
(2) staging early stage disease
(3) post-treatment surveillance

A multidisciplinary panel of experts reviewed meta-analyses and systematic reviews published in the [18]F-FDG PET literature before March 2006 and made recommendations for the use of [18]F-FDG PET in oncology[34]:

(1) The panel found little evidence to support the use of [18]F-FDG PET for the diagnosis of breast carcinoma.
(2) [18]F-FDG PET should routinely be added to the conventional work-up in detecting metastatic or recurrent breast cancer in those patients clinically suspected of metastases or recurrence.

## Case Presentations

### *Case II.4.1*

#### History

This 60-year-old woman was referred for evaluation of hematochezia to the colorectal surgeon. Subsequent body CT revealed no abdominopelvic abnormality but showed a right lower lobe lung mass. She was referred to $^{18}$F-FDG PET/CT imaging for staging (Fig. II.4.1A, B).

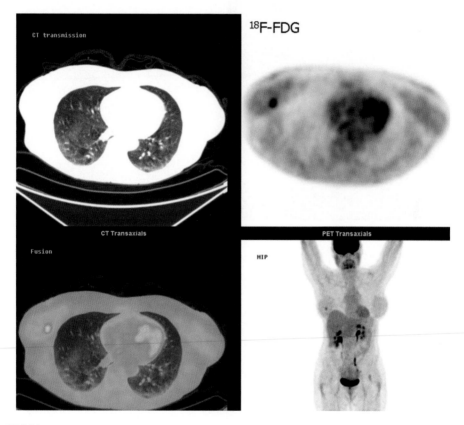

**Fig. II.4.1A**

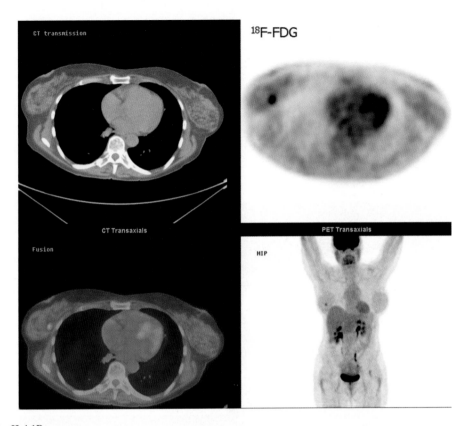

**Fig. II.4.1B**

## Findings

The 20 × 14 mm lung mass is a venous anomaly as it connects to the right atrium. It shows no
[18]F-FDG uptake (Fig. II.4.1A, lung windowing on CT). Incidental finding on the same section
is of a focal area of intense [18]F-FDG uptake within the right breast, corresponding to a 13 ×
13 mm soft tissue mass on CT (Fig. II.4.1B, soft tissue windowing on CT). No other abnormal
areas of intense [18]F-FDG uptake are seen in the bowel or elsewhere.

## Discussion

Given the history of no known primary tumor and no other [18]F-FDG-avid foci the abnormal
tracer uptake in the right breast is highly suggestive of an incidentally detected primary breast
cancer. On clinical examination, a 15 mm palpable right breast mass was discovered. The
biopsy revealed lobular breast carcinoma confirmed immunohistologically. The patient
subsequently underwent a curative mastectomy.

Most breast cancers are detected during screening (physical examination and mammography). [18]F-FDG PET/CT is considered unsuitable for the primary diagnosis of primary breast
cancer due to a low spatial resolution and suboptimal performance in small tumors. Incidental
detection of breast cancer has been reported in patients with other primary malignancies, such
as colorectal, lung, lymphoma, and carcinoid tumors.[35] In a retrospective study reviewing 2,360
[18]F-FDG PET/CT reports, 44 unexpected malignancies were found.[36] Three of the five

incidental breast lesions identified on [18]F-FDG PET/CT were primary malignant tumors. One lesion was only detected on the CT part of the study and was not [18]F-FDG-avid, with a final diagnosis of lobular carcinoma, whereas the other two were [18]F-FDG-avid infiltrating ductal carcinomas. Of the two additional [18]F-FDG-avid foci, one was a fibroadenoma, and, in the other patient, no abnormality was detected.[36]

This case illustrates a focal [18]F-FDG-avid incidental breast lesion, with no evidence of a primary tumor that was suspected and diagnosed as primary breast cancer.

**Diagnosis**

Right breast cancer, incidentally diagnosed.

## Case II.4.2

### History

This 60-year-old woman was diagnosed with invasive ductal carcinoma of the left breast 5 years earlier and underwent wide local excision and axillary dissection followed by adjuvant radiation and chemotherapy. She initially presented with rising Ca 15-3 serum levels. A diagnostic CT of the chest, abdomen, and pelvis revealed no metastases. Her tumor markers continued to rise over the next 3 months, and she was referred to [18]F-FDG PET/CT imaging for detection of recurrence (Fig. II.4.2A–C). Subsequently, she had further chemotherapy and was referred to [18]F-FDG PET/CT imaging for restaging (Fig. II4.2D–E).

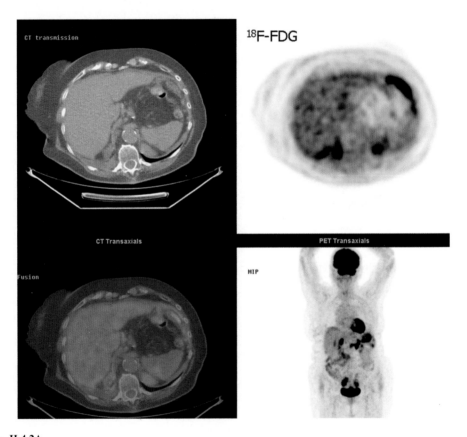

**Fig. II.4.2A**

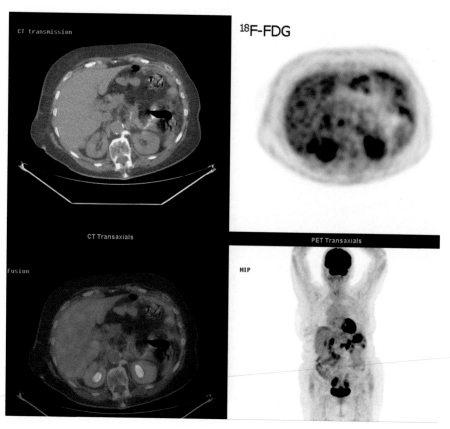

**Fig. II.4.2B**

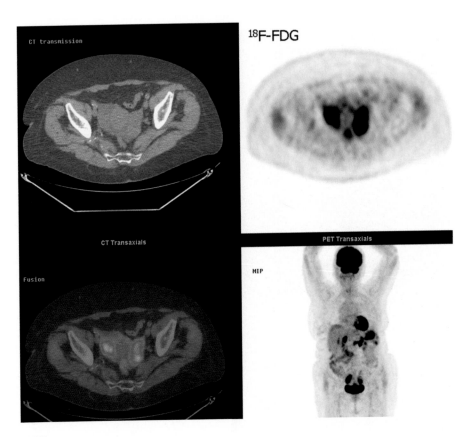

Fig. II.4.2C

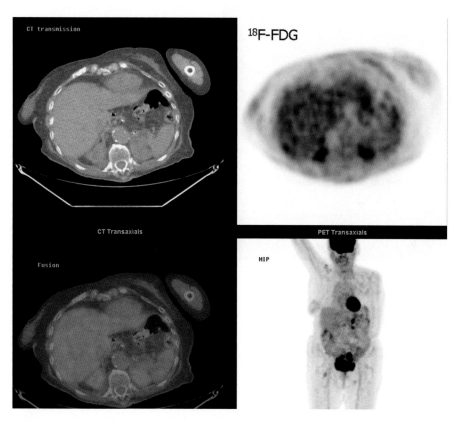

**Fig. II.4.2D**

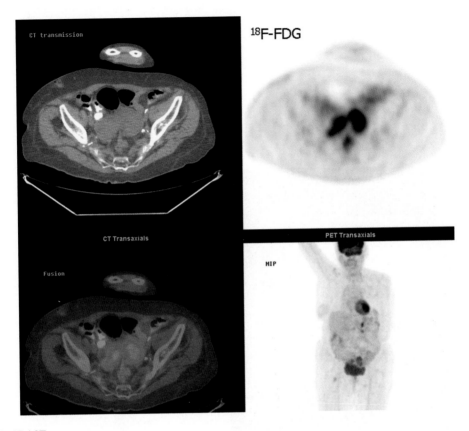

**Fig. II.4.2E**

## Findings

Focal areas of intense $^{18}$F-FDG uptake are seen in the left upper abdomen and posterior to liver, corresponding on CT to a 41 × 11 mm nodule in the greater omentum (SUVmax 7.8) (Fig. II.4.2A) and a 13 × 13 mm peritoneal nodule (SUVmax 5.9) (Fig. II.4.2B). These findings were consistent with metastases. In the pelvis, focal areas of intense $^{18}$F-FDG uptake correspond on CT to right 45 × 26 mm (SUVmax 13.5) and left 52 × 23 mm (SUVmax 12.1) adnexal masses which are also suspicious for metastases (Fig. II.4.2C).

Following therapy, there is no $^{18}$F-FDG uptake or CT abnormality at the sites of previously detected peritoneal and omental disease (Fig. II.4.2D). The bilateral adnexal lesions show less $^{18}$F-FDG uptake (SUVmax reduced to 7.8 in the right ovary and 8.2 in the left ovary) and have decreased in size on CT, now measuring 41 × 17 mm on the right and 47 × 18 mm on the left (Fig. II.4.2E).

## Discussion

These findings are consistent with metastatic breast cancer to peritoneum and suggestive of ovarian metastases, further histologically confirmed by ovarian biopsy. Following treatment, $^{18}$F-FDG PET/CT demonstrated complete resolution of the peritoneal and omental metastases and partial resolution of the ovarian disease, indicating only a partial response to chemotherapy. Consequently, alternative chemotherapy was given, which controlled the disease.

Ovarian metastases are encountered in one of five women with breast cancer.[37] Patients with breast cancer have an increased risk of both primary and secondary ovarian neoplasms, and this risk is even higher in the subset of patients with BRCA mutations.[37] Ovarian metastases are difficult to diagnose clinically, unless they are associated with peritoneal spread. The colon and stomach are the most common primary tumors with ovarian metastases, followed by the breast, lung, and contralateral ovary. In a series of 54 patients with breast cancer and adnexal masses on ultrasound, half of them were due to breast metastases and half were primary ovarian cancer.[38] The presence of ovarian metastases is a poor prognostic sign. Aggressive therapy is used for palliation. Differentiation between primary and metastatic ovarian carcinoma is important to determine the most accurate therapy and patient prognosis.

This case illustrates the role of $^{18}$F-FDG PET/CT in the diagnosis of distant metastases of breast cancer in the omentum, peritoneum, and ovaries with partial response to therapy on follow-up studies.

## Diagnosis

1. Metastatic breast cancer to omentum, peritoneum, and ovaries.
2. Partial response to therapy.

## Case II.4.3

### History

This 72-year-old woman was diagnosed with carcinoma of the right breast T2N1 grade 2 disease 3 years earlier and was treated with chemo- and radiotherapy. She presented with chest infection. CT of the thorax and abdomen revealed a focal low-density lesion in the right lobe of the liver and a lytic skeletal lesion. Prior to possible further chemotherapy, she was referred to $^{18}$F-FDG PET/CT imaging for restaging (Fig. II.4.3A–C).

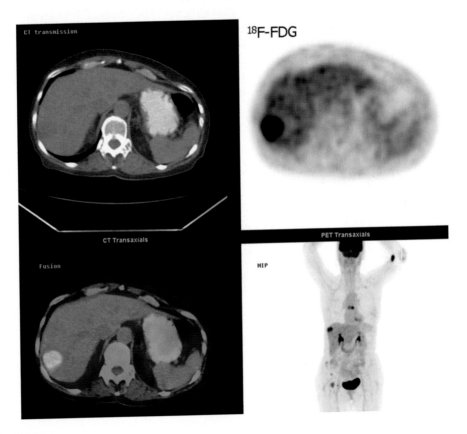

**Fig. II.4.3A**

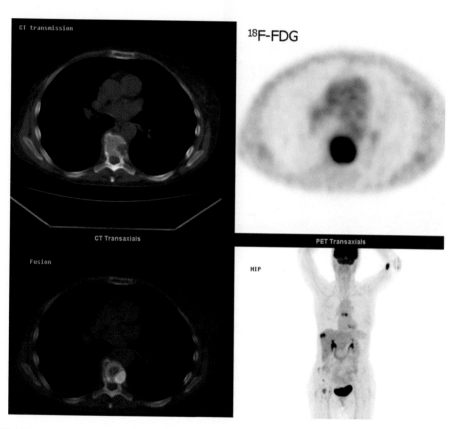

**Fig. II.4.3B**

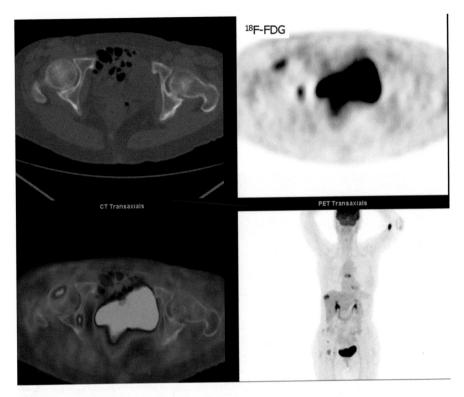

**Fig. II.4.3C**

## Findings

A focal area of intense ${}^{18}$F-FDG uptake is identified in the right lobe of the liver, corresponding to the $35 \times 31$ mm hypodense hepatic lesion on CT (Fig. II.4.3A) consistent with a
metastasis. Another focus of intense ${}^{18}$F-FDG uptake is identified in the left side of the T8
vertebral body (Fig. II.4.3B) corresponding to a lytic metastasis. Two additional intense
areas of ${}^{18}$F-FDG uptake are seen in the right femoral head and right acetabulum
(Fig. II.4.3C) with no corresponding CT abnormality.

## Discussion

These findings are consistent with metastatic breast cancer to the right hepatic lobe and T8
vertebra. The ${}^{18}$F-FDG-avid foci in the right femoral head and acetabulum are worrisome
for early skeletal metastases. A follow-up CT confirmed these lesions to be progressive lytic
metastases.
   ${}^{18}$F-FDG PET/CT has been used for the detection and follow-up of skeletal metastases
with a wide range of sensitivities, higher in osteolytic and significantly lower in osteoblastic
lesions.[15,16] In patients with suspected recurrence of breast cancer, increased ${}^{18}$F-FDG
uptake was found in 94% of osteolytic, 82% of mixed, and 61% of osteoblastic skeletal
lesions, with no corresponding morphologic changes on CT in up to 15% of these sites. On
follow-up after therapy, all lesions became ${}^{18}$F-FDG negative, and nine of them became
osteoblastic on CT, suggesting the presence of a healing process.[15] Although the absence of

morphologic changes on CT as described earlier poses a diagnostic dilemma, it is hypothesized that, in the early stages of metastatic skeletal disease, metabolic abnormalities on [18]F-FDG precede morphologic changes depicted on CT.

More than 50% of patients with breast cancer develop hepatic metastases. Usually, this is a late finding, when metastases are already present in other organs and the patients are treated with chemotherapy. Approximately 5% of patients with breast cancer will develop only hepatic metastases. These lesions will potentially benefit from resection. Detecting extra-hepatic metastases is therefore clinically important, excluding potential surgical resection. The accuracy of [18]F-FDG PET for the detection and monitoring of hepatic metastases in breast cancer patients has not been assessed. [18]F-FDG PET has been shown to be superior to CT for the detection of hepatic metastases larger than 10 mm from colon cancer. Moreover, when positive, [18]F-FDG PET may help to characterize equivocal CT lesions. In a study assessing a large variety of tumors, [18]F-FDG PET/CT was more accurate than contrast-enhanced CT for both colorectal and noncolorectal malignancies in the detection of metastatic hepatic disease.[39] The sensitivity and specificity of [18]F-FDG PET/CT was 96 and 75% versus 84 and 25% for contrast-enhanced CT, comparable in colorectal and noncolorectal primary tumors. However, only few breast cancer patients were enrolled in this study.[39]

This case illustrates the role of [18]F-FDG PET/CT in the diagnosis of an equivocal CT finding in the liver as a metastatic lesion. In addition, focal [18]F-FDG-avid skeletal lesions in patients with recurrent metastatic breast cancer may represent early skeletal metastases despite no corresponding morphologic changes on CT.

## Diagnosis

1. Solitary hepatic metastasis.
2. Lytic bone metastasis in T8 vertebral body.
3. Early bone metastases in the right femoral head and acetabulum.

## Case II.4.4 (DICOM Images on DVD)

### History

This 70-year-old woman had a past history of left invasive ductal breast carcinoma treated with conserving surgery and postsurgical radiotherapy to breast and axilla 20 years earlier. She presented with a left brachial plexopathy. Clinical examination found an excoriating mass in the nipple with further suspicious nodules below the clavicle. She was referred for [18]F-FDG PET/CT (Fig. II.4.4A–D) to further investigate the plexopathy, as she could not tolerate an MRI owing to claustrophobia.

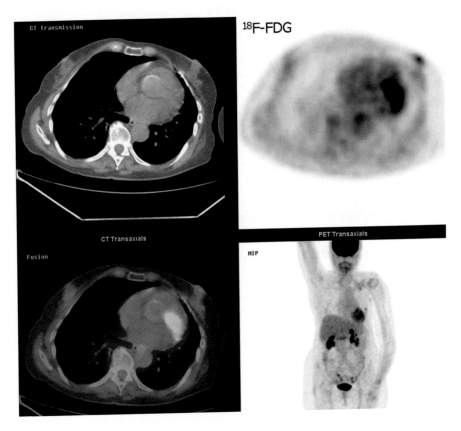

Fig. II.4.4A

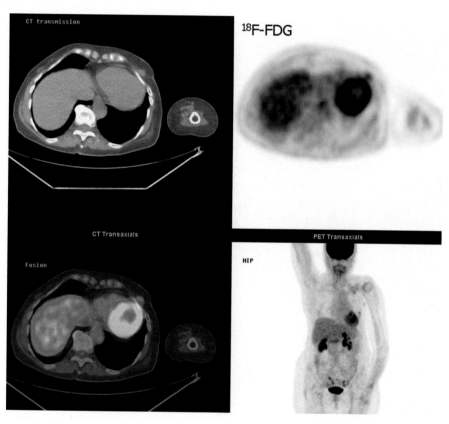

**Fig. II.4.4B**

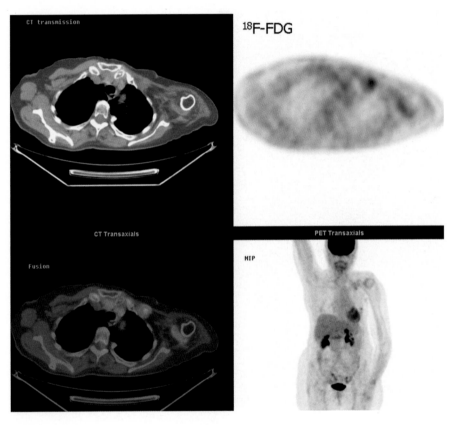

**Fig. II.4.4C**

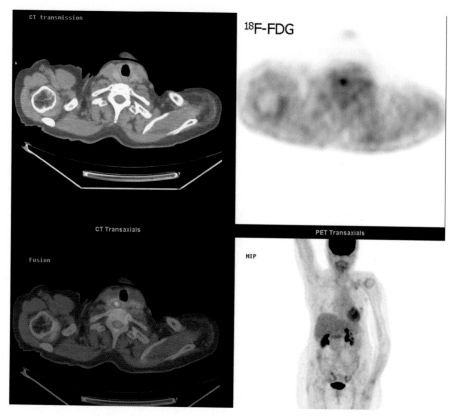

**Fig. II.4.4D**

### Findings

There is a superficial focus of intense $^{18}$F-FDG uptake in the left breast with an SUVmax of 2.8, which, on CT, corresponds to a lesion in the left nipple measuring $18 \times 5$ mm (Fig. II.4.4A), suspicious for tumor. Inferiorly, there is another focus of intense $^{18}$F-FDG uptake corresponding on CT to a soft tissue nodule, $12 \times 8$ mm in size, in the left anterior chest wall abutting the left 3rd rib (Fig. II.4.4B), suspicious for a tumor deposit as well. An additional $^{18}$F-FDG-avid focus is localized to an infraclavicular $17 \times 13$ mm soft tissue nodule on CT (Fig. II.4.4C). A focus of intense $^{18}$F-FDG uptake (SUVmax 3.3) is demonstrated in the lower pole of the right lobe of the thyroid gland (Fig. II.4.4D).

### Discussion

The findings are consistent with local recurrence of breast cancer around the left nipple and a regional metastasis in the chest wall, accounting for the clinical complaints of left brachial plexopathy. This was confirmed histopathologically. There is incidental uptake in the right thyroid lobe suspicious for malignancy, confirmed by image-guided biopsy as a synchronous primary thyroid tumor.

Studies have shown that thyroid diseases are common among women with breast cancer.[39,40] Breast and thyroid tumors are both more common in females, and both peak in the postmenopausal age group. Thyroid stimulating hormone (TSH) receptors are abundant in breast tissue, whereas estrogen may influence the development, physiology, and pathology of the thyroid gland. Japanese women who consume diets rich of seaweed have a low incidence of breast cancer, and iodine-rich seaweed was found to inhibit the development of these tumors. In addition, increased level of thyroid peroxidase has been associated with significantly improved prognosis in breast cancer patients.[40] Many forms of thyroid disease, including nodular hyperplasia, hyperthyroidism, thyroiditis, nontoxic goiter, and thyroid cancer have been identified in association with breast cancer.[40,41] As in this case, a focal [18]F-FDG-avid lesion in the thyroid of patients with documented breast cancer should raise the suspicion for a second primary thyroid tumor.

**Diagnosis**

1. Locally recurrent left breast cancer with regional metastases to the left chest wall.
2. Synchronous right thyroid papillary cancer.

**Follow-Up**

The image-guided biopsy confirmed a recurrent left breast carcinoma and a synchronous thyroid primary papillary tumor.

**Clinical Report: Body [18]F-FDG PET/CT (for DVD cases only)**

Indication

Restaging for breast cancer.

History

This 70-year-old woman had a past history of left invasive ductal breast carcinoma treated with conserving surgery and postsurgical radiotherapy to breast and axilla 20 years earlier. She presented with a left brachial plexopathy. Clinical examination found an excoriating mass in the nipple with further suspicious nodules below the clavicle. She was referred for [18]F-FDG PET/CT to further investigate the plexopathy, as she could not tolerate an MRI owing to claustrophobia.

Procedure

The patient was fasted for over 4 h and had a normal blood glucose level prior to [18]F-FDG injection. The PET acquisition was performed using a PET/CT scanner with a low-dose CT for anatomical correlation and attenuation correction. Oral CT contrast was administered. PET emission images were started approximately 60 min after IV injection of 400 MBq (10.8 mCi) of [18]F-FDG and covered the area from the base of the skull through the upper thighs.

Findings

*Quality of the study*: The quality of the study is good. There is physiologic distribution of the radiopharmaceutical in the brain, myocardium, bowel, liver, and renal collecting system.
*Brain*: Within normal range.

*Head and neck*: A focus of moderate ${}^{18}$F-FDG uptake is seen in the lower pole of the right thyroid gland.

*Chest*: A focus of intense ${}^{18}$F-FDG uptake is seen in the left breast, corresponding on CT to a 18 × 5 mm left nipple mass. The infraclavicular 17 × 13 mm soft tissue mass on CT also shows intense ${}^{18}$F-FDG uptake. Inferiorly, there is another focus of intense ${}^{18}$F-FDG uptake corresponding on CT to a 12 × 8 mm soft tissue nodule in the left anterior chest wall abutting the left 3rd rib.

*Abdomen*: No foci of abnormal ${}^{18}$F-FDG uptake are identified. CT of the abdomen shows an 11 mm oval low-density lesion in the right lobe of liver, consistent with a simple liver cyst and a partially calcified 29 mm abdominal aortic aneurysm.

*Pelvis*: Within normal range.

*Musculoskeletal*: Degenerative changes are seen in the skeleton.

Impression

1. Intense ${}^{18}$F-FDG uptake in the left nipple, infraclavicular lymph node, and chest wall nodule are suspicious for local breast cancer recurrence with regional spread causing the plexopathy. Biopsy of the infraclavicular mass appears to be the best site for histopathological analysis.
2. The focality and intensity of the right thyroid ${}^{18}$F-FDG uptake is concerning for malignancy given the history of a known primary breast cancer. An ultrasound to confirm this lesion and subsequent guided biopsy is recommended for further evaluation.

## *Case II.4.5*

### History

This 58-year-old woman was diagnosed with carcinoma of the right breast 4 years earlier and underwent a mastectomy followed by radiotherapy. She presented with symptoms and signs of left brachial plexopathy. MRI of the cervical spine and brachial plexus were unrevealing, and she was referred to [18]F-FDG PET/CT imaging for restaging (Fig. II.4.5A–C).

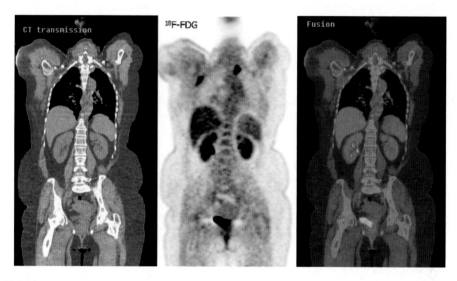

**Fig. II.4.5A**

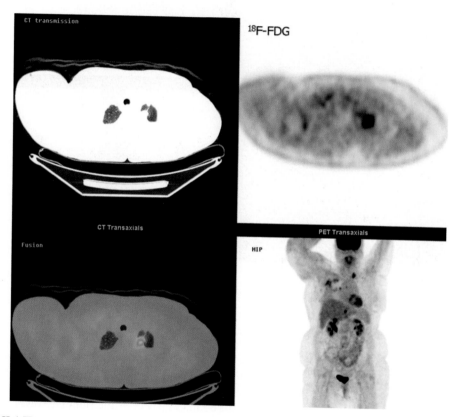

**Fig. II.4.5B**

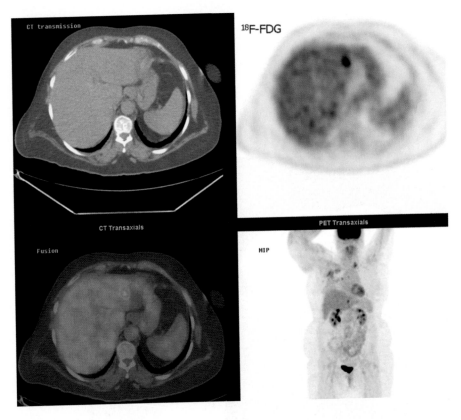

**Fig. II.4.5C**

**Findings**

A focal area of intense $^{18}$F-FDG uptake is identified in the apex of the left lung corresponding to a 17 × 13 mm pleural-based soft tissue nodule on CT (Fig. II.4.5A coronal, Fig. II.4.5B transaxial images) consistent with a metastasis. An additional area of diffuse abnormal $^{18}$F-FDG uptake is seen in the antero-lateral aspect of the right chest wall (Fig. II.4.5A), consistent with tumor recurrence at the primary site. Another focus of intense $^{18}$F-FDG uptake is seen in the left hepatic lobe (Fig. II.4.5C).

**Discussion**

These findings are consistent with recurrent breast cancer to right chest wall, metastases in segment II of the liver, and in the right pleura.

Dedicated breast MRI is gaining a major role in the diagnosis and management of breast cancer and is often used for the differentiation of post-therapy changes from recurrent breast cancer with sensitivity, specificity, and accuracy values of 100, 89, and 95%, respectively, and a negative predictive value of 100%.[24] MRI is highly sensitive, and, due to its higher resolution, it is more sensitive than $^{18}$F-FDG imaging for detection of breast lesions, particularly after surgery, as well as for diagnosis of axillary lymph node involvement. MRI can provide high spatial resolution images of the brachial plexus and axilla, but its diagnostic accuracy can be limited in the presence of diffusely infiltrating tumors, which often cannot be differentiated from scarring or radiation-induced fibrosis. In 10 patients suspected of having loco-regional metastases that were imaged with MRI and [18]F-FDG PET, MRI imaging was diagnostic in five of nine patients with tumor and was indeterminate in four, whereas [18]F-FDG PET correctly identified all nine patients diagnosed with metastatic disease.[42] In 10 patients suspected of loco-regional disease, MRI imaging was diagnostic in 5 and indeterminate in 4, whereas [18]F-FDG PET correctly identified all patients diagnosed with metastatic disease.[42] [18]F-FDG PET has a dominant contribution in differentiating between metastatic and benign brachial plexopathy in patients with breast cancer.[43]

In addition, as a whole-body examination, [18]F-FDG PET/CT can also detect unsuspected lesions outside the breast and axilla and may lead to a change in patient management. Although the identification of additional foci of metastatic disease with [18]F-FDG PET does not always change the clinical management of patients who would be treated with chemotherapy anyway, most also receive local therapy for palliation of symptoms of brachial plexopathy. These patients may respond to local therapy, but may have subsequent disease progression at other sites. Therefore, it is important to diagnose unsuspected distant metastases with [18]F-FDG PET, which will also facilitate the assessment of response to systemic therapy.

This case illustrates the use of [18]F-FDG PET/CT for the diagnosis of loco-regional recurrent breast cancer to the chest wall, a pulmonary metastasis, and a distant unsuspected hepatic metastasis. In this case, [18]F-FDG PET/CT was superior to MRI not only by allowing the detection of a distant hepatic metastasis, but also the detection of local recurrence.

## Diagnosis

1. Right chest wall breast cancer recurrence.
2. Solitary hepatic metastasis.
3. Right apical lung metastasis causing brachial plexopathy.

## Case II.4.6 (DICOM Images on DVD)

### History

This 60-year-old woman was diagnosed with carcinoma of the left breast 4 years earlier and underwent a mastectomy and adjuvant chemotherapy. She presented with increasing right-sided back pain. MRI of the spine was unrevealing. She was referred for further evaluation with $^{18}$F-FDG PET/CT imaging (Fig. II.4.6A–F). Subsequently, she completed five cycles of chemotherapy. Response to therapy was assessed with a follow-up $^{18}$F-FDG PET/CT study (Fig. II.4.6G–J).

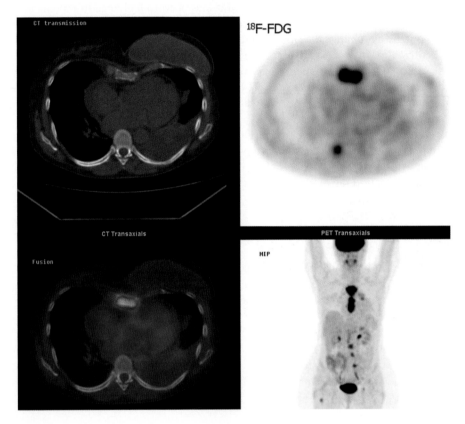

Fig. II.4.6A

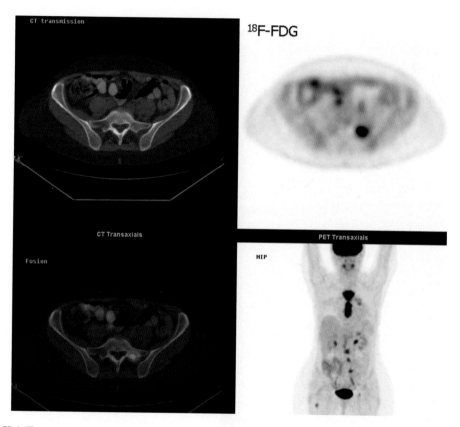

**Fig. II.4.6B**

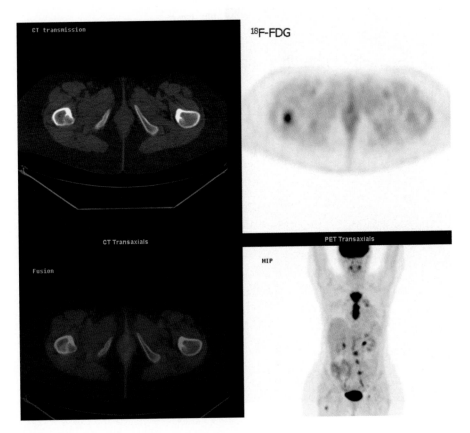

**Fig. II.4.6C**

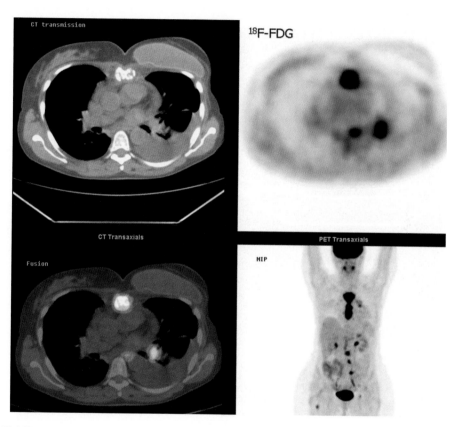

Fig. II.4.6D

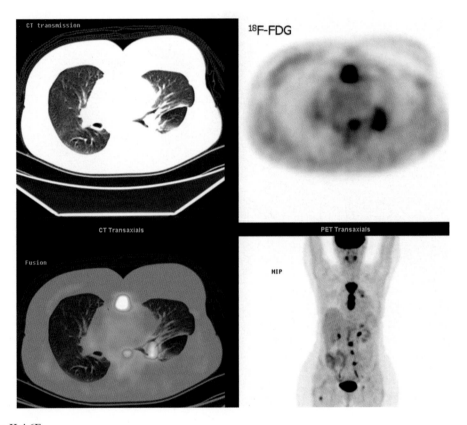

**Fig. II.4.6E**

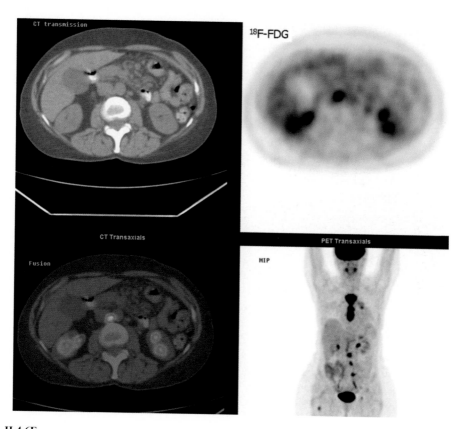

**Fig. II.4.6F**

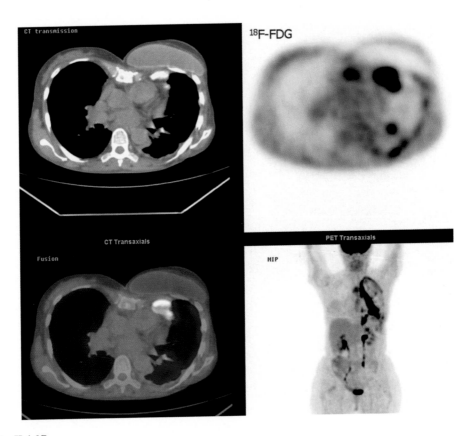

Fig. II.4.6G

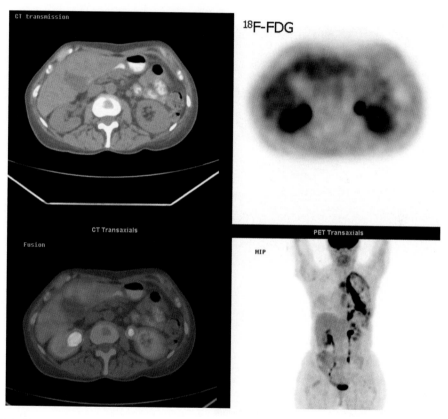

**Fig. II.4.6H**

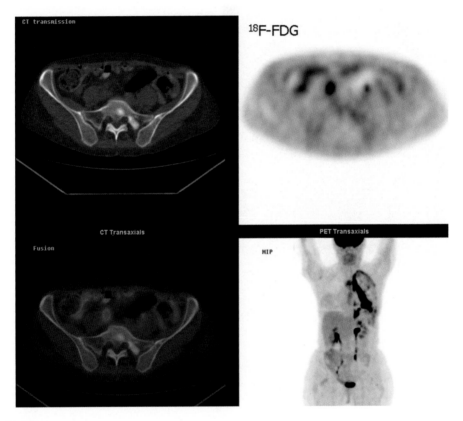

**Fig. II.4.6I**

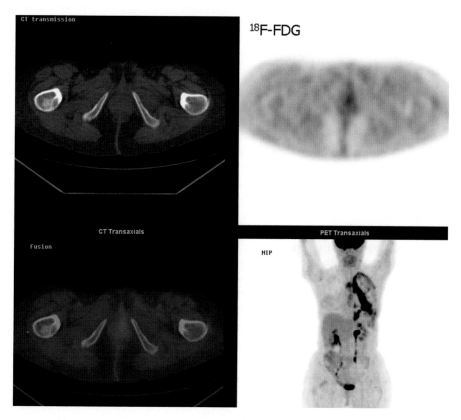

**Fig. II.4.6 J**

**Findings**

Focal areas of intense $^{18}$F-FDG uptake are identified in the right 9th posterior rib (SUVmax 5.2) and sternum (SUVmax 14) (Fig. II.4.6A), L3, and L4 (MIP and DICOM) corresponding on CT to osteolytic lesions and consistent with skeletal metastases. Other focal areas of intense $^{18}$F-FDG uptake are seen in the left sacral wing (Fig. II.4.6B), the right proximal femur (Fig. II.4.6C), and left acetabulum (MIP, DICOM) with no corresponding abnormalities on CT assessed with bone windows, suggesting early skeletal metastases. Additional areas of intense $^{18}$F-FDG uptake are seen in an inferior mediastinal mass and in the left lung corresponding on CT to a 12 × 5 mm lymph node (Fig. II.4.6D) and a 20 × 23 mm left lung mass with associated pleural effusion (Fig. II.4.6E). In the upper abdomen a focal area of increased $^{18}$F-FDG uptake corresponds on CT to a 10 × 8 mm aorto-caval lymph node (Fig. II.4.6F). There is a left breast implant.

Following completion of chemotherapy, there is intense $^{18}$F-FDG uptake circumferentially around the left lung corresponding on CT to post-talc pleurodesis with calcifications (Fig. II.4.6G), most likely representing an inflammatory process. $^{18}$F-FDG uptake in the sternum has decreased in intensity (SUVmax 10.9) (Fig. II.4.6G), and the CT now shows increased sclerosis, suggesting reparative bone healing at this site. Furthermore, no $^{18}$F-FDG uptake is now seen in the previously involved aorto-caval node (Fig. II.4.6H), left sacral wing (Fig. II.4.6I), and right proximal femur (Fig. II.4.6 J). The corresponding CT shows new focal areas of sclerosis at the sacrum (Fig. II.4.6I) and right proximal femur (Fig. II.4.6 J), L3, L4, L5, and left acetabulum (DICOM), consistent with bone healing.

## Discussion

These findings are consistent with metastatic breast cancer to abdominal lymph node, skeleton, lung, and pleura. Following therapy, there is partial response in sites of disease in the soft tissues and skeleton.

[18]F-FDG PET imaging allows the monitoring of extensive metastatic disease with a single imaging procedure. It has been used to monitor response to therapy in patients with breast cancer.[18]F-FDG PET has a prognostic accuracy of 90% for predicting patient outcome.[29] In a prospective study, sequential [18]F-FDG PET correctly predicted response to therapy in all patients, whereas conventional imaging performed after three cycles of chemotherapy was less accurate.[30] Beriolo-Riedinger and colleagues[31] have recently assessed the predictive value of decreasing [18]F-FDG uptake in breast cancer patients treated with neoadjuvant chemotherapy. Forty-seven women with newly diagnosed nonmetastatic tumors were assessed with [18]F-FDG PET at baseline and before the second course of chemotherapy. A decrease below 60% of the baseline SUVmax differentiated between complete and noncomplete responders with an accuracy of 87%.[31]

Du and colleagues[15] followed up patients with skeletal metastases. Sequential [18]F-FDG PET/CT studies revealed a gradual osteoblastic process in [18]F-FDG-avid osteolytic lesions after effective treatment. These lesions also became rapidly [18]F-FDG negative. On the other hand, in [18]F-FDG-avid osteoblastic lesions, persistent tracer uptake during treatment in association with an increase in size and disease progression on CT. Persistent [18]F-FDG-avid skeletal metastases have a major impact on prognosis. There are significant differences in survival between patients with and without persistent [18]F-FDG-avid skeletal metastases.[14]

This case illustrates the use of [18]F-FDG PET/CT for monitoring response to therapy in metastatic breast cancer.

## Diagnosis

1. Metastatic breast cancer to abdominal lymph nodes, skeleton, lung, and pleura.
2. Good response to therapy in left lung and pleura.
3. Partial response to therapy in skeleton.

## Follow-Up

The patient had thoracocentesis, and fluid analysis confirmed breast cancer recurrence. Talc pleurodesis was performed. After completing five cycles of chemotherapy, response to treatment was assessed with a follow-up [18]F-FDG PET/CT. [18]F-FDG uptake in the sternum has reduced in intensity. There is no [18]F-FDG uptake seen in the previously involved left sacral wing, the right proximal femur, and a metastatic aorto-caval node. The corresponding CT shows new focal areas of sclerosis in the left sacral wing and right proximal femur due to bone healing. Overall, these findings are consistent with partial response to therapy.

**Clinical Report: Body $^{18}$F-FDG PET/CT (for DVD cases only)**

Indication

Restaging for breast cancer.

History

This 60-year-old woman was diagnosed with carcinoma of the left breast 4 years earlier and underwent a mastectomy followed by adjuvant chemotherapy. MRI of the spine was unrevealing. She was referred for further evaluation with $^{18}$F-FDG PET/CT. Subsequently, she completed five cycles of chemotherapy, and response to therapy was assessed with a follow-up $^{18}$F-FDG PET/CT study.

Procedure

The patient was fasted over 4 h and had a normal blood glucose level prior to $^{18}$F-FDG injection. The $^{18}$F-FDG PET acquisition was performed using a PET/CT scanner with a low-dose CT being used for anatomical correlation and attenuation correction. Oral contrast was administered. PET emission images were started approximately 60 min after IV injection of 400 MBq (10.8 mCi) of $^{18}$F-FDG and covered the area from the base of the skull through the upper thighs.

Findings

   *Quality of study*: The quality of the study is good. There is physiologic distribution of the radiopharmaceutical in the brain, bowel, liver, and renal collecting system.
   *Brain*: Within normal range.
   *Head and neck*: Within normal range.
   *Chest*: Focal areas of intense $^{18}$F-FDG uptake are identified in the right 9th posterior rib and sternum corresponding to osteolytic lesions on CT. Additional areas of intense $^{18}$F-FDG uptake are seen in an inferior mediastinal mass and in the left lung corresponding on CT to a 12 × 5 mm lymph node and a 20 × 23 mm left lung mass abutting the bifurcation of the left upper and lower lobe bronchi. On CT, there is also left pleural effusion of moderate volume with associated passive atelectasis of the left lower lobe. A left breast implant is seen.
   *Abdomen*: In the upper abdomen, a linear area of increased $^{18}$F-FDG uptake corresponds on CT to a 10 × 8 mm cluster of aorto-caval lymph nodes. There are additional areas of intense $^{18}$F-FDG uptake in L3 and L4 vertebral bodies, which on CT correspond to mixed lytic and sclerotic lesions.
   *Pelvis*: A focal area of intense $^{18}$F-FDG uptake is seen in the left sacral wing and the left posterior acetabulum with no corresponding abnormality on CT.
   *Lower limbs*: A focal area of intense $^{18}$F-FDG uptake is seen in the right proximal femur with no corresponding CT abnormality.

Impression

1. $^{18}$F-FDG-avid left lung mass, ipsilateral $^{18}$F-FDG-avid lymphadenopathy and non-$^{18}$F-FDG-avid left pleural effusion, consistent with malignancy. This is likely to be a

recurrent breast cancer, and thoracocentesis with fluid cytological analysis may be the easiest confirmatory method.

2. Focal areas of intense [18]F-FDG uptake are identified in the right 9th posterior rib, sternum, L3, and L4 corresponding on CT to osteolytic lesions, consistent with established skeletal metastases. Other focal areas of intense [18]F-FDG uptake seen in the left sacral wing, left posterior acetabulum, and right proximal femur with no corresponding CT abnormalities are suggestive of early skeletal metastases.

**Acknowledgments**  The authors are thankful to Prof. Peter J. Ell for critically reviewing this chapter.

# References

1. Ries LAG, Melbert D, Krapacho M, Mariotto A, Miller BA, Feuer EJ, Clegg L, Horner MJ, Howlader N, Eisner MP, Reichman M, Edwards BK (eds). *SEER Cancer Statistics Review, 1975–2004*. Bethesda, MD:National Cancer Institute, http://seer.cancer.gov/csr/19752004/, posted to the SEER web site 2007.
2. http://www.cancer.gov/cancertopics/pdq/treatment/breast/HealthProfessional/page4/.
3. Esserman L. Integration of imaging in the management of breast cancer. *J Clin Oncol* 2005; 23:1601–1602.
4. Avril N, Adler LP. F-18 Fluorodeoxyglucos positron emission tomography imaging for primary breast cancer and loco-regional staging. *PET Clinics* 2006;1:1–14.
5. Eubank WB. Diagnosis of recurrent and metastatic disease using F-18 fluorodeoxyglucose-positron emission tomography. *PET Clinics* 2006;1:15–24.
6. Quon A, Gambhir SS. FDG-PET and beyond: Molecular breast cancer imaging. *J Clin Oncol* 2005;23:1664–1673.
7. Ell PJ. The contribution of PET/CT to improved patient management. *Br J Radiol* 2006;79:32–36.
8. Scheidhauer K, Walter C, Seedmann MD. FDG PET and other imaging modalities in the primary diagnosis of suspicious breast lesions. *Eur J Nucl Med Mol Imaging* 2004;31(Suppl. 1):S70–S79.
9. Wahl RL, Siegel BA, Coleman R, Gatsonis CG. A prospective multicentre study of axillary nodal staging by positron emission tomography in breast cancer: A report of the staging breast cancer with PET study group. *J Clin Oncol* 2004;22:277–285.
10. Aarsvold JN, Alzaraki NP. Update on detection of sentinel lymph nodes in patients with breast cancer. *Semin Nucl Med* 2005;35:116–128.
11. Iagaru A, Masamed R, Keesara H, Conti PS. Breast MRI and [18]F FDG PET/CT in the management of breast cancer. *Ann Nucl Med* 2007;21:33–38.
12. Tafra L. Positron emission tomography (PET) and mammography (PEM) for breast cancer: importance to surgeons. *Ann Surg Oncol* 2007;14:3–13.
13. Eubank WB, Mankoff DA. Evolving role of positron emission tomography in breast cancer imaging. *Semin Nucl Med* 2005;35:84–99.
14. Fogelman I, Cook G, Israel O, Van der Wall H. Positron emission tomography and skeletal metastases. *Semin Nucl Med* 2005;35:135–142.
15. Du Y, Cullum I, Illidge TM, Ell PJ. Fusion of metabolic function and morphology: Sequential [[18]F] Fluorodeoxyglucose positron-emission tomography/computed tomography studies yield new insights into the natural history of skeletal metastases in breast cancer. *J Clin Oncol* 2007;25: 3440–3447.
16. Nakai T, Okuyama C, Kubota T, Yamada K, Ushijima Y, Taniike K, Suzuki T,Nishimura T. Pitfalls of FDG-PET for the diagnosis of osteoblastic skeletal metastases in patients with breast cancer. *Eur J Nucl Med Mol Imaging* 2005;32:1253–1258.
17. Zangheri B, Messa C, Picchio M, Gianolli L, Landoni C, Fazio F. PET/CT and breast cancer. *Eur J Nucl Med Mol Imaging* 2004;31(Suppl.1): S135–S142.
18. Tatsumi M, Cohade C, Mourtzikos KA, Fishman EK, Wahl RL. Initial experience with FDG-PET/CT in the evaluation of breast cancer. *Eur J Nucl Med Mol Imaging* 2006;33:254–262.
19. Weir L, Worsley D, Bernstein V. The value of FDG positron emission tomography in the management of patients with breast cancer. *Breast J* 2005;11:204–209.
20. Isasi CR, Moadel RM, Blaufox MD. A meta-analysis of FDG-PET for the evaluation of breast cancer recurrence and metastases. *Breast Cancer Res Treat* 2005;90:105–112.
21. Suárez M, Pérez-Castejón MJ, Jiménez A, Romper M, Ruiz G, Montz R, Carreras JL. Early diagnosis of recurrent breast cancer with FDG-PET in patients with progressive elevation of serum tumor markers. *Q J Nucl Med* 2002;46:113–121.
22. Eubank WB, Mankoff DA, Bhattacharya M, Gralow J, Linden H, Ellis G, Lindsley S, Austin-Seumour M, Livingston R. Impact of [18]-Fluorodeoxyglucose PET on defining the extent of disease and management of patients with recurrent or metastatic breast cancer. *Am J Roentgenol* 2004;183: 479–486.
23. Fueger BJ, Weber WA, Quon A, Crawford TL, Allen-Auerbach MS, Halpern BS, Ratio O, Phelps ME, Czernin J. Performance of 2-deoxy-2-[F-18]fluoro-d-glucose positron emission tomography and integrated PET/CT in restaged breast cancer patients. *Mol Imag Biol* 2005;7:369–376.

24. Radan L, Ben-Haim S, Bar-Shalom R, Guralnik L, Israel O. The role of FDG-PET/CT in suspected recurrence of breast cancer. *Cancer* 2006;107:2545–2551.
25. Belli P, Constantini M, Romani M, Marano P, Pastore G. Magnetic resonance imaging in breast cancer recurrence. *Breast Cancer Res Treat* 2002;73:223–235.
26. Goerres GW, Michel SCA, Fehr MK, Kaim AH, Steinert HC, Seifert B, von Schulthess GK, Kubik-Hoch RA. Follow-up of women with breast cancer: Comparison between MRI and FDG PET. *Eur Radiol* 2003;13:1635–1644.
27. Kostakoglu L, Goldsmith SJ. 18F-FDG PET evaluation of the response to therapy for lymphoma and breast for breast, lung, and colorectal carcinoma. *J Nucl Med* 2003;44:224–239.
28. Biersack HJ, Bender H, Palmedo H.FDG-PET in monitoring therapy of breast cancer. *Eur J Nucl Med Mol Imaging* 2004;31(Suppl. 1):S112–S117.
29. Vranjesevic D, Filmont JE, Meta J, Silverman DH, Phelps ME, Rao J, Valk PE, Czernin J. Whole-body (18)F-FDG PET and conventional imaging for predicting outcome in previously treated breast cancer patients. *J Nucl Med* 2002;43:325–329.
30. Schwartz JD, Bader M, Jenicke L, Hemminger G, Jänicke F, Avril N. Early prediction of response to chemotherapy in metastatic breast cancer using sequential [18]F-FDG PET. *J Nucl Med* 2005; 46:1144–1150.
31. Berriolo-Riedinger A, Touzery C, Riedinger J-M, Toubeau M, Coudert B, Arnould L, Boichot C, Cochet A, Fumoleau P, Brunotte F. [18F]FDG-PET predicts complete pathological response of breast cancer to neoadjuvant chemotherapy. *Eur J Nucl Med Mol Imaging* 2007;34:1915–1924.
32. Heron DE, Beriwal S, Avril N. FDG-PET and PET/CT in radiation therapy simulation and management of patients who have primary and recurrent breast cancer. *PET Clinics.* 2006;1:39–49.
33. Podoloff DA, Advani RH, Allred C, Benson AB, Brown E, Burstein HJ, Carlson RW, Coleman RE, Czuczman MS, Delbeke D, Edge SB, Ettinger DS, Grannis FW, Hillner BE, Hoffman JM, Keil K, Komaki R, Larson SM, Mankoff DA, Rozenzweig KE, Skibber JM, Yahalom J, Yu JM, Zelenetz AD. NCCN task force report: Positron emission tomography (PET/Computed tomography (CT) scanning in cancer. *J Natl Compr Canc Netw* 2007;5 (Suppl 1): S1–S22. www/nccn.org/professionals/physician_gls/f_guidelines.asp
34. Fletcher JW, Djulbegovic B, Soares HP, Siegel BA, Lowe VJ, Lyman GH, Coleman E, Wahl R, Paschold JC, Avril N , Einhorn LH, Suh WW, Samson D, Delbeke D,Gorman M, Shields AF. Recommendations for the Use of FDG (fluorine-18, (2-[18F]Fluoro-2-deoxy-D-glucose) Positron emission tomography in oncology. *J Nucl Med* 2008;49:480–508.
35. Agress H, Cooper BZ. Detection of clinically unexpected malignant and premalignant tumors with whole-body FDG PET:Histopathologic comparison. *Radiology* 2004;230:417–422.
36. Even-Sapir E, Lerman H, Gutman M, Lievshitz G, Zuriel L, Polliack A, Inbar M, Metser U. The presentation of malignant tumours and pre-malignant lesions incidentally found on PET-CT. *Eur J Nucl Med Mol Imaging* 2006;33:541–552.
37. Pickel H, Reich O. Ovarian metastases of breast cancer. *CME Journal of Gynecologic Oncology* 2004;9:129–132.
38. Hann LE, Lui DM, Shi W, Bach AM, Selland D-L, Castiel M. Adnexal masses in women with breast cancer: US findings with clinical and histopathologic correlation. *Radiology* 2000;216:242–247.
39. Chua SC, Groves AM, Kayani I, Menezes L, Gacinovic S, Du Y, Bomanji JB, Ell PJ. The impact of [18]F-FDG PET/CT in patients with hepatic metastases. *Eur J Nucl Med Mol Imaging* 2007;34:1906–1914.
40. Turken O, NarIn Y, DemIrbas S, Onde ME, Sayan O, KandemIr EG, Yaylac IM, Ozturk A. Breast cancer in association with thyroid disorders. *Breast Cancer Res* 2003;5:R110–R113.
41. Agarwal DP, Soni TP, Sharma OP, Sharma S. Synchronous malignancies of breast and thyroid gland: A case report and review of literature. *J Cancer Res Ther* 2007;3:172–173.
42. Hathaway PB, MAnkoff DA, MAravilla KR, Austin-Seymour MM, Ellis GK, Gralow JR, Cortese AA, Hayes CE, Moe RE. Value of combined FDG PET and MR imaging in the evaluation of suspected recurrent local-regional breast cancer:Preliminary experience. *Radiology* 1999;210:807–814.
43. Juweid ME, Cheson BD. Positron-emission tomography and assessment of cancer therapy. *N Engl J Med* 2006;354:496–507.

# Chapter II.5
# Colorectal Cancer

Dominique Delbeke and Ronald C. Walker

## Introduction

Colorectal cancer (CRC) is the third most common cause of malignancy in both men and women. The incidence rate has decreased over the last two decades partially due to an increase in screening. The American Cancer Society (ACS) estimates that there are approximately 149,000 new cases of CRC per year and approximately 50,000 patients per year die from this disease in the USA, representing 10% of new cases and 8% of all cancer deaths. Approximately 70–80% of patients are treated with curative intent, mostly by surgery. Chemotherapy alone, or in combination with radiation (for rectal cancer), is given before or after surgery to most patients whose tumor has penetrated the bowel wall or spread to lymph nodes. The overall survival at 1 and 5 years is 82 and 64%, respectively. The 5-year survival is 90% for localized stage, 68% when there is regional spread, and 10% when there are distant metastases.[1]

## [18]F-FDG PET and PET/CT for Screening and Diagnosis of Colorectal Carcinoma

The diagnosis of CRC is based on colonoscopy and biopsy. The ACS recommends yearly screening for CRC of asymptomatic individuals over the age of 50 with fecal occult blood test and flexible sigmoidoscopy every 5 years.[2]

In 2008, the American College of Radiology (ACR), the ACS, and the US Multisociety Task Force on CRC (composed of the three gastroenterology societies: the American Gastroenterology Association, American Society for Gastrointestinal Endoscopy, and American College of Gastroenterology) reviewed a broad range of screening modalities for CRC including various forms of stool tests, flexible sigmoidoscopy, colonoscopy, barium enema, and computed tomography (CT) colonography.[3] Examinations designed to both prevent and detect cancer are encouraged, and CT colonography (virtual colonoscopy) is one of the newly recommended screening tests.

D. Delbeke (✉)
Department of Radiology and Radiological Sciences, Vanderbilt University Medical Center,
Nashville, TN, USA
e-mail: dominique.delbeke@vanderbilt.edu

D. Delbeke, O. Israel (eds.), *Hybrid PET/CT and SPECT/CT Imaging*,
DOI 10.1007/978-0-387-92820-3_7, © Springer Science+Business Media, LLC 2010

Although [18]F-fluorodeoxyglucose positron emission tomography ([18]F-FDG PET) is not routinely used for screening or diagnosing CRC, it is not uncommon to detect this malignancy incidentally on whole body studies performed for other indications.

[18]F-FDG uptake, which is normally present in the gastrointestinal tract, can occasionally be difficult to differentiate from a malignant lesion. Mild-to-moderate diffuse colonic uptake has been associated with a normal colonoscopy, segmental intense uptake can be due to colitis, and focal uptake can be associated with benign adenomas and premalignant and malignant lesions. Incidental detection of unexpected focal areas of [18]F-FDG uptake located in the gastrointestinal tract, unlikely related to the known primary, is seen in 3–5% of patients. More than 50% of these unexpected lesions need further attention, including newly diagnosed asymptomatic CRC and tubular or villous adenomas and, less frequently, metastases. Therefore, in spite of [18]F-FDG imaging not being recommended as a routine tool for detection or screening for precancerous or malignant colonic neoplasms, the identification of focal colon uptake should not be ignored.[4–7]

# [18]F-FDG PET and PET/CT in the Initial Staging of Colorectal Carcinoma

The preoperative staging with imaging modalities is usually limited because most patients will need to undergo colectomy to prevent intestinal obstruction and bleeding. The extent of the disease can be evaluated during surgery with excision of pericolonic and mesenteric lymph nodes along with peritoneal exploration. Preoperative [18]F-FDG imaging may be helpful in the detection of distant metastases and will cancel surgery in patients with increased surgical risk. It may also be helpful as a baseline evaluation prior to neoadjuvant chemotherapy in patients with advanced stage disease. [18]F-FDG imaging is a powerful tool for assessment of the response to therapy.

# [18]F-FDG PET and PET/CT for Assessment of Recurrent Colorectal Carcinoma

## Detection and Restaging of Recurrence

Most CRCs are detected early and treated surgically with curative intent. A recent retrospective review of 1,838 patients who underwent curative resection of non-metastatic CRC with a minimum follow-up of 3 years reported an overall recurrence rate of 16.4%, with a local recurrence rate of 8.5%, with or without systemic metastases.[8]

For patients who present with isolated liver metastases, hepatic resection is the only curative therapy but has been associated with significant morbidity and mortality.[9] The poor prognosis of extrahepatic metastases is considered a contraindication to hepatic resection.[10] Therefore, accurate non-invasive detection of inoperable disease with imaging modalities plays a pivotal role in selecting patients who would benefit from surgery.

A number of studies have demonstrated the role of [18]F-FDG PET as a metabolic imaging modality for detecting recurrent or metastatic CRC. Overall, the sensitivity of [18]F-FDG PET is in the 90% range, with a specificity greater than 70%, both superior to CT. A meta-analysis of 11 clinical reports and 577 patients determined that the sensitivity and specificity of [18]F-FDG PET for detecting recurrent CRC were 97 and 76%, respectively.[11] A comprehensive review of the [18]F-FDG PET literature (including 2,244 patients) reported a weighted average sensitivity and specificity of 94 and 87%, respectively, compared to 79 and 73% for CT.[12] False-negative [18]F-FDG PET findings have been reported with mucinous adenocarcinoma.[13,14] The performance of [18]F-FDG PET for detection of hepatic and extrahepatic metastases, local recurrence, and relapsed disease in patients with rising carcinoembryonic antigen (CEA) levels and negative CT studies is discussed with the patient cases at the end of this chapter. The presence of extrahepatic disease has a significant effect on the management of these patients. [18]F-FDG PET is currently the most sensitive non-invasive modality to detect and localize extrahepatic disease in patients with CRC.[15]

Fused PET/CT images are especially important in the abdomen and pelvis, in order to clarify and precisely localize non-specific [18]F-FDG uptake to the stomach, small bowel and colon, and the urinary tract. In a study of 204 patients including 34 gastrointestinal tumors, investigators at Rambam Medical Center[16] concluded that PET/CT improved the diagnostic accuracy in approximately 50% of patients as compared to PET stand-alone. Fusion images improved characterization of equivocal lesions as either definitely benign in 10% or definitely malignant in 5% of sites. It precisely defined the anatomic location of malignant FDG uptake in 6% and led to retrospective lesion detection on PET or CT in 8%. The results of PET/CT images impacted on the management of 14% of patients, including 20% of all patients in this study with gastrointestinal tumors. Changes in management of patients with CRC included guided colonoscopy with biopsy for local recurrence, guided biopsy to metastatic lymph nodes, guided surgery and referred patients to chemotherapy. Similar conclusions were found in a study of 173 patients performed at Vanderbilt University, including 24 with CRC.[17] In an additional study of 45 patients with CRC [18]F-FDG PET/CT increased the interpretation accuracy and certainty of lesion localization, decreasing the frequency of equivocal lesions by 50% as compared to PET alone, with a subsequent increase by 25% in the number of definite locations and in the overall correct staging from 78 to 89% of patients.[18]

Selzner et al.[19] have compared contrast-enhanced CT and non-enhanced PET/CT in 76 patients referred for restaging prior to resection of hepatic metastases. For detection of hepatic metastases, the two modalities had similar sensitivities of 95 and 91%, respectively. However, for evaluation of patients who had a prior hepatic resection, PET/CT had a specificity of 100% compared to only 50% for contrast-enhanced CT. For local recurrence and extrahepatic metastases, PET/CT demonstrated superior sensitivity (~90% range) compared to contrast-enhanced CT (50–60%). The performance of PET/contrast-enhanced CT has also been compared to PET/low-dose CT.[20,21] PET/low-dose CT was superior to stand-alone contrast-enhanced CT in 50% of patients by detection of additional metastases and change therapy in 10% of patients. PET/contrast-enhanced CT had a further incremental value to PET/low-dose CT in 72% of patients mainly by providing correct segmental localization of hepatic metastases and thus changing the management in 42% of patients. For nodal staging of patients with rectal cancer, the accuracy of PET/contrast-enhanced CT was slightly superior than that of PET/low-dose CT (79% versus 70%), with no statistical significance.

## Impact on Management and Cost Analysis in Patients with Recurrent Disease

In a meta-analysis of the literature, [18]F-FDG PET imaging changed the management in 29% (102/349) of patients.[11] A comprehensive review of the [18]F-FDG PET literature has reported a weighted average change of management related to [18]F-FDG PET findings in 32% of 915 patients.[12]

In a survey-based study of 60 referring oncologists, surgeons, and generalists, [18]F-FDG PET had a major impact on the management of CRC patients and contributed to a change in clinical stage in 42% (80% upstaged and 20% downstaged) and a change in the clinical management in over 60%. As a result of the PET findings, physicians avoided major surgery in 41% of patients for whom surgery was the intended treatment.[22]

In a prospective study of 51 patients evaluated for resection of hepatic metastases, clinical management decisions based on conventional diagnostic methods were changed in 20% of patients based on the findings on [18]F-FDG PET imaging, especially by detecting unsuspected extrahepatic disease.[23] A meta-analysis assessing the performance of [18]F-FDG PET in patients with hepatic metastases demonstrated its higher specificity when compared to CT (96% versus 84%) for detection of hepatic metastases and higher sensitivity than CT (91% versus 61%) for detection of extrahepatic metastases. [18]F-FDG PET changed the management of 31% of patients (range 20–58%).[24] [18]F-FDG PET also improves prognostic stratification in patients with recurrent CRC.[25] In that study, two groups of symptomatic patients were studied: patients with a residual structural lesion suggestive of recurrent tumor and patients with potentially resectable pulmonary or hepatic metastases. Data were similar in both groups. [18]F-FDG PET detected additional sites of disease in 48 and 44% of patients, and a change in planned management was documented in 66 and 49%, respectively. These management plans were implemented in 96% of patients. Follow-up data showed progressive disease in 60 and 66% of patients with additional lesions detected by [18]F-FDG PET compared with conventional imaging, and in 36 and 39% of patients with no additional lesions detected by PET.

Although survival is not an endpoint for a diagnostic test, Strasberg et al.[26] have estimated the survival of patients who underwent [18]F-FDG PET imaging in their preoperative evaluation for resection of hepatic metastases. The overall 3-year survival was 77%, with a lower confidence limit of 60%, higher than the range of 30–64% in previously published series. In patients undergoing [18]F-FDG imaging prior to hepatic resection, the 3-year disease-free survival rate was 40%, again higher than that usually reported. This same group of investigators[27] recently reported the 5-year survival after resection of metastases from CRC. The 5-year survival rate was 30% by pooling the data of 19 studies with a total of 6,090 patients and appeared not to have changed over time. These results were compared to their group of 100 patients with hepatic metastases, who were preoperatively staged for resection with curative intent with the addition of [18]F-FDG imaging. The 5-year survival rate improved to 58%, thus indicating the ability to define a subgroup of patients with a better prognosis. The main contribution was in detecting occult disease, leading to a reduction of futile surgeries.

Another study investigated the role of [18]F-FDG PET in addition to conventional diagnostic methods compared to conventional diagnostic methods alone for selection of patients with metastatic CRC for surgery.[28] The percent of futile surgery was lower if [18]F-FDG PET was included in the presurgical evaluation (19% versus 28%). However, for patients ultimately undergoing surgical treatment, the overall survival at 3 years was similar, 60% versus 51%.

Including [18]F-FDG PET in the evaluation of patients with recurrent CRC has been shown to be cost-effective in studies using clinical evaluation of effectiveness with modeling of costs and studies using decision tree sensitivity analysis.[29,30]

# $^{18}$F-FDG Imaging for Monitoring Therapy Response of Colorectal Carcinoma

## Systemic Chemotherapy

$^{18}$F-FDG imaging has an important role in monitoring patients with advanced stage CRC that is associated with poor prognosis. Systemic chemotherapy with 5-fluorouracil has demonstrated effective palliation and improved survival, although response rates are only 10–20% in patients with advanced disease.[31] More recently, chemotherapeutic agents such as irinitecan and oxiplatin have been shown to improve survival in combination with 5-fluorouracil-based therapies. In a study of 18 patients with hepatic metastases, Findley et al.[32] were able to discriminate responders from non-responders after 4–5 weeks of chemotherapy with fluorouracil by measuring $^{18}$F-FDG uptake before and during therapy.

Several studies have compared detection of hepatic metastases in patients with and without preoperative adjuvant chemotherapy.[33–36] Both PET and CT were shown to have a lower sensitivity for detection of hepatic metastases after chemotherapy ranging from 49 to 62% for $^{18}$F-FDG imaging compared to 65–92% for CT. CT is slightly more sensitive than $^{18}$F-FDG especially for small lesions. Normalization of FDG uptake in hepatic metastases after chemotherapy was followed by complete histopathological response in only 15% of lesions.[37] Therefore, curative resection should not be deferred based on $^{18}$F-FDG imaging.

## Radiation Therapy

For patients with rectal carcinoma, systemic chemotherapy with 5-fluorouracil in combination with radiotherapy has been shown to improve survival. $^{18}$F-FDG PET/CT fusion images have the potential to provide better maps than CT alone for field and dose modulation of radiation therapy, including for patients with CRC.[38]

After treatment of these patients, radiation-induced inflammation and necrosis make the differential diagnosis of post-radiation changes from residual tumor difficult with ultrasound, CT, and MRI.[39] Increased $^{18}$F-FDG uptake immediately following radiation may be due to inflammatory changes and is not always associated with residual tumor. The time course of post-radiation $^{18}$F-FDG activity has not been studied systematically. It is, however, generally accepted that increased $^{18}$F-FDG activity at 6 months after completion of radiation therapy most likely represents tumor recurrence. A case-controlled study of 60 $^{18}$F-FDG studies performed at 6 months following external beam radiation therapy for rectal cancer found a sensitivity of 84% and specificity of 88% for detection of local pelvic recurrence.[40] In a study of 15 patients with locally advanced rectal carcinoma, Guillem et al.[41] demonstrated that $^{18}$F-FDG imaging performed before and 4–5 weeks after completion of preoperative radiation and 5-fluorouracil-based chemotherapy had the potential to assess the pathological response. The same authors further demonstrated that $^{18}$F-FDG imaging could predict long-term outcome after a median follow-up of 42 months.[42] The mean percent decrease in SUVmax was 69% for patients free from recurrence and 37% for patients with recurrence.

## Regional Therapy to the Liver

Hepatic metastases can be treated with regional therapy to the liver. A variety of regional treatment modalities for hepatic metastases have been investigated, including chemotherapy administered through the hepatic artery using infusion pumps, selective chemoembolization, cryoablation, alcohol and radiofrequency ablation, and radioembolization using $^{90}$Y-microspheres.[43] Monitoring regional therapy to malignant hepatic lesions is discussed in Chapter II.7.

## Summary

Evaluation of patients with known or suspected recurrent CRC is now an accepted indication for $^{18}$F-FDG PET/CT, with complementary information provided by the PET and CT components of the study and unique, incremental information added by fused images. The most common indications for $^{18}$F-FDG PET/CT in patients with CRC are for diagnosis of recurrence and for preoperative N and M restaging of known recurrence considered to be resectable. $^{18}$F-FDG PET/CT is also of value for differentiation of post-treatment changes from recurrent tumor, differentiation of benign from malignant lesions such as indeterminate lymph nodes, hepatic and pulmonary lesions, and evaluation of patients with rising tumor markers and no other evidence of active malignancy. Addition of $^{18}$F-FDG PET/CT to the evaluation of these patients reduces overall treatment costs by accurately differentiating between patients who will benefit from surgical procedures from those who will not.

  Although initial staging at the time of diagnosis is often performed during colectomy, $^{18}$F-FDG PET/CT is now commonly performed preoperatively. It is particularly useful if $^{18}$F-FDG PET shows metastases and unnecessary surgery can be avoided. Screening for recurrence in patients at high risk has also been advocated, as has been monitoring patient response to therapy. Both these clinical indications for $^{18}$F-FDG imaging in patients with CRC need further evaluation in large studies.

# Guidelines and Recommendations for the Use of $^{18}$F-FDG PET and PET/CT

The National Comprehensive Cancer Network (NCCN) has incorporated $^{18}$F-FDG PET and PET/CT in its practice guidelines and management algorithms for a variety of malignancies including CRC.[44] The use of $^{18}$F-FDG PET (PET/CT where available) is recommended in the following clinical scenarios:

(1) Initial staging if conventional imaging studies are equivocal for metastatic disease
(2) Rising CEA levels or suspicious symptoms for occult recurrence unless other imaging tests are diagnostic
(3) Restaging of recurrent CRC if curative resection is considered

  $^{18}$F-FDG PET is not indicated:

(1) For restaging after non-surgical treatment of metastatic disease
(2) For post-treatment surveillance

A multidisciplinary panel of experts assessed meta-analyses and systematic reviews published in the $^{18}$F-FDG PET literature before March 2006 and made recommendations for the use of $^{18}$F-FDG PET in oncology[45]:

(1) The panel found little evidence to support the use of $^{18}$F-FDG PET for the diagnosis of CRC.

(2) $^{18}$F-FDG PET should be used routinely in addition to conventional imaging in the preoperative diagnostic workup of patients with potentially resectable hepatic metastases from CRC.

(3) $^{18}$F-FDG PET should be performed following the conventional workup, especially if CEA levels are increased and the results of this workup are negative. PET can also be used to differentiate between local relapse and postsurgical scars.

# Case Presentations

## *Case II.5.1( DICOM Images on DVD)*

### History

This 81-year-old man presented with a recurrent fibrohistiocytoma of the right upper chest, recently biopsied. A chest radiograph revealed a right lower lobe mass. Biopsy demonstrated an adenocarcinoma. He was referred for preoperative assessment with [18]F-FDG PET/CT (Fig. II.5.1A–D).

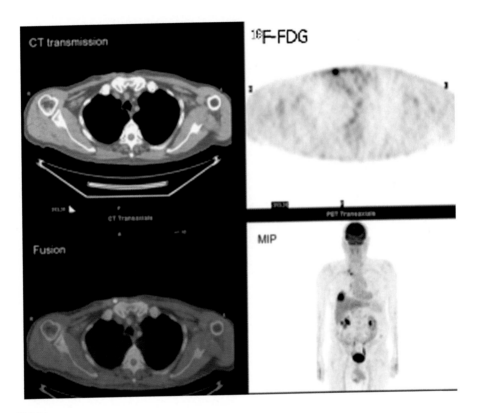

Fig. II.5.1A

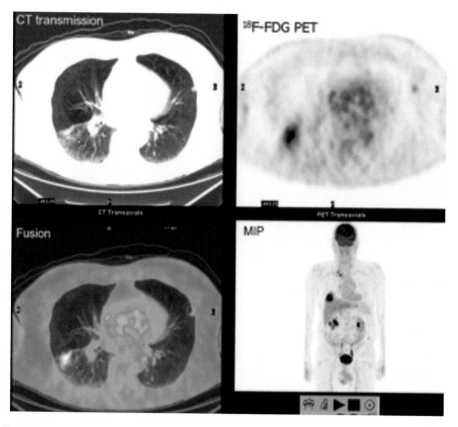

**Fig. II.5.1B**

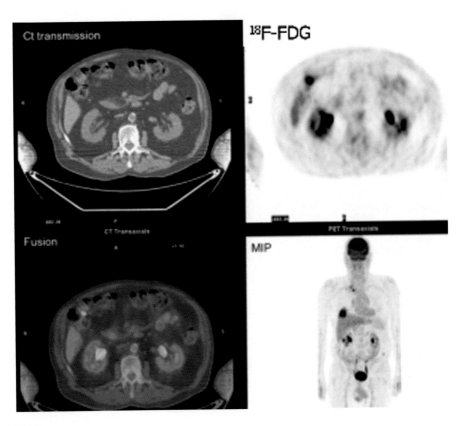

**Fig. II.5.1C**

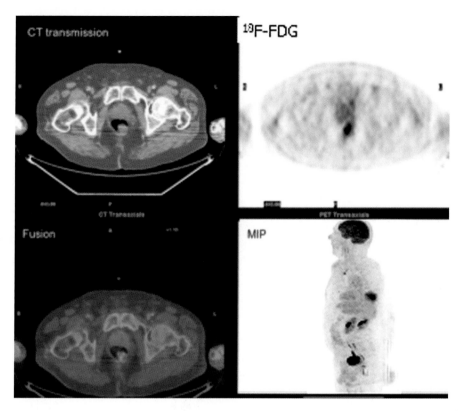

**Fig. II.5.1D**

**Findings**

Two focal areas of intense [18]F-FDG uptake in the anterior upper right hemithorax correspond to soft tissue stranding anterior to the proximal third of the right clavicle (Fig. II.5.1A). Given the patient's history of recurrent malignant fibrohistiocytoma in this region, these foci are consistent with local recurrence. A large focus of intense [18]F-FDG uptake corresponding to a 74 × 41 mm infiltrative mass is identified in the lateral aspect of the lower lobe of the right lung (maximum intensity projection [MIP] images). A 7 mm nodular density is present within the anterolateral aspect of the left upper lobe and demonstrates mild [18]F-FDG uptake (Fig. II.5.1B). There is intense focal [18]F-FDG uptake corresponding to an approximately 20 mm soft tissue mass within the transverse colon at the hepatic flexure (Fig. II.5.1C). An additional focus of mild-to-moderate [18]F-FDG uptake corresponds to an exophytic lesion, 20 × 20 mm in size, in the distal rectum (Fig. II.5.1D). Additional CT findings are seen on the DICOM images (DVD) and described in the clinical report.

**Discussion**

These findings are consistent with the known recurrent malignant fibrohistiocytoma and right lower lobe adenocarcinoma. The 7 mm left lung nodule has mild uptake. It is at the size limit of PET resolution and suffers from partial volume averaging artifact being smaller than twice the resolution of the PET system. Any uptake in a structure less than twice the resolution of the PET system is worrisome for malignancy. The degree and focality of uptake in the transverse colon and rectum are very concerning for a malignant or pre-malignant etiology. The patient underwent colonoscopy with biopsies. The lesion in the transverse colon was proven to represent moderately differentiated adenocarcinoma and the polyp resected from the rectum was a tubulovillous adenoma with high-grade dysplasia.

Agress and Cooper[4] reviewed [18]F-FDG PET studies of 1,750 patients with known or suspected malignancies. The authors found 58 unexpected focal areas of [18]F-FDG uptake unlikely to be related to the known primary tumor in 3.3% of patients. Forty-two lesions were pathologically confirmed: 71% were malignant or premalignant lesions, including adenoma and carcinoma of the colon. Similar data were published by Kamel and coworker who reviewed 3,281 patients,[5] Gutman et al. in 1,716 patients,[6] and Israel and coworkers in 4,390 patients.[7]

The sensitivity of [18]F-FDG imaging is highly dependent on both the size of the lesion, with up to 72% sensitivity for lesions greater than 10 mm in diameter, and the degree of dysplasia, reaching up to 89% for carcinoma and up to 76% for high-grade and 36% for low-grade degrees of dysplasia.[46] The sensitivity of [18]F-FDG imaging is lower for flat (sessile) premalignant lesions.[47]

**Diagnosis**

1. Recurrent malignant fibrohistiocytoma.
2. Lung adenocarcinoma, right lower lobe.
3. Possible small metastasis in the left lung.
4. Transverse colon carcinoma.
5. Rectal high-grade tubular adenoma.

**Clinical Report: Body [18]F-FDG PET/CT (for DVD cases only)**

Indication

Initial staging of non-small cell lung carcinoma.

History

The patient is an 81-year-old make with a history of recurrent fibrohistiocytoma of the right upper chest, which had been diagnosed 2 years earlier by excisional biopsy and followed by wide excision. The patient presented with a recurrent chest wall lesion, confirmed as recurrence at biopsy. A preoperative chest x-ray revealed a lung mass in the right lower lobe. Subsequent bronchoscopy with biopsy was consistent with adenocarcinoma, and the patient now presents for initial staging.

Procedure

The fasting blood glucose level was 93 mg/dl. A dose of 480 MBq (13.0 mCi) of [18]F-FDG was administered intravenously in the right antecubital fossa. After a distribution time of 65 min, whole body low-dose CT without intravenous contrast was acquired to correct for attenuation and for anatomic localization, followed by PET images acquired over the head, neck, thorax, abdomen, and pelvis. The patient was positioned with the arms to the torso's sides.

Findings

> *Quality of the study*: The quality of this study is good.
>
> *Head and neck*: There is physiologic distribution of the radiopharmaceutical in the brain and in the lymphoid and glandular tissues of the neck.
>
> *Chest*: Two focal areas of intense $^{18}$F-FDG uptake correspond to soft tissue stranding immediately anterior to the proximal third of the right clavicle. Given the patient's history, these areas of uptake are most consistent with local recurrence of malignant fibrohistiocytoma. A large focus of intense $^{18}$F-FDG uptake corresponds to a 74 × 41 mm infiltrative mass within the lateral aspect of the right lower lobe. A 7 mm nodular density is present within the anterolateral sub-pleural portion of the left upper lobe and demonstrates a mild degree of $^{18}$F-FDG uptake. Two sub-centimeter nodules are identified within the apex of the right lung on CT, below the PET resolution. There is mild pulmonary emphysema, old granulomatous disease in the mediastinum, and a small pericardial effusion.
>
> *Abdomen and pelvis*: There is an area of focal, high-intensity $^{18}$F-FDG uptake corresponding to an approximately 20 mm soft tissue mass in the transverse colon at the level of the hepatic flexure. Another focus of mild-to-moderate degree of $^{18}$F-FDG uptake corresponds to an exophytic 20 × 20 mm lesion within the distal rectum. There are multiple small gallstones and vascular calcifications in the aorta and its branches demonstrated on CT.
>
> *Musculoskeletal*: There are degenerative changes in the spine.

Impression

1. Intense $^{18}$F-FDG uptake in a right lower lobe mass, consistent with the known lung adenocarcinoma.
2. A small, 7 mm, nodular opacification within the anterolateral portion of the left upper lobe with mild $^{18}$F-FDG uptake, suggestive of metastasis.
3. Two sub-centimeter nodules in the apex of the right lung on CT, below the PET resolution.
4. Two focal areas of intense $^{18}$F-FDG uptake in soft tissue stranding anterior to the right clavicle, consistent with the known recurrent malignant fibrohistiocytoma.
5. Intense focal $^{18}$F-FDG uptake, corresponding to a 20 mm lesion in the transverse colon at the hepatic flexure and a focus of moderate uptake, corresponding to an exophytic 20 mm lesion in the distal rectum. The differential diagnosis includes malignancy versus benign polyp; correlation with colonoscopy is recommended.
6. Additional CT findings are described earlier.

## Case II.5.2

### History

This 63-year-old male presented with anal carcinoma. A biopsy revealed a moderately differentiated adenocarcinoma. CT demonstrated a large lesion in the left lobe of the liver. The patient was referred to PET/CT for initial staging (Fig. II.5.2A–D).

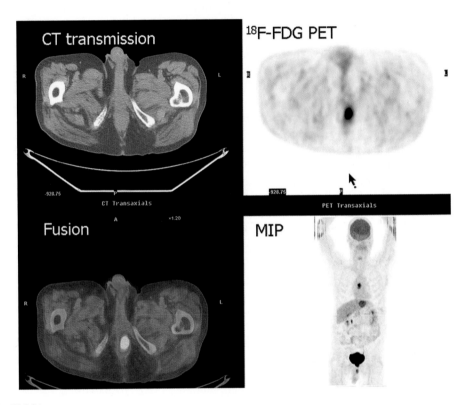

**Fig. II.5.2A**

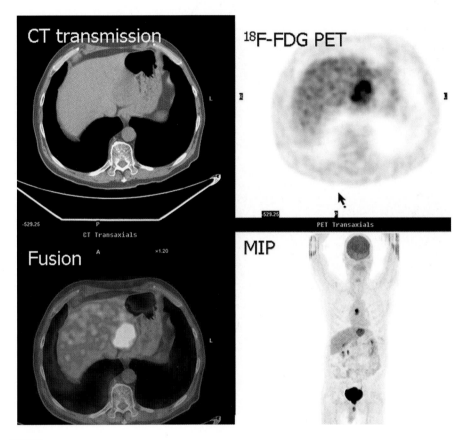

**Fig. II.5.2B**

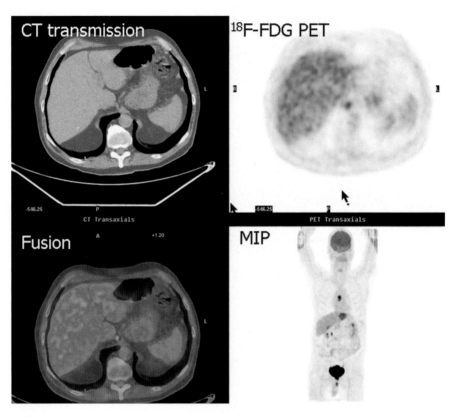

Fig. II.5.2C

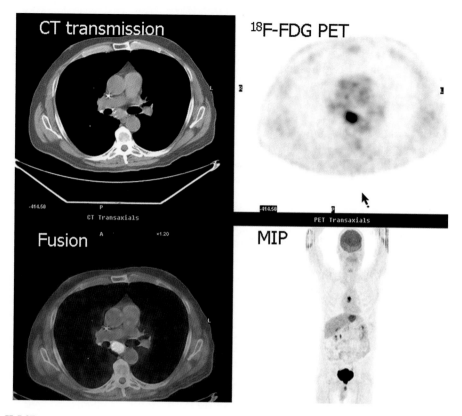

**Fig. II.5.2D**

### Findings

Focal intense $^{18}$F-FDG uptake is seen in the rectum corresponding to thickening of the anus, consistent with the known primary tumor (Fig. II.5.2A). There is a 57 × 47 mm hypodense lesion in the left lobe of the liver seen on CT, which demonstrated intense $^{18}$F-FDG uptake, indicating a hepatic metastasis (Fig. II.5.2B). In addition, a small focus of uptake is seen in the right para-aortic/peri-esophageal region corresponding to a sub-centimeter lymph node retrospectively seen also on CT (Fig. II.5.2C) and a larger focus of uptake in the subcarinal mediastinum corresponding to a 17 × 25 mm lymph node or nodal conglomerate (Fig. II.5.2D), each consistent with metastasis.

### Discussion

$^{18}$F-FDG uptake in the anus represents the known primary tumor. As there was evidence of distant hepatic and extrahepatic metastases, surgical cure was not an option and the patient was referred for chemotherapy. PET/CT allowed precise localization of the distribution of extrahepatic disease, with the full extent of this disease seen on CT only in retrospect.

Several studies have evaluated the usefulness of $^{18}$F-FDG PET for staging patients with known or suspected primary CRC. $^{18}$F-FDG PET imaging identified almost all primary carcinomas. Both $^{18}$F-FDG and CT had equally low sensitivities for detection of loco-regional lymph node involvement, with a sensitivity of approximately 30% each. However,

[18]F-FDG PET was superior to CT for detection of hepatic metastases, with sensitivity and specificity greater than 90%, compared to 38 and 97%, respectively. [18]F-FDG PET changed the treatment modality in 8% of patients and the extent of surgery in 13%.[48] False-positive [18]F-FDG findings include abscesses, fistulas, diverticulitis, and adenomas.

**Diagnosis**

1. Primary rectal adenocarcinoma.
2. Hepatic metastasis in the left lobe.
3. Evidence of extrahepatic nodal metastases in the right para-aortic/distal peri-esophageal region and in the subcarinal mediastinum, seen on CT only in retrospect.

## Case II.5.3

### History

This 74-year-old male was diagnosed with colon carcinoma 9 months earlier and subsequently treated with an ileocolic resection. He was referred to PET/CT for evaluation of a hepatic lesion detected on CT performed for restaging (Fig. II.5.3).

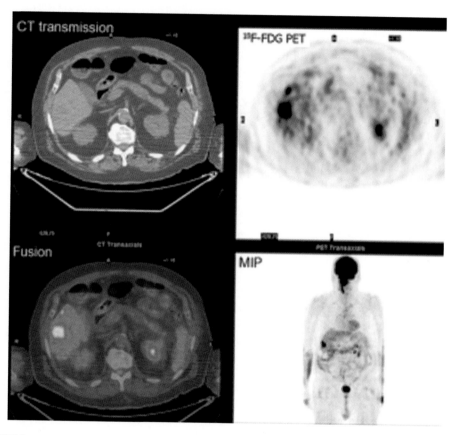

**Fig. II.5.3**

### Findings

There is a focus of intense $^{18}$F-FDG uptake corresponding to a 25 mm hypodense lesion seen in the right lobe of the liver on CT. In addition, there is a second focus of intense $^{18}$F-FDG uptake anterior to the first lesion. There is physiological uptake in the glandular and lymphoid tissue of the neck and motion artifact of the head and neck region, best appreciated on the anterior maximum intensity projection (MIP) image. There is mild linear uptake along the sternum (seen on MIP), corresponding to a prior sternotomy and coronary artery bypass grafting evident on CT (not shown). There is no evidence of extrahepatic metastases.

**Discussion**

The findings are consistent with two hepatic metastases in segment 6 of the liver. In the absence of extrahepatic lesions, this patient is a candidate for resection. For patients who present with isolated liver metastases, hepatic resection is the only curative therapy, but this procedure is associated with significant morbidity and mortality.[9] The poor prognosis of extrahepatic metastases represents a contraindication to hepatic resection.[10] Therefore, accurate non-invasive detection of inoperable disease plays a pivotal role in selecting patients who would benefit from surgery.

A meta-analysis comparing non-invasive imaging methods (ultrasound [US], CT, MRI, and $^{18}$F-FDG PET) for the detection of hepatic metastases from colorectal, gastric, and esophageal cancers demonstrated that, at an equivalent specificity of 85%, $^{18}$F-FDG PET had the highest sensitivity (90%) compared to MRI (76%), CT (72%), and US (55%).[49] A subsequent meta-analysis, including studies that performed MRI with gadolinium and superparamagnetic iron oxide particle (SPIO) enhancement, came to similar conclusions for a patient-based analysis.[50] For a lesion-based analysis, $^{18}$F-FDG PET had the highest sensitivity of 76% compared to 66% for unenhanced MRI and 64% for CT. Both gadolinium- and SPIO-enhanced MRI were superior to non-enhanced MRI. SPIO-MRI was the most sensitive technique, with a sensitivity of 90% for detection of lesions greater than 10 mm, compared to 76% for $^{18}$F-FDG PET. In patients with CRC, the sensitivity of $^{18}$F-FDG PET for detection of hepatic metastases was compared to that of multiphase CT, using intraoperative ultrasound as reference standard for lesions of different sizes.[28] The overall sensitivity was similar for PET (71%) and CT (72%); both modalities missed approximately 30% of smaller lesions but resulted in a change of management in 7% of patients. One study compared mangafodipir-trisodium-enhanced hepatic MRI with $^{18}$F-FDG for detection of liver metastases in patients with colorectal and pancreatic cancer.[51] On a per-patient analysis, MRI and $^{18}$F-FDG showed sensitivities of 97 and 93%, positive predictive values of 100 and 90%, and accuracies of 97 and 85%, respectively. On a per-lesion analysis, MRI and $^{18}$F-FDG showed sensitivities of 81 and 67%, positive predictive values of 90 and 81%, and accuracies of 76 and 64%, respectively. $^{18}$F-FDG imaging provided additional information regarding the presence of extrahepatic disease and was therefore useful in initial staging. However, significantly more and smaller (sub-centimeter) hepatic metastases were detected on MRI than on $^{18}$F-FDG PET.

Valk et al.[52] compared the sensitivity and specificity of $^{18}$F-FDG and CT for detection of metastases in specific anatomic locations and found that $^{18}$F-FDG PET was more sensitive than CT in all locations except the lung, where the two modalities were equivalent. The greatest differences between PET and CT were found in the abdomen, pelvis, and retroperitoneum, where over one-third of PET-positive lesions were negative by CT. PET was more specific than CT in all locations except the retroperitoneum, but less significant than for the sensitivity.

In a prospective study of 51 patients prior to resection of hepatic metastases, clinical management decisions based on conventional diagnostic methods were changed in 20% of patients based on the findings of $^{18}$F-FDG imaging, especially due to detection of unsuspected extrahepatic disease.[23]

**Diagnosis**

1. Two hepatic metastases.
2. No evidence of extrahepatic disease.

## *Case II.5.4 (DICOM Images on DVD)*

### History

This 69-year-old male has a history of sigmoid colon carcinoma treated with sigmoidectomy 2 years earlier. One year later, he had tumor recurrence in the liver and underwent resection of the left hepatic lobe. At surgery metastatic lymph nodes were found, and lymph node dissection was also performed. The patient then received chemotherapy and was referred to [18]F-FDG PET/CT for restaging (Fig. II.5.4A–C). Figure II.5.4C is not corrected for attenuation correction (no AC).

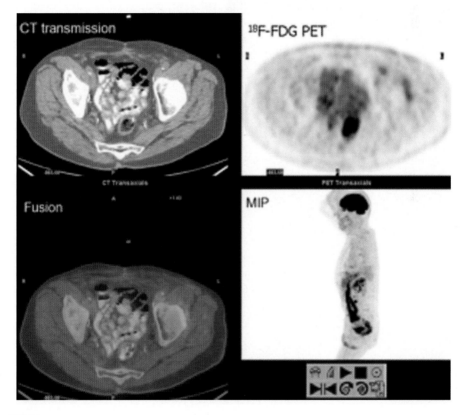

**Fig. II.5.4A**

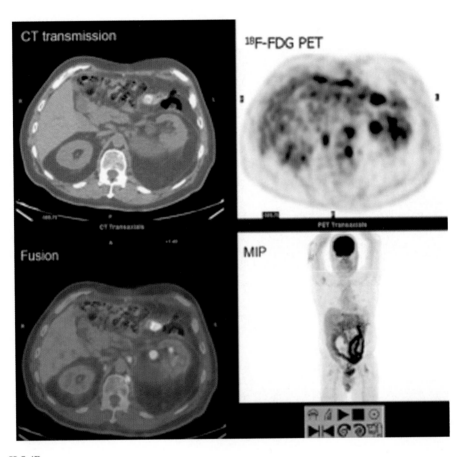

**Fig. II.5.4B**

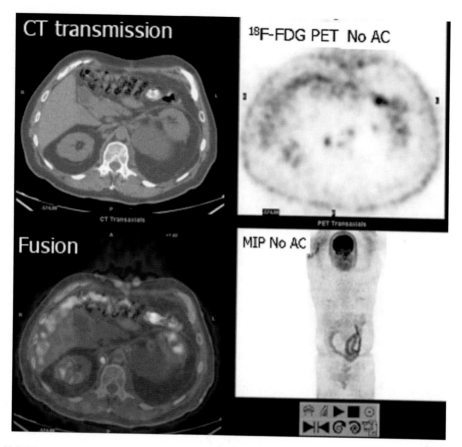

**Fig. II.5.4C**

## Findings

There is a focus of intense $^{18}$F-FDG uptake corresponding to the surgical anastomosis in the sigmoid colon (Fig. II.5.4A). The anastomosis can be identified on CT by the presence of staples. There are also three foci of uptake corresponding to sub-centimeter lymph nodes on CT in the left retrocrural, left para-aortic, and right retrocaval regions.

There is intense uptake throughout much of the GI tract, seen on both the attenuation corrected (Fig. II.5.4B) and the non-attenuation corrected (Fig. II.5.4C) images.

Examination of the CT component of the study (see DICOM images on the DVD) reveals a 12 cm fluid collection on the left, felt to represent a post-surgical lymphocele, resulting in displacement of the left kidney anteriorly and in mild hydronephrosis. There is an exophytic left renal cyst.

## Discussion

The findings indicate local recurrence and metastatic disease in superior retroperitoneal lymph nodes. Since the patient was no longer a candidate for surgery with curative intent, he was referred to further chemotherapy.

Several studies have compared [18]F-FDG PET and CT for detection of local recurrence. CT was equivocal in most cases, whereas the accuracy of [18]F-FDG PET imaging exceeded 90%. In the largest study including 76 patients comparing [18]F-FDG PET and CT for differentiation of scar from local recurrence, the accuracy was 95 and 65%, respectively.[53] In addition, [18]F-FDG detected metastases in normal size lymph nodes seen on CT. PET/CT improved retrospective detection of lesions on both the PET and the CT images and improved their accurate characterization as either benign or malignant. PET/CT also allowed more precise anatomic localization of the [18]F-FDG-avid foci. In this case study, sub-centimeter retroperitoneal lymph nodes were retrospectively identified on CT after being characterized as malignant by PET because of their [18]F-FDG avidity. [18]F-FDG uptake in the sigmoid colon could be precisely localized to the region of the anastomosis, therefore characterized as malignant since the surgical insult was remote.

Diffuse bowel uptake is also seen in this patient. The uptake is intense and fairly homogenous, and seen on both the attenuation corrected (AC) and the non-attenuation corrected (non-AC) images. The major differential diagnosis for diffuse bowel uptake includes normal variation, malignancy such as peritoneal carcinomatosis with diffuse bowel wall tumor implant, ischemic gut, diverticulitis, inflammatory bowel disease, and enterocolitis, especially in the context of myeloablative chemotherapy in association with bone marrow transplantation. The presence of GI contrast can, at times, produce an AC artifact from a combination of "over-correction" and peristalsis occurring in the interim between the CT and the PET acquisition of the images. This can result in misregistration between the two components of the PET/CT. If the uptake in the bowel is also seen on the non-AC image, as in this case, the GI contrast given for the diagnostic CT is not the source for artefactual GI tract uptake on PET/CT. In this case, the most likely cause for the bowel uptake was enterocolitis.

### Diagnosis

1. Local recurrence at the surgical anastomosis.
2. Metastases to retroperitoneal lymph nodes.

### Clinical Report: Body [18]F-FDG PET/CT (for DVD cases only)

Indication

Restaging of colon cancer.

History

This 69-year-old male with a history of adenocarcinoma in the sigmoid colon, status post-sigmoidectomy 2 years earlier followed by chemotherapy, was found to have recurrent metastatic disease to the liver, treated with left hepatic resection. At surgery, metastatic lymph nodes were found, and the patient also underwent lymph node dissection. The patient then received additional chemotherapy and is now referred for restaging by [18]F-FDG PET/CT.

Procedure

The patient is to receive a diagnostic, contrast-enhanced CT study of the chest, abdomen, and pelvis immediately after the PET/CT scan and, therefore, oral contrast was administered prior to $^{18}$F-FDG administration. The fasting blood glucose level was 85 mg/dl at the time of injection of the radioisotope; 470 MBq (12.8 mCi) of $^{18}$F-FDG was administered intravenously via the right antecubital vein. After a distribution time of 90 min, a whole body low-dose CT without IV contrast was acquired for attenuation correction and for anatomic localization, followed by PET imaging over the brain, neck, thorax, abdomen, and pelvis. The patient was positioned with his arms above the head.

Findings

*Quality of the study*: The quality of the study is good.

*Head and neck*: There is physiologic distribution of $^{18}$F-FDG in the cortex of the brain and in the glandular and lymphoid tissue of the neck.

*Chest*: There is physiologic uptake in the myocardium. The lungs are clear.

*Abdomen and pelvis*: There are several foci of intense $^{18}$F-FDG uptake within multiple retroperitoneal lymph nodes. Two of these lymph nodes are at the level of the mid-pole of the right kidney. Four lymph nodes are located in the left periaortic region at the same level and caudal to it. The largest lymph node is located caudally anterior to the left renal vein and measures 14 × 9 mm. There is a large 127 × 107 mm fluid collection that is not $^{18}$F-FDG avid on the left, which most likely represents a postsurgical lymphocele. This lesion has resulted in displacement of the left kidney anteriorly and in subsequent mild left hydronephrosis.

An exophytic left renal cyst is noted. There is intense $^{18}$F-FDG uptake corresponding to the anastomotic site in the sigmoid colon. There is also increased $^{18}$F-FDG uptake along the lateral margin of the distal sigmoid colon. In addition, there appears to be some wall thickening associated with intense $^{18}$F-FDG uptake within the rectum.

*Musculoskeletal*: There is a small amount of $^{18}$F-FDG uptake seen within the muscles of the right shoulder, which is likely inflammatory in etiology. Mild degenerative changes are seen throughout the spine with no abnormal $^{18}$F-FDG uptake.

Impression

1. Increased $^{18}$F-FDG uptake at the site of the previous sigmoid anastomosis and along the lateral margin of the distal sigmoid. In addition, there is bowel wall thickening and $^{18}$F-FDG uptake in the rectum, consistent with residual viable malignant disease.
2. Multiple borderline-sized periaortic and retroperitoneal $^{18}$F-FDG-avid lymph nodes consistent with metastases.
3. Large fluid collection in the left perinephric space, suggesting a postsurgical lymphocele. This has resulted in anterior displacement of the left kidney and mild hydronephrosis.
4. For additional anatomic detail, refer to the report of the diagnostic, contrast-enhanced CT examinations of the chest, abdomen, and pelvis performed on the same day as the PET/CT.
5. Incidental findings include (a) surgical changes from a partial left hepatectomy, recto-sigmoid surgery, and prostatectomy; (b) stable scarring in the left lower lobe; and (c) left subclavian venous infusion port in place.

## Case II.5.5

### History

This 56-year-old patient has a history of rectal carcinoma treated with surgical resection. He presented with rising CEA levels. CT of the abdomen and pelvis was negative. The patient was referred for $^{18}$F-FDG PET/CT imaging (Fig. II.5.5).

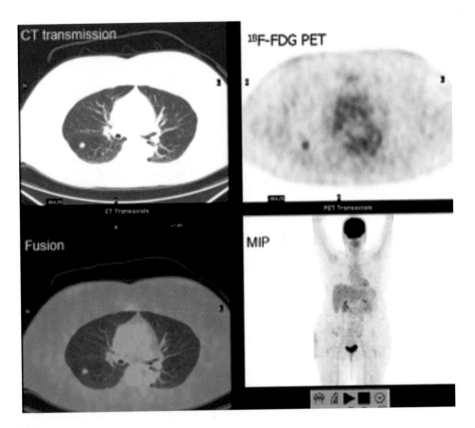

**Fig. II.5.5**

### Findings

There is a focus of moderate $^{18}$F-FDG uptake corresponding to an 8 mm nodule in the lower lobe of the right lung. No additional foci of abnormal uptake are seen (Fig. II.5.5).

### Discussion

$^{18}$F-FDG uptake in this sub-centimeter lung nodule is suspicious for metastasis in a patient with a history of rectal carcinoma. Biopsy was recommended and confirmed the diagnosis. This example illustrates the value of PET/CT as a whole body imaging technique, allowing detection of metastases in unsuspected locations that are not always imaged with conventional workup.

The measurement of serum levels of CEA may be used to monitor patients for recurrence with a sensitivity of 59% and specificity of 84%. However, an elevated CEA level does not localize recurrent tumor. Flanagan et al.[55] reported the use of $^{18}$F-FDG PET in 22 patients with unexplained elevation of serum CEA levels after resection of colorectal carcinoma, with no abnormal findings on conventional workup, including CT. Sensitivity and specificity of $^{18}$F-FDG PET for detection of tumor recurrence were 100 and 71%, respectively. Valk et al.[52] reported a sensitivity of 93% and specificity of 92% in a similar group of 18 patients. In both studies, PET correctly demonstrated tumor in two-thirds of patients with rising CEA levels and negative CT scans. Pooled data from published studies demonstrate that $^{18}$F-FDG PET detects tumor in 84% of patients with rising CEA levels and a negative conventional workup. Surgical resection is possible in 26% of these patients.

**Diagnosis**

Pulmonary metastasis in the right lower lobe.

## Case II.5.6

### History

A 38-year-old male diagnosed with colon cancer 1 year previously presented with rising serum CEA levels. A recent CT demonstrated several large hypodense lesions in the liver. The patient was referred for $^{18}$F-FDG PET/CT prior to considering surgery (Fig. II.5.6).

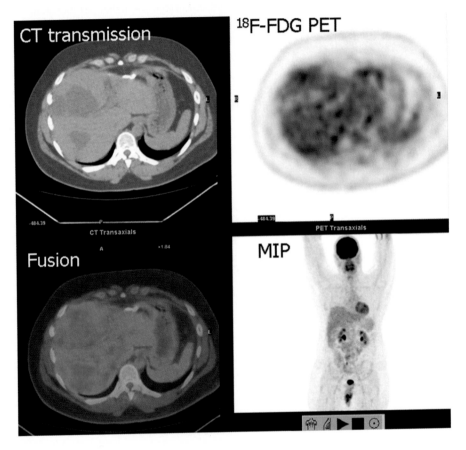

**Fig. II.5.6**

### Findings

CT shows several large hypodense lesions in the right lobe of the liver, with no corresponding abnormal $^{18}$F-FDG uptake (Fig. II.5.6).

### Discussion

The CT abnormalities are greater than 1 cm in diameter, therefore well within the resolution of PET, and yet do not demonstrate increased $^{18}$F-FDG uptake. When there is discordance between compelling laboratory and CT evidence for metastases and negative PET findings, it is essential to review the histological features of the tumor. Biopsy of the liver revealed metastatic mucinous adenocarcinoma with signet ring features. Adenocarcinoma from various primary sources can have large mucinous components, as was the case in this patient, and can be false negative on [18]F-FDG PET. The patient underwent partial right hepatectomy. This study also demonstrates the complementary nature of PET/CT; in this example, metastases were seen on CT but not on PET.

A meta-analysis of 11 clinical reports determined that the sensitivity and specificity for [18]F-FDG PET for detection of recurrent CRC are 97 and 76%, respectively. These values are superior to that of CT, which has a sensitivity and specificity of 86 and 58%, respectively, for detection of extrahepatic recurrence.[11] However, false-negative [18]F-FDG studies have been reported with mucinous adenocarcinoma. Whiteford et al.[13] reported that the sensitivity of [18]F-FDG PET for detection of mucinous adenocarcinoma is significantly lower than for non-mucinous adenocarcinoma, 58 and 92%, respectively. These investigators also reported that [18]F-FDG PET detected tumor in 60% (15/25) of patients with mucinous carcinoma (11 colorectal, 8 gastroesophageal, 2 pancreatic, 3 lung, and 1 breast) and postulated that the low sensitivity of [18]F-FDG PET for detection of mucinous adenocarcinoma might be due to the relative hypocellularity of these tumors. Similar low sensitivity of 41% has been reported in a subsequent series of 22 patients.[14]

**Diagnosis**

Mucinous adenocarcinoma metastatic to the liver seen on CT but not on [18]F-FDG PET.

# References

1. American Cancer Society. *Cancer facts and figures,* 2008. Atlanta, Georgia.
2. Smith RA, Cokkinides V, Eyre HJ. American Cancer Society Guidelines for the early detection of cancer, 2004. *CA Cancer J Clin* 2004;54:41–52.
3. McFarland EG, Levin B, Lieberman DA, Pickhardt PJ, Johnson CD, Glick SN, Brooks D, Smith RA. Revised colorectal screening guidelines: Joint effort of the American Cancer Society, U.S. Multisociety Task Force on Colorectal Cancer, and American College of Radiology. *Radiology* 2008;248: 717–720.
4. Agress H, Cooper BZ. Detection of clinically unexpected malignant and premalignant tumors with whole-body FDG PET: Histopathologic comparison. *Radiology* 2004;230: 417–422.
5. Kamel EM, Thumshirn M, Truninger K, Schiesser M, Fried M, Padberg B, Schneiter D, Stoeckli SJ, von Schulthess GK, Stumpe KDM. Significance of incidental 18F-FDG accumulations in the gastrointestinal tract in PET/CT: Correlation with endoscopic and histopathological results. *J Nucl Med* 2004;45:1804–1810.
6. Gutman F, Alberini JL, Wartski M, Vilain D, Le Stanc E, Sarandi F, Corone C, Tainturier C, Pecking AP. Incidental colonic focal lesions detected by FDG PET/CT. *Am J Roentgenol* 2005;185:495–500.
7. Israel O, Yefremov N, Bar-Shalom R, Kagana O, Frenkel A, Keidar Z, Fischer D. PET/CT detection of unexpected gastrointestinal foci of 18F-FDG uptake: Incidence, localization patterns, and clinical significance. *J Nucl Med* 2005;46:758–762.
8. Yun HR, Lee LJ, Park JH, Cho YK, Cho YB, Lee WY, Kim HC, Chun HK, Yun SH. Local recurrence after curative resection in patients with colon and rectal cancers. *Int J Colorectal Dis* 2008;23:1081–1087.
9. Helling TS, Blondeau B. Anatomic segmental resection compared to major hepatectomy in the treatment of liver neoplasms. *HPB (Oxford)* 2005;7:222–225.
10. Hughes KS, Simon R, Songhorabodi S, Adson MA, Ilstrup DM, Fortner JG, Maclean BJ, Foster JH, Daly JM, Fitzherbert D et al. Resection of liver for colorectal carcinoma metastases: A multi-institutional study of indications for resection. *Surgery* 1988;103:278–288.
11. Huebner RH, Park KC, Shepherd JE, Schwimmer J, Czernin J, Phelps ME, Gambhir SS. A meta-analysis of the literature for whole-body FDG PET detection of colorectal cancer. *J Nucl Med* 2000;41: 1177–1189.
12. Gambhir SS, Czernin J, Schimmer J, Silverman DHS, Coleman RE, Phelps ME. A tabulated review of the literature. *J Nucl Med* 2001;42 (suppl):9S–12S.
13. Whiteford MH, Whiteford HM, Yee LF, Ogunbiyi OA, Dehdashti F, Siegel BA, Birnbaum EH, Fleshman JW, Kodner IJ, Read TE. Usefulness of FDG-PET scan in the assessment of suspected metastatic or recurrent adenocarcinoma of the colon and rectum. *Dis Colon Rectum* 2000;43:759–767; discussion 767–770.
14. Berger KL, Nicholson SA, Dehadashti F, Siegel BA. FDG PET evaluation of mucinous neoplasms: Correlation of FDG uptake with histopathologic features. *Am J Roentgenol* 2000;174:1005–1008.
15. Yang YY, Fleshman JW, Strasberg SM. Detection and management of extrahepatic colorectal cancer in patients with resectable liver metastases. *J Gastrointest Surg* 2007;11:929–944.
16. Bar-Shalom R, Yefremov N, Guralnik L, Gaitini D, Frenkel A, Kuten A, Altman H, Keidar Z, Israel O. Clinical performance of PET/CT in the evaluation of cancer: Additional value for diagnostic imaging and patient management. *J Nucl Med* 2003;44:1200–1209.
17. Roman CD, Martin WH, Delbeke D. Incremental value of fusion imaging with integrated PET-CT in oncology. *Clin Nucl Med* 2005;30:470–477.
18. Cohade C, Osman M, Leal J, Wahl RL. Direct comparison of FDG PET and PET-CT imaging in colorectal carcinoma. *J Nucl Med* 2003;44:1797–1803.
19. Selzner M, Hany TF, Wildbrett P, McCormack L, Kadry Z, Clavien P-A. Does the novel PET/CT imaging modality impact on the treatment of patients with metastatic colorectal cancer of the liver? *Ann Surg* 2004;240:1027–1034.
20. Soyka JD, Veit-Haibach P, Strobel K, Breitenstein S, Tschopp A, Mende KA, Perez Lago M, Hany TF. Staging pathways in recurrent colorectal carcinoma: Is contrast-enhanced 18F-FDG PET/CT the diagnostic tool of choice? *J Nucl Med* 2008;49:354–361.
21. Tateishi U, Maeda T, Morimoto T, Miyake M, Arai Y, Kim EE. Non-enhanced CT versus contrast-enhanced CT in integrated PET/CT studies for nodal staging of rectal cancer. *Eur J Nucl Med Mol Imaging* 2007;34:1627–1634.

23. Ruers TJ, Langenhoff BS, Neeleman N, Jager GJ, Strijk S, Wobbes T, Corstens FHM, Oyen WJG. Value of positron emission tomography with [F-18] fluorodeoxyglucose in patients with colorectal liver metastases: A prospective study. *J Clin Oncol* 2002;20:388–395.

24. Wiering B, Krabbe PF, Jager GJ, Oyen WJ, Ruers TJ. The impact of fluor-18-deoxyglucose-positron emission tomography in the management of colorectal liver metastases. *Cancer* 2005;15;104:2658–2670.

25. Scott AM, Gunawardana DH, Kelley B, Stuckey JG, Byrne AJ, Ramshaw JE, Fulham MJ. PET changes management and improves prognostic stratification in patients with recurrent colorectal cancer: Results of a multicenter prospective study. *J Nucl Med* 2008;49:1451–1457.

26. Strasberg SM, Dehdashti F, Siegel BA, Drebin JA, Linehan D. Survival of patients evaluated by FDG PET before hepatic resection for metastatic colorectal carcinoma: A prospective database study. *Ann Surg* 2001;233:320–321.

27. Fernandez FG, Drebin JA, Linehan DC, Dehdashti F, Siegel BA, Strasberg SM. Five-year survival after resection of hepatic metastases from colorectal cancer in patients screened by positron emission tomography with F-18 fluorodeoxyglucose (FDG-PET). *Ann Surg* 2004;240:438–447; discussion 447–450.

28. Wiering B, Krabbe PF, Dekker HM, Oyen WJ, Ruers TJ. The role of FDG-PET in the selection of patients with colorectal liver metastases. *Ann Surg Oncol* 2007;14:771–779.

29. Gambhir SS, Valk P, Shepherd J, Hoh C, Allen M, Phelps ME. Cost effective analysis modeling of the role of FDG-PET in the management of patients with recurrent colorectal cancer. *J Nucl Med* 1997;38:90P.

30. Park KC, Schwimmer J, Sheperd JE, Phelps ME, Czernin JR, Schiepers C, Gambhir SS. Decision analysis for the cost-effective management of recurrent colorectal cancer. *Ann Surg* 2001;233:310–319.

31. Venook A. Critical evaluation of current treatments in metastatic colorectal cancer. *Oncologist* 2005;10:250–261.

32. Findlay M, Young H, Cunningham D, Iveson A, Cronin B, Hickish T, Pratt B, Husband J, Flower M, Ott R. Noninvasive monitoring of tumor metabolism using fluorodeoxyglucose and positron emission tomography in colorectal cancer liver metastases: Correlation with tumor response to fluorouracil. *J Clin Oncol.* 1996;14:700–708.

33. Akhurst T, Kates TJ, Mazumdar M, Yeung H, Riedel ER, Burt BM, Blumgart L, Jarnagin W, Larson SM, Fong Y. Recent chemotherapy reduces the sensitivity of [18F]fluorodeoxyglucose positron emission tomography in the detection of colorectal metastases. *J Clin Oncol* 2005;23:8713–8716.

34. Takahashi S, Kuroki Y, Nasu K, Nawano S, Konishi M, Nakagohri T, Gotohda N, Saito N, Kinoshita T. Positron emission tomography with F-18 fluorodeoxyglucose in evaluating colorectal hepatic metastasis down-staged by chemotherapy. *Anticancer Res* 2006;26:4705–4711.

35. Carnaghi C, Tronconi MC, Rimassa L, Tondulli L, Zuradelli M, Rodari M, Doci R, Luttmann F, Torzilli G, Rubello D, Al-Nahhas A, Santoro A, Chiti A. Utility of 18F-FDG PET and contrast-enhanced CT scan in the assessment of residual liver metastasis from colorectal cancer following adjuvant chemotherapy. *Nucl Med Rev Cent East Eur* 2007;10:12–15.

36. Lubezky N, Metser U, Geva R, Nakache R, Shmueli E, Klausner JM, Even-Sapir E, Figer A, Ben-Haim M. The role and limitations of 18-fluoro-2-deoxy-D-glucose positron emission tomography (FDG-PET) scan and computerized tomography (CT) in restaging patients with hepatic colorectal metastases following neoadjuvant chemotherapy: Comparison with operative and pathological findings. *J Gastrointest Surg* 2007;11:472–478.

37. Tan MC, Linehan DC, Hawkins WG, Siegel BA, Strasberg SM. Chemotherapy-induced normalization of FDG uptake by colorectal liver metastases does not usually indicate complete pathologic response. *J Gastrointest Surg* 2007;11:1112–1119.

38. Anderson C, Koshy M, Staley C, Esiashvili N, Ghavidel S, Fowler Z, Fox T, Esteves F, Landry J, Godette K. PET-CT fusion in radiation management of patients with anorectal tumors. *Int J Radiat Oncol Biol Phys* 2007;69:155–162.

39. Kahn H, Alexander A, Ratinic J, Nagle D, Fry R. Preoperative staging of irradiated rectal cancers using digital rectal examination, computed tomography, endorectal ultrasound, and magnetic resonance imaging does not accurately predict T0, N0 pathology. *Dis Colon Rectum* 1997;40:140–144.

40. Moore HG, Akhurst T, Larson SM, Minsky BD, Mazumdar M, Guillem JG. A case controlled study of 18-fluorodeoxyglucose positron emission tomography in the detection of pelvic recurrence in previously irradiated rectal cancer patients. *J Am Coll Surg* 2003;197:22–28.

41. Guillem J, Calle J, Akhurst T, Tickoo S, Ruo L, Minsky BD, Gollub MJ, Klimstra DS, Mazumdar M, Paty PB, Macapinlac H, Yeung H, Saltz L, Finn RD, Erdi Y, Humm J, Cohen AM, Larson S.

Prospective assessment of primary rectal cancer response to preoperative radiation and chemotherapy using 18-Fluorodeoxyglucose positron emission tomography. *Dis Colon Rectum* 2000;43:18–24.

42. Guillem JG, Moore HG, Akhurst T, Klimstra D, Ruo L, Mazumdar M, Minsky B, Saltz L, Wong W, Larson S. Sequential preoperative fluorodeoxyglucoise-Positron emission tomography assessment of response to preoperative chemoradiation: A means for determining longterm outcomes of rectal cancer. *J Am Coll Surg* 2004;199:1–7.

43. Lin M, Shon IH, Wilson R, D'Amours SK, Schlaphoff G, Lin P. Treatment response in liver metastases following 90Y SIR-spheres: An evaluation with PET. *Hepatogastroenterology* 2007;54:910–912.

44. Podoloff DA, Advani RH, Allred C, Benson AB 3rd, Brown E, Burstein HJ, Carlson RW, Coleman RE, Czuczman MS, Delbeke D, Edge SB, Ettinger DS, Grannis FW Jr, Hillner BE, Hoffman JM, Kiel K, Komaki R, Larson SM, Mankoff DA, Rosenzweig KE, Skibber JM, Yahalom J, Yu JM, Zelenetz AD. NCCN task force report: Positron emission tomography (PET/Computed tomography (CT) scanning in cancer. *J Natl Compr Canc Netw* 2007;5(Suppl 1): S1–S22. www/nccn.org/professionals/physician_gls/f_guidelines.asp

45. Fletcher JW, Djulbegovic B, Soares HP, Siegel BA, Lowe VA, Lyman GH, Coleman RE, Wahl R, Paschold JC, Avril N, Einhorn LH, Suh WW, Samson D, Delbeke D, Gorman M, Shields AF. Recommendations for the use of FDG (fluorine-18, (2-[18F]Fluoro-2-deoxy-D-glucose) positron emission tomography in oncology. *J Nucl Med* 2008;49:480–508.

46. Van Kouwen MC, Nagengast FM, Jansen JB, Oyen WJ, Drenth JP. 2-(18F)-fluoro-2-deoxy-D-glucose positron emission tomography detects clinical relevant adenomas of the colon: A prospective study. *J Clin Oncol* 2005;23: 3713–3717.

47. Friedland S, Soetikno R, Carlisle M, Taur A, Kaltenbach T, Segall G. 18-Fluorodeoxyglucose positron emission tomography has limited sensitivity for colonic adenomas and early stage colon cancer. *Gastrointest Endosc* 2005;61:305–400.

48. Kantorova I, Lipska L, Belohlavek O, Visokai V, Trubač M, Schneiderová M. Routine 18F-FDG PET preoperative staging of colorectal cancer: Comparison with conventional staging and its impact on treatment decision making. *J Nucl Med* 2003;44:1784–1788.

49. Kinkel K, Lu Y, Both M, Warren RS, Thoeni RF. Detection of hepatic metastases from cancers of the gastrointestinal tract by using noninvasive imaging methods (US, CT, MRimaging, PET) : A meta-analysis. *Radiology* 2002;224:748–756.

50. Bipat S, van Leeuwen MS, Comans EF, Pijl ME, Bossuyt PM, Zwinderman AH, Stoker J. Colorectal liver metastases: CT, MR imaging, and PET for diagnosis – meta-analysis. *Radiology*. 2005;237:123–131.

51. Sahani DV, Kalva SP, Fischman AJ, Kadavigere R, Blake M, Hahn PF, Saini S. Detection of liver metastases from adenocarcinoma of the colon and pancreas: Comparison of mangafodipir trisodium-enhanced liver MRI and whole-body FDG PET. *AJR Am J Roentgenol* 2005;185:239–246.

52. Valk PE, Abella-Columna E, Haseman MK, Pounds TR, Tesar RD, Myers RW, Greiss HB, Hofer GA. Whole-body PET imaging with F-18-fluorodeoxyglucose in management of recurrent colorectal cancer. *Arch Surg*1999;134:503–511.

53. Schiepers C, Penninckx F, De Vadder N, Merckx E, Mortelmans L, Bormans G, Marchal G, Filez L, Aerts R. Contribution of PET in the diagnosis of recurrent colorectal cancer: Comparison with conventional imaging. *Eur J Surg Oncol* 1995;21:517–522.

54. Flanagan FL, Dehdashti F, Ogunbiyi OA, Siegel BA. Utility of FDG PET for investigating unexplained plasma CEA elevation in patients with colorectal cancer. *Ann Surg* 1998;227:319–323.

# Chapter II.6
# $^{18}$F-FDG PET/CT in Tumors of the Gastrointestinal Tract: Esophageal and Gastric Cancer and Gastrointestinal Stromal Tumors (GIST)

Rachel Bar-Shalom and Ludmila Guralnik

## $^{18}$F-FDG Imaging in Esophageal Cancer

### *Introduction*

Esophageal cancer is the eighth leading cause of cancer with a worldwide estimate of more than 400,000 new cases annually. It is the third most common gastrointestinal malignancy, with a highly variable incidence in different geographic locations. While in the United States and Western Europe less than 5/100,000 individuals suffer from this disease, its incidence is steadily increasing over recent years in these countries.[1–3]

Overall, esophageal cancer is a highly aggressive tumor with poor prognosis and a low 5-year survival rate of less than 50% even when diagnosed at an early stage.[4,5] Local spread to surrounding tissues and lymph nodes occurs often, as well as to distant metastatic sites, involving most commonly cervical, supraclavicular, and abdominal lymph nodes, the liver, lungs, bones, and adrenals. Esophageal cancer may uncommonly spread to sites such as the peritoneum, brain, muscles, thyroid, and pancreas.[1,6] Surgery is the only therapeutic option for cure in patients with early stage disease. Resection rates range between 19 and 64% and are associated with a relatively high morbidity and mortality.[1] Up to 50% of patients with esophageal cancer present with locally advanced unresectable disease or distant metastases[2] and are treated with combined chemo–radiotherapy regimens either before or after surgery, with the aim to improve survival or to enable potentially curative treatment.[2] Accurate assessment of extent of disease and response to treatment are important for decisions regarding patient management. At present, a multimodality approach is recommended to enable optimized, individually tailored treatment of esophageal cancer.

Diagnostic tools for evaluation of esophageal cancer include mainly endoscopic ultrasound (EUS), EUS-guided fine needle aspiration (EUS-FNA), and computed tomography (CT). $^{18}$F-FDG imaging, with positron emission tomography (PET)/CT in recent years, has been shown to be of complementary value for assessment of this malignancy at presentation for staging, in evaluation of response to neoadjuvant therapy, and for detection of recurrence.[1,2,6–8]

R. Bar-Shalom (✉)
Department of Nuclear Medicine, Rambam Health Care Campus, B. and R. Rappaport School of Medicine, Technion—Israel Institute of Technology, Haifa, Israel
e-mail: r_bar_shalom@rambam.health.gov.il

D. Delbeke, O. Israel (eds.), *Hybrid PET/CT and SPECT/CT Imaging*,
DOI 10.1007/978-0-387-92820-3_8, © Springer Science+Business Media, LLC 2010

## $^{18}$F-FDG Imaging for Staging of Esophageal Cancer

Accurate staging of esophageal carcinoma needs to define tumor size and location, loco-regional lymph node involvement, and the presence of distant metastases. Tumor (T) stage is defined by the degree of tumor invasion through the layers of the esophageal wall, with T1–2 disease confined to the submucosa or muscularis propria, T3 involving the adventitia, and T4 invading into adjacent extramural structures.[6] Nodal (N) stage defines the absence (N0) or presence (N1) of metastases in loco-regional lymph nodes in the route of the primary esophageal lymphatic drainage. The location of loco-regional nodal metastases varies according to the site of the primary tumor in the esophagus. For cervical esophageal tumors, these include scalene, internal jugular, and supraclavicular lymph nodes; for cancer in the thoracic esophagus they include periesophageal and subcarinal nodes; and for tumors in the distal esophagus or the gastroesophageal (GE) junction regional lymphatic metastases drain to lower periesophageal, diaphragmatic, pericardial, left gastric, and celiac lymph nodes.[6] M stage indicates the presence (M1) or absence (M0) of distant metastatic spread, with M1a and M1b defining non-regional nodal or organ involvement, respectively.[6]

EUS is the most accurate modality for T staging, defining the depth of the invasion of the esophageal wall and detecting loco-regional lymph node metastases.[2] In the presence of esophageal stenosis, the performance of EUS is limited both for assessment of esophageal wall invasion and of celiac and gastro-hepatic lymph nodes, liver, adrenals, and perito-neum.[1,5] EUS is also of limited value in differentiating between malignant and inflammatory processes in lymph nodes, as well as for identifying distant metastatic sites.[1,2,7] CT is the modality routinely used for assessment of nodal and distant involvement, limited by the use of size-based criteria to define abnormal lymph nodes, and has an overall accuracy of 50–60%.[1]

Although most esophageal cancers demonstrate high $^{18}$F-FDG uptake on pre-therapy studies,[2,6] $^{18}$F-FDG PET has been used for T staging only on a limited scale, in patients in whom EUS and CT cannot adequately assess the primary tumor.[2] Pre-therapy $^{18}$F-FDG imaging provides data of prognostic significance, with higher uptake within the primary tumor predicting worse prognosis.[2]

A meta-analysis of 12 studies reported a low overall accuracy, ranging between 46 and 61%, for assessment of loco-regional N stage by $^{18}$F-FDG PET, with sensitivity and specificity of 51 and 84%, respectively.[2,6] This relatively low sensitivity is attributed to factors such as masking of nodal $^{18}$F-FDG uptake by high intensity adjacent activity in the primary tumor, or in physiologically tracer-avid organs as well as by the inability of PET to detect microscopic nodal disease.[6,9] While the superiority of EUS over $^{18}$F-FDG PET for T staging has been demonstrated, the comparative role of these imaging modalities for nodal staging is less clear.[2,7]

The use of PET/CT improves the diagnosis of clinically significant tracer uptake in the vicinity of the primary $^{18}$F-FDG-avid tumor or adjacent to physiologic sites of increased activity.[9,10] In a prospective study comparing pre-surgical loco-regional lymph node staging by PET/CT to side-by-side review of PET and CT, PET/CT correctly defined 67% of false-negative and 38% of false-positive sites on PET.[10]

At initial staging of esophageal cancer, the main advantage of $^{18}$F-FDG imaging over conventional imaging is its ability to accurately detect distant metastases. $^{18}$F-FDG imaging may detect distant metastases not diagnosed by other modalities, mainly located in bone, liver, and cervical nodes, in 4–28% of patients, for a high specificity of

82–99%.[1,2,6,7] $^{18}$F-FDG PET has been reported to significantly impact management of 6–40% patients with newly diagnosed esophageal cancer, mainly by excluding patients from futile surgery.[7,11,12] PET/CT has been shown to have a further incremental value over side-by-side review of stand-alone PET and CT, inducing a change in management of an additional 11% of patients.[7]

Differentiating between non-regional nodal (M1a) and distant organ metastatic spread (M1b) is important. Although it indicates a worse prognosis than N1 disease, patients with M1a disease have a somewhat better outcome than those with M1b disease.[6] Although challenging, both EUS and PET/CT can be helpful in solving such clinical dilemmas.[6] In spite of the high specificity of $^{18}$F-FDG imaging for M staging of esophageal cancer, confirmation of PET positive sites is warranted prior to cancelling a potentially curable procedure.[6,13]

For detection of distant metastases, $^{18}$F-FDG PET showed a pooled sensitivity and specificity of 67 and 97%, respectively, in summarized data of 12 studies,[13] superior to CT and EUS, leading to a change in pre-therapy staging in 19% of patients.[13] A more limited contribution than previously described for initial staging has been reported for $^{18}$F-FDG PET in a recent prospective study of 199 patients considered for curative surgery of esophageal cancer.[14] PET detected previously unrecognized distant metastases and upstaged disease in only 4% of patients, all with advanced disease, and prevented futile surgery in 3%.[14] This relatively low benefit of PET was attributed to the extensive pre-operative evaluation by conventional protocol preceding the performance of PET, and to the prospective nature of the study evaluating a wide range of disease stages.[14]

Wallace and colleagues[15] compared the cost-effectiveness of six different pre-operative staging strategies of esophageal cancer, using CT, EUS with FNA (EUS + FNA), thoracoscopy and laparoscopy (TL), and PET. The combined CT and EUS + FNA strategy was associated with the lowest cost. However, the combination of PET with EUS + FNA, although slightly more expensive, provided the most effective pre-surgical staging measured in quality-adjusted-life years. This highest efficiency was mainly due to the higher sensitivity of PET for detecting distant metastases as well as the ability to perform biopsy for tissue diagnosis, thus reducing the rate of false-positive studies, subsequently resulting in improved selection of patients for surgery. Staging by $^{18}$F-FDG imaging provides more accurate prognostic data than CT. The survival rate of patients with only local disease on PET was significantly higher when compared to that of patients with distant $^{18}$F-FDG-avid metastases, 60% versus 20%, respectively.[16] In addition, synchronous malignancies can be found in 2–6% of patients with newly diagnosed esophageal cancer, and PET/CT, when performed at presentation, has the whole-body capabilities to detect second primary tumors that occur mainly in the region of the head and neck, lung, and colon.[6,7,14]

## $^{18}$F-FDG Imaging for Monitoring Response to Treatment of Esophageal Cancer

Neoadjuvant chemo-radiotherapy of locally advanced esophageal cancer aims at reducing the volume of the primary tumor and at eradicating micrometastases, thus enabling further complete resection. Patients who respond to neoadjuvant treatment have a higher chance to benefit from surgical resection.

After treatment, anatomic imaging modalities cannot accurately differentiate between viable tumor and residual fibrotic mass. The sensitivity and specificity of CT for predicting pathologic response to neoadjuvant therapy ranges between 33–55% and 50–70%, respectively.[3] [18]F-FDG PET can specifically detect viable residual tumor and can therefore assess response of both the primary tumor and of nodal metastatic disease. Metabolic response on [18]F-FDG PET, assessed by percent of change in standardized uptake value (SUV) or by a single point SUV measurement after treatment, has been found as an accurate predictor of response.[1,3,6,13,17] [18]F-FDG PET is more accurate than CT and equivalent to EUS for assessing response, with a joint sensitivity of approximately 85% for these modalities versus 54% for CT.[7,18]

In assessing response to treatment, [18]F-FDG imaging may be impaired by false-positive uptake in sites of reactive inflammation, post-treatment esophagitis, and ulceration.[6] False-negative results may occur in the presence of microscopic nodal metastases or in tumors with low initial [18]F-FDG avidity (more frequent in adenocarcinoma than in squamous cell carcinoma), and in cervical and abdominal lymph node metastases as compared with thoracic and peritumoral nodes.[3] A low performance of [18]F-FDG PET/CT has been reported in a recent study assessing response to neoadjuvant therapy in 88 patients planned for surgical resection. PET was unable to predict the presence of residual pathologic disease in the primary tumor or loco-regional lymph nodes.[19] Overall, multimodality assessment of esophageal cancer using PET/CT in combination with EUS-FNA has been suggested as the optimal strategy to evaluate treatment response and for directing further clinical decisions.[3]

## [18]F-FDG Imaging for Diagnosis of Recurrent Esophageal Cancer

Detection of recurrent esophageal cancer by conventional anatomic imaging modalities such as CT, EUS, and MRI is suboptimal due to the limitations of these modalities in differentiating between treatment-related structural changes and recurrent cancer. [18]F-FDG imaging can specifically identify viable tumor tissue even within a region of scar and fibrosis. PET/CT provides the precise localization of increased [18]F-FDG uptake and enables the diagnosis of active tumor within regions of post-therapy distorted anatomy, mainly in the cervical and abdomino-pelvic region.[9] [18]F-FDG imaging allowed detection of recurrent esophageal cancer in approximately one of four patients, in sites not seen on CT, or outside the field of conventional follow-up protocols.[6,20] PET/CT is valuable mainly for the detection of recurrent esophageal carcinoma in regional and distant sites.[21] [18]F-FDG PET/CT had a sensitivity, specificity, and accuracy of 93, 76, and 87%, respectively, for detecting all sites of recurrence in 56 patients with a suspected recurrent cancer of the esophagus assessed after definitive treatment.[21] Intensity of uptake at the site of recurrence and its extent on PET/CT were independent prognostic factors for overall survival.[21] PET/CT improved the specificity and accuracy of stand-alone PET for detecting esophageal cancer from 59 and 83% to 81 and 90%, respectively, with impact on further management of 10% of patients.[9]

## [18]F-FDG Imaging in Gastric Cancer

### Introduction

Gastric cancer is the second most frequent cause for malignancy-related death worldwide, with higher incidence in the Far East, where it represents the most frequent type of malignant tumor.[22] Most tumors are adenocarcinomas, often associated with *Helicobacter pylori* infection. The intestinal tumor subtype forms gland-like structures and affects mainly elderly patients, while the non-intestinal diffuse type is poorly differentiated and related to a genetic pre-disposition.[23,24]

The only effective curative therapy in patients with cancer of the stomach is complete resection of the primary tumor and of adjacent lymph nodes, which is possible in only a small fraction of patients, since advanced stage disease is found at presentation in about 80% of cases.[22] EUS and CT are the main imaging modalities for pre-operative staging and follow-up. Limiting factors of these imaging modalities are related to their ability to diagnose metastatic disease in small lymph nodes or peritoneal spread.[22]

Only relatively scarce literature data report on the use of $^{18}$F-FDG imaging in gastric carcinoma. $^{18}$F-FDG PET is useful for pre-therapy assessment of the presence of distant metastatic spread, involving mainly the liver, lungs, adrenals, ovaries, and skeleton. $^{18}$F-FDG imaging is of limited value for T staging as well as for assessment of loco-regional lymph node involvement.[22] $^{18}$F-FDG PET may have potential advantages for assessing early response to chemotherapy,[22] which may in turn enable stratification of therapy according to the individual patient response. This may become of increased clinical significance with the development of new treatment strategies, including endoscopic mucosal resection and aggressive systemic neoadjuvant and adjuvant treatment protocols.[22]

## $^{18}$F-FDG Imaging for Diagnosis and Staging of Gastric Cancer

The use of $^{18}$F-FDG imaging for diagnosis of gastric cancer is limited by the variable degree of tracer uptake, with overall reported sensitivity and detectability rates ranging between 48 and 94%.[22,25,26] Uptake of $^{18}$F-FDG in a gastric tumor is related to the depth of invasion and to the histological subtype of the gastric tumor, with lower tracer avidity described in diffusely growing and mucous-containing malignancies. Histological subtypes such as mucinous, signet ring cell and non-solid, poorly differentiated carcinoma have lower $^{18}$F-FDG-avidity as compared with papillary or tubular adenocarcinoma.[22,24–26]

Accurate tumor, nodes, metastases (TNM) staging is highly important for providing the patient with the most appropriate and potentially effective treatment, as well as for avoiding futile, invasive, or toxic therapy.[22] Accurate T staging with good definition of tumor invasion through and beyond the gastric wall is the most significant factor in determining the further treatment approach. EUS is the modality of choice for this purpose, with a diagnostic accuracy of 78–93%.[22] CT plays at present a limited role, but may be more efficient with the introduction of advanced techniques. The use of $^{18}$F-FDG imaging for T staging of gastric cancer has not yet been demonstrated.

Precise anatomic lymph node localization is important for pre-operative staging, since surgical exploration differs according to the involvement of specific nodal groups.[22] CT is currently the modality of choice for nodal staging in gastric carcinoma. $^{18}$F-FDG imaging can detect malignant involvement of small lymph nodes or exclude the presence of suspected malignancy in enlarged nodes. $^{18}$F-FDG PET has been reported to have a lower sensitivity but higher specificity than CT for detecting metastatic spread to various nodal stations.[27] As with esophageal cancer, $^{18}$F-FDG imaging may be limited in the assessment of nodes adjacent to an $^{18}$F-FDG-avid primary tumor, as is the case with perigastric nodes or those located along the left gastric and common hepatic artery or celiac trunk.[22] Careful assessment of hybrid PET/CT images solves most of these difficulties. Also, the nodes of highest clinical significance are those located remote from the primary tumor. These nodal stations can be efficiently detected by [18]F-FDG imaging.[22] At present, only limited systematic literature data regarding the performance of [18]F-FDG PET for nodal staging of gastric cancer have been published.

The main advantage of [18]F-FDG imaging over CT in staging of gastric cancer is its ability to detect distant metastases because of its high sensitivity and contrast, and its whole-body scanning range. Distant metastases commonly involve lymph nodes in the supraclavicular region or are located in the abdomen, in peripancreatic nodes distal to the stomach, and adjacent to the head of the pancreas, as well as in mesenteric and para-aortic stations. Distant metastases in solid organs are less frequent.[22] [18]F-FDG imaging is the most sensitive non-invasive diagnostic modality for assessment of hepatic metastases from colorectal, gastric, and esophageal cancer.[28] [18]F-FDG PET is also highly accurate for detecting lung and lymph node metastases and is more sensitive than CT for detection of peritoneal carcinomatosis[22] in spite of its overall poor sensitivity for the detection of peritoneal or pleural carcinomatosis and bone metastases.[23]

## [18]F-FDG Imaging for Monitoring Response to Treatment of Gastric Cancer

Since most gastric cancers are not measurable on CT, it is difficult to use this modality for assessing local response to treatment. [18]F-FDG uptake was shown to predict early response of cancer of the stomach to pre-operative chemotherapy.[29] In a prospective evaluation of 35 patients with [18]F-FDG-avid, locally advanced gastric carcinoma, changes in tracer uptake before and at 14 days after initiation of neoadjuvant chemotherapy predicted the histologic response at 3 months of therapy, with a sensitivity and specificity of 77 and 86%, respectively.[29] A metabolic response, defined as a greater than 35% reduction in SUV in the tracer uptake of the primary tumor, indicated a 2-year survival rate of 90% as compared with 25% in metabolic non-responders.[29]

The possibility to tailor treatment plans according to early metabolic response was further assessed in a prospective trial of 110 patients with locally advanced adenocarcinoma of the gastroesophageal junction.[30] Responders on PET after 2 weeks of neoadjuvant therapy completed 12 weeks of chemotherapy before proceeding to surgery, while non-responders were operated without any further systemic treatment. Major histologic response with less than 10% residual tumor on pathology was found in 58% of metabolic responders but in none of the non-responders. Response on PET was also associated with a significant better overall and event-free median survival.[30]

## [18]F-FDG Imaging for Diagnosis of Recurrent Gastric Cancer

Recurrent gastric carcinoma has a poor prognosis but may respond to chemo- or radio-therapy if diagnosed with a small tumor load. CT is limited in areas of treatment-related structural changes, at the site of the anastomosis, or in areas of bowel loop adhesions.[22] Equivocal findings on CT can be further clarified assessing their $^{18}$F-FDG avidity.[22,31–34] On the other hand, limiting factors for the use of $^{18}$F-FDG imaging in diagnosis of recurrent gastric cancer are related to low $^{18}$F-FDG uptake in certain tumor types and small size of recurrent or metastatic sites.[22]

# $^{18}$F-FDG Imaging in Gastrointestinal Stromal Tumors

## Introduction

Gastrointestinal stromal tumor (GIST) is a stromal or connective tissue tumor that arises from the interstitial cells of Cajal (ICC), considered as the pacemaker cells of the gastrointestinal tract (GIT).[35–38] Although a rare tumor, less than 1% of all gastrointestinal malignancies, it is the most common mesenchymal tumor of the GIT, representing 5% of all sarcomas, with an estimated annual incidence of 10–20 cases per million.[35–37] Accurate data regarding the true incidence and prevalence of GIST are still limited, as the origin and differentiation of this tumor have been clarified only recently.[35] The distinct feature of this tumor is the expression of the KIT protein, a transmembrane tyrosine kinase receptor. A gain-of-function mutation in the KIT gene, with activation of tyrosine kinase and subsequent uncontrolled cell proliferation, is considered the early crucial event promoting tumor development.[36] This genomic characterization has led to the development of novel molecularly targeted therapy of GIST, imatinib mesylate (Gleevec®), a KIT-receptor selective tyrosine kinase inhibitor.[36]

GIST presents with a wide clinical spectrum ranging from benign, incidentally detected nodules, to large symptomatic malignant tumors.[37,38] It is most common in the stomach (40–70%), followed by the small intestine (20–40%), and colon and rectum (5–15%) and is less frequent in the esophagus, omentum, mesentery, and retroperitoneum.[36] Metastatic disease is found in up to 50% of patients at presentation, almost exclusively intra-abdominal and involving mainly the liver and peritoneum.[36]

The malignant potential of GIST is variable, and the precise definition of its malignancy criteria is still evolving.[36,37] While all GIST tumors are considered to have some malignant potential, the only certain indication today of its degree of malignancy is the presence of metastatic spread at initial diagnosis. Tumor size and mitotic index are also considered to represent predicting factors of tumor malignancy.[35,36,39]

Complete aggressive surgery is the treatment of choice in patients with localized GIST and should include resection of the primary tumor en bloc with normal soft tissue or bowel margins. A higher median survival rate was reported in patients who underwent complete resection of GIST, 46 months, as compared with only 21 months for incomplete resection.[37] While radio- and chemotherapy are ineffective in unresectable, locally advanced, or metastatic disease,[36,37] Gleevec® is a new highly effective treatment, inducing early and durable response.[35,36] Up to 80% of patients show some response or stable disease, with only 11–14% showing drug resistance and tumor progression.[36] Response is usually durable for periods ranging from several months to a few years before the development of secondary drug resistance.[36] The use of this drug in a neoadjuvant and adjuvant setting after complete macroscopic resection of a malignant GIST or its metastases is currently under investigation.[36]

## $^{18}$F-FDG Imaging at Initial Diagnosis of GIST

Since most GIST are submucosal endophytic tumors growing parallel to the bowel lumen, with overlying mucosal necrosis and ulceration, tissue diagnosis by endoscopy may be difficult and is often obtained only during surgery.[36] CT and MRI are used for delineation of the extension of the primary tumor and its metastatic spread, and demonstrate, as a rule, slightly enhancing lesions with areas of necrosis. Accurate assessment of poorly defined tumors may be difficult on CT, such as bowel, peritoneum, or bone metastases.[36]

There are only scarce literature data regarding the role of $^{18}$F-FDG PET at the initial diagnosis and staging of GIST. $^{18}$F-FDG uptake in GIST is widely variable, generally of moderate to high intensity, with a wide range of SUV values between 2 and 24.8.[39,40] A significant correlation between the intensity of $^{18}$F-FDG uptake and the malignant potential of GIST, as defined by conventional accepted criteria of size, mitotic rate, and the presence of metastases, has been reported.[39] Metabolic information provided by $^{18}$F-FDG imaging may be clinically significant in the setting of adjuvant treatment or follow-up after surgery.

False-positive $^{18}$F-FDG-avid sites are related to physiologic uptake in the region of the gastroesophageal junction and the ascending colon. False-negative lesions have been described in metastases with a newly acquired mutation of the KIT gene, leading to tumor resistance to treatment.[41]

Hybrid PET/CT has an incremental value for imaging of GIST, with CT detecting more lesions than PET and guiding the planning of surgical procedures.[38]

## $^{18}$F-FDG Imaging for Monitoring Response to Treatment of GIST

CT and MRI are routinely used for follow-up after surgery and for monitoring response to Gleevec® therapy. Decrease in lesion size, which is indicative of tumor response, occurs, if at all, only late after therapy, as the reduction of the viable tumor cell fraction may be masked by intratumoral bleeding, accumulation of necrotic or fibrotic tissue, and myxoid degeneration of the tumor.[36,40] Morphologic imaging is therefore performed only at 2–3 months after initiation of therapy. In contrast, GIST response to Gleevec® is associated with a rapid reduction in $^{18}$F-FDG uptake reported to occur within a few hours or days after the institution of Gleevec® treatment,[36] thus preceding changes in conventional response criteria by several weeks.[36]

A pre-treatment study is mandatory in order to allow accurate assessment of the tumor response to Gleevec®. Metabolic response reflected by decreased $^{18}$F-FDG uptake 1–2 months after therapy has been found to be predictive of patient outcome and progression-free survival (PFS).[38,40,42] The definition of response on CT is more difficult since response may be reflected by changes of small range in tumor size and density.[42] Preliminary data indicate, however, that the metabolic response measured by $^{18}$F-FDG uptake may not reflect complete pathologic response and should not be used to exclude surgical resection of $^{18}$F-FDG-negative residual masses after treatment.[43]

While Gleevec® is at present the only treatment option in metastatic GIST and early assessment of response to Gleevec® may not be crucial in this group of patients, future expansion of Gleevec® therapy indications to the neoadjuvant setting will demand the need of an early assessment of response in order to enable efficient selection of responding patients for surgery.[40]

Long-term follow-up is mandatory for all patients with GIST since metastases may appear even decades after initial treatment.[37] Overall recurrence rates of 76 and 64% have been reported in gastric and intestinal GIST, respectively.[37] Recurrence occurs mainly at the primary site, in the liver, and peritoneum. CT has been shown to detect more metastatic lesions than $^{18}$F-FDG PET before therapy, with 20% of lesions 1–4.7 cm in diameter seen only on CT.[44] PET/CT was of value in the assessment of 34 patients with GIST, most of them after surgery or Gleevec® therapy, mainly for delineation of the whole extent of disease and for directing further surgical procedures.[38]

## Guidelines and Recommendations for the Use of $^{18}$F-FDG PET and PET/CT in Esophageal Cancer

The National Comprehensive Cancer Network (NCCN) has incorporated $^{18}$F-FDG PET and PET/CT in the evaluation and management algorithm of a variety of malignancies including esophageal cancer.[45] The use of $^{18}$F-FDG PET (PET/CT where available) is recommended in the following clinical scenarios:

(1) For initial staging if there is no evidence of distant metastatic disease by conventional imaging.
(2) To monitor pre-operative neoadjuvant chemoradiation therapy.

A multidisciplinary panel of experts reviewed meta-analyses and systematic reviews published in the FDG-PET literature before March 2006 and made recommendations for the use of $^{18}$F-FDG PET in oncology.[46] The panel concluded that $^{18}$F-FDG PET should routinely be used as an additional tool for staging esophageal cancer.

# Case Presentations

## Case II.6.1 (DICOM Images on DVD)

### History

This 46-year-old man presenting with dysphagia and weight loss was diagnosed with poorly differentiated carcinoma of the distal esophagus. CT demonstrated prominent thickening of the distal esophagus, an enlarged gastro-hepatic lymph node with central necrosis, a small lung nodule in the right middle lobe, mild mediastinal (retrocaval, left pre-vascular, and subcarinal) lymphadenopathy, and a well-circumscribed small sclerotic lesion in the right iliac wing. PET/CT was performed for initial staging (Fig. II.6.1A–C).

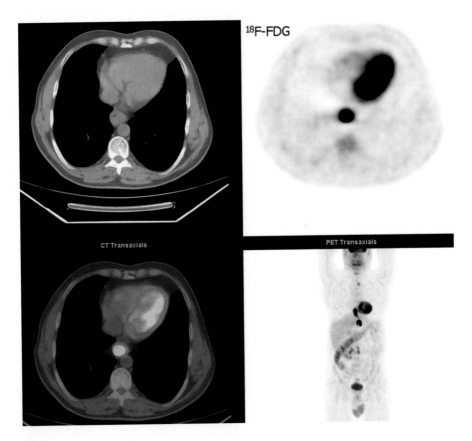

Fig. II.6.1A

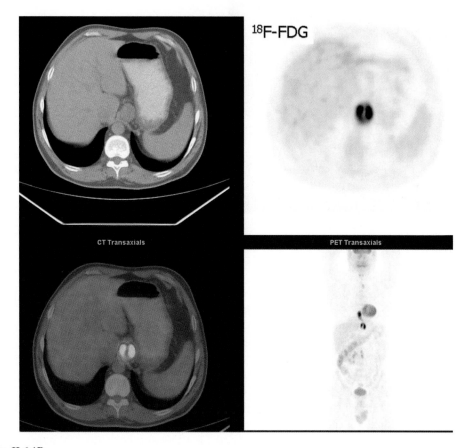

**Fig. II.6.1B**

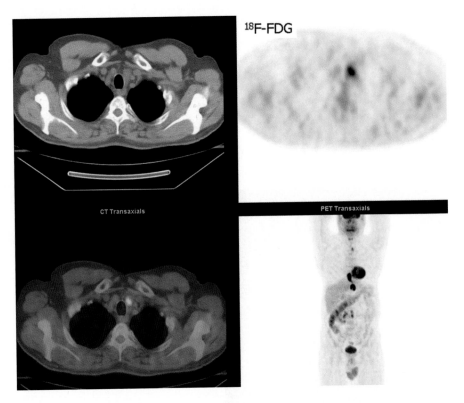

**Fig. II.6.1C**

## Findings

There is intense [18]F-FDG uptake within the prominently thickened wall of the distal esophagus with eccentric lumen, consistent with the primary carcinoma (Fig. II.6.1A). An additional focus of intense uptake with a central photon deficient area is seen in the mid-upper abdomen, corresponding to a 28 × 20 mm enlarged hypodense lymph node at the level of the gastro-hepatic ligament (Fig. II.6.1B). A small focus of moderately increased [18]F-FDG uptake is seen in a 1.8 × 1 cm left pretracheal lymph node at the level of the thoracic inlet, retrospectively identified on CT (Fig. II.6.1C). There is another small focus of uptake corresponding to a 4 mm left paratracheal lymph node more inferiorly and just anterior to the esophagus (not shown). There is no abnormal [18]F-FDG uptake in the lungs, mediastinum, and skeleton. The area of increased [18]F-FDG uptake in the right paramedian mid-abdomen corresponds to a horseshoe kidney with crossed ectopia of the left kidney (maximum intensity projection [MIP]).

## Discussion

Highly intense [18]F-FDG uptake in the distal thoracic esophagus is consistent with the known primary tumor. Although [18]F-FDG PET is of limited value for T staging, the intensity of [18]F-FDG uptake within the primary tumor has been reported to be a predictor of prognosis, with tumors showing at presentation SUVmax higher than 6.6 having a shorter survival as compared with tumors with lower uptake.[7]

A loco-regional metastasis in an enlarged, partially necrotic lymph node at the level of the gastro-hepatic ligament was detected on both PET and CT, defining N1 disease. In tumors involving the lower thoracic esophagus, it may be challenging but very important, to differentiate between nodal metastases in the gastro-hepatic ligament, considered regional nodal spread (N1), and celiac lymph node involvement, which is defined as distant, non-regional disease (M1a), rendering the tumor as non-resectable.[6]

In present case, CT had initially identified only N1 disease involving gastro-hepatic ligament nodes. The additional $^{18}$F-FDG-avid focus located on PET/CT in a mildly enlarged left pretracheal lymph node represents a distant, previously unrecognized non-regional lymph node metastasis (M1a), thus defining the patient as having stage IVA disease. The patient was spared previously planned surgery and received chemotherapy. He died with progressive disease12 months later.

The main advantage of $^{18}$F-FDG imaging in the initial staging of esophageal cancer is the potential detection of previously unrecognized distant metastases, thus obviating futile surgery in patients with advanced disease. In a prospective study of 91 patients with cancer of the esophagus considered for surgical resection, $^{18}$F-FDG PET was more accurate than CT for M staging detecting previously unsuspected distant metastases in 17% of patients.[15] In a more recent study of 74 patients with potentially resectable esophageal cancer, $^{18}$F-FDG PET had a sensitivity of 74% for detecting distant metastases in supraclavicular and retroperitoneal lymph nodes as compared to only 47% for combined CT and EUS assessment.[11] $^{18}$F-FDG imaging upstaged 15% and downstaged 7% of patients, changing management in 22% of the study population.[11] Duong and colleagues[12] compared planning of the therapeutic strategy in esophageal cancer before and after performing $^{18}$F-FDG PET in 68 patients. PET results had an impact on the management of 40% of patients, mainly by avoiding initially planned curative surgery.

## Diagnosis

1. Carcinoma of the distal esophagus.
2. Loco-regional metastatic adenopathy at the level of the gastro-hepatic ligament.
3. Distant non-regional left pretracheal lymph node metastasis.

## Clinical Report: Body FDG-PET/CT (for DVD cases only)

Indication

Initial staging of poorly differentiated carcinoma of the distal esophagus.

History

This 46-year-old man presenting with dysphagia and weight loss was diagnosed with poorly differentiated carcinoma of the distal esophagus. CT demonstrated prominent thickening of the distal esophagus, an enlarged gastro-hepatic lymph node with central necrosis, a small lung nodule in the right middle lobe, mild mediastinal (retrocaval, left pre-vascular, and subcarinal) lymphadenopathy, and a well-circumscribed small sclerotic lesion in the right iliac wing. PET/CT was performed for initial staging.

Procedure

The fasting blood glucose level was 76 mg/dl. $^{18}$F-FDG, 666 MBq (18 mCi), was administered intravenously in the right antecubital fossa. After an uptake time of 120 min and
administration of oral contrast, just prior to starting the study, whole-body low-dose CT
was acquired to correct for attenuation and anatomic localization, followed by PET
images acquired over the neck, thorax, abdomen, and pelvis. The patient was positioned
with arms up.


Findings

*Quality of the study*: The quality of this study is good.

*Neck*: There is physiologic $^{18}$F-FDG uptake in lymphoid and glandular tissues of the
  neck and in both vocal cords.

*Chest*: There is intense physiologic myocardial uptake. There is a large focus of intense
  $^{18}$F-FDG uptake within the prominently thickened wall of the distal esophagus with
  eccentric lumen, consistent with the known primary tumor. There is a focus of
  moderately increased $^{18}$F-FDG uptake in an 18 × 10 mm left pretracheal lymph
  node at the level of the thoracic inlet, most probably consistent with a distant
  lymph node metastasis. There is another small focus of uptake corresponding to a
  4 mm left paratracheal lymph node more inferiorly and just anterior to the esophagus,
  also consistent with a metastasis.
  In addition, there are several small mediastinal lymph nodes in the retrocaval, left
  pre-vascular, and subcarinal region, the latter being the largest, with no $^{18}$F-FDG
  uptake. There is a 3 mm lung nodule in the right middle lobe with no FDG uptake.

*Abdomen and pelvis*: There is a large focus of intense uptake with a photon deficient
  center, in a 28 × 20 mm enlarged hypodense lymph node at the level of the gastro-
  hepatic ligament, consistent with a loco-regional lymph node metastasis.
  An additional area of inhomogenous $^{18}$F-FDG uptake is seen in the right paramedian
  mid-abdomen, corresponding to a horseshoe kidney with crossed ectopia of the left
  kidney. The prostate is moderately enlarged, with no significant $^{18}$F-FDG uptake.

*Musculoskeletal*: A sclerotic bone island is seen in the right iliac wing, with no significant
  $^{18}$F-FDG uptake.


Impression

1. Distal esophageal carcinoma.
2. Loco-regional metastatic adenopathy at the gastro-hepatic ligament.
3. Distant left pre- and paratracheal lymph node metastases.
4. Additional CT findings as described earlier.

## Case II.6.2

### History

This 74-year-old asymptomatic male presented with a history of adenocarcinoma of the distal esophagus treated with total esophagectomy with gastric pull-through 4 years earlier. $^{18}$F-FDG PET/CT was performed to assess the possibility of recurrence (Fig. II.6.2).

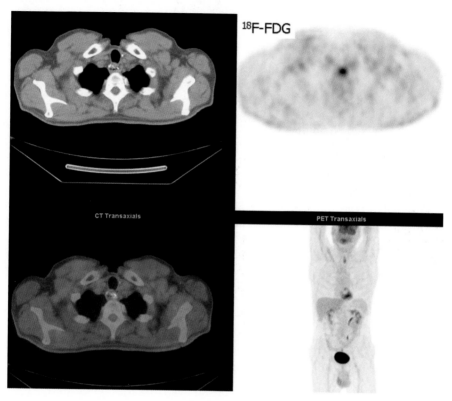

Fig. II.6.2

### Findings

There is a focus of moderately increased $^{18}$F-FDG uptake at the posterior, midline aspect of the thoracic inlet, localized on PET/CT to the upper anastomosis without a corresponding anatomic lesion on CT.

### Discussion

Focal $^{18}$F-FDG uptake at the site of the anastomosis in a patient with a history of esophageal cancer should be considered suspicious of local recurrence. Most recurrences of esophageal cancer occur within the first 2 years after diagnosis.[21] Since there was no clinical or other imaging evidence for recurrent disease, the focus of increased $^{18}$F-FDG activity was considered equivocal, and further diagnostic endoscopic investigation with biopsy of the anastomosis was recommended. The patient refused endoscopy and was followed clinically and by CT, with no evidence for recurrent cancer during a follow-up of 24 months. The focus of [18]F-FDG uptake was therefore considered to be due to physiologic [18]F-FDG uptake within the intrathoracic displaced stomach or, less probably, due to a transient benign inflammatory process at this site.

Detection of local recurrence of esophageal cancer is challenging in the presence of post-therapy structural distortion, or when small foci of disease occur in distant or loco-regional sites. Flamen and colleagues[20] evaluated the role of [18]F-FDG PET for diagnosis of recurrence after curative resection in 41 patients with esophageal cancer. [18]F-FDG PET had a sensitivity of 100% for the diagnosis of perianastomotic recurrence, but its specificity of 50% was significantly lower than that for distant metastases of 93%. False-positive increased [18]F-FDG uptake was found at sites of progressive anastomotic stenosis requiring repetitive endoscopic dilatation. In a recent study of 56 patients with previously treated esophageal squamous cell carcinoma, [18]F-FDG PET/CT was found to play a significant role for detecting recurrence, with a sensitivity, specificity, and accuracy for diagnosis of local recurrence of 97, 50, and 84%, for regional recurrence of 89, 82, and 87%, and for distant metastases of 91, 93, and 91%, respectively.[21] Six of nine false-positive sites were located at the site of the esophago-gastric anastomosis and in a gastric pull-up, representing gastroesophageal reflux or a post-surgical reactive inflammation.

In the present case, PET/CT allowed for the precise localization of the focus of increased [18]F-FDG activity to the anastomotic site at the level of the thoracic inlet. In a study of 41 patients with esophageal cancer, most of them assessed after surgery, [18]F-FDG PET/CT had an incremental value over separate assessment of PET and CT in 22% of suspicious sites.[9] While [18]F-FDG imaging has a high sensitivity for diagnosis and accurate whole-body staging of symptomatic recurrent esophageal cancer, its role in the surveillance of asymptomatic patients is still to be determined.[20]

**Diagnosis**

Increased focal [18]F-FDG uptake at the site of the upper anastomosis, most probably due to physiologic gastric uptake or a mild inflammatory process.

## Case II.6.3 (DICOM Images on DVD)

### History

This is a 72-year-old man diagnosed with poorly differentiated gastric carcinoma in the body of the stomach. Chest and abdomino-pelvic CT were negative, except for a prominent thickening of the gastric wall at the level of the fundus and along the lesser curvature of the gastric body, and thickening of the cecal wall of unclear significance. $^{18}$F-FDG PET/CT was performed for staging before surgery (Fig. II.6.3A, B). A repeated PET/CT study was performed for restaging 7 months later (Fig. II.6.3C, D).

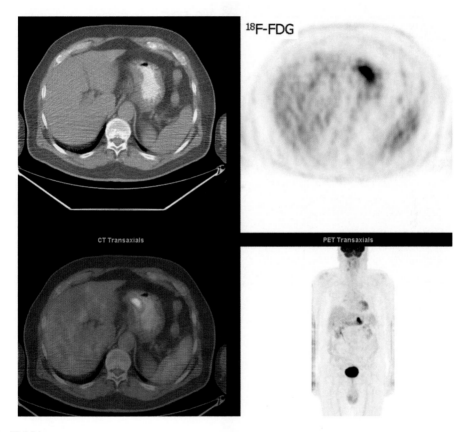

Fig. II.6.3A

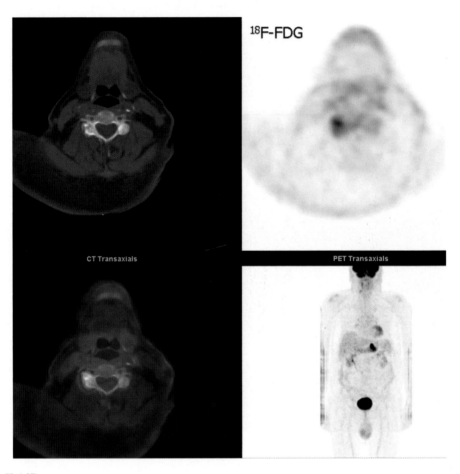

Fig. II.6.3B

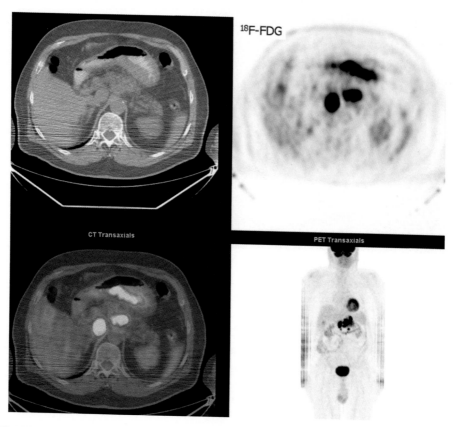

Fig. II.6.3C

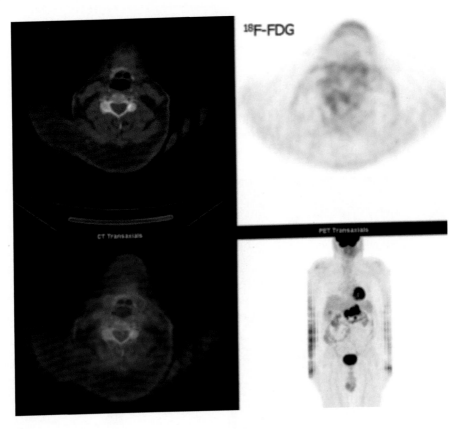

**Fig. II.6.3D**

## Findings

There is prominent abnormal [18]F-FDG uptake in the thickened wall of the lesser curvature of the gastric body (Fig. II.6.3A), consistent with the known primary tumor. An additional focus of abnormal [18]F-FDG uptake is seen in the right upper cervical region localized by fused PET/CT images to degenerative changes seen on CT in the right facet joint of C-4 (Fig. II.6.3B). There is no abnormal [18]F-FDG uptake in the caecum.

The patient refused surgery. A repeated [18]F-FDG PET/CT study was performed for restaging 7 months later (Fig. II.6.3C, D) and showed significant disease progression in the primary gastric tumor, which increased in intensity of [18]F-[18]F-FDG uptake and in tumor size on CT, and multiple new foci of abnormal [18]F-FDG uptake in the upper abdomen, corresponding to loco-regional and distant lymphadenopathy in gastro-hepatic, celiac, and left retroperitoneal lymph nodes (Fig. II.6.3C). The focus of [18]F-FDG uptake previously seen in the C-4 vertebra has decreased significantly in intensity (Fig. II.6.3D).

## Discussion

At presentation, the findings are consistent with an [18]F-FDG-avid primary gastric carcinoma (in the body of the stomach), with no evidence for loco-regional or distant metastatic disease. The majority of patients with gastric cancer presents with advanced disease at initial diagnosis, mainly with metastases to lymph nodes. Solid distant metastases are infrequent at initial presentation, but may involve the liver, lungs, adrenals, bones, and ovaries.[22] $^{18}$F-FDG imaging was found useful for the diagnosis of distant metastases in gastric cancer. Yoshioka and colleagues[23] assessed 42 patients with advanced, metastatic, or recurrent gastric carcinoma and found that $^{18}$F-FDG PET was highly accurate for detection of nodal, liver, and lung metastases (75–86%). This modality had, however, a lesion-based accuracy of only 57% for diagnosis of bone metastases, although in a small number of patients. Bone scintigraphy had a higher sensitivity than $^{18}$F-FDG PET for defining the whole extent of skeletal involvement, in spite of the $^{18}$F-FDG-avidity of osteolytic lesions demonstrated on radiography.[23]

The focus of increased $^{18}$F-FDG uptake in the neck may be suspicious for metastasis in a cervical lymph node or in the spine on PET-only evaluation. PET/CT provides the anatomic landmarks needed for precise location of this suspicious lesion and its characterization in view of the corresponding structural changes on CT. The increased $^{18}$F-FDG uptake in the cervical spine is attributed to an inflammatory reaction related to degenerative changes. This is confirmed on the follow-up PET/CT study on which vertebral uptake resolved, while the malignant foci of tracer uptake in the primary tumor showed progression, and in new regional and non-regional nodal metastases became evident. Degenerative spinal disease may demonstrate increased $^{18}$F-FDG uptake, related probably to the presence of an inflammatory reaction. In a retrospective review of PET/CT studies of 150 patients with known or suspected malignancy, $^{18}$F-FDG uptake in areas of degenerative disk and facet disease was observed in 22% of cases, with highly intense uptake in 11%.[33] The severity of PET findings correlated with the severity of degenerative disease as graded by CT.

## Diagnosis

1. Primary gastric cancer.
2. Degenerative cervical spine disease.
3. No evidence of metastatic disease.

## Clinical Report: Body FDG-PET/CT (for DVD cases only)

Indication

Initial staging of poorly differentiated gastric carcinoma.

History

The patient is a 72-year-old man with poorly differentiated gastric carcinoma in the body of the stomach diagnosed by biopsy on gastroscopy. Chest and abdomino-pelvic CT were negative, except for prominent thickening of the gastric wall at the level of the fundus and along the lesser curvature of the gastric body, and thickening of the caecal wall of unclear significance. The patient was referred for staging before surgery.

Procedure

Oral contrast was administered prior to the study. The fasting blood glucose level was 77 mg/dl. $^{18}$F-FDG, 444 MBq (12 mCi), was administered intravenously, in the right hand. After 90 min distribution time, a whole-body low-dose CT scan was acquired to correct for attenuation and anatomic localization, followed by PET images acquired over the neck, thorax, abdomen, and pelvis. The patient was positioned with arms along the torso.

Findings

*Quality of the study*: The quality of this study is good.

*Neck*: There is physiologic $^{18}$F-FDG uptake in the occipital cerebral cortex and in lymphoid and glandular tissues in the neck. There is a mild diffuse enlargement of the thyroid on CT with no increased $^{18}$F-FDG uptake. A focus of moderately increased $^{18}$F-FDG uptake is seen in the right upper cervical region, corresponding to degenerative changes seen on CT within the right facet joint of C4.

*Chest*: Mild $^{18}$F-FDG uptake is seen in both lung hila with no corresponding findings on CT, representing benign tracer activity in a chronic granulomatotic process or in antracotic nodes in this 72-year-old past smoker patient.

On CT there is an enlarged calcified retrocaval pretracheal lymph node showing no $^{18}$F-FDG uptake. In addition, a pacemaker implanted in the left chest wall with the distal end of the electrode within the right ventricle is demonstrated, with no $^{18}$F-FDG uptake.

*Abdomen and pelvis*: There is a focal area of intense $^{18}$F-FDG uptake in the thickened wall of the lesser curvature of the gastric body, consistent with the known primary gastric tumor. There is no increased $^{18}$F-FDG uptake in the cecum.

Additional findings on CT include a 50 mm cortical cyst in the lower pole of the left kidney, significant atheromatotic plaques in the wall of the abdominal aorta and its branches, and mild prostatic hypertrophy, with no uptake of $^{18}$F-FDG.

*Musculoskeletal*: Facetal arthropathy is seen on CT along several cervical vertebra beside C-4 and in the lumbar spine at the level of L4-S1, with no abnormally increased $^{18}$F-FDG uptake.

Impression

1. Focal intense $^{18}$F-FDG uptake in the thickened wall of the lesser curvature of the gastric body, consistent with the primary gastric cancer.
2. Focus of moderately increased $^{18}$F-FDG uptake in degenerative changes in the right facet joint of C-4.
3. No evidence for local or distant metastases.
4. Mildly increased $^{18}$F-FDG uptake in pulmonary hila, consistent with a benign inflammatory or granulomatotic process.
5. Additional CT findings described above.

## Case II.6.4

### History

This is a 62-year-old man, assessed at 12 months after proximal gastrectomy and distal esophagectomy for adenocarcinoma of the gastroesophageal junction. The patient was referred to $^{18}$F-FDG PET/CT for assessment of persistent elevation of serum tumor markers (CA19-9) over several months. The patient had no complaints, and a CT study performed 3 month prior to current examination was negative except for a stable known left lower lung infiltrate related to chronic bronchiectases (Fig. II.6.4A–C).

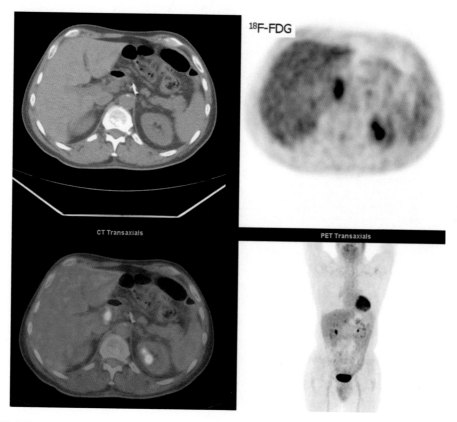

Fig. II.6.4A

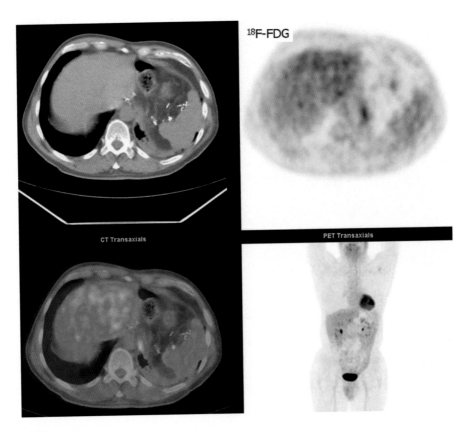

Fig. II.6.4B

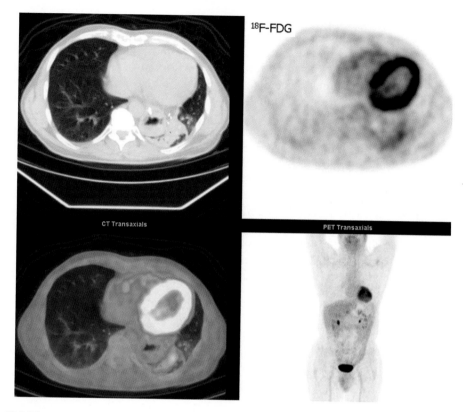

**Fig. II.6.4C**

## Findings

A focal area of high $^{18}$F-FDG uptake is seen in the upper right paramedian abdomen corresponding to a 22 × 20 mm lymph node in the porta hepatic region, adjacent to, but not involving, the residual gastric wall (Fig. II.6.4A). After review of the PET/CT images, this lymph node was retrospectively identified on the prior diagnostic CT.

An additional focus of moderately intense $^{18}$F-FDG uptake is seen in the upper abdomen, in the left para-vertebral region, corresponding to the stomach at its new, post-surgical location, pulled to its anastomosis with the esophagus (Fig. II.6.4B). An area of diffuse, moderately increased $^{18}$F-FDG uptake is also seen in a lung infiltrate in the posterior aspect of the left lower lobe (Fig. II.6.4C).

## Discussion

The focus of intense $^{18}$F-FDG uptake in the right upper abdomen was consistent with metastatic adenopathy in a porta hepatic lymph node. Following the diagnosis of metastatic disease, the patient was referred to chemotherapy. The focus of increased activity in the left upper abdomen, located to the gastric wall, was considered to be of equivocal significance. Although most likely representing physiologic uptake in the stomach in its new location after surgery, an inflammatory gastric process or local recurrence could not be excluded. No endoscopic verification of this site was performed, and there was no evidence of local disease on further clinical and imaging follow-up.

The increased $^{18}$F-FDG uptake located to the lower lobe of the left lung was considered to represent an inflammatory lung infiltrate in a region of known chronic bronchiectases.

The patient did not respond to chemotherapy and presented 7 months later with widespread metastatic disease with abdominal adenopathy, omental cake, peritoneal spread, and ascitis.

De Potter and colleagues[31] reported a sensitivity and specificity of 70 and 69%, respectively, for $^{18}$F-FDG PET diagnosis of recurrence in 33 patients with gastric carcinoma assessed after curative surgical resection. $^{18}$F-FDG PET results were of prognostic significance, with a longer mean survival in PET-negative recurrent gastric cancer as compared with PET-positive patients. $^{18}$F-FDG PET was the only indicator of widespread metastatic disease in 3 out of 18 patients (17%) with suspected recurrent gastric cancer, all three presenting with rising serum tumor markers and negative conventional imaging.[32] PET/CT is of value in assessment of cancer patients with unexplained elevated tumor markers.[34] In present patient, therapy-related structural changes made interpretation of findings on both the PET and CT components of the study difficult. PET/CT enabled early precise diagnosis of a regional nodal metastasis.

### Diagnosis

1. Adenocarcinoma of the gastro-esophgeal junction with nodal metastasis in the porta hepatic region.
2. Physiologic gastric wall $^{18}$F-FDG uptake in the stomach at its new location after surgery.
3. Inflammatory left lower lobe lung infiltrate.

## Case II.6.5

### History

This 33-year-old man was diagnosed with a para-rectal GIST of intermediate risk of malignancy, on rectoscopy performed due to perianal pain. CT demonstrated a large heterogenous, right para-rectal pelvic mass with blurring of the adjacent fat and several small retroperitoneal and mesenteric lymph nodes. $^{18}$F-FDG PET/CT was performed for staging (Fig. II.6.5A).

The tumor was considered locally advanced, unresectable, and systemic treatment with Gleevec$^®$ (400 mg/day) was administered. A repeated $^{18}$F-FDG PET/CT was performed after 4 months of treatment, to assess response prior to a decision regarding further surgical resection (Fig. II.6.5B).

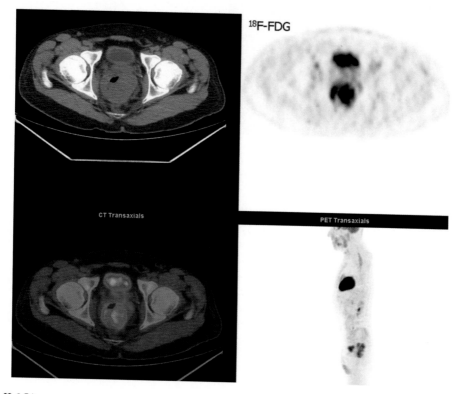

Fig. II.6.5A

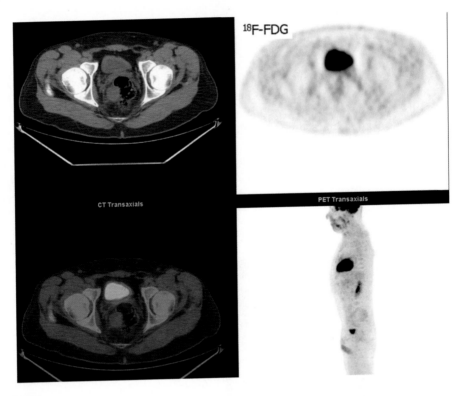

Fig. II.6.5B

## Findings

The baseline pre-treatment PET/CT study (Fig. II.6.5A) demonstrates a site of intense, heterogenous [18]F-FDG uptake in the posterior pelvis corresponding to a large 50 × 45 mm right para-rectal mass, consistent with the known GIST. No other foci of abnormal [18]F-FDG uptake suspicious for metastases are seen.

On the follow-up post-treatment PET/CT study (Fig. II.6.5B), there is no [18]F-FDG uptake in the 28 × 20 mm right para-rectal residual mass, which has significantly decreased in size on CT as compared with the pre-treatment study, consistent with a good metabolic response.

## Discussion

The findings on the initial [18]F-FDG PET/CT study demonstrate a large GIST tumor with intense [18]F-FDG uptake and no evidence of distant metastases. Although assessment of GIST at presentation is routinely performed with CT, intensity of [18]F-FDG correlates with the malignant potential of the tumor. Documentation of [18]F-FDG avidity is important to further monitor response to treatment.[36,39] In 10 patients with gastric GIST and no evidence of metastases scheduled for surgical resection, all primary tumors were [18]F-FDG-avid, but with a wide variability in intensity, with SUV ranging between 2 and 10.6.[39] There was a significant correlation between FDG uptake and the mitotic rate and Ki67-index, but not with the size of tumor.[39]

In present case, $^{18}$F-FDG PET/CT performed after Gleevec® treatment demonstrated a complete metabolic response in the presence of a residual mass on CT. The patient was referred to surgery, which consisted of anterior resection with ileostomy. The tumor mass was resected, with no evidence of mitoses but showing close margins. On follow-up, recurrence in rectal anastomosis was diagnosed 11 months later. The patient was stable under Gleevec® treatment for 3 months.

Surgical resection is the primary curative treatment of GIST. Before the era of Gleevec®, non-resectability carried a poor prognosis, with a mortality rate of 83%.[35] Gleevec® is the first effective systemic drug for advanced GIST and the first model of effective molecular-targeted treatment of a solid tumor. A response rate of about 50% was reported with an oral daily dose of 400–1000 mg, with partial response in about 70% of patients with metastatic disease.[36] $^{18}$F-FDG imaging indicated complete or partial response to Gleevec® in 13 of 17 patients with FDG-avid GIST assessed 8 days after initiation of therapy, with a reduction in SUV of 80 and 30%, respectively.[40] CT showed response in only 10 patients at a median follow-up of 8 weeks.[40] $^{18}$F-FDG PET can also assess late response of GIST to Gleevec®. Choi and colleagues[42,44] compared FDG-PET and CT at 2 months after treatment and observed a decrease of 65% in SUVmax, while reduction in tumor size on CT was only of 13%. A decrease of 99% in SUVmax was found in 70% of patients with stable disease by traditional tumor response criteria on CT.[44] The use of lower thresholds with only small changes in tumor size and density had better predictive values, and a modification of the definition of response criteria on CT has been suggested.[42]

$^{18}$F-FDG PET results after treatment can predict prognosis of patients with GIST. A 1 year PFS rate of 92% was reported in PET responders compared with only 12% in non-responders, when assessed 8 days after initiation of therapy.[40] A rapid decline in $^{18}$F-FDG uptake after treatment may, however, reflect the tumorostatic effect of therapy and not the actual destruction of viable tumor cells.[43] In a literature review of 37 patients who performed PET after neoadjuvant treatment with Gleevec® before surgical resection, a complete metabolic response on PET correlated with pathologic response in only 6 of 23 patients as compared with 31 of 36 on CT.[43] Surgical resection of $^{18}$F-FDG-negative residual masses is therefore important and patient surveillance should be performed using both PET and CT at short intervals.

## Diagnosis

1. $^{18}$F-FDG-avid para-rectal primary GIST with no evidence for metastatic spread.
2. Complete metabolic response to treatment with Gleevec® on $^{18}$F-FDG PET in the presence of a partial response with a residual para-rectal mass on CT.

## Case II.6.6

### History

This 61-year-old woman presented with a new 12 cm in diameter mesenteric para-cecal adenopathy on a follow-up CT and no clinical symptoms, 14 months after wedge resection of the stomach and splenectomy due to GIST. $^{18}$F-FDG PET/CT was performed to assess and restage suspected recurrence (Fig. II.6.6A–D).

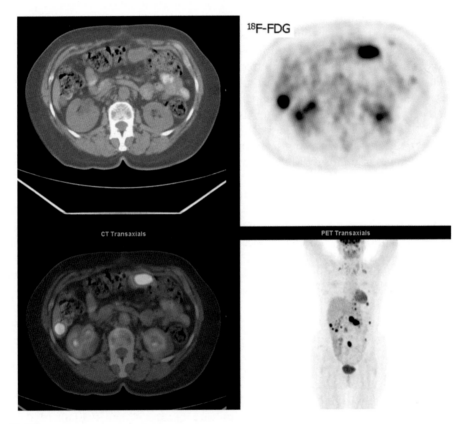

Fig. II.6.6A

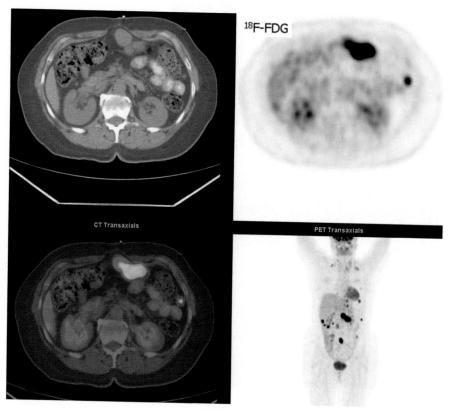

Fig. II.6.6B

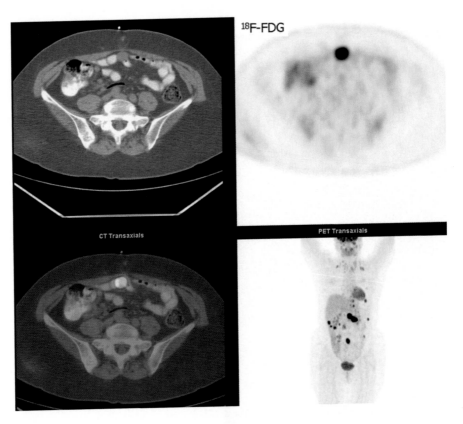

Fig. II.6.6C

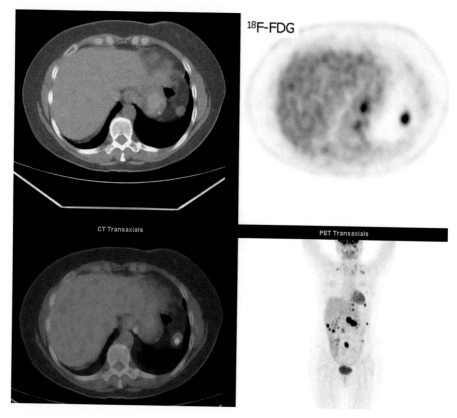

**Fig. II.6.6D**

## Findings

Multiple foci of intense $^{18}$F-FDG uptake corresponding to multiple omental and peritoneal lesions of variable size are seen in the abdomen. There are two adjacent large foci of intense $^{18}$F-FDG uptake in the left paramedian upper abdomen, corresponding to two large omental masses, 31 × 26 and 38 × 20 mm in diameter, located anterior to the transverse colon (Fig. II.6.6A, B). There is an additional small focus of intense FDG uptake within an 8 × 8 mm omental node, at the left lateral aspect of the upper abdomen, near the descending colon (Fig. II.6.6B). A focus of intense uptake is seen in the anterior aspect of the mid-lower abdomen, within a 16 × 13 mm omental mass adherent to small bowel loops (Fig. II.6.6C), and in an 18 × 18 mm left subdiaphragmatic node (Fig. II.6.6D). A focus of abnormal $^{18}$F-FDG uptake in the left upper abdomen, corresponding to a 14 × 17 mm left para-esophageal soft tissue density, most probably represents a peritoneal node at the level of the gastroesophageal junction (Fig. II.6.6D). There is no abnormal $^{18}$F-FDG uptake in the para-cecal adenopathy, the referral cause of the patient to PET/CT.

Several foci of mildly increased $^{18}$F-FDG uptake seen in the shoulder girdle bilaterally and at the left paramedian upper abdomen (seen on MIP) represent physiologic uptake in brown fat.

## Discussion

PET/CT findings are consistent with a widespread metastatic disease within omental and peritoneal nodes. Treatment with Gleevec® was administered with good response. The patient has no evidence for active disease for 14 months with a negative follow-up PET/CT.

In spite of complete resection of the primary tumor, recurrence is diagnosed in the majority of GIST patients, mainly during the first 2 years. Metastases may, however, appear even at more than 10 years after initial diagnosis, and long-term follow-up is therefore important.[37]

CT has been reported to detect more lesions than [18]F-FDG PET both before therapy and during follow-up.[38] In a study of 34 patients assessed by PET/CT and CT for staging or restaging after treatment, [18]F-FDG PET detected 66 lesions as compared to 96 detected by contrast-enhanced CT.[38] FDG uptake in GIST lesions is variable. Heterogenous uptake and areas of absent tracer activity are typically seen within large, partially necrotic lesions.[38]

The exclusive involvement of abdomino-pelvic sites with GIST, the limitations of CT in identifying small peritoneal lesions, and the large variability of [18]F-FDG uptake within these lesions underscore the significance of PET/CT for defining the presence of active GIST, localization of lesions, and surgical planning.[38]

## Diagnosis

1. Recurrent GIST within multiple [18]F-FDG-avid omental and peritoneal metastases.
2. Physiologic [18]F-FDG uptake in brown fat in the shoulder girdle and around the large vessels in the left paramedian upper abdomen.

# References

1. Plukker JT, van Westreenen HL. Staging in oesophageal cancer. *Best Pract Res Clin Gastroenterol* 2006;20:877–891.
2. Bombardieri E. The added value of metabolic imaging with FDG-PET in oesophageal cancer: prognostic role and prediction of response to treatment. *Eur J Nucl Med Mol Imaging* 2006;33:753–758.
3. Das A, Chak A. Reassessment of patients with esophageal cancer after neoadjuvant therapy. *Endoscopy* 2006;381:S13–17.
4. Cerfolio RJ, Bryant AS. Maximum standardized uptake values on positron emission tomography of esophageal cancer predicts stage, tumor biology, and survival. *Ann Thorac Surg* 2006;82:391–395.
5. McDonough PB, Jones DR, Shen KR, Shen R, Northup P, Hernandez A, White G, Kahaleh M, Shami V. Does FDG-PET add information to EUS and CT in the initial management of esophageal cancer? A prospective single center study. *Am J Gastroenterol* 2007;65:AB136–AB136.
6. Bruzzi JF, Munden RF, Truong MT, Marom EM, Sabloff BS, Gladish GW, Iyer RB, Pan T-S, Macapinlac HA, Erasmus JJ. PET/CT of esophageal cancer: Its role in clinical management. *Radiographics* 2007;27:1635–1652.
7. Wong WL, Chambers RJ. Role of PET/CT in the staging and restaging of thoracic oesophageal cancer and gastro-oesophageal cancer: A literature review. *Abdom Imaging* 2008;33:183–190.
8. Meyers BF, Downey RJ, Decker PA, Keenan RJ, Siegel BA, Cerfolio RJ, Landreneau RJ, Reed CE, Balfe DM, Dehdashti F, Ballman KV, Rusch VW, Putnam JB Jr; American College of Surgeons Oncology Group Z0060. The utility of positron emission tomography in staging of potentially operable carcinoma of the thoracic esophagus: Results of the american college of surgeons. Oncology Group Z0060 trial. *J Thorac Cardiovasc Surg* 2007;133:738–745.
9. Bar-Shalom R, Guralnik L, Tsalic M, Leiderman M, Frenkel A, Gaitini D, Ben-Nun A, Keidar Z, Israel O. The additional value of PET/CT over PET in FDG imaging of oesophageal cancer. *Eur J Nucl Med Mol Imaging* 2005;32:918–924.
10. Yuan S, Yu Y, Chao KS, Fu Z, Yin Y, Liu T, Chen S, Yang X, Yang G, Guo H Yu J. Additional value of PET/CT over PET in assessment of locoregional lymph nodes in thoracic esophageal squamous cell cancer. *J Nucl Med* 2006;47:1255–1259.
11. Flamen P, Lerut A, Van Cutsem E, De Wever W, Peeters M, Stroobants S, Dupont P, Bormans G, Hiele M, De Leyn P, Van Raemdonck D, Coosemans W, Ectors N, Haustermans K, Mortelmans L. Utility of positron emission tomography for the staging of patients with potentially operable esophageal carcinoma. *J Clin Oncol* 2000;18:3202–3210.
12. Duong CP, Demitriou H, Weih L, Thompson A, Williams D, Thomas RJ, Hicks RJ. Significant clinical impact and prognostic stratification provided by FDG-PET in the staging of oesophageal cancer. *Eur J Nucl Med Mol Imaging* 2006;33:759–769.
13. Ott K, Weber W, Siewert JR. The importance of PET in the diagnosis and response evaluation of esophageal cancer. *Dis Esophagus* 2006;19:433–442.
14. van Westreenen HL, Westerterp M, Sloof GW, Groen H., Bossuyt PMM, Jager PL, Comans EF, van Dullemen HM, Fockens P, Stoker J, van der Jagt EJ, van Lanschot JJB, Plukker JT. Limited additional value of positron emission tomography in staging oesophageal cancer. *Br J Surg* 2007;94:1515–1520.
15. Wallace MB, Nietert PJ, Earle C, Krasna MJ, Hawes RH, Hoffman BJ, Reed CE. An analysis of multiple staging management strategies for carcinoma of the esophagus: computed tomography, endoscopic ultrasound, positron emission tomography, and thoracoscopy/laparoscopy. *Ann Thorac Surg* 2002;74:1026–1032.
16. Luketich JD, Friedman DM, Weigel TL, Meehan MA, Keenan RJ, Townsend DW, Meltzer CC. Evaluation of distant metastases in esophageal cancer: 100 consecutive positron emission tomography scans. *Ann Thorac Surg* 1999;68:1133–1136
17. Siersema PD. Pathogenesis, diagnosis and therapeutic possibilities of esophageal cancer. *Curr Opin Gastroenterol* 2007;23:456–461.
18. Westerterp M, van Westreenen HL, Reitsma JB, Hoekstra OS, Stoker J, Fockens P, Jager PL, Van Eck-Smit BLF, Plukker JT, van Lanschot JJB, Sloof GW. Esophageal cancer: CT, endoscopic US, and FDG PET for assessment of response to neoadjuvant therapy – systematic review. *Radiology* 2005;236:841–851.
19. Bruzzi JF, Swisher SG, Truong MT, Munden RF, Hofstetter WL, Macapinlac HA, Correa AM, Mawlawi O, Ajani JA, Komaki RR, Fukami N, Erasmus JJ. Detection of interval distant metastases:

Clinical utility of integrated CT-PET imaging in patients with esophageal carcinoma after neoadjuvant therapy. *Cancer* 2007;109:125–134.

20. Flamen P, Lerut A, Van Cutsem E, Cambier JP, Maes A, De Wever W, Peeters M, De Leyn P, Van Raemdonck D, Mortelmans L. The utility of positron emission tomography for the diagnosis and staging of recurrent esophageal cancer. *J Thorac Cardiovasc Surg* 2000;120:1085–1092.

21. Guo H, Zhu H, Xi Y, et al. Diagnostic and prognostic value of 18F-FDG PET/CT for patients with suspected recurrence from squamous cell carcinoma of the esophagus. *J Nucl Med* 2007;48:1251–1258.

22. Lim JS, Yun MJ, Kim MJ, Hyung WJ, Park M-S, Choi J-Y, Kim T-S, Lee JD, Noh SH, Kim KW. CT and PET in stomach cancer: Preoperative staging and monitoring of response to therapy. *Radiographics* 2006;26:143–156.

23. Yoshioka T, Yamaguchi K, Kubota K, Saginoya T, Yamazaki T, Ido T, Yamaura G, Takahashi H, Fukuda H, Kanamaru R. Evaluation of 18F-FDG PET in patients with metastatic or recurrent gastric cancer. *J Nucl Med* 2003;44:690–699.

24. Wu MS, Yang KC, Shun CT, Hsiao TJ, Lin C-C, Wang H-P, Chuang S-M, Lee W-J, Lin J-T. Distinct clinicopathologic characteristics of diffuse- and intestinal-type gastric cancer in Taiwan. *J Clin Gastroenterol* 1997;25:646–649.

25. Yamada A, Oguchi K, Fukushima M, Imai Y, Kadoya M. Evaluation of 2-deoxy-2-[18F]fluoro-D-glucose positron emission tomography in gastric carcinoma: Relation to histological subtypes, depth of tumor invasion, and glucose transporter-1 expression. *Ann Nucl Med* 2006;20:597–604.

26. Chen J, Cheong JH, Yun MJ, Kim J, Lim JS, Hyung WJ, Noh SH. Improvement in preoperative staging of gastric adenocarcinoma with positron emission tomography. *Cancer* 2005;103:2383–2390.

27. Kim SK, Kang KW, Lee JS, Kim HK, Chang HJ, Choi JY, Lee JH, Ryu KW, Kim Y-W, Bae J-M. Assessment of lymph node metastases using 18F-FDG PET in patients with advanced gastric cancer. *Eur J Nucl Med Mol Imaging* 2006;33:148–155.

28. Kinkel K, Lu Y, Both M, Warren RS, Thoeni, RF. Detection of hepatic metastases from cancers of the gastrointestinal tract by using noninvasive imaging methods (US, CT, MR imaging, PET): A meta-analysis. *Radiology* 2002;224:748–756.

29. Ott K, Fink U, Becker K, Stahl A, Dittler H-J, Busch R, Stein H, Lordick F, Link T, Schwaiger M, Siewert J-R, Weber WA. Prediction of response to preoperative chemotherapy in gastric carcinoma by metabolic imaging: Results of a prospective trial. *J Clin Oncol* 2003;21:4604–4610.

30. Lordick F, Ott K, Krause BJ, Weber WA, Becker K, Stein HJ, Lorenzen S, Schuster T, Wieder H, Herrmann K, Bredenkamp R, Höfler H, Fink U, Peschel C, Schwaiger M, Siewert JR. PET to assess early metabolic response and to guide treatment of adenocarcinoma of the oesophagogastric junction: The MUNICON phase II trial. *Lancet Oncol* 2007;8:797–805.

31. De Potter T, Flamen P, Van Cutsem E, Penninckx F, Filez L, Bormans G, Maes A, Mortelmans L. Whole-body PET with FDG for the diagnosis of recurrent gastric cancer. *Eur J Nucl Med Mol Imaging* 2002;29:525–529.

32. Jadvar H, Tatlidil R, Garcia AA, Conti PS. Evaluation of recurrent gastric malignancy with [F-18]-FDG positron emission tomography. *Clin Radiol* 2003;58:215–221.

33. Rosen RS, Fayad L, Wahl RL. Increased 18F-FDG uptake in degenerative disease of the spine: characterization with 18F-FDG PET/CT. *J Nucl Med* 6;47:1274–1280.

34. Radan L, Ben-Haim S, Bar-Shalom R, Guralnik L, Israel O. The role of FDG-PET/CT in suspected recurrence of breast cancer. *Cancer* 2006;107:2545–2551

35. Nilsson B, Bümming P, Meis-Kindblom JM, Odén A, Dortok A, Gustavsson B, Sablinska K, Kindblom L-G. Gastrointestinal stromal tumors: The incidence, prevalence, clinical course, and prognostication in the preimatinib mesylate era – a population-based study in western Sweden. *Cancer* 2005;103:821–829.

36. Joensuu H, Fletcher C, Dimitrijevic S, Silberman S, Roberts P, Demetri G. Management of malignant gastrointestinal stromal tumors. *Lancet Oncol* 2002;3:655–664.

37. Pidhorecky I, Cheney RT, Kraybill WG, Gibbs JF. Gastrointestinal stromal tumors: Current diagnosis, biologic behavior, and management. *Ann Surg Oncol* 2000;7:705–712.

38. Goerres GW, Stupp R, Barghouth G, Hany TG, Pestalozzi B, Dizendorf E, Schnyder P, Luthi F, von Schulthess JK, Leyvraz S. The value of PET, CT and in-line PET/CT in patients with gastrointestinal stromal tumors: Long-term outcome of treatment with imatinib mesylate. *Eur J Nucl Med Mol Imaging* 2005;32:153–162.

39. Kamiyama Y, Aihara R, Nakabayashi T, Mochiki E, Asao T, Kuwano H, Oriuchi N, Endo K. 18F-fluorodeoxyglucose positron emission tomography: Useful technique for predicting malignant potential of gastrointestinal stromal tumors. *World J Surg* 2005;29:1429–1435.

40. Stroobants S, Goeminne J, Seegers M, Dimitrijevic S, Dupont P, Nuyts J, Martens M, van den Borne B, Cole P, Sciot R, Dumez H, Silberman S, Mortelmans L, van Oosterom A.18FDG-Positron emission tomography for the early prediction of response in advanced soft tissue sarcoma treated with imatinib mesylate (Gleevec$^{®}$). *Eur J Cancer* 2003;39:2012–2020

41. Grimpen F, Yip D, McArthur G, Waring P, Goldstein D, Loughrey M, Beshay V, Chong G. Resistance to imatinib, low-grade FDG-avidity on PET, and acquired KIT exon 17 mutation in gastrointestinal stromal tumor. *Lancet Oncol* 2005;6:724–727.

42. Choi H, Charnsangavej C, Faria SC, Macapinlac HA, Burgess MA, Patel SR, Chen LL, Podoloff DA, Benjamin RS. Correlation of computed tomography and positron emission tomography in patients with metastatic gastrointestinal stromal tumor treated at a single institution with imatinib mesylate: proposal of new computed tomography response criteria. *J Clin Oncol* 2007;25:1753–1459.

43. Goh BK, Chow PK, Chuah KL, Yap WM, Wong WK. Pathologic, radiologic and PET scan response of gastrointestinal stromal tumors after neoadjuvant treatment with imatinib mesylate. *Eur J Surg Oncol* 2006;32:961–963.

44. Choi H, Charnsangavej C, de Castro Faria S, Tamm EP,. Benjamin RS, Johnson MM, Macapinlac HA, Podoloff DA. CT evaluation of the response of gastrointestinal stromal tumors after imatinib mesylate treatment: A quantitative analysis correlated with FDG PET findings. *AJR Am J Roentgenol* 2004;183:1619–1628.

45. Podoloff DA, Ball DW, Ben-Josef E, Benson AB, Cohen SJ, Coleman RE, Delbeke D, Ho M, Ilson DH, Kalemkerian GP, Lee RJ, Loeffler JS, Macapinlac HA, Morgan RJ, Siegel BA, Singhal S, Tyler DS, Wong RJ. NCCN Task Force: Clinical Utility of PET in a Variety of Tumor Types Task Force. J Natl Compr Canc Netw 2009;7 Suppl 2: S1–S23. www.nccn.org/professionals/physician_gls/f_guide lines.asp

46. Fletcher JW, Djulbegovic B, Soares HP, Siegel BA, Lowe VJ, Lyman GH, Coleman E, Wahl R, Paschold JC, Avril N, Einhorn LH, Suh WW, Samson D, Delbeke D, Gorman M, Shields AF. Recommendations for the use of FDG (fluorine-18, (2-[$^{18}$F]Fluoro-2-deoxy-D-glucose) positron emission tomography in oncology. *J Nucl Med* 2008; 49:480–508.

# Chapter II.7
# Hepatobiliary and Pancreatic Malignancies

Dominique Delbeke and Ronald C. Walker

## Hepatobiliary Neoplasms

A variety of benign and malignant tumors occur in the liver. The most common benign hepatic tumors are cysts followed by cavernous hemangiomas. Focal nodular hyperplasia and adenomas more often affect women on oral contraceptives, whereas fatty infiltration and regenerating nodules more commonly occur in patients with cirrhosis. Abscesses and angiomyolipomas are uncommon. Among malignant tumors, metastases to the liver from various primaries, often multifocal, occur 20 times more often than primary hepatocellular carcinoma (HCC). Although many tumors may metastasize to the liver, this occurs mainly in colorectal, gastric, pancreatic, lung, and breast carcinoma. Ninety percent of malignant primary hepatic tumors are of epithelial origin and include HCC and cholangiocarcinoma.

HCCs represent 90% of primary epithelial hepatic tumors. They arise from malignant transformation of hepatocytes. HCC is often encountered in association with chronic hepatic diseases, such as viral hepatitis and cirrhosis, or in patients exposed to carcinogens. HCC metastasizes mainly to regional lymph nodes, the lungs, and skeleton.

Cholangiocarcinoma arises from biliary cells and represents only 10% of primary epithelial hepatic tumors. About 20% of the patients who develop cholangiocarcinoma have predisposing conditions, including sclerosing cholangitis, ulcerative colitis, Caroli's disease, choledocal cyst, infestation by the fluke *Clonorchis sinensis*, cholelithiasis, or exposure to Thorotrast (an early radiographic vascular contrast agent), among others. Approximately 50% of cholangiocarcinomas occur in the liver, with the other half arising in the extra hepatic biliary tree. These tumors are often unresectable at the time of diagnosis and have a poor prognosis. Intrahepatic cholangiocarcinomas can be further subdivided in two categories: the peripheral type arising from the interlobular biliary duct and the hilar type (Klatskin's tumor), which arises from the main hepatic duct or its bifurcation. Cholangiocarcinoma can further develop into three different morphological types: infiltrating sclerosing lesions (which are most common), exophytic lesions, and polypoid intraluminal masses. Malignant tumors that arise along the extra, hepatic bile ducts are usually diagnosed early because they cause biliary obstruction. Tumors arising near the hilum of the liver have a worse prognosis due to their direct extension to the liver. Distant metastases occur late in the course of disease and most often affect the lungs.

D. Delbeke (✉)
Department of Radiology and Radiological Sciences, Vanderbilt University Medical Center, Nashville, TN, USA
e-mail: dominique.delbeke@vanderbilt.edu

D. Delbeke, O. Israel (eds.), *Hybrid PET/CT and SPECT/CT Imaging*,
DOI 10.1007/978-0-387-92820-3_9, © Springer Science+Business Media, LLC 2010

Mesenchymal tumors such as angiosarcoma and epithelioid angioendothelioma (both of endothelial origin) and primary lymphoma are relatively rare malignancies that can affect the liver.

Carcinoma of the gallbladder is uncommon and associated with cholelithiasis in 75% of the cases. These are insidious tumors, unsuspected clinically, and often discovered incidentally at surgery. They frequently spread to the liver and can perforate the wall of the gallbladder, metastasizing to the abdomen. Distant metastases affect the lungs, pleura, and diaphragm.

## Pancreatic Neoplasms

Pancreatic carcinoma usually arises from the pancreatic ducts. These are the third most common malignant tumor of the gastrointestinal tract (GIT) and the fifth leading cause of cancer-related mortality. Most tumors arise in the head of the pancreas, with patients presenting with bile duct obstruction, pain, and jaundice. Carcinoma of the ampulla of Vater may be difficult to differentiate from tumors arising from the head of the pancreas. Tumors of the body and the tail of the pancreas are more insidious and are typically detected at advanced stages. Prognosis of pancreatic carcinoma is extremely poor, with most patients dying within 2 years of diagnosis. Surgical resection is the only potentially curative approach. Only 3% of newly diagnosed patients will survive 5 years. Pancreatico-duodenectomy improves 5-year survival to over 20%, with 2–3% mortality in carefully selected patients. Adverse prognostic factors include high histological grade, capsular infiltration, and the presence of lymphatic vessel and perineural invasion.

Acinar cell carcinomas comprise less than 1–2% of all pancreatic malignancies and have a poor prognosis, similar to ductal cell cancer. Cystic neoplasms can arise in the pancreas and differentiation of benign from malignant etiology is critical.

Islet cell and other endocrine tumors make up a small fraction of all pancreatic neoplasms and are most often located in the body and tail of the pancreas. They are usually slowly growing tumors and can be associated with other endocrine abnormalities. This topic is addressed in another chapter.

## Imaging of Hepatobiliary and Pancreatic Neoplasms

Various imaging modalities are available for evaluation of hepatobiliary and pancreatic neoplasms. In addition, some of these tumors are associated with elevated serum levels of tumor markers, which play an important role in evaluation of this group of malignancies, such as alpha-fetoprotein used for screening patients at risk for HCC and Ca 19-9 for surveillance of patients with pancreatic carcinoma.

Transabdominal ultrasound (US) is a valuable screening technique, inexpensive, portable, sensitive for assessing the presence of bile duct dilatation and able to detect hepatic lesions as small as 1 cm. Ultrasound can also guide biopsy and drainage procedures. Its limitations include poor sensitivity of about 50% for detection of small hepatic lesions, below 1 cm in diameter, and for diagnosis of regional lymphadenopathy as compared to computed tomography (CT) and magnetic resonance imaging (MRI).

Endoscopic US is sensitive for detection of choledocolithiasis and pancreatic masses. However, it is highly operator-dependent, requires sedation, and is associated with significant morbidity. In addition, its limited field of view makes it inappropriate for the purpose of staging.

Imaging of hepatic lesions using CT and MRI is based on the dual perfusion of the liver. Most of the blood flow to the normal hepatic parenchyma is derived from the portal vein, whereas nearly all of the blood flow to hepatic neoplasms is derived from the hepatic artery. Therefore, various lesions enhance at different times following administration of contrast material, either during the "hepatic arterial phase" or the "portal venous phase." The correlation of maximum enhancement with the phase of hepatic perfusion is helpful in the differential diagnosis of the lesion. Typically, hypervascular lesions such as HCC or metastases of carcinoid, islet cell tumor, malignant pheochromocytoma, renal cell carcinoma, sarcoma, melanoma, and breast cancer may be visualized during the arterial phase of enhancement or before contrast administration. Hypovascular metastases from colorectal carcinoma and most other solid tumors are best visualized during the portal venous phase of enhancement. Cavernous hemangiomas are best characterized using dynamic imaging with the appearance of "puddling" of contrast in the dependent portions of the lesion on delayed images. In summary, a triple phase helical CT should be performed on all patients referred for evaluation of hepatic lesions to allow optimal detection and characterization.

MRI has a similar sensitivity to CT for detection of focal hepatic lesions following the development of a multitude of pulse sequences to characterize them. Gadolinium chelate contrast agents are used like the intravenous CT contrast agents. They are rapidly leaving the vascular space and reach equilibrium throughout the extracellular fluid compartment after approximately 3 min. MR cholangiopancreatography (MRCP) permits non-invasive visualization of the biliary tree without administration of contrast agents. Although MRCP does not provide the resolution of percutaneous transhepatic cholangiography (PTC) or endoscopic retrograde cholangiopancreatography (ERCP), it can demonstrate intraluminal filling defects and luminal narrowing.

Cholangiopancreatography, via PTC and ERCP, remains the procedure of choice for high-resolution assessment of the anatomy of the biliary tree following direct injection of contrast material. However, they are invasive techniques. Both techniques offer the advantage of allowing interventional procedures, such as stent placement, in the same setting as the imaging procedure. PTC demonstrates the intrahepatic ducts better while ERCP better depicts the extrahepatic ducts.

Functional scintigraphic imaging can help to characterize hepatic lesions. $^{99m}$Tc-labeled red blood cells (RBC) scintigraphy images the blood pool and is highly accurate in differentiating cavernous hemangiomas from other lesions. $^{99m}$Tc-sulfur colloid accumulation in hepatic Kupffer cells allows characterization of focal nodular hyperplasia. $^{131}$I-metaiodobenzylguanidine (MIBG) can be used to image neuroendocrine tumors and their metastases. $^{111}$In-octreotide accumulates in a variety of neuroendocrine tumors and may also help characterize other pathologic processes such as lymphoma, sarcoidosis, and autoimmune diseases. $^{67}$Gallium, $^{201}$Thallium, $^{99m}$Tc-methoxyisobutyl isonitriles (MIBI), and radiolabeled monoclonal antibodies are poor imaging agents for hepatic lesions due to high physiological hepatic background activity.

Positron emission tomography (PET) with $^{18}$F-fluorodeoxyglucose ($^{18}$F-FDG) has become an established modality for assessment of these malignancies.[1] There is only a paucity of data available at the time of writing this chapter regarding the incremental diagnostic utility of integrated $^{18}$F-FDG PET/CT in hepatobiliary and pancreatic neoplasms, but initial results as well as studies on other types of malignancy indicated a significant additional value from combined metabolic and structural assessment.[2] It needs to be emphasized that for evaluation of the liver, multiphase contrast-enhanced CT and MRI are the optimal modalities to characterize hepatic lesions and should be performed in addition to hybrid PET/CT imaging.

## Hepatic Metastases

On US, hepatic metastases can appear hypo- or hyperechoic, with a mixed echogenicity, or even cystic, relative to the normal hepatic echotexture. Isoechoic metastases may be missed. CT is at present the conventional method for screening of the liver at many institutions. Metastases may be better seen during the arterial or portal venous phase after contrast injection or, rarely, prior to contrast injection depending on their vascularity, etiology, and predominant source of blood supply.

## $^{18}$F-FDG PET/CT Imaging of Hepatic Metastases

A first meta-analysis comparing non-invasive imaging methods including US, CT, MRI, and $^{18}$F-FDG PET for the detection of hepatic metastases from colorectal, gastric, and esophageal cancers demonstrated that at an equivalent specificity of 85%,$^{18}$F-FDG PET had the highest sensitivity of 90% compared to 76% for MRI, 72% for CT, and 55% for US.[3] A subsequent meta-analysis included MRI studies with Gadolinium and superparamagnetic iron oxide particle (SPIO) enhancement.[4] SPIO MRI had a 90% sensitivity compared to 76% for $^{18}$F-FDG PET for lesions greater than 1 cm. A study comparing sensitivity of $^{18}$F-FDG PET with multiphase CT with intraoperative US as reference standard for lesions of different sizes showed that the overall sensitivity of $^{18}$F-FDG PET and CT was similar (71 and 72%, respectively). Both $^{18}$F-FDG PET and CT missed approximately 30% of smaller lesions and led to a change of management in 7% of patients.[5]

## Hepatocellular Carcinoma

Differentiation of low-grade HCC from hepatic adenoma can be difficult even on core biopsy. A capsule is often present in small HCC but is seldom found in large tumors. Invasion of the portal vein is often present, especially with large HCCs, though invasion of the inferior vena cava and hepatic vein occurs in only 5% of the cases. HCC can undergo hemorrhage and necrosis or demonstrate fatty metamorphosis. The presence of these characteristics on imaging studies is suggestive of HCC, but high-resolution techniques are required for successful detection. Although lesions larger than 3 cm in diameter may be visualized by CT and US with sensitivity in the range of 80–90%, smaller lesions may be difficult to distinguish from the surrounding hepatic parenchyma, especially in patients with cirrhosis and regenerating nodules, with sensitivity decreasing to 50%. Between 70 and 90% of HCC have $^{67}$Gallium uptake greater than the normal liver, and scintigraphy with this tracer has been used in conjunction with standard $^{99m}$Tc-sulfur colloid scintigraphy to differentiate HCC from regenerating nodules in cirrhotic patients[6]. $^{67}$Gallium scintigraphy has low performance for lesions less than 2–3 cm in diameter.

Fibrolamellar carcinoma, a low-grade malignant tumor accounting for 6–25% of HCC, occurs in younger patients without underlying cirrhosis. An avascular scar that may contain calcifications characterizes these tumors in contrast to focal nodular hyperplasia, which exhibits a vascular scar without calcifications.

## $^{18}$F-FDG PET/CT for Diagnosis and Staging of HCC

Differentiated hepatocytes have a relatively high glucose-6-phosphatase activity. Although experimental studies have shown that glycogenesis decreases and glycolysis increases during carcinogenesis, the accumulation of $^{18}$F-FDG in HCC is variable due to varying degrees of glucose-6-phosphatase activity in these tumors.[7,8] Dynamic studies have reported an elevated phosphorylation kinetic constant (k3) in virtually all malignant tumors, including HCC. The dephosphorylation kinetic constant (k4) is low in metastatic lesions and in cholangiocarcinomas, thus resulting in intralesional accumulation of $^{18}$F-FDG. But k4 is similar to k3 for HCC that do not accumulate $^{18}$F-FDG.[9,10] HCC can exhibit three $^{18}$F-FDG uptake patterns: activity that is higher, equal to, or lower than the hepatic background. $^{18}$F-DG imaging detects only 50–70% of HCC, but has a sensitivity greater than 90% for other malignant primary as well as hepatic metastases.[11,12] All benign tumors, including focal nodular hyperplasia, adenoma, and regenerating nodules, demonstrate $^{18}$F-FDG uptake of similar intensity to the normal liver, except for rare abscesses with granulomatous inflammation. A correlation was found between the degree of $^{18}$F-FDG uptake measured by the standard uptake value (SUV) and k3, and the grade of malignancy.[10,11] Therefore, $^{18}$F-FDG imaging may have a prognostic significance in the evaluation of patients with HCC. Tumors that accumulate $^{18}$F-FDG tend to be moderately to poorly differentiated and are associated with markedly elevated alpha-fetoprotein levels.[13,14]

$^{18}$F-FDG imaging is of limited value in assessment of focal hepatic lesions in patients with chronic hepatitis C because of both the low sensitivity for detection of HCC and the high prevalence of HCC in this population of patients.[15,16] Teefey and colleagues[17] prospectively compared the diagnostic performance of CT, MRI, US, and $^{18}$F-FDG PET for detection of HCC or cholangiocarcinoma in 25 liver transplant candidates. Explanted liver specimens were examined histologically to determine presence and type of lesion. The sensitivities were as follows: US 89%, CT 60%, MRI 53%, PET 0%. In patients with HCC that accumulate $^{18}$F-FDG, PET can accurately detect unsuspected regional and distant metastases, as with other tumors. In some cases, $^{18}$F-FDG PET is the only imaging modality that can demonstrate the tumor and its metastases.[11] In a study of 91 patients, despite the low sensitivity of 64% of $^{18}$F-FDG imaging for detection of HCC, the results of PET had a significant impact on management in 28% of patients due to detection of unsuspected metastases in high-risk patients, including liver transplant candidates, and monitoring response to liver-directed therapy.[18]

## $^{11}$C-Acetate Imaging of HCC

$^{11}$C-Acetate is a marker of membrane lipid synthesis and is a promising PET radiopharmaceutical for evaluation of malignancies with limited $^{18}$F-FDG avidity such as HCC. Neoplastic cells incorporate acetate into lipids rather than into aminoacids or $CO_2$ as a necessary condition for cell proliferation.

Possible biochemical pathways that lead to accumulation of [11]C-acetate in tumors include entry into the Krebs cycle from acetyl coenzyme A (acetyl CoA) or as an intermediate metabolite; esterification to form acetyl CoA as a major precursor in β-oxidation for fatty acid synthesis; combining with glycine in heme synthesis; and through citrate for cholesterol synthesis. Among these possible metabolic pathways, participation in free fatty acid (lipid) synthesis is believed to be the dominant method of incorporation into tumors.

[11]C-Acetate PET has been evaluated in patients with HCC. Ho and colleagues[19] used both [18]F-FDG and [11]C-acetate PET imaging to study 57 patients with various hepatobiliary neoplasms. For the 23 patients with HCC, the sensitivity of [18]F-FDG and [11]C-acetate imaging was 47 and 87%, respectively, with a combined sensitivity of 100%. Well-differentiated tumors tended to be [11]C-acetate-avid, whereas poorly differentiated tumors tended to be [18]F-FDG-avid. Other malignant tumors were [18]F-FDG-avid but not [11]C-acetate-avid. Benign tumors were not [11]C-acetate-avid except for mild uptake in focal nodular hyperplasia. The complimentarity of [11]C-acetate and [18]F-FDG has been confirmed in a larger series of 121 patients, as well as the impact on management.[20] [18]F-fluorocholine is another promising PET tracer for HCC.[21]

## Cholangiocarcinoma

Cholangiocarcinomas are often missed on CT because of their small size and isodensity to the normal hepatic parenchyma. This occurs in most hilar tumors and 25% of peripheral tumors, and in these cases the location and degree of biliary ductal dilatation suggest the location of the tumor. When the tumor is detected on CT, it most often appears as a nonspecific hypodense mass. Delayed retention of contrast material is characteristic and must be differentiated from the retention pattern of a cavernous hemangioma. A central scar or calcification is seen in 25–30% of the cases. On MRI, these tumors are usually hypointense on T1-weighted and hyperintense on T2-weighted images. The central scar is best seen as a hypointense structure on T2-weighted images. After gadolinium administration, there is early peripheral and progressive concentric enhancement, similar to CT. MRI may demonstrate tumors not seen on CT and is best utilized as a problem-solving tool.

MRCP used as an adjunct to conventional MRI may provide additional information regarding the extension of hilar cholangiocarcinoma. PTC and ERCP are usually not indicated for peripheral tumors, but they can demonstrate most hilar cholangiocarcinomas and are superior to CT for evaluation of the intraductal extent of the tumor. ERCP/PTC is the procedure of choice to demonstrate the infiltrating/sclerosing tumor. Typically, a malignant stricture tapers irregularly and is associated with proximal ductal dilatation. The differential diagnosis from sclerosing cholangitis, one of the preexisting conditions, may be difficult. Some tumors are seen as intraluminal defects, but mucin, blood clots, calculi, an air bubble, or biliary sludge may have a similar appearance. ERCP/PTC is often performed at the same time as a biliary drainage procedure.

## *[18]F-FDG PET/CT for Diagnosis and Staging of Cholangiocarcinoma*

There is preliminary evidence that [18]F-FDG imaging may be useful in diagnosis and management of small cholangiocarcinomas in patients with sclerosing cholangitis.[22] Anderson and colleagues[23] reviewed 36 consecutive patients who underwent [18]F-FDG

PET for suspected cholangiocarcinoma due to either a nodular mass larger than 1 cm in diameter or the presence of an infiltrating lesion. The sensitivity of [18]F-FDG imaging for nodular morphology was 85% but decreased to only 18% for the infiltrating pattern. Sensitivity for detection of metastases was 65% with false negatives in patients with carcinomatosis and false positives in the presence of primary sclerosing cholangitis with superimposed acute cholangitis. A significant percent of patients had also [18]F-FDG uptake along the tract of a biliary stent, probably due to a foreign body inflammatory reaction. [18]F-FDG PET led to a change in surgical management in 30% of patients, mainly due to detection of unsuspected metastases.

The clinical usefulness of [18]F-FDG imaging in the differential diagnosis of bile duct cancer is also related to the site of primary disease. Although helpful in cases of intrahepatic and common bile duct cancers, [18]F-FDG imaging is less optimal in perihilar cholangio-carcinoma.[24,25] However, [18]F-FDG PET is of definite value in detection of unsuspected distant metastases. A study of 126 patients with biliary cancer confirmed an overall sensitivity of 78% for cholangiocarcinoma.[26]

## Gallbladder Carcinoma

Unsuspected gallbladder carcinoma is discovered incidentally in 1% of patients undergoing routine cholecystectomy. With most cholecystectomies being currently performed laparoscopically, occult gallbladder carcinoma has been associated with reports of seeding of laparoscopic trocar sites.[27,28]

## *[18]F-FDG PET/CT for Diagnosis and Staging of Gallbladder Carcinoma*

Increased [18]F-FDG uptake has been demonstrated in gallbladder carcinoma[29] and found of value in identifying recurrence at the site of the surgical incision, while CT could not differentiate scar tissue from malignant recurrence.[30] The sensitivity of [18]F-FDG imaging for detection of gallbladder carcinoma ranges between 78 and 86%.[23,26,31] The reported sensitivity of [18]F-FDG PET for detection of extrahepatic metastases is of approximately 50%.[23]

## *[18]F-FDG PET/CT Monitoring Therapy of Hepatic Tumors*

Hepatic metastases can be treated with systemic chemotherapy or regional therapy to the liver. Because the majority of patients with HCC have advanced-stage tumors and/or underlying cirrhosis with impaired hepatic reserve, surgical resection is often not possible.

There are a variety of procedures to administer regional therapy to hepatobiliary tumors, including chemotherapy administered through the hepatic artery using an infusion pump, selective chemoembolization, radiofrequency ablation (RFA), cryoablation, alcohol ablation, and radiolabeled [90]Y-microspheres.[32–34]

In patients treated with hepatic artery chemoembolization, [18]F-FDG imaging is more accurate than retention of lipiodol on CT to predict the presence of residual viable tumor. Residual [18]F-FDG uptake in some lesions can help guide further regional therapy.[35,36,37]

RFA and [90]Y-microspheres radioembolization are now the interventional techniques of choice for patients with unresectable hepatic metastases and HCC. RFA is indicated for patients with a limited number of hepatic metastases measuring less than 5 cm in diameter. It is usually performed percutaneously guided by US or CT. Anatomic imaging modalities, including MRI, have limited ability to differentiate between residual tumor and treatment-related changes in the liver. Contrast enhancement and morphological changes at the periphery of the ablative necrosis can occur and persist for as long as 3 months following RFA, due to the treatment-induced hyperthermia and subsequent tissue regeneration.[38] Preliminary data suggest that [18]F-FDG imaging may be more accurate than CT for detection of recurrence.[39–43] However, other studies have reported the presence of [18]F-FDG uptake in the inflammatory rim of the treatment bed, with a difficult differential diagnosis between tracer uptake related to treatment-induced inflammatory changes and recurrent/residual tumor.[43,44] A study in an animal model suggests that [18]F-FDG imaging should be performed immediately after the ablative procedure, before an inflammatory response has occurred, to detect residual tumor and avoid interference from inflammatory uptake.[45]

Wong and colleagues[46,47] have compared changes on [18]F-FDG imaging, CT, and MRI with changes in serum carcinoembryonic antigen (CEA) levels following intra-arterial hepatic radioembolization with [90]Y-microspheres. They found a significantly superior correlation between changes in serum levels of CEA and changes in [18]F-FDG uptake as compared to changes seen on CT or MRI following treatment.

These preliminary data suggest that [18]F-FDG imaging may monitor the efficacy of regional therapy to the liver. However, more studies with larger numbers of patients are needed to confirm these findings.

## Pancreatic Cancer

The suspicion for pancreatic cancer is often raised when either a pancreatic mass or dilatation of the biliary or pancreatic ducts are detected by US or CT. CT is superior to US in detecting a pancreatic mass and also in assessing its vascular involvement and invasion of adjacent organs. The reported diagnostic accuracy of CT for both detection of pancreatic cancer and establishing the resectability status ranges between 85 and 95%.[48,49] Interpretation of CT may be difficult in the setting of mass-forming pancreatitis or other equivocal findings, such as enlargement of the head of the pancreas without definite signs of malignancy.[50,51] Small hepatic and peritoneal metastases are also difficult to detect on CT.[48]

Endoscopic US has a higher sensitivity than CT for detection of pancreatic carcinoma and offers the possibility of guiding tissue diagnosis with fine needle aspiration (FNA) biopsy.[49]

Due to its high resolution of ductal structures, ERCP has an accuracy of 80–90% for differentiating benign from malignant pancreatic processes, including the differential diagnosis of tumor from chronic pancreatitis. Limitations of ERCP include false-negative studies when the tumor does not originate from the main duct, a 10% technical failure rate, and up to 8% morbidity related mainly to iatrogenic pancreatitis. Principal advantages of ERCP include its ability to perform FNA biopsy and other interventional procedures (e.g., sphincterotomy or stent placement). Although

FNA biopsy may provide a tissue diagnosis, this technique suffers from significant sampling error.[52,53]

## $^{18}$F-FDG PET/CT for Preoperative Diagnosis of Pancreatic Carcinoma

Delbeke[54] published a review of the role of PET imaging in the evaluation of pancreatic carcinoma. Most malignancies, including pancreatic carcinoma, demonstrate increased glucose utilization.[55–56] The summary of the literature published in 2001 reported average sensitivity and specificity of 94 and 90%, respectively.[59] All studies have reported relatively high sensitivity, between 85 and 100%, specificity of 67–99%, and accuracy of 85–93% for $^{18}$F-FDG PET imaging in the differential diagnosis of benign from malignant pancreatic masses. Most studies also suggest an improved accuracy compared to CT. These results are similar to the findings of Rose and colleagues,[60] who reported a sensitivity of 92% and specificity of 85% for $^{18}$F-FDG imaging compared to 65 and 62%, respectively, for CT. These studies suggest that $^{18}$F-FDG imaging may represent a useful add-on diagnostic tool in evaluation of patients with suspected pancreatic cancer, especially when CT results are inconclusive.

$^{18}$F-FDG imaging may be limited in the evaluation of pancreatic cancer due to a high incidence of glucose intolerance and diabetes exhibited by patients with pancreatic pathology. Elevated serum glucose levels result in decreased $^{18}$F-FDG uptake in tumors due to competitive inhibition. Some investigators have suggested various methods to correct or compensate the measured SUV based on serum glucose levels at the time of the radiopharmaceutical injection.[61–64] Several studies have demonstrated a lower sensitivity in hyperglycemic compared to euglycemic patients.[64–66] In a study of 106 patients with a prevalence of disease of 70%, Zimny and colleagues[66] found that $^{18}$F-FDG PET had a sensitivity of 98%, specificity 84%, and accuracy of 93% in a subgroup of euglycemic patients compared to 63, 86, and 68%, respectively, in hyperglycemic patients. Conversely, other investigators noted no variation in the accuracy of $^{18}$F-FDG PET based on serum glucose levels.[67,68]

Both glucose and $^{18}$F-FDG are substrates for cellular mediators of inflammation. Some benign inflammatory lesions, including chronic active pancreatitis with or without abscess formation, can accumulate $^{18}$F-FDG and lead to false-positive interpretations.[69] Nonetheless, $^{18}$F-FDG PET was able to detect pancreatic carcinoma in the setting of chronic pancreatitis with a sensitivity of 92% and a negative predictive value of 87%.[70] False-positive studies are frequent in patients with elevated C-reactive protein and/or acute pancreatitis, decreasing the specificity to as low as 50%.[64] Correlation of the C-reactive protein level with the $^{18}$F-FDG imaging patterns is recommended in this clinical setting. For cystic and intraductal papillary mucinous tumors, the sensitivity and specificity of $^{18}$F-FDG PET ranges from 80 to 94%, both superior to CT and MRCP.[71]

Studies on a small number of patients suggest that the degree of $^{18}$F-FDG uptake in pancreatic malignancies has an inverse prognostic impact. Nakata and colleagues[72] noted an inverse correlation between SUV and survival in 14 patients with pancreatic adenocarcinoma. Patients with an SUV higher than 3.0 had a mean survival of 5 months compared to 14 months in those with an SUV of less than 3.0. Zimny and colleagues[73] performed a multivariate analysis on 52 patients, including SUV and accepted prognostic factors, to determine the prognostic value of $^{18}$F-FDG PET. The median survival of patients with SUV higher than 6.1 was 5 months as compared to 9 months for patients with an SUV below 6.1. Multivariate analysis revealed that SUV and Ca 19-9 were independent factors for prognosis. In an additional study of 118 patients, survival was significantly influenced by tumor stage and grade, and SUV.[74]

[18]F-FDG imaging is complementary to CT in the evaluation of patients with pancreatic masses and in the diagnosis of suspected pancreatic carcinoma. In view of the decreased sensitivity of [18]F-FDG imaging in patients with hyperglycemia, PET acquisition should be performed under controlled metabolic conditions and preferably in the absence of acute inflammatory abdominal disease.

## [18]F-FDG PET/CT for Staging of Pancreatic Carcinoma

In the TNM staging system for pancreatic cancer, Stage I disease is confined to the pancreas. Stage II disease is characterized by extrapancreatic extension (T stage), Stage III by lymph node involvement (N stage), and Stage IV by distant metastases (M stage). T staging can only be evaluated with anatomical imaging modalities, which demonstrate best the relationship between the tumor, adjacent organs, and vascular structures. Functional imaging modalities can obviously not replace anatomical imaging in the assessment of local tumor resectability. [18]F-FDG imaging is not superior to contrast-enhanced CT for N staging, but more accurate for M staging.[75] False-positive interpretations occur in patients with intrahepatic cholestasis with dilated bile ducts and in inflammatory granulomas.[76]

## [18]F-FDG PET/CT in the Post-therapy Setting

Preliminary data suggest that [18]F-FDG imaging is useful for assessment of tumor response to neo-adjuvant therapy and for diagnosis of recurrent disease following resection.[60] [18]F-FDG imaging may be particularly useful for evaluation of an equivocal CT abnormality in the resection bed that is difficult to differentiate between surgical- or radiation-induced fibrosis, for evaluation of new hepatic lesions that may be too small to biopsy, and for restaging of patients with rising serum tumor marker levels and a negative conventional work-up.

## Impact of [18]F-FDG PET/CT on Management of Patients with Pancreatic Carcinoma

Delbeke and colleagues[75] reported a series of 65 patients in whom that the addition of [18]F-FDG PET to CT altered the surgical management in 41% of the patients, either by detection of CT-occult pancreatic carcinoma in 27% of patients or by identification of unsuspected distant metastases in 14%. The addition of [18]F-FDG PET to CT was also helpful in defining the benign nature of equivocal findings seen on CT. [18]F-FDG imaging allows the selection of the optimal surgical approach in patients with pancreatic carcinoma.

Kalady and colleagues[77] reviewed the performance of [18]F-FDG PET in patients with suspected periampullary malignancy. Despite a high sensitivity of 88% and specificity of 86% of [18]F-FDG PET compared to CT, which had a sensitivity of 90% and specificity of

62%, $^{18}$F-FDG imaging did not change clinical management in most patients previously evaluated by CT. $^{18}$F-FDG-PET missed over 10% of patients with periampullar malignancies and did not provide the anatomical detail necessary to define resectability.

## Limitations of $^{18}$F-FDG Imaging

Metabolic tumor detectability depends on the size of the lesion and the degree of radiotracer uptake, as well as on the surrounding background uptake and intrinsic resolution of the imaging system. Small lesions may yield false-negative results because of partial volume averaging which leads to underestimation of the uptake in small lesions,which are below twice the resolution of the imaging system, such as a small ampullary carcinoma, cholangiocarcinoma of the infiltrating type, miliary carcinomatosis, or necrotic lesions with a thin viable rim. The low relative uptake can lead to falsely classifying these lesions as benign instead of malignant.

The sensitivity of $^{18}$F-FDG PET for detection of mucinous adenocarcinoma is lower than for other histological subtypes of adenocarcinoma, 41–58% versus 92%, respectively, probably because of the relative hypocellularity of mucinous tumors.[78] Other tumors with a high rate of non $^{18}$F-FDG-avidity are differentiated neuroendocrine tumors and HCC. The high incidence of glucose intolerance and diabetes exhibited by patients with pancreatic pathology represents a potential limitation of $^{18}$F-FDG imaging in the diagnosis of pancreatic cancer, since low SUV values and false-negative $^{18}$F-FDG studies occur in hyperglycemic patients.

The high uptake of $^{18}$F-FDG in activated macrophages, neutrophils, fibroblasts, and granulation tissue is responsible for the $^{18}$F-FDG avidity of inflammatory tissue. Mild to moderate $^{18}$F-FDG uptake early after radiation therapy, along recent or in infected incisions, biopsy sites, drainage tubes and catheters, and colostomy can lead to errors in interpretation if the history is not known. Some inflammatory lesions, especially those containing granulomatous tissue, may be markedly $^{18}$F-FDG-avid and misinterpreted for malignancies. This relates mainly to abscesses and other acute processes such as cholangitis, cholecystitis, and chronic active pancreatitis with or without abscess formation. False-positive studies are frequent in patients with elevated C-reactive protein and/or acute pancreatitis with a specificity as low as 50%.[66]

## Summary

Various single photon emission computed tomography (SPECT) and PET radiopharmaceuticals are used for characterization of hepatic neoplasms. $^{18}$F-FDG imaging can differentiate malignant from benign hepatic lesions, with the exception of false-negative results in HCC, infiltrating cholangiocarcinoma, and false-positive inflammatory lesions. $^{18}$F-FDG imaging is not helpful in identifying HCC in patients with cirrhosis and regenerating nodules. In patients with primary malignant hepatic tumors that accumulate $^{18}$F-FDG, this test can identify unexpected distant metastases (although, as with other imaging modalities, miliary carcinomatosis is often false negative). $^{18}$F-FDG imaging is promising for monitoring patient response to therapy, including regional therapy to the liver, but larger studies are necessary to verify the initial reports.

$^{18}$F-FDG imaging is of value for the preoperative diagnosis of pancreatic carcinoma in patients with suspected cancer in whom CT fails to identify a discrete tumor mass or in whom biopsy is non-diagnostic. $^{18}$F-FDG imaging is also useful for M staging and restaging of pancreatic carcinoma due to improved detection of CT-occult metastatic disease, preventing futile attempts at complete surgical extirpation. $^{18}$F-FDG imaging can accurately differentiate treatment-induced changes from recurrence and holds promise for monitoring response to neo-adjuvant chemo-radiation therapy.

Because SPECT and PET imaging are complementary to morphological imaging with CT, integrated SPECT/CT and PET/CT studies provide optimal diagnostic tools.

# Guidelines and Recommendations for the Use of $^{18}$F-FDG PET and PET/CT

The National Comprehensive Cancer Network (NCCN) has incorporated $^{18}$F-FDG PET and PET/CT in the practice guidelines and management algorithm of a variety of malignancies including hepatobiliary and pancreatic malignancies. The use of $^{18}$F-FDG PET (PET/CT where available) may be helpful in the following clinical scenarios: 1) As adjunctive diagnostic tool for evaluating patients with suspected pancreatic cancer, especially when CT and biopsy are inconclusive; 2) In HCC recurrence assessment and evaluation of response to liver-directed therapy, as additional treatment options may be available for localized disease; 3) Improved detection of recurrence and response assessment in pancreatic and biliary cancers is less likely to be of clinical benefit, given the limited efficacy of available treatments.[79]

A multidisciplinary panel of experts reviewed meta-analyses and systematic reviews published in the FDG PET literature before March 2006 and made recommendations for the use of FDG PET in oncology.[80] The panel concluded that for pancreatic cancer $^{18}$F-FDG PET should be added to conventional imaging in selected patients whose conventional imaging findings are inconclusive.

In 2000, the European consensus designated $^{18}$F-FDG imaging as an established modality for differentiation of benign from malignant pancreatic masses.[81]

## Case Presentations

### Case II.7.1 (DICOM Images on DVD)

#### History

A 65-year-old male presented with acute cholecystitis and underwent laparoscopic cholecystectomy. A nodule estimated to be 30–40 mm in size was seen on the surface of the liver
lateral to the falciform ligament; a biopsy revealed poorly differentiated HCC in the setting
of cirrhosis. Alpha-fetoprotein plasma levels were elevated. Triple phase CT revealed a
nodular contour of the liver, with hypertrophy of the left and caudate lobes, and three sub-
centimeter low-density lesions in the right lobe of the liver with no definite enhancing
masses. There was also aorto-caval lymphadenopathy. The patient was referred for
dual tracer ($^{18}$F-FDG and $^{11}$C-acetate) PET/CT for initial staging (Fig. II.7.1A–D).
Figure II.7.1A displays the slice from the arterial phase of the contrasted CT corresponding to the PET slice and demonstrating the largest of the three low-density
lesions.

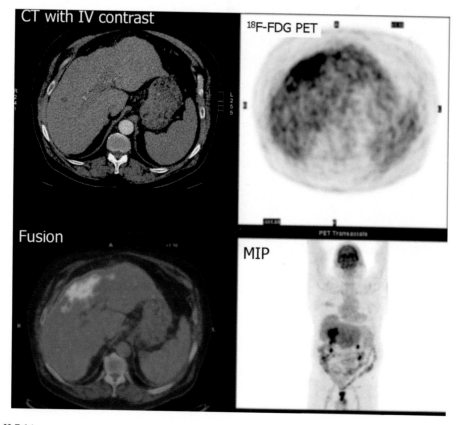

**Fig. II.7.1A**

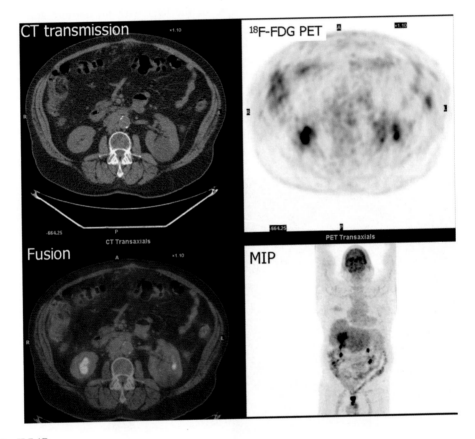

Fig. II.7.1B

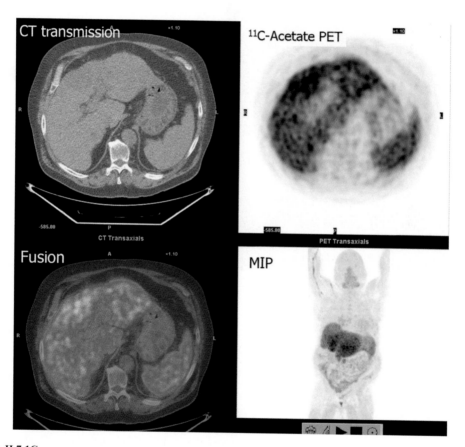

**Fig. II.7.1C**

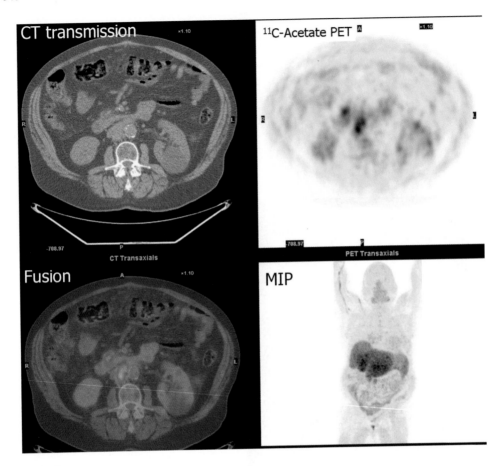

**Fig. II.7.1D**

**Findings**

$^{18}$F-FDG PET/CT images reveal a poorly delineated area of intense uptake lateral to the falciform ligament in the right lobe of the liver (Fig. II.7.1A). There is no abnormal $^{18}$F-FDG uptake in the left lobe of the liver or in the retroperitoneal adenopathy (Fig. II.7.1B).

$^{11}$C-acetate PET/CT images demonstrate moderate uptake matching the $^{18}$F-FDG uptake in the right lobe hepatic lesion as well as additional moderate uptake in the lobulated left lobe of the liver indicating involvement of the left lobe of the liver (Fig. II.7.1C). Unlike the $^{18}$F-FDG images, there is $^{11}$C-acetate uptake in the retroperitoneal adenopathy consistent with extrahepatic metastases (Fig. II.7.1D).

There is no abnormal $^{18}$F-FDG or $^{11}$C-acetate uptake in the sub-centimeter hypodense lesions seen on the contrast-enhanced CT, but they are at the limit of PET resolution (Fig. II.7.1A, C). Because the malignant neoplasm is isodense, the small lesions are probably hepatic cysts.

Multiple sub-centimeter pulmonary nodules are seen on CT but do not demonstrate either $^{18}$F-FDG nor $^{11}$C-acetate uptake, though they are below PET resolution. The pattern of these pulmonary nodules on CT is most consistent with pulmonary metastases (see DICOM images).

## Discussion

These findings are consistent with HCC in both the right and the left lobe of the liver with retroperitoneal and potentially pulmonary metastases. Therefore, the patient was not a surgical candidate and was referred for experimental therapy.

This case illustrates the complimentarity of CT, [18]F-FDG, and [11]C-acetate imaging. CT is the best modality for detection of sub-centimeter pulmonary metastases that are often below PET resolution. Although most HCC enhance on the arterial phase of the contrast-enhanced CT, the large HCC in this case is isodense to normal hepatic parenchyma, illustrating the limitations of CT for evaluation of hepatic masses. Involvement of the right lobe of the liver with HCC is better seen on the [18]F-FDG images, while involvement of the left lobe and the retroperitoneal metastatic adenopathy is better visualized on the [11]C-acetate images.

The accumulation of [18]F-FDG in HCC is variable due to the differing amounts of glucose-6-phosphatase present in individual tumors. [18]F-FDG accumulation in HCC is greater than in normal hepatic parenchyma in approximately 50–70% of patients. It has been associated with high levels of alpha-fetoprotein and poorly differentiated tumors. [11]C-acetate accumulates in well-differentiated HCC. The combined sensitivity for detection of HCC using both tracers is greater than 95%. HCCs are heterogenous tumors, with different portions of a tumors being either [18]F-FDG- or [11]C-acetate-avid, according to their level of differentiation. A study of dual tracer PET/CT in the evaluation of HCC demonstrated a positive correlation between the specific tracer avidity of the primary tumor and its metastases, although some metastases are seen with only one of the tracers. Dual tracer PET/CT leads to a change in management of patients with metastatic HCC, 19% of which were only [11]C-acetate-avid. Dual tracer PET/CT was found to be more effective than single tracer PET/CT in identifying patients for curative therapy. Both tracers are complimentary and have incremental value compared to either used alone.[20]

## Diagnosis

1. HCC accumulating [18]F-FDG and [11]C-acetate
2. Retroperitoneal metastases [18]F-FDG negative and [11]C-acetate avid
3. Suspected sub-centimeter pulmonary metastases seen on CT only

## Clinical Report: Body [18]F-FDG and [11]C-Acetate PET/CT (for DVD cases only)

Indication

Initial staging of HCC.

History

A 65-year-old male presented with acute cholecystitis and underwent laparoscopic chole-cystectomy. A nodule estimated to be 30–40 mm in size was seen on the surface of the liver lateral to the falciform ligament. Biopsy revealed poorly differentiated HCC in the setting of cirrhosis. Alpha-fetoprotein plasma levels were elevated. Triple phase CT revealed a nodular contour of the liver, hypertrophy of the left and caudate lobes, and three subcentimeter low-density lesions in the right lobe of the liver, but no definite enhancing masses. There was also aorto-caval adenopathy.


## Procedure

The $^{11}$C-acetate study was performed first followed by the $^{18}$F-FDG study. Approximately 15 min after the IV administration of 1,473 MBq (39.8 mCi) of $^{11}$C-acetate in the antecubital fossa, low-dose CT transmission images were acquired to correct for attenuation and to provide anatomic localization. PET images were then acquired from the vertex of the brain through the proximal femori, in one acquisition, with the arms up. DICOM fusion PET/CT images with and without attenuation correction were reviewed along with PET-only, CT-only, and 3D MIP images.

Next, $^{18}$F-FDG PET/CT imaging was performed. The fasting blood glucose level was 93 mg/dl at the time of injection of the radiopharmaceutical. $^{18}$F-FDG, 555 MBq (15.0 mCi), was administered IV in right antecubital fossa. After 65 min distribution time, a whole-body low-dose CT without intravenous contrast was acquired to correct for attenuation and to provide anatomic localization, followed by $^{18}$F-FDG PET images acquired from the vertex of the brain through the proximal femori, with the arms up. DICOM fusion PET/CT images with and without attenuation correction were reviewed.


## Findings

*Quality of the study*: The quality of this study is good.

*Head and neck*: There is physiologic distribution of the radiopharmaceutical in the cerebral cortex and lymphoid and glandular tissues of the neck. Within the right maxillary sinus is a soft tissue density, which demonstrates severely increased $^{18}$F-FDG uptake. This lesion does not demonstrate increased $^{11}$C-acetate uptake and is most consistent with an inflammatory process.

*Chest*: No abnormal $^{18}$F-FDG or $^{11}$C-acetate uptake is seen in the chest. Multiple sub-centimeter nodules are identified in both lungs on CT, below the PET resolution. There is aneurysmal dilatation of the ascending aorta to approximately 49 × 48 mm. The aortic arch is aneurysmal measuring approximately 59 mm in maximum transaxial diameter. There are diffuse vascular calcifications along the wall of the aorta and its branches, including the coronary arteries. The heart is enlarged.

*Abdomen and pelvis*: On the $^{18}$F-FDG images there is intense $^{18}$F-FDG metabolism within sub-segment eight of the liver. The lesion measures approximately 78 mm in its axial diameter. This lesion is also $^{11}$C-acetate positive. In addition, on the $^{11}$C-acetate images there is diffusely increased activity within the left lobe of the liver indicating involvement by HCC that is not demonstrated on the $^{18}$F-FDG images. The liver is enlarged and demonstrates a nodular contour. There is a conglomerate mass of aorto-caval lymph nodes which measures 54 × 30 mm. These nodes demonstrate increased $^{11}$C-acetate uptake although they are not $^{18}$F-FDG-avid.

The patient is status post cholecystectomy. The spleen is enlarged measuring approximately 165 mm. There is a large cyst within the left kidney, approximately 60 mm. There are colonic diverticulae. There is aneurysmal dilatation of the distal abdominal aorta measuring 31 × 32 mm, with bilateral extension into the iliac arteries, measuring approximately 22 mm on the right and 27 mm on the left.

*Musculoskeletal*: There are degenerative changes in the spine.

Disclaimers

Lesions less than 5 mm in diameter are below the resolution of PET. Lesions between 5 and 10 mm are detected with a lower sensitivity in the range of 50–80% than that reported for larger lesions. The technique used for a whole-body PET study is not optimal for evaluation of the brain, which is also not always entirely in the field of view.

Impression

1. Findings consistent with HCC in the right lobe ($^{11}$C-acetate $+$/$^{18}$F-FDG $+$) and left lobe ($^{11}$C-acetate $+$/$^{18}$F-FDG $-$) of the liver
2. Retroperitoneal metastases ($^{11}$C-acetate $+$/$^{18}$F-FDG $-$)
3. Multiple sub-centimeter bilateral pulmonary nodules ($^{11}$C-acetate $-$/$^{18}$F-FDG $-$) below PET resolution, concerning for metastatic disease. Follow-up CT of the chest is recommended within 3 months
4. Aneurysmal dilatation of the ascending aorta, aortic arch, distal abdominal aorta, and bilateral iliac arteries
5. Vascular calcifications consistent with atherosclerotic disease within the aorta and its branches, including the coronary arteries
6. Left renal cyst
7. For additional anatomical detail, please refer to diagnostic contrast-enhanced examination of the abdomen previously performed

## *Case II.7.2*

### History

A 44-year-old male presented with jaundice and epigastric pain. ERCP demonstrated irregular intrahepatic bile ducts with an equivocal mass in the porta hepatis. A biliary stent was placed in the common bile duct. Brushings were negative for malignancy. Outside CT, MRI, and MRCP also reported an ill-defined mass-like lesion in the left lobe of the liver with neoplastic and inflammatory etiologies in the differential considerations. The patient was referred to the authors' institution. A triple phase contrast-enhanced CT of the abdomen revealed dilated intrahepatic bile ducts and an ill-defined, low-density mass in the left lobe of the liver with mild marginal enhancement, 50 × 36 mm in size. A biliary stent was in place. Porto-caval adenopathy was also present (Fig. II.7.2A). A CT-guided core biopsy revealed poorly differentiated cholangiocarcinoma. The patient was referred to [18]F-FDG PET/CT for initial staging. (Fig. II.7.2B–D).

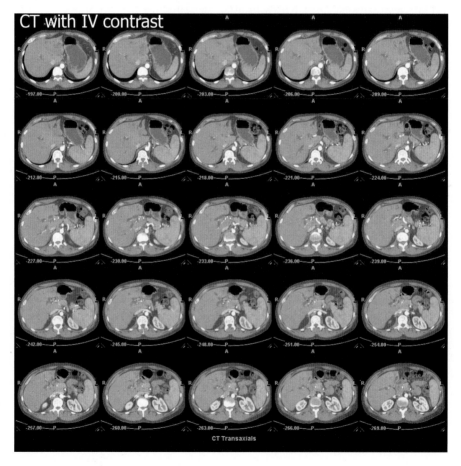

**Fig. II.7.2A**

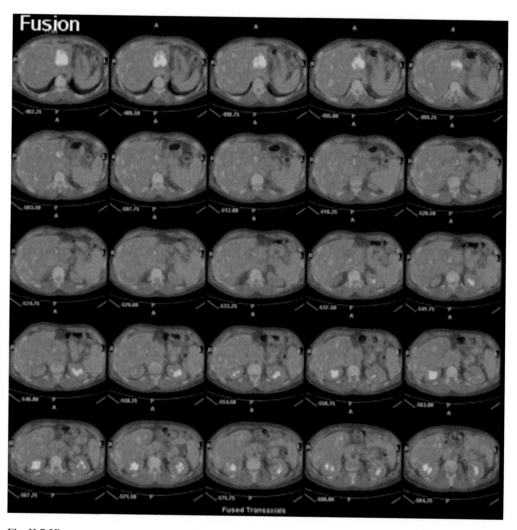

**Fig. II.7.2B**

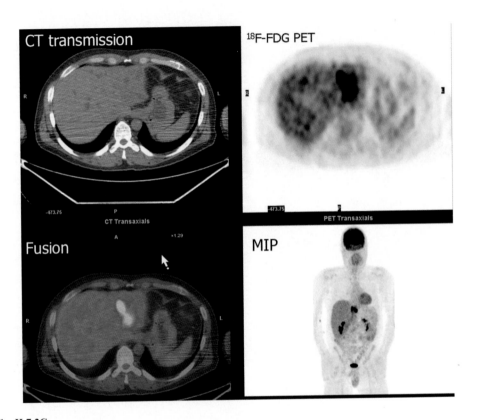

Fig. II.7.2C

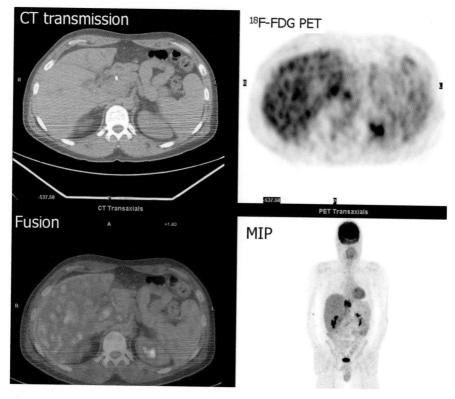

**Fig. II.7.2D**

## Findings

There is a large area of intense $^{18}$F-FDG uptake in the left lobe of the liver consistent with cholangiocarcinoma (Fig. II.7.2B, C). In addition there are foci of moderate $^{18}$F-FDG uptake corresponding to the adenopathy in the porta hepatis seen on CT, consistent with metastases (Fig. II.7.2B, D).

## Discussion

Endoscopic US was performed. FNA biopsy of the porto-caval lymph nodes was non-diagnostic. One month later, exploratory laparoscopy with peritoneal biopsy revealed metastatic cholangiocarcinoma. This case illustrates the difficulty in obtaining a diagnosis when multiple imaging modalities are highly suggestive for but not diagnostic of malignancy, and biopsy of limited invasiveness (e.g., brushing and FNA biopsy) is non-diagnostic. $^{18}$F-FDG PET/CT was helpful in supporting a diagnosis of metastatic malignancy, with the fusion images allowing precise localization of $^{18}$F-FDG uptake to anatomical abnormalities in the left lobe of the liver and in porta hepatis lymphadenopathy.

Cholangiocarcinoma is a relatively rare tumor with 17,000 cases reported annually in the United States. The majority of these tumors are unresectable at the time of presentation but slow growing, and patients may therefore survive for years. Distant metastases are relatively rare, although 50% of patients will have loco-regional nodal involvement.

CT diagnosis of cholangiocarcinoma can be difficult because the majority of these lesions are isodense to liver. The point at which intrahepatic ductal dilatation begins or where hepatic atrophy is identified can imply the location of the tumor. MRI can be helpful at times with a hypointense central scar identified on T2-weighted images in approximately 25–30% of cases.[82]

[18]F-FDG imaging can be of value in diagnosis and management of patients with suspected cholangiocarcinoma and sclerosing cholangitis.[22] Unlike HCC, which may have variable degrees of glucose-6-phosphatase activity and may not accumulate [18]F-FDG, cholangiocarcinomas do accumulate [18]F-FDG. However, false-negative results are not uncommon because of the frequently diffuse infiltrating pattern of this tumor.[23] The sensitivity for tumors with a nodular morphology is 85%, but only 18% for infiltrating tumors. Peritoneal carcinomatosis can result in false-negative [18]F-FDG studies while cholangitis can account for false-positive studies. Inflammatory changes along the tract of a biliary stent can lead to false-positive interpretation for tumor as well. Despite these limitations, [18]FDG PET can induce a change in surgical management in up to 30% of patients with cholangiocarcinoma because of detection of unsuspected metastases.

### Diagnosis

1. Cholangiocarcinoma in the left lobe of the liver
2. Nodal metastases in the porta hepatis

## Case II.7.3

### History

A 44-year-old female presented with epigastric discomfort. Abdominal US revealed a 30 × 20 mm lesion in the gallbladder. Contrast-enhanced CT of the abdomen and pelvis confirmed these findings and also revealed retroperitoneal adenopathy (Fig. II.7.3A). The patient was referred to $^{18}$F-FDG PET/CT for initial staging (Fig. II.7.2B–D).

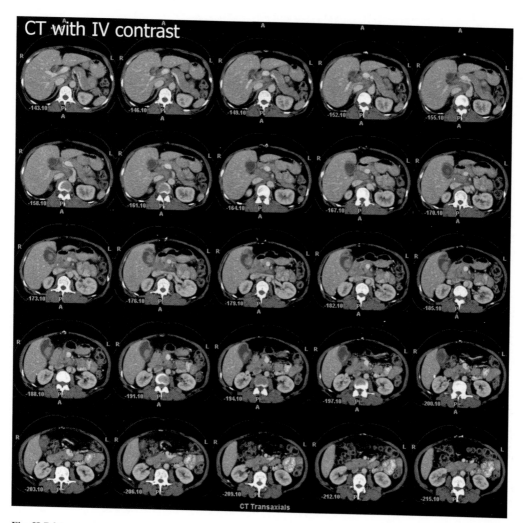

Fig. II.7.3A

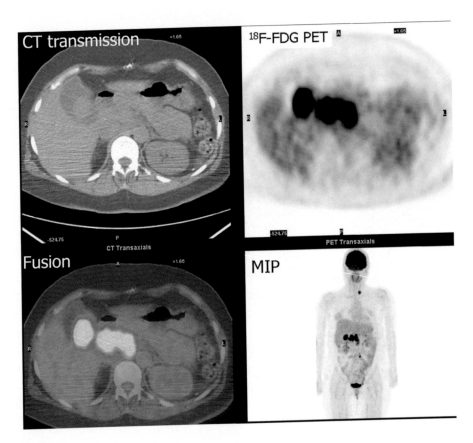

Fig. II.7.3B

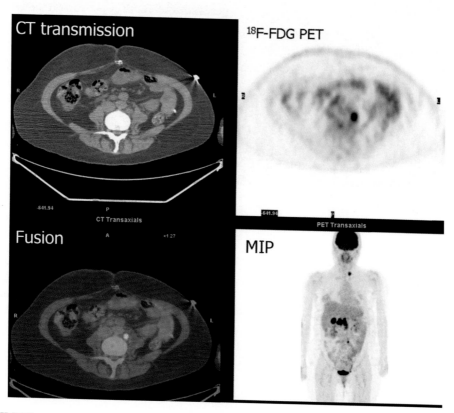

**Fig. II.7.3C**

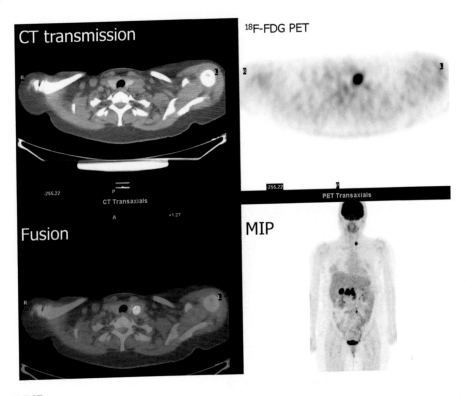

**Fig. II.7.3D**

## Findings

There is intense [18]F-FDG uptake corresponding to a sessile lesion arising from the gall-bladder wall, consistent with malignancy. In addition, there is intense [18]F-FDG uptake corresponding to a conglomerate of enlarged lymph nodes extending from the gallbladder fossa to the celiac axis and superior mesenteric artery (Fig. II.7.3B). There is also intense [18]F-FDG uptake corresponding to two left periaortic lymph nodes below the level of the kidneys measuring up to 17 mm in greatest axial diameter (Fig. II.7.3C) and in a left supraclavicular lymph node 20 mm in greatest axial diameter (Fig. II.7.3D), indicating additional metastases.

## Discussion

These findings are consistent with gallbladder carcinoma with distant metastases. PET/CT demonstrated that the patient was not a surgical candidate, and she was referred to medical oncology for chemotherapy. The lymph nodes detected by [18]F-FDG imaging in the left supraclavicular and left periaortic region could be easily missed on CT alone, but the combination of PET/CT is diagnostic of distant meta-static disease.

Gallbladder carcinoma is often discovered incidentally and is usually metastatic at the time of diagnosis. Peritoneal spread is common but can be below PET resolution.

**Diagnosis**

1. Gallbladder carcinoma
2. Metastatic lymph nodes in the porta hepatic
3. Left periaortic metastatic lymph node at the pelvic inlet
4. Left supraclavicular metastatic lymph node

## Case II.7.4 (DICOM Images on DVD)

### History

A 53-year-old male presented with jaundice and epigastric pain. CT revealed intra- and extra hepatic ductal dilatation and a 39 × 22 mm pancreatic lesion and an intrahepatic non-enhancing 25 mm lesion adjacent to the inferior vena cava (IVC) (Fig. II.7.4A). ERCP was performed with a stent placed from the common bile duct to the duodenum, spanning the region of obstruction. FNA biopsy of the pancreatic lesion was non-diagnostic. The patient was referred to [18]F-FDG PET/CT for initial staging (Fig. II.7.4B–D).

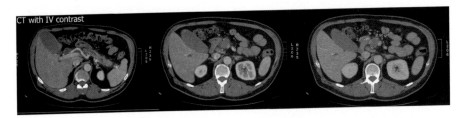

**Fig. II.7.4A**

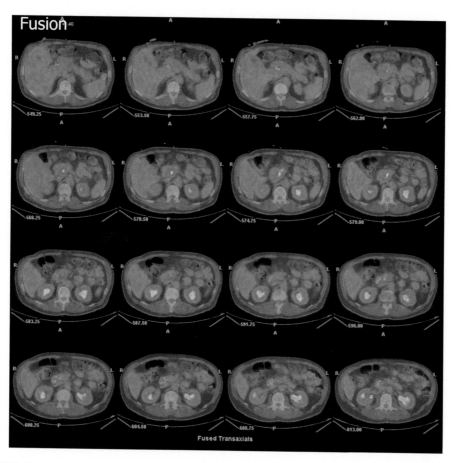

Fig. II.7.4B

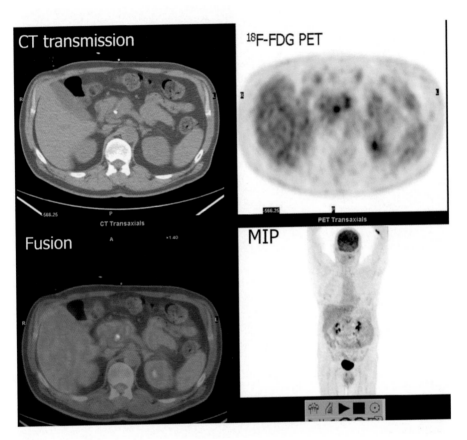

Fig. II.7.4C

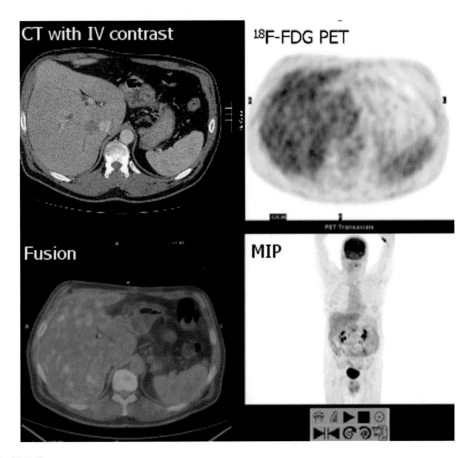

**Fig. II.7.4D**

**Findings**

There is intense $^{18}$F-FDG uptake corresponding to the mass in the head of the pancreas consistent with malignancy (Fig. II.7.4B). There is a stent in the common duct seen on CT with $^{18}$F-FDG uptake along the stent (Fig. II.7.4B,C), probably due to inflammatory changes. These two areas of increased tracer uptake are in close vicinity to each other and can be differentiated with the help of fused images. The contrast-enhanced CT (upper left) demonstrates the hypodense lesion in the liver adjacent to the IVC with no abnormal $^{18}$F-FDG uptake, most probably consistent with a benign lesion (Figure II.7.4D).

**Discussion**

These findings are consistent with carcinoma of the head of the pancreas. The patient underwent explorative laparotomy. The pancreatic tumor was found to be unresectable, encasing the gastroduodenal and hepatic arteries and the portal vein. Hepato-jejunostomy and biliary bypass procedures were performed. Tissue biopsy obtained at surgery confirmed the diagnosis of adenocarcinoma in the pancreas and hamartoma of the liver.

The typical initial evaluation of a pancreatic neoplasm includes CT and endoscopic US with biopsy. CT has an accuracy of 70% for diagnosis of pancreatic cancer and a positive predictive value of non-resectability of 90%. ERCP is another means of evaluating the pancreas, with an accuracy of 80–90% in differentiating benign from malignant masses. ERCP has an approximately 10% technical failure rate and up to 8% morbidity, primarily due to iatrogenic pancreatitis. Endoscopic US allows FNA biopsy, but is non-diagnostic in up to 30% of cases due to sampling errors. $^{18}$F-FDG imaging is very helpful for diagnosis of pancreatic cancer for these indeterminate patients.

Diagnosis of pancreatic malignancy can also be difficult in patients with mass-forming pancreatitis and in cases of enlargement of the pancreatic head without a definite mass. $^{18}$F-FDG imaging has a sensitivity of 85–100%, a specificity of 67–99%, and an accuracy of 85–93% for preoperative diagnosis of pancreatic carcinoma. $^{18}$F-FDG imaging is particularly useful in determining the presence of metastatic disease, which can significantly alter patient management.

## Diagnosis

1. Pancreatic carcinoma
2. Benign hepatic lesion

## Clinical Report: Body $^{18}$F-FDG PET/CT (for DVD cases only)

Indication

Initial staging for pancreatic carcinoma.

History

A 53-year-old male presented with jaundice and epigastric pain. CT revealed intra- and extra hepatic ductal dilatation and a 39 × 22 mm pancreatic lesion. In addition, there was an intrahepatic non-enhancing 25 mm lesion adjacent to the inferior vena cava. ERCP was performed, and a stent was placed from the common bile duct to the duodenum. FNA biopsy of the pancreatic lesion was non-diagnostic. The patient is referred to $^{18}$F-FDG PET/CT for initial staging.

Procedure

The fasting blood glucose level was 120 mg/dl. $^{18}$F-FDG, 400 MBq (10.8 mCi), was administered IV in the left antecubital fossa. After 65 min distribution time, a whole-body low-dose CT without intravenous contrast was acquired to correct for attenuation and for anatomic localization, followed by $^{18}$F-FDG PET images acquired over the head, neck, thorax, abdomen, and pelvis with the arms up.

Findings

*Quality of the study*: The quality of this study is good.
*Head and neck*: There is physiologic distribution of the radiopharmaceutical in the cerebral cortex and lymphoid and glandular tissues of the neck.
*Chest*: No abnormal $^{18}$F-FDG uptake is seen in the chest.

*Abdomen and pelvis*: On the $^{18}$F-FDG images, there is intense $^{18}$F-FDG uptake within the head of the pancreas corresponding to the patient's known mass. This lesion is poorly delineated on the non-contrasted CT. There is also $^{18}$F-FDG uptake around a biliary stent. There is no $^{18}$F-FDG uptake in the hepatic lesion adjacent to the inferior vena cava seen on the prior contrast-enhanced CT of the liver.

*Musculoskeletal*: There are degenerative changes in the spine.

Impression

1. Focal region of markedly increased $^{18}$F-FDG uptake in the head of the pancreas with a corresponding mass on CT, consistent with a malignant neoplasm.
2. Focal area of moderately increased FDG uptake corresponding to the biliary stent, most probably related to inflammatory changes.
3. No evidence of abnormal $^{18}$F-FDG uptake within the patient's liver hamartoma.

## Case II.7.5

### History

A 76-year-old male presented with jaundice. ERCP was performed with a stent placed. An outside CT demonstrated an equivocal lesion at the bifurcation of the bile ducts. The patient was referred for a repeat triple phase CT with contrast (Fig. II.7.5A, B) and for $^{18}$F-FDG PET/CT for initial staging (Fig. II.7.5C, D).

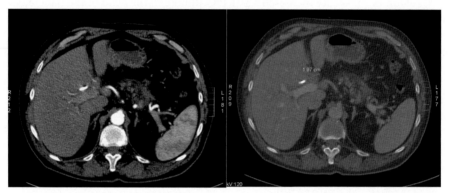

CT arterial phase          CT delayed phase

**Fig. II.7.5A**

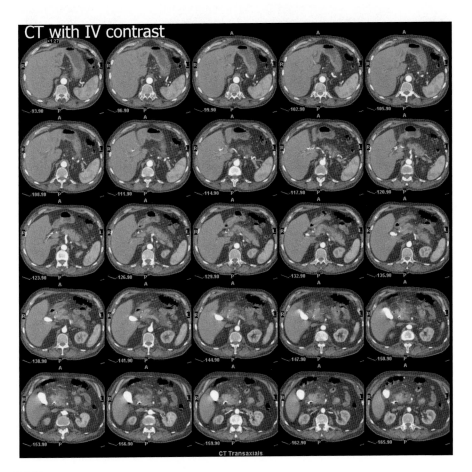

**Fig. II.7.5B**

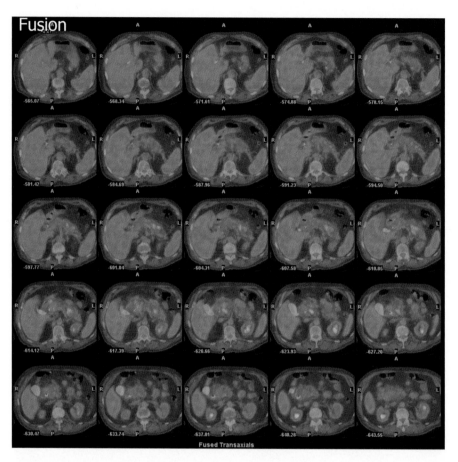

**Fig. II.7.5C**

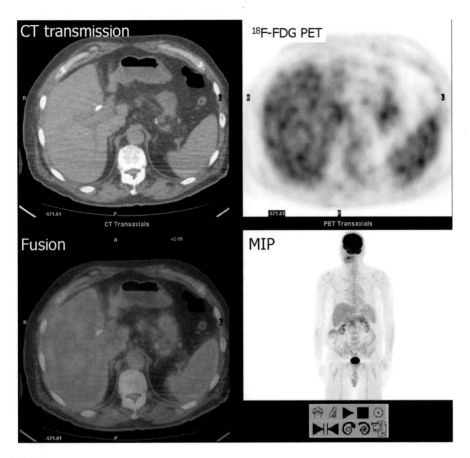

**Fig. II.7.5D**

## Findings

Contrast-enhanced CT demonstrates an ill-defined soft tissue mass inferior to the portal vein along the medial segment of the left lobe of the liver (Fig. II.7.5A). A biliary stent is seen in the common bile duct and the duodenum, and there is contrast in the gallbladder (Fig. II.7.5A, B).

Sequential fused $^{18}$F-FDG PET/CT images (Fig. II.7.5C) demonstrate diffuse $^{18}$F-FDG uptake in the pancreas corresponding to stranding around the pancreas on CT, most consistent with acute iatrogenic pancreatitis after ERCP. A selected PET/CT slice at the level of the porta hepatis demonstrates mild $^{18}$F-FDG uptake in the lesion seen on CT (Fig. II.7.5D).

## Discussion

Klatskin's tumor is a type of cholangiocarcinoma arising at the junction of the right and left hepatic ducts. Patients present with jaundice early in the course of disease when the lesion is small and therefore difficult to detect on imaging studies, often at the limit of resolution of PET. In this case, $^{18}$F-FDG PET could be considered false negative as the lesion is above

PET resolution and the degree of uptake in the lesion is very mild. False-negative findings on [18]F-FDG PET are common with Klatskin's tumors. Fused PET/CT is critical for reaching an accurate diagnosis.

This case also illustrates the typical diffuse pattern of [18]F-FDG uptake in acute pancreatitis that was confirmed clinically in this patient.

**Diagnosis**

1. Klatskin's cholangiocarcinoma diagnosed only by PET/CT
2. Acute iatrogenic pancreatitis after ERCP

## Case II.7.6

### History

This 49-year-old male was referred for evaluation of a 20 × 10 mm hypodense lesion in the inferior aspect of the right lobe of the liver seen on an outside CT. US excluded a simple cyst. The patient was referred for $^{99m}$Tc-RBC scintigraphy, including a SPECT/low-dose CT (Fig. II.7.6).

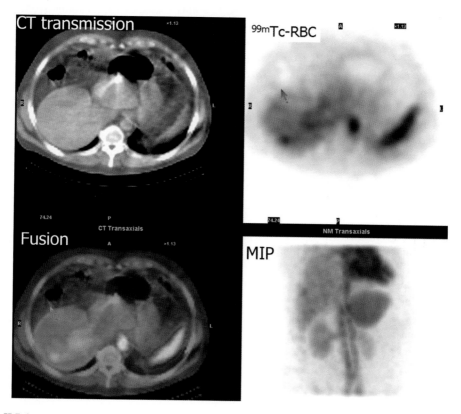

**Fig. II.7.6**

### Findings

On the anterior view of the MIP image (lower right), a small focus of uptake is seen in the right lobe of the liver. On the transaxial slices, the focus of uptake corresponds to an equivocal lesion on the CT transmission in the location described in the outside CT report (Fig. II.7.6).

### Discussion

These findings are consistent with a benign liver hemangioma. As the patient was asymptomatic, his treating physician decided to electively follow him as needed.

Space-occupying lesions in the liver are always concerning for malignant tumors, especially in patients with a history of cancer. In patients without known malignancies, the most common benign lesions are hepatic cysts, hemangiomas, focal nodular hyperplasia, and adenomas. Simple cysts are the most common benign hepatic lesions. On CT, cysts have a density close to that of water ($-15 < HU > +15$).

Hemangioma is the second most common benign tumor of the liver. It is characterized by sluggish perfusion and increased activity on delayed blood pool imaging. On CT, they are hypodense in the early porto-venous phase of the study, demonstrating progressive enhancement beginning at the periphery that moves centrally on delayed images. Therefore, characterization of hemangiomas requires dynamic and delayed imaging. Small hemangiomas are more difficult to characterize with CT, sometimes indistinguishable from small primary or metastatic lesions.

$^{99m}$Tc-RBC scintigraphy is commonly used to differentiate cavernous hemangiomas from other lesions. $^{99m}$Tc-RBC is a blood pool imaging tracer and is helpful to evaluate the vascularity of the lesion, similar to intravenous contrast agents used for CT and MRI. There is progressive visualization of hemangiomas over time, and images are typically acquired as long as 2 h after administration of the radiopharmaceutical. The specificity of $^{99m}$Tc-RBC for the diagnosis of liver hemangioma is extremely high, but the sensitivity is high only for lesions larger than 2.5 cm. With SPECT, the sensitivity for smaller lesions improves. SPECT/CT is very helpful for localization of the lesions and correlation with diagnostic CT. It is also of use for evaluation of lesions adjacent to structures with high uptake such as blood vessels, heart, spleen, or renal blood pool.

**Diagnosis**

Small hemangioma in the right lobe of the liver.

## Case II.7.7

### History

This 49-year-old female presented with epigastric discomfort. An outside US reported a pancreatic mass. She was referred for contrast-enhanced CT, which demonstrated a 38 × 44 mm exophytic mass arising from the left lobe of the liver with a central scar suspicious for focal nodular hyperplasia (Fig. II.7.7A). She was referred for a $^{99m}$Tc-sulfur colloid scintigraphy, with SPECT/CT imaging performed with a very low-dose CT (Fig. II.7.7B).

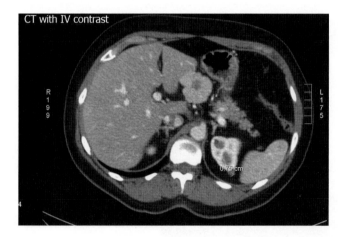

**Fig. II.7.7A**

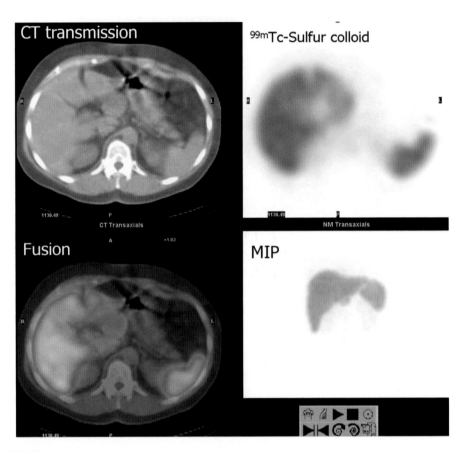

**Fig. II.7.7B**

## Findings

On $^{99m}$Tc-sulfur colloid SPECT/CT, the exophytic lesion arising from the left lobe of the liver is demonstrated on the MIP image. The selected slice through the lesion demonstrates sulfur colloid uptake in the lesion consistent with focal nodular hyperplasia.

## Discussion

A biopsy confirmed focal nodular hyperplasia in this patient.

The patient's age and gender are important as malignant tumors are more common in males and benign tumors in female. For the middle-aged female, the more common hepatic tumors are cavernous hemangioma, focal nodular hyperplasia, adenoma, and fibrolamellar HCC. Characterization of hemangioma has been discussed in case II.7.6 and HCC in case II.7.1. Among the benign hepatic neoplasms, it is important to differentiate an adenoma from focal nodular hyperplasia because an adenoma can rupture with life-threatening hemorrhage whereas focal nodular hyperplasia does not. Focal nodular hyperplasia appears typically as a solitary mass detected incidentally in asymptomatic young women. Histologically, the tumor has a thin capsule with a small central fibrous scar and numerous bile ducts. It contains all types of hepatic cells, including Kupffer cells. Focal nodular

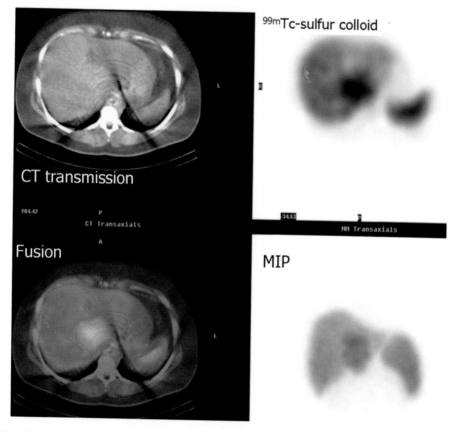

Fig. II.7.7C

hyperplasia and adenoma have characteristic CT features related to vascularity (both enhance during the arterial phase post-contrast), hemorrhage (suggesting adenoma), fat content (adenomas are usually hypodense on non-contrast images because they contain fat), and central scar (the central scar of focal nodular hyperplasia enhances on the delayed images post-contrast).[83]

$^{99m}$Tc-sulfur colloid is removed from the circulation by the reticuloendothelial system. Therefore, in the liver, it is a marker for the Kupffer cells. Most space-occupying lesions in the liver, including adenoma and malignancies, do not usually contain Kupffer cells but focal nodular hyperplasia does. Therefore, $^{99m}$Tc-sulfur colloid uptake is helpful for characterization of focal nodular hyperplasia. $^{99m}$Tc-sulfur colloid uptake in focal nodular hyperplasia can be less than that of normal hepatic parenchyma, as in this case, but still clearly present. Between 40 and 70% of focal nodular hyperplasia lesions show normal or increased uptake (Fig. II.7.7C). Scintigraphy is more specific than CT for characterization of focal nodular hyperplasia.

SPECT/CT allows precise identification and localization of the lesion and evaluation of the degree of uptake, especially if it is exophytic and not clearly localized in the liver as in the above case (Fig. II.7.7C).


**Diagnosis**

Focal nodular hyperplasia.

## Case II.7.8

### History

A 70-year-old male was diagnosed with sigmoid adenocarcinoma 2 years prior to the current examination with metastases to the liver and lung. He was treated with sigmoidectomy and multiple cycles of chemotherapy. A recent CT demonstrated resolution of the pulmonary metastases but persistent low densities in the liver. Palliative regional treatment to the liver with $^{90}$Y-microspheres (SIRSpheres®, Sirtex Medical, Inc) was considered. The patient was referred for restaging with $^{18}$F-FDG PET/CT before and monitoring response 4 months after therapy with 50 mCi $^{90}$Y-microspheres injected into the right hepatic artery with MIP images displayed for each study (Fig. II.7.8).

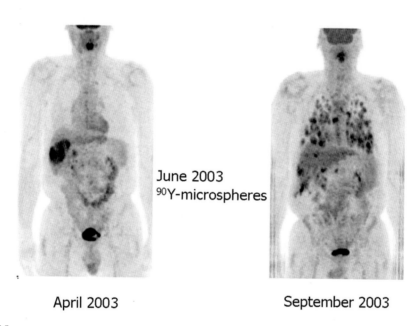

June 2003
$^{90}$Y-microspheres

April 2003        September 2003

Fig. II.7.8

### Findings

On the baseline study, there are two large foci of uptake in the right lobe of the liver, measuring 72 × 48 mm and 20 mm in diameter, respectively, consistent with metastases (Fig. II.7.8, left). There is no evidence of abnormal uptake in the lungs and no evidence of pulmonary metastases on CT (not shown). On the 4 month follow-up study, the findings in the right lobe of the liver have markedly improved. However, there are new bilateral innumerable $^{18}$F-FDG-avid pulmonary metastases, in addition to new metastases in the left lobe of the liver, retroperitoneum, and sternum (Fig. II.7.8, right).

## Discussion

Hepatic metastases can be treated with either regional therapy to the liver or systemic chemotherapy. A variety of procedures to administer regional therapy to hepatic metastases have been described, including radiolabeled $^{90}$Y-microspheres.[32,33,34] There are 2 types of $^{90}$Y-labeled microspheres, $^{90}$Y integrated into a glass matrix (TheraSpheres® manufactured by MDS Nordion) or $^{90}$Y attached to resin beads with diameters from 15 to 35 μm (SIRSpheres® manufactured by Sirtex Medical, Inc). Regional therapy with $^{90}$Y-microspheres is a palliative treatment for patients with unresectable hepatic metastases. $^{18}$F-FDG imaging can demonstrate partial response to therapy in the right lobe of the liver where the microspheres were delivered. However, in this patient, systemic chemotherapy did not eradicate extrahepatic metastases. Although there was no evidence of pulmonary metastases by imaging (CT and PET) at restaging, undetectable microscopic disease probably persisted and progressed over time.

Preliminary data suggest that $^{18}$F-FDG imaging may be able to effectively monitor the efficacy of regional therapy to hepatic metastases, but these data need to be confirmed. For example, Wong and colleagues[46,47] have compared $^{18}$F-FDG imaging, CT, MRI, and serum levels of CEA for monitoring of the therapeutic response of hepatic metastases to $^{90}$Y-glass microspheres. They found that the changes on $^{18}$F-FDG PET imaging demonstrated superior and significant correlation with changes in serum CEA levels following therapy compared to CT or MRI.

## Diagnosis

1. Partial palliative regional therapy to hepatic metastases with $^{90}$Y-microspheres documented by $^{18}$F-FDG PET
2. Progression of metastases in the lungs, retroperitoneum, and sternum

# References

1. Townsend DW, Beyer T, Bloggett TM. PET/CT scanners: A hardware approach to image fusion. *Semin Nucl Med* 2003;33:193–204.
2. Czernin J (ed). PET/CT: Imaging structure and function. *J Nucl Med* 2004;45(Suppl 1):1S–103S.
3. Kinkel K, Lu Y, Both M, Warren RS, Thoeni RF. Detection of hepatic metastases from cancers of the gastrointestinal tract by using noninvasive imaging methods (US, CT, MR imaging, PET) : A meta-analysis. *Radiology* 2002;224:748–756.
4. Bipat S, van Leeuwen MS, Comans EF, Pijl ME, Bossuyt PM, Zwinderman AH, Stoker J. Colorectal liver metastases: CT, MR imaging, and PET for diagnosis – meta-analysis. *Radiology* 2005;237: 1230–1231.
5. Wiering B, Ruers TJ, Krabbe PF, Dekker HM, Oyen WJ. Comparison of multiphase CT, FDG-PET and intra-operative ultrasound in patients with colorectal liver metastases selected for surgery. *Ann Surg Oncol* 2007;14:818–826.
6. Oppenheim BE. Liver imaging. In Sandler MP, Coleman RE, Wackers FTJ et al. (eds): *Diagnostic Nuclear Medicine*. Baltimore, MD:Williams and Wilkins, 1996, pp 749–758.
7. Weber G, Cantero A. Glucose-6-phosphatase activity in normal, precancerous, and neoplastic tissues. *Cancer Res* 1955;15:105–108.
8. Weber G, Morris HP. Comparative biochemistry of hepatomas. III. Carbohydrate enzymes in liver tumors of different growth rates. *Cancer Res* 1963;23:987–994.
9. Messa C, Choi Y, Hoh CK, Jacobs EL, Glaspy JA, Rege S, Nitzsche E, Huang SC, Phelps ME, Hawkins RA. Quantification of glucose utilization in liver metastases: parametric imaging of FDG uptake with PET. *J Comput Assist Tomogr* 1992;16:684–689.
10. Torizuka T, Tamaki N, Inokuma T, Magata Y, Sasayama S, Yonekura Y, Tanaka A, Yamaoka Y, Yamamoto K, Konishi J. In vivo assessment of glucose metabolism in hepatocellular carcinoma with FDG-PET. *J Nucl Med* 1995;36:1811–1817.
11. Khan MA, Combs CS, Brunt EM, Lowe VJ, Wolverson MK, Solomon H, Collins BT, Di Bisceglie AM. Positron emission tomography scanning in the evaluation of hepatocellular carcinoma. *J Hepatol* 2000;32:792–797.
12. Delbeke D, Martin WH, Sandler MP, Chapman WC, Wright JK Jr, Pinson CW. Evaluation of benign vs. malignant hepatic lesions with positron emission tomography.*Arch Surg* 1998;133:510–515.
13. Iwata Y, Shiomi S, Sasaki N, Jomura H, Nishiguchi S, Seki S, Kawabe J, Ochi H. Clinical usefulness of positron emission tomography with fluorine-18-fluorodeoxiglucose in the diagnosis of liver tumors. *Ann Nucl Med* 2000;14:121–126.
14. Trojan J, Schroeder O, Raedle J, Baum RP, Herrmann G, Jacobi V, Zeuzem S. Fluorine-18 FDG positron emission tomography for imaging of hepatocellular carcinoma. *Am J Gastroenterol* 1999;94:3314–3319.
15. Schroder O, Trojan J, Zeuzem S, Baum RP. Limited value of fluorine-18-fluorodeoxyglucose PET for the differential diagnosis of focal liver lesions in patients with chronic hepatitis C virus infection. *Nuklearmedizin* 1998;37:279–285.
16. Liangpunsakul S, Agarwal D, Horlander JC, Kieff B, Chalasani N. Positron emission tomography for detecting occult hepatocellular carcinoma in hepatitis C cirrhotics awaiting for liver transplantation. *Transplant Proc* 2003;35:2995–2997.
17. Teefey SA, Hildeboldt CC, Dehdashti F, Siegel BA, Peters MG, Heiken JP, Brown JJ, McFarland EG, Middleton WD, Balfe DM, Ritter JH. Detection of primary hepatic malignancy in liver transplant candidates: prospective comparison of CT, MR imaging, US, and PET. *Radiology* 2003;226:533–542.
18. Wudel LJ, Delbeke D, Morris D, Rice M, Washington MK, Shyr Y, Pinson CW, Chapman WC. The role of FDG-PET imaging in the evaluation of hepatocellular carcinoma. *Amer Surg* 2003;69:117–126.
19. Ho CL, Yu SC, Yeung DW.[11]C-Acetate PET imaging in hepatocellular carcinoma and other liver masses. *J Nucl Med* 2003;44:213–221.
20. Ho CL, Shen S, Young DWC, Cheng TKC. Dual tracer PET/CT in the evaluation of hepatocellular carcinoma. *J Nucl Med* 2007;48:902–909.
21. Talbot JN, Gutman F, Fartoux L, Grange JD, Ganne N, Kerrou K, Grahek D, Montravers F, PouponR, Rosmorduc O.PET/CT in patients with hepatocellular carcinoma using [(18)F]fluorocholine: Preliminary comparison with [(18)F]FDG PET/CT. *Eur J Nucl Med Mol Imaging* 2006;33:1285–1289.

22. Keiding S, Hansen SB, Rasmussen HH, Gee A, Kruse A, Roelsgaard K,Tage-Jensen U, Dahlerup JF. Detection of cholangiocarcinoma in primary sclerosing cholangitis by positron emission tomography. *Hepatology* 1998;28:700–706.

23. Anderson CA, Rice MH, Pinson CW, Chapman WC, Ravi RS, Delbeke D. FDG PET imaging in the evaluation of gallbladder carcinoma and cholangiocarcinoma. *J Gastrointest Surg* 2004;8:90–97.

24. Kim YJ, Yun M, Lee WJ, Kim KS, Lee JD. Usefulness of 18F-FDG PET in intrahepatic cholangio-carcinomas. *Eur J Nucl Med Mol Imaging* 2003;30:1467–1472.

25. Moon CM, Bang S, Chung JB, Park SW, Song SY, Yun M, Lee JD. Usefulness of (18)F-fluorodeox-yglucose positron emission tomography in differential diagnosis and staging of cholangiocarcinomas. *J Gastroenterol Hepatol* 2008;23:759–765.

26. Corvera CU, Blumgart LH, Akhurst T, DeMatteo RP, D'Angelica M, Fong Y, Jarnagin WR. 18F-fluorodeoxyglucose positron emission tomography influences management decisions in patients with biliary cancer. *J Am Coll Surg* 2008;206:57–65.

27. Drouard F, Delamarre J, Capron JP. Cutaneous seeding of gallbladder cancer after laparoscopic cholecystectomy. *N Engl J Med* 1991;325:1316.

28. Weiss SM, Wengert PA, Harkavy SE. Incisional recurrence of gallbladder cancer after laparoscopic cholecystectomy. *Gastrointest Endosc* 1994;40:244–246.

29. Hoh CK, Hawkins RA, Glaspy JA, Dahlbom M, Tse NY, Hoffman EJ, Schiepers C, Choi Y, Rege S, Nitzsche E, et al. Cancer detection with whole-body PET using 2-[18F]fluoro-2-deoxy-D-glucose. *J Comput Assist Tomogr* 1993;17:582–589.

30. Lomis KD, Vitola JV, Delbeke D, Snodgrass SL, Chapman WC, Wright JK, Pinson CW. Recurrent gallbladder carcinoma at laparoscopy port sites diagnosed by PET scan: Implications for primary and radical second operations. *Am Sur* 1997;63:341–345.

31. Rodríguez-Fernández A, Gómez-Río M, Llamas-Elvira JM, Ortega-Lozano S, Ferrón-Orihuela J, Ramia-Angel J, Mansilla-Roselló A, Martínez-del-Valle M, Ramos-Font C. Positron-emission tomo-graphy with fluorine-18-fluoro-2-deoxy-D-glucose for gallbladder cancer diagnosis. *Am J Surg* 2004;188:171–175.

32. Gray B, Van Hazel G, Hope M, Burton M, Moroz P, Anderson J, Gebski V. Randomized trial of Sir-spheres plus chemotherapy vs chemotherapy alone for treating patients with liver metastases from primary large bowel cancer. *Ann Oncol* 2001;12:1711–1720.

33. Atassi B, Bangash AK, Bahrani A, Pizzi G,Lewandowski RJ, Ryu RK,Sato KT, Gates VL, Mulcahy MF, Kulik L, Miller F, Yaghmai V,Murthy R, Larson A, Omary RA, Salem R. Multimodality imaging following 90Y radioembolization: A comprehensive review and pictorial essay. *Radiographics* 2008;28:81–99.

34. Kalva SP, Thabet A, Wicky S. Recent advances in transarterial therapy of primary and secondary liver malignancies. *Radiographics.* 2008;28:101–117.

35. Torizuka T, Tamaki N, Inouma T, Magata Y, Yonekura Y, Tanaka A, Yamaoka Y, Yamamoto K, Konishi J. Value of fluorine-18-FDG PET to monitor hepatocellular carcinoma after interventional therapy. *J Nucl Med* 1994;35:1965–1969.

36. Nagata Y, Yamamoto K, Hiraoka M, Abe M, Takahashi M, Akuta K, Nishimura Y, Jo S, Masunaga S, Kubo S et al. Monitoring liver tumor therapy with [18F]FDG positron emission tomography. *J Comput Assist Tomogr* 1990;14:370–374.

37. Vitola JV, Delbeke D, Meranze SG, Mazer MJ, Pinson CW. Positron emission tomography with F-18-fluorodeoxyglucose to evaluate the results of hepatic chemoembolization. *Cancer* 1996;78:2216–2222.

38. Linamond P, Zimmerman P, Raman SS, Kadell BM, Lu DSK. Interpretation of CT and MRI after radiofrequency ablation of hepatic malignancies. *Am J Roentgenol* 2003;181:1635–1640.

39. Langenhoff BS, Oyen WJ, Jager GJ, Strijk SP, Wobbes T, Corstens FHM, Ruers TJM. Efficacy of fluorine-18-deoxyglucose positron emission tomography in detecting tumor recurrence after local ablative therapy for liver metastases: A prospective study. *J Clin Oncol* 2002;20:4453–4458.

40. Anderson GS, Brinkmann F, Soulen MC, Alavi A, Zhuang H. FDG positron emission tomography in the surveillance of hepatic tumors treated with radiofrequency ablation. *Clin Nucl Med* 2003;28:192–197.

41. Ludwig V, Hopper OW, Martin WH, Kikkawa R, Delbeke D. FDG-PET surveillance of hepatic metastases from prostate cancer following radiofrequency ablation-Case report. *Am Surg* 2003; 69:593–598.

42. Donckier V, Van Laetham JL, Goldman S, Van Gansbeke D, Feron P, Ickx B, Wikler D, Gelin M. Fluorodeoxyglucose positron emission tomography as a tool for early recognition of incomplete tumor destruction after radiofrequency ablation for liver metastases. *J Surg Oncol* 2003;84:215–223.

43. Veit P, Antoch G, Stergar H, Bockisch A, Forsting M, Kuehl H. Detection of residual tumor after radiofrequency ablation of liver metastasis with dual-modality PET/CT: Initial results. *Eur Radiol* 2006;16:80–87.

44. Barker DW, Zagoria RJ, Morton KA, Kavanagh PV, Shen P. Evaluation of liver metastases after radiofrequency ablation: Utility of FDG PET and PET/CT. *Am J Roentgenol* 2005;184:1096–1102.

45. Antoch G, Vogt FM, Veit P, Freudenberg LS, Blechschmid N, Dirsch O, Bockisch A, Forsting M, Debatin JF, Kuehl H. Assessment of liver tissue after radiofrequency ablation: Findings with different imaging procedures. *J Nucl Med* 2005;46:520–525.

46. Wong CY, Salem R, Raman S, Gates VL, Dworkin HJ. Evaluating 90Y-glass microsphere treatment response of unresectable colorectal liver metastases by [18F]FDG PET: a comparison with CT or MRI. *Eur J Nucl Med Mol Imag* 2002;29:815–820.

47. Wong CY, Salem R, Qing F, Wong KT, Barker D, Gates V, Lewandowski R, Hill EA, Dworkin HJ, Nagle C. Metabolic response after intraarterial 90Y-glass microsphere treatment for colorectal liver metastases: Comparison of quantitative and visual analysis by 18F-FDG PET. *J Nucl Med* 2004;45:1892–1897.

48. Vargas R, Nino-Murcia M, Trueblood W, Jeffrey RB Jr. MDCT in Pancreatic adenocarcinoma: prediction of vascular invasion and resectability using a multiphasic technique with curved planar reformations. *AJR Am J Roentgenol* 2004;182:419–425.

49. DeWitt J, Devereaux B, Chriswell M, McGreevy K, Howard T, Imperiale TF, Ciaccia D, Lane KA, Maglinte D, Kopecky K, LeBlanc J, McHenry L, Madura J,. Aisen A, Cramer H, Cummings O, Sherman S. Comparison of endoscopic ultrasonography and multidetector computed tomography for detecting and staging pancreatic cancer. *Ann Intern Med* 2004;141:753–763.

50. Johnson PT, Outwater EK. Pancreatic carcinoma versus chronic pancreatitis: dynamic MR imaging. *Radiology* 1999;212:213–218.

51. Lammer J, Herlinger H, Zalaudek G, Hofler H. Pseudotumorous pancreatitis. *Gastrointest Radiol* 1995;10:59–67.

52. Brandt KR, Charboneau JW, Stephens DH, Welch TJ, Goellner JR. CT- and US-guided biopsy of the pancreas. *Radiology* 1993;187:99–104.

53. Chang KJ, Nguyen P, Erickson RA, Durbin TE, Katz KD. The clinical utility of endoscopic ultrasound-guided fine-needle aspiration in the diagnosis and staging of pancreatic carcinoma. *Gastrointest Endosc* 1997;45:387–393.

54. Delbeke D. Pancreatic tumors: Role of imaging in the diagnosis, staging, decision making and treatment. *J Hepato-Biliary-Pancreatic Surg* 2004;11:4–10.

55. Flier JS, Mueckler MM, Usher P, Lodish HF. Elevated levels of glucose transport and transporter messenger RNA are induced by ras or src oncogenes. *Science* 1987;235:1492–1495.

56. Monakhov NK, Neistadt EL, Shavlovskil MM, Shvartsman AL, Neĭfakh SA. Physiochemical properties and isoenzyme composition of hexokinase from normal and malignant human tissues. *J Natl Cancer Inst* 1978; 61:27–34.

57. Higashi T, Tamaki N, Honda T, Torizuka T, Kimura T, Inokuma T, Ohshio G, Hosotani R, Imamura M, Konishi J. Expression of glucose transporters in human pancreatic tumors compared with increased F-18 FDG accumulation in PET study. *J Nucl Med* 1997;38:1337–1344.

58. Reske S, Grillenberger KG, Glatting G, Port M, Hildebrandt M,Gansauge F, Beger H-G. Overexpression of glucose transporter 1 and increased F-18 FDG uptake in pancreatic carcinoma. *J Nucl Med* 1997;38:1344–1348.

59. Gambir SS, Czernin J, Schimmer J, Silverman D, Coleman RE, Phelps ME. A tabulatedsummary of the FDG PET literature. *J Nucl Med* 2001;42 (Suppl):1S–93S.

60. Rose DM, Delbeke D, Beauchamp RD, Chapman WC, Sandler MP, Sharp KW, Richards WO, Wright JK, Frexes ME, Pinson CW, Leach SD. 18Fluorodeoxyglucose – positron emission tomography (18FDG – PET) in the management of patients with suspected pancreatic cancer. *Ann of Surg* 1990;229:729–738.

61. Wahl RL, Henry CA, Ethrer SP. Serum glucose: effects on tumor and normal tissue accumulation of 2-[F-18]-fluoro-2-deoxy-D-glucose in rodents with mammary carcinoma. *Radiology* 1992;183:643–647.

62. Lindholm P, Minn H, Leskinen-Kallio S, Bergman J, Ruotsalainen U, Joensuu H. Influence of the blood glucose concentration on FDG uptake in cancer – a PET study. *J Nucl Med* 1993;34:1–6.

63. Diederichs CG, Staib L, Glatting G, Beger HG, Reske SN. FDG PET: Elevated plasma glucose reduces both uptake and detection rate of pancreatic malignancies. *J Nucl Med* 1998;39:1030–1033.

64. Diederichs CG, Staib L, Vogel J, Glasbrenner B,Glatting G, Brambs H-J, Beger H G, Reske SN. Values and limitations of FDG PET with preoperative evaluations of patients with pancreatic masses. *Pancreas* 2000;20:109–116.

65. Stollfuss JC, Glatting G, Friess H, Kocher F, Berger HG, Reske SN. 2-(Fluorine-18)-fluoro-2-deoxy-D-glucose PET in detection of pancreatic cancer: Value of quantitative image interpretation. *Radiology* 1995;195:339–344.

66. Zimny M, Bares R, Faß J, Adam G,Cremerius U, Dohmen B, Klever P, Sabri O, Schumpelick V, Buell U. Fluorine-18 fluorodeoxyglucose positron emission tomography in the differential diagnosis of pancreatic carcinoma: a report of 106 cases. *Eur J Nucl Med* 1997;24:678–682.

67. Ho CL, Dehdashti F, Griffeth LK, Buse PE, Balfe Dennis M, Siegel BA. FDG-PET evaluation of indeterminate pancreatic masses. *Comput Assist Tomogr* 1996;20:363–369.

68. Friess H, Langhans J, Ebert M, Beger HG, Stollfuss J, Reske SN, Büchler MW. Diagnosis of pancreatic cancer by 2[F-18]-fluoro-2-deoxy-D-glucose positron emission tomography. *Gut* 1995;36:771–777.

69. Shreve PD. Focal fluorine-18 fluorodeoxyglucose accumulation in inflammatory pancreatic disease. *Eur J Nucl Med* 1998;25:259–264.

70. van Kouwen M, Jansen JB, van Goor H, de Castro S, Oyen WJ, Drenth JP. FDG-PET is able to detect pancreatic carcinoma in chronic pancreatitis. *Eur J Med Mol Imaging* 2005;32:399–404.

71. Sperti C, Bissoli S, Pasquali C, Frison L, Liessi G, Chierichetti F, Pedrazzoli S.18-Fluorodeoxyglucose positron emission tomography enhances computed tomography diagnosis of malignant intraductal papillary mucinous neoplasms of the pancreas. *Ann Surg* 2007;246:932–939.

72. Nakata B, Chung YS, Nishimura S, Nishihara T, Sakurai Y, Sawada T, Okamura T, Kawabe J, Ochi H, Sowa M.18F-fluorodeoxyglucose positron emission tomography and the prognosis of patients with pancreatic carcinoma. *Cancer* 1997;79:695–699.

73. Zimny M, Fass J, Bares R, Cremerius O, Sabri P, Buechin V, Schumpelick U, Buell M. Fluorodeoxyglucose positron emission tomography and the prognosis of pancreatic carcinoma. *Scand J Gastroenterol* 2000;35:883–888.

74. Sperti C, Pasquali C, Chierichetti F, Ferronato A, Decet G, Pedrazzoli S. 18-Fluorodeoxyglucose positron emission tomography in predicting survival of patients with pancreatic carcinoma. *J Gastrointest Surg* 2003;7:953–959.

75. Delbeke D, Rose M, Chapman WC, Rose M, Chapman WC, Pinson CW, Wright JK, Beauchamp DR, Leach S. Optimal interpretation of F-18FDG Imaging of FDG PET in the diagnosis, staging and management of pancreatic carcinoma. *J Nucl Med* 1999;40:1784–1792.

76. Frolich A, Diederichs CG, Staib L, Vogel J, Beger HG, Reske SN. Detection of liver metastases from pancreatic cancer using FDG PET. *J Nucl Med* 1999;40:250–255.

77. Kalady MF, Clary BM, Clark LA, Gottfried M, Rohren EM, Coleman RE,Pappas TN, DS Tyler, Clinical utility of positron emission tomography in the diagnosis and management of periampullary neoplasms. *Ann Surg Oncol* 2002;9:799–806.

78. Whiteford MH, Whiteford HM, Yee LF, Ogunbiyi OA, Dehdashti F, Siegel BA, Birnbaum EH, Fleshman JW, Kodner IJ, Read TE. Usefulness of FDG-PET scan in the assessment of suspected metastatic or recurrent adenocarcinoma of the colon and rectum. *Dis Colon Rectum* 2000;43:759–767; discussion 767–770.

79. Podoloff DA, Ball DW, Ben-Josef E, Benson AB, Cohen SJ, Coleman RE, Delbeke D, Ho M, Ilson DH, Kalemkerian GP, Lee RJ, Loeffler JS, Macapinlac HA, Morgan RJ, Siegel BA, Singhal S, Tyler DS, Wong RJ. NCCN Task Force: Clinical Utility of PET in a Variety of Tumor Types Task Force. *J Natl Compr Canc Netw* 2009;7 Suppl 2:S1–S23. www.nccn.org/professionals/physician_gls/f_guidelines.asp

80. Fletcher JW, Djulbegovic B, Soares HP, Siegel BA, Lowe VJ, Lyman GH, Coleman E, Wahl R, Paschold JC, Avril N, Einhorn LH, Suh WW, Samson D, Delbeke D, Gorman M, Shields AF. Recommendations for the Use of FDG(fluorine-18, (2-[$^{18}$F]Fluoro-2-deoxy-D-glucose) positron emission tomography in oncology. *J Nucl Med* 2008;49:480–508.

81. Reske SN, Kotzerke J. FDG-PET for clinical use. Results of the 3rd German interdisciplinary consensus conference, Onko-PET III, 21 July and 19 September 2000. *Eur J Nucl Med* 2001;28:1707–1723.

82. Guthrie JA, Ward J, Robinson PJ. Hilar cholangiocarcinomas: T2-weighted spin-echo and gadolinium-enhanced FLASH MR imaging. *Radiology* 1996;201:347–351.

83. Hussain SM, Terkivatan T, Zondervan PE, Lanjouw E, de Rave S, Ijzermans JN, de Man RA. Focal nodular hyperplasia: Findings at state-of-the-art MR imaging, US, CT and pathologic analysis. *Radiographics* 2004;24:3–17. http://radiographics.rsnajnls.org/cgi/content/full/24/1/3

# Chapter II.8
# Gynecological Tumors

Farrokh Dehdashti and Barry A. Siegel

## Introduction

Gynecological cancers as a group comprise approximately 11% of female cancer.[1] In the United States, it is estimated that nearly 80,720 women will be diagnosed in 2009 with gynecological cancers and that approximately 28,120 women will die as a result of these cancers (accounting for 10% of all cancer-related deaths in women). Gynecological cancers are typically diagnosed by history, physical examination, and selected imaging studies. There has been an increasing use of PET using [18]F-fluorodeoxyglucose (FDG) for staging and restaging of these cancers, as well as for assessing response to therapy.[2]

## Cervical Cancer

In the United States, cervical cancer is the third most common gynecological cancer, with an estimated 11,270 new cases and 4,070 deaths expected in 2009.[1] Squamous cell carcinomas represent over 90% of cervical cancers. Adenocarcinomas and adenosquamous carcinomas account for most of the remaining cases.

## [18]F-FDG PET/CT in Staging Cervical Cancer

Cervical cancers initially spread locally and then through lymphatic channels before metastasizing to distant organs. Like other gynecological neoplasms, cervical cancer is staged in accordance with the International Federation of Gynecology and Obstetrics (FIGO) system. Lymph node status is not included in this staging system, despite the fact that the status of pelvic and para-aortic lymph nodes is an important determinant of prognosis in patients with locally advanced disease and guides treatment planning in patients undergoing radiation therapy. Since carcinoma of the uterine cervix initially grows locally, the clinical staging of this cancer has relied on careful physical examination (including examination under anesthesia), and traditionally only selective radiological examinations have been used. More recently, [18]F-FDG PET has been recognized to improve evaluation of this cancer.

F. Dehdashti (✉)
Professor of Radiology, Mallinckrodt Institute of Radiology, Washington University School of Medicine, St. Louis, Missouri, USA
e-mail: dehdashtif@mir.wustl.edu

D. Delbeke, O. Israel (eds.), *Hybrid PET/CT and SPECT/CT Imaging*,
DOI 10.1007/978-0-387-92820-3_10, © Springer Science+Business Media, LLC 2010

A systematic review of 15 published studies up through 2003 demonstrated pooled sensitivity and specificity for detection of pelvic nodal metastases of 79 and 99%, respectively, for PET; the corresponding values for MRI were 72 and 96%, respectively.[3] Pooled sensitivity for CT was 47%. The pooled specificity was not available. The pooled sensitivity and specificity of PET for para-aortic lymph node metastases were 84 and 95%, respectively.[3] Based on these promising results, in January 2005, the United States Centers for Medicare and Medicaid Services approved coverage for use of [18]F-FDG PET in initial staging of patients with newly diagnosed cervical cancer who have no evidence of extra-pelvic metastatic disease on CT or MRI. More recent studies with [18]F-FDG PET/CT have demonstrated further advantages by comparison to PET as a stand-alone modality.[4,5]

Some investigators have found that [18]F-FDG PET may not be ideal in evaluating early cervical cancer, in particular for detection of metastases in lymph nodes less than 5 mm in size. Wright and colleagues prospectively studied 59 patients with stages IA–IIA cervical cancer prior to surgery.[6] The patient-based analysis demonstrated a sensitivity of 53%, specificity of 90%, positive predictive value (PPV) of 71%, and negative predictive value (NPV) of 80% for PET detection of pelvic lymph node metastasis. The sensitivity was 25%, specificity 98%, PPV 50%, and NPV 93% for detection of para-aortic lymph node metastases. Chou and colleagues[7] prospectively studied 60 patients with stage IA2–IIA cervical cancer who were MRI negative for lymph node metastases prior to surgery. The sensitivity, specificity, PPV, NPV, and accuracy for detecting metastatic disease in pelvic lymph nodes with PET were 10, 94, 25, 84, and 80%, respectively. In a more recent study employing PET/CT, Sironi and coworkers[8] evaluated 47 patients with stage IA–IB cervical carcinoma prior to surgery. The sensitivity, specificity, PPV, NPV, and accuracy were 72, 99.7, 81, 99.5, and 99.3%, respectively.

## [18]F-FDG PET/CT in Directing Therapy in Cervical Cancer

Treatment of patients with locally advanced cervical cancer includes a combination of radio- and chemotherapy. [18]F-FDG PET/CT is increasingly used to delineate the target volume for radiation treatment planning. Fused PET/CT images can be used to differentiate tumor from adjacent normal structures more reliably and, thus, allow for delivery of higher doses of radiation to the tumor while decreasing radiation dose to normal structures. Lin and colleagues[9] recently demonstrated that [18]F-FDG PET-based treatment planning allows for improved dose coverage of the tumor without significantly increasing the dose to the bladder and rectum.

## [18]F-FDG PET/CT in Predicting Prognosis in Cervical Cancer

Size of the primary tumor and the presence of lymph node metastases are important prognostic factors in patients with cervical carcinoma.[10,11] Miller and Grigsby[12] demonstrated that tumor volume measured on [18]F-FDG PET, using a 40% count threshold, was predictive of survival in cervical cancer. [18]F-FDG uptake of the primary tumor at diagnosis is also a sensitive biomarker of prognosis in cervical cancer. Kidd and colleagues[13] studied 287 patients with stage IA2 through IVB cervical cancer who underwent pretreatment [18]F-FDG PET. A Cox proportional hazards model for death from cervical cancer was used to evaluate tumor histology, lymph node metastases, tumor volume, and $SUV_{max}$.

The investigators found the $SUV_{max}$ of the primary tumor to be the only significant independent prognostic factor. The overall survival rates at 5 years were 95% for patients with $SUV_{max}$ of 5.2 or less, 70% for those with $SUV_{max}$ >5.2, and 44% for those with $SUV_{max}$ >13.3. Increasing $SUV_{max}$ was associated with persistent abnormal [18]F-FDG uptake in the cervix on 3-month [18]F-FDG PET studies in patients who received curative chemoradiation. The extent of lymph node involvement by PET is also highly predictive of prognosis.[14]

## [18]F-FDG PET/CT in Post-therapy Monitoring of Cervical Cancer

Several investigators have demonstrated that [18]F-FDG PET after completion of therapy is useful in evaluating clinically asymptomatic patients as well as those with clinically suspected disease. Chung and colleagues[15] demonstrated that the sensitivity, specificity, and accuracy of [18]F-FDG PET/CT for detecting disease recurrences were 90.3, 81.0, and 86.5%, respectively. Results of [18]F-FDG PET/CT studies changed the management of 12 patients (23%). The 2-year disease-free survival rate of patients with negative PET/CT for recurrence was significantly better than that of patients with positive PET/CT (85.0% vs. 10.9%). Yen and colleagues demonstrated that, in recurrent cervical cancer, the benefits of [18]F-FDG PET exceed those of CT/MRI, owing to the ability of PET to identify extra-pelvic metastases with higher sensitivity and specificity.[16]

While the best time interval to perform [18]F-FDG PET/CT following therapy is not well established, it has been demonstrated that a study performed at 3 months after completion of therapy is highly accurate in determining long-term survival in patients with advanced cervical cancer treated by chemoradiation.[17,18]

## Ovarian Cancer

In the United States ovarian cancer is the second most common gynecological cancer, with an estimated 21,550 new cases and 14,600 deaths expected in 2009.[1] Nearly 90% of ovarian cancers are epithelial in origin and arise from the cells on the surface of the ovary. The remaining 10% are germ cell and stromal tumors. Ovarian cancer typically has vague symptoms that are often ignored, and the disease is therefore usually diagnosed at advanced stage. Prognosis is strongly related to the stage of disease at diagnosis. While early stage disease has a very good prognosis, advanced disease carries poor prognosis. Ovarian cancer spreads early by implantation on both parietal and visceral peritoneum before spreading through lymphatics and involving inguinal, pelvic, para-aortic, and mediastinal lymph nodes. The serum tumor marker CA-125 is elevated in nearly 80% of patients with advanced ovarian cancer and is therefore widely used to assess effectiveness of therapy and to detect tumor recurrence. Abnormal marker levels often precede clinical and radiologic signs of disease recurrence.

## [18]F-FDG PET/CT in Diagnosis and Staging of Ovarian Cancer

Because ovarian cancer typically presents as an adnexal mass, differentiating between their benign or malignant etiology is very important. Adnexal masses go undetected until the patient develops signs and symptoms. Transvaginal ultrasonography (TVUS) has a 90% sensitivity and is considered the imaging method of choice for detecting and evaluating adnexal masses.[19] [18]F-FDG PET is limited for evaluating adnexal masses because they are often cystic in nature and because physiologic uptake of [18]F-FDG can occur in normal ovaries in premenopausal patients. Lerman and colleagues[20] reported increased ovarian uptake of [18]F-FDG (SUV 5.7 ± 1.5) in premenopausal women without known ovarian malignancy, including a few patients with oligomenorrhea, while the majority were at the mid-phase of the ovulatory cycle. They reported that a threshold ovarian SUV of 7.9 separated benign from malignant lesions with sensitivity, specificity, accuracy, PPV, and NPV of 57, 95, 85, 80, and 86%, respectively. Whereas earlier studies have demonstrated that [18]F-FDG PET is limited in differentiating benign from malignant adnexal masses, more recent reports using PET/CT suggest its possible role in this clinical setting.[21] Castellucci and coworkers demonstrated that the sensitivity, specificity, NPV, PPV, and accuracy of [18]F-FDG PET/CT were 87, 100, 81, 100, and 92%, respectively, compared with 90, 61, 78, 80, and 80%, respectively, for TVUS.[23] Ovarian cancer is typically staged by exploratory laparotomy at the time of tumor debulking. CT and/or MRI have been accepted as useful imaging modalities for preoperative staging ovarian cancer. Recent studies have demonstrated that [18]F-FDG PET may be useful as an adjunct to diagnostic CT for staging ovarian cancer. Yoshida and colleagues[22] found that [18]F-FDG PET has a higher diagnostic accuracy than CT (87% vs. 53%) in preoperative staging of patients with suspected ovarian cancer using histology as the "gold standard" reference. Castellucci and coworkers[23] demonstrated that [18]F-FDG PET/CT was concordant with final pathological staging in 69% of patients as compared to 53% for CT alone. More data are needed to better define the role of PET in initial staging of ovarian cancer.

## [18]F-FDG PET/CT in Assessment of Response to Therapy in Ovarian Cancer

Standard treatment of advanced ovarian cancer includes aggressive cytoreductive surgery followed by platinum/taxane-based chemotherapy. Despite an often initial good response to this therapy, most patients will subsequently die of progressive disease.[24] Recently, neoadjuvant chemotherapy followed by surgical debulking has been used in order to improve outcome. This, however, can only be achieved in patients with complete or nearly complete response to neoadjuvant therapy.[25] CT and MRI are limited in detecting response early after initiation of therapy. Moreover, these modalities are limited in distinguishing residual tumor from necrosis or fibrosis. [18]F-FDG PET/CT has been used in a limited fashion in this clinical setting. Avril and colleagues[26] demonstrated that overall survival showed a significant correlation with changes in tumor tracer uptake after the first and third cycles of chemotherapy, but not with conventional clinical or CA-125 response criteria. A higher rate of complete tumor resections was achieved in metabolic responders (defined as 20% reduction in SUV after the first cycle and 50% after the third cycle) compared with non-responders, and macroscopically tumor-free surgery was achieved in 33% of metabolic responders compared with only 13% of non-responders. Metabolic responders had longer median overall survival than non-responders.

## [18]F-FDG PET/CT in Detection of Recurrent Ovarian Cancer

Several studies have shown that [18]F-FDG PET/CT is superior to conventional imaging and measurement of CA-125 in detecting recurrent ovarian cancer. A recent systematic review of six published studies that assessed patients with clinical suspicion for recurrent ovarian cancer calculated a pooled sensitivity and specificity of 90 and 86%, respectively, for

$^{18}$F-FDG PET, 68 and 58%, respectively, for conventional imaging, and 81 and 83%, respectively, for CA-125 measurement.[3] Three studies evaluated $^{18}$F-FDG PET in patients with negative conventional imaging and CA-125 measurements in whom surveillance studies were used to detect recurrent or persistent ovarian cancer. The pooled sensitivity and specificity of $^{18}$F-FDG PET were 54 and 73%, respectively.[3] Another three studies evaluated patients with rising CA-125 levels and negative or equivocal conventional imaging studies. The pooled sensitivity and specificity of $^{18}$F-FDG PET were 96 and 80%, respectively.[3] It appears that $^{18}$F-FDG imaging is highly effective as a diagnostic tool in patients with rising CA-125 levels and negative or equivocal CT. $^{18}$F-FDG PET/CT has been shown to be very useful in early detection of recurrent disease that is suitable for surgical resection.[27–29]

## Endometrial Cancer

Endometrial cancer is the most common gynecologic cancer in the United States, with an estimated 42,160 new cases and 7,780 deaths expected in 2009.[1] Two different clinico-pathological subtypes are recognized: the more-common estrogen-related (type I, endometrioid) and the non-estrogen related (type II, non-endometrioid). Endometrial cancer is staged and treated surgically. There are limited reports of the use of $^{18}$F-FDG imaging for diagnosis of primary endometrial cancer. One of the potential limitations of $^{18}$F-FDG PET is related to $^{18}$F-FDG accumulation in benign processes such as menstrual bleeding and leiomyoma.[30,31] Horowitz and colleagues[32] reported that the sensitivity of PET for detection of primary endometrial cancer was 84%. They also reported that the sensitivity and specificity of PET for detection of lymph node metastases were 60 and 98%, respectively. Recently, Suzuki and coworkers demonstrated that PET has a sensitivity of 97% for detection of primary tumor vs. 83% for CT/MRI.[33] The sensitivity, specificity, PPV, and NPV for prediction of pelvic lymph node metastases were 0, 100, 0, and 81%, respectively, for PET and 40, 86, 40, and 86%, respectively, for CT/MRI. For detection of para-aortic lymph node metastases, the sensitivity, specificity, PPV, and NPV were 0, 100, 0, 95%, respectively, for PET and 100, 94.4, 50, and 100%, respectively, for CT/MRI. All the retroperitoneal lymph node metastases were microscopic, and PET was unable to detect any of the involved lymph nodes. The sensitivity of $^{18}$F-FDG PET for detection of extra-uterine lesions, excluding retroperitoneal lymph nodes, was superior to that of CT/MRI (83% vs. 67%), while there was no difference in the specificity between the modalities (100%). This study demonstrated that the diagnostic ability of $^{18}$F-FDG imaging may be limited if PET is used alone while $^{18}$F-FDG PET/CT may have a potential role in the preoperative staging of endometrial cancer.

Evaluation of endometrial cancer after therapy typically includes physical examination, evaluation of the serum tumor markers CA-125 or CA-19.9, and selected imaging. All of these methods are limited in early detection of recurrent disease. However, PET has been shown to be beneficial for detection of recurrent endometrial cancer, particularly in asymptomatic patients.[34,35]

## Summary

$^{18}$F-FDG PET/CT is a very useful adjunct to CT/MRI in initial staging of cervical cancer. It not only provides information about the extent of disease, it is also used to direct radio-therapy and predict prognosis. In ovarian cancer, $^{18}$F-FDG PET/CT plays an important role in detecting recurrent disease in patients with rising tumor markers and equivocal or negative CT/MRI. The role of [18]F-FDG PET/CT in endometrial cancer is evolving and may be of clinical significance mainly in the post-therapy evaluation of these patients.

# Guidelines and Recommendations for the Use of [18]F-FDG PET and PET/CT

The National Comprehensive Cancer Network (NCCN) has incorporated [18]F-FDG PET and PET/CT in the practice guidelines and management algorithm of a variety of malignancies including cervical cancer.[36] The use of [18]F-FDG PET (PET/CT where available) is recommended 1) For initial staging and restaging of cervical cancer; 2) For evaluation of recurrent ovarian cancer in patients with rising CA-125 levels. 3) In uterine cancer, the reported impact of PET on management is not substantial.

# Case Presentations

## *Case II.8.1 (DICOM Images on DVD)*

### History

This 74-year-old woman presented with FIGO stage IIb squamous cell carcinoma of the cervix. She was referred for initial staging with $^{18}$F-FDG PET/CT (Fig. II.8.1A–F).

$^{18}$F-FDG

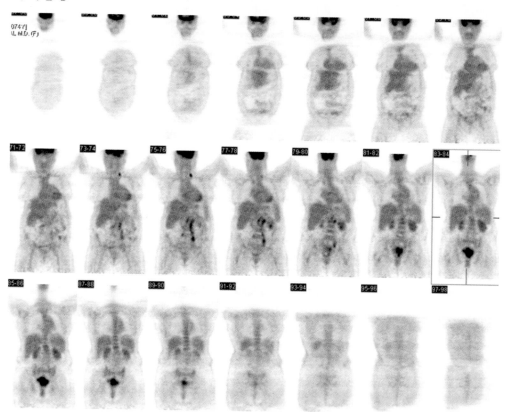

Fig. II.8.1A

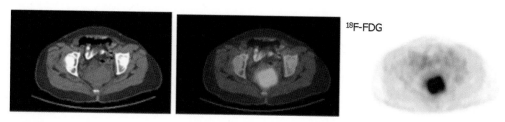

Fig. II.8.1B

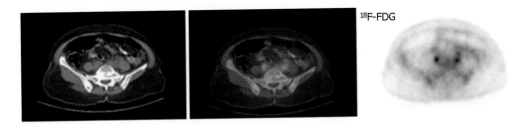

Fig. II.8.1C

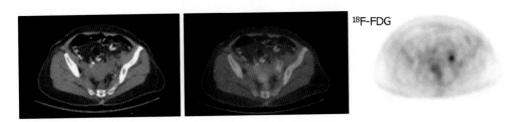

Fig. II.8.1D

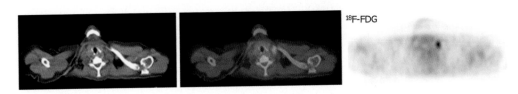

Fig. II.8.1E

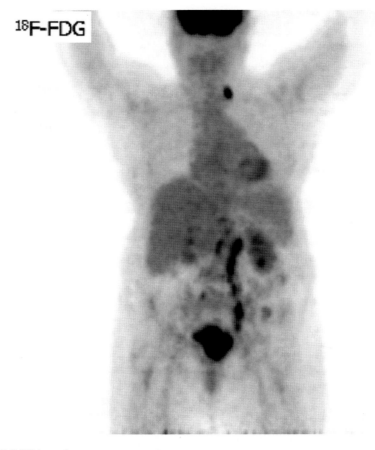

¹⁸F-FDG

**Fig. II.8.1F (MIP image)**

## Findings

Intense ¹⁸F-FDG activity is noted in the cervical mass, most consistent with the known primary cancer (Fig. II.8.1A, B, F). Multiple foci of increased uptake are noted in retro-peritoneal para-aortic lymph nodes, predominantly on the left side, with the largest measuring 17 × 14 mm (Fig. II.8.1A, C, F). The lymphadenopathy extends to the aortic bifurcation with increased tracer activity noted in multiple left common iliac and left external iliac lymph nodes (Fig. II.8.1A, D, F). There also is intense ¹⁸F-FDG activity in a left supraclavicular lymph node measuring 16 × 13 mm (Fig. II.8.1A, E, F). Additional CT findings are seen on the DICOM images and described in the clinical report.

## Discussion

The pattern of lymph node involvement in this patient is typical for metastatic cervical cancer. Lymph node involvement, which is the most common form of metastatic disease in cervical cancer, typically begins in the pelvis extending to the para-aortic and ultimately the left supraclavicular lymph nodes. The extent of lymph node involvement has been shown to be of prognostic significance and is inversely related to survival. Grigsby and colleagues[14] studied 101 patients with newly diagnosed cervical cancer and demonstrated that the lymph node status determined by [18]F-FDG PET is predictive of progression-free and overall survival in patients with cervical cancer. [18]F-FDG PET evidence of lymph node involvement was a better predictor of the 2-year disease-free survival than the CT findings. Based on pelvic lymph node status on imaging studies, the 2-year disease-free survival was 84% for CT–/PET–, 64% for CT–/PET+, and 48% for CT+/PET+ patients. Based on the status of the para-aortic nodes on imaging studies, the 2-year disease-free survival was 78% for CT–/PET–, 31% for CT–/PET+, and 14% for CT+/PET+ patients. The finding of PET+ supraclavicular lymph nodes was indicative of dismal prognosis and none of such patients survived 2 years. They also found that the PET-determined status of the para-aortic nodes was the strongest predictor of survival in a multivariate logistic regression analysis.

**Diagnosis**

Metastatic cervical cancer (regional and distant disease).

**Clinical Report: Body [18]F-FDG PET/CT (for DVD cases only)**

Indication

Initial staging of carcinoma of the cervix.

History

The patient presented with complaint of post-menopausal bleeding. A cervical mass was found, and the biopsy showed moderately to poorly differentiated squamous cell carcinoma of the cervix. The patient stated that the bleeding began about 1 month ago, but she did not require blood transfusion. There was no trouble with her urination including hematuria. She has experienced no lower extremity or groin swelling or pain in her back or pain radiating to her legs. The patient now presents for initial staging.

Procedure

After oral administration of MD-Gastroview[TM] and intravenous administration of 500 MBq (13.5 mCi) of [18]F-FDG, non-contrast CT images were obtained for attenuation correction and fusion. A series of PET images were then obtained beginning approximately 60 min after injection of [18]F-FDG. The patient's fasting blood glucose level, measured before injection of [18]F-FDG, was 97 mg/dL. The imaged area spanned from the skull base to the upper thighs. The patient was positioned with arms up.

Before administration of [18]F-FDG, intravenous access was established for patient hydration. In addition, a 16-French Foley catheter was inserted into the urinary bladder using standard aseptic technique. Furosemide, 20 mg, was administered by slow intravenous injection approximately 20 min after the injection of [18]F-FDG. At the conclusion of the procedure, the intravenous line and Foley catheter were removed without incident. The patient tolerated the procedure well, without apparent complications.

Findings

*Quality of the study*: The quality of this study is good.

*Head and neck*: There is physiologic distribution of the radiopharmaceutical in the cerebral cortex and lymphoid and glandular tissues of the neck. There is a mucosal retention cyst in the left maxillary sinus. There is intense $^{18}$F-FDG uptake within left supraclavicular lymph nodes, with the largest measuring $16 \times 13$ mm.

*Chest*: There is mild cardiomegaly with biatrial enlargement. Calcifications of the aorta and coronary arteries are noted. No pulmonary nodule is seen.

*Abdomen and pelvis*: There is intense $^{18}$F-FDG activity within the cervical mass (approximately 81 mm in greatest diameter), consistent with the patient's known primary cancer. There are multiple foci of increased $^{18}$F-FDG uptake in retroperitoneal para-aortic lymph nodes, predominantly on the left side with the largest measuring $17 \times 14$ mm. The lymphadenopathy extends to the aortic bifurcation, with increased $^{18}$F-FDG uptake also noted in multiple left common iliac and left external iliac lymph nodes. Multiple diverticula are noted in the sigmoid colon. Multiple anterior body wall collateral vessels are noted.

*Musculoskeletal*: Extensive degenerative disc disease is noted, more prominent at L1/L2 and L5/S1. Grade 2 anterolisthesis is noted at L5 on S1. Mild T11 and L1 compression deformities are seen. Diffusely increased $^{18}$F-FDG uptake is noted intramedullary within the axial and proximal appendicular bones, consistent with bone marrow hyperplasia due to anemia related to bleeding.

Impression

1. Intense $^{18}$F-FDG uptake corresponding to the cervical mass, consistent with cervical carcinoma.
2. Intense $^{18}$F-FDG uptake within left supraclavicular, para-aortic, and pelvic lymph nodes, consistent with lymph node metastases.

## *Case II.8.2*

### History

This 60-year-old woman presented with FIGO stage IIIb squamous cell carcinoma of the cervix. She is referred to $^{18}$F-FDG PET/CT for initial staging (Fig. II.8.2A–E).

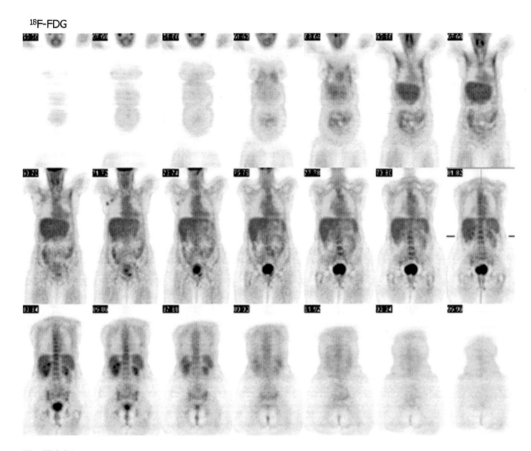

Fig. II.8.2A

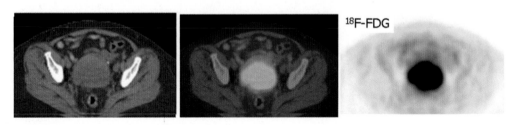

Fig. II.8.2B

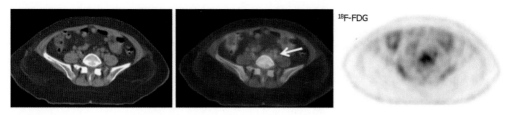

**Fig. II.8.2C**

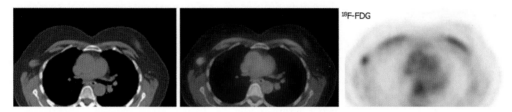

**Fig. II.8.2D**

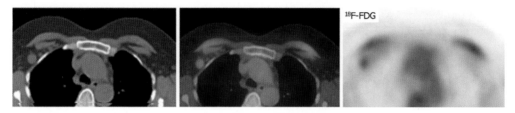

**Fig. II.8.2E**

### Findings

There is intense $^{18}$F-FDG uptake within the cervical mass, most consistent with the known primary cancer (Fig. II.8.2A, B). In addition, abnormal $^{18}$F-FDG uptake is noted in a 4 mm left common iliac lymph node (arrow, Fig. II.8.2C). Increased tracer uptake is also seen in two enlarged (19 and 15 mm) right axillary lymph nodes (Fig. II.8.2A, D, E).

### Discussion

$^{18}$F-FDG uptake in the cervix is consistent with the known primary cervical cancer. The uptake within the small left common iliac lymph node is highly suspicious for a metastasis.

More recent studies with PET/CT have demonstrated the superiority of this imaging modality for detection of lymph node metastases. One study has demonstrated that MRI has a lower sensitivity than $^{18}$F-FDG PET/CT for detection of lymph node metastases. The sensitivity, specificity, and accuracy rates for detecting metastatic lymph nodes were 30, 93, and 73%, respectively, for MRI, and 58, 93 and 85%, respectively, for PET/CT.[4] A recent study demonstrated that $^{18}$F-FDG PET/CT had a PPV of 75%, NPV of 96%, sensitivity of 75%, and specificity of 96% for detection of pelvic lymph node metastases in 27 patients who underwent radical surgery.[5] For para-aortic nodal disease in 119 patients, PET/CT showed a PPV of 94%, NPV of 100%, sensitivity of 100%, and specificity of 99%. For distant metastases, [18]F-FDG PET/CT had a PPV of 63%, NPV of 100%, sensitivity of 100%, and specificity of 94%.

The uptake within the axillary lymph nodes in this patient is a highly atypical pattern for metastatic cervical cancer. Biopsy of an axillary lymph node demonstrated abundant mixed polymorphous lymphocytes but no evidence of carcinoma. In general, abnormal [18]F-FDG PET findings that would potentially lead to a change in management need to be confirmed by biopsy. Although the axillary lymph node foci were highly unlikely to be related to cervical cancer, the physician opted to biopsy one of the lymph nodes. The finding of a probable pelvic lymph node metastasis did not change patient management but affected patient's prognosis, as described in case II.8.1.

**Diagnosis**

1. Primary cervical squamous cell carcinoma.
2. Metastatic disease in a left pelvic lymph node.
3. Benign hypermetabolic [18]F-FDG-avid right axillary lymph nodes.

## Case II.8.3

### History

This 27-year-old woman presented with a newly diagnosed FIGO stage IIb poorly differentiated squamous cell carcinoma of the cervix. She began to have lower abdominal pain and bleeding approximately a month and a half prior to current examination and was referred to $^{18}$F-FDG PET/CT for staging (Fig. II.8.3A–C). Subsequently, chemoradiation treatment was initiated and a follow-up PET/CT study was thereafter performed (Fig. II.8.3D–F).

## $^{18}$F-FDG

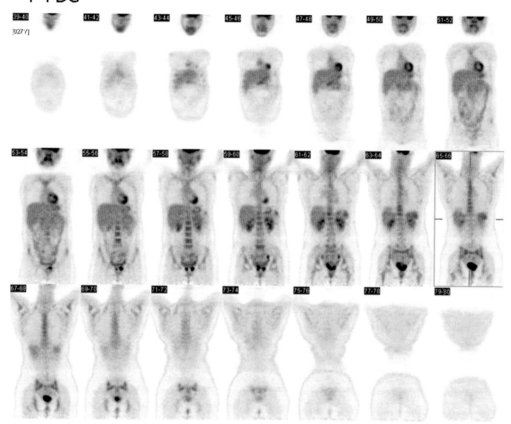

Fig. II.8.3A

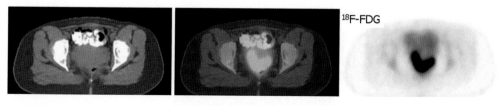

Fig. II.8.3B

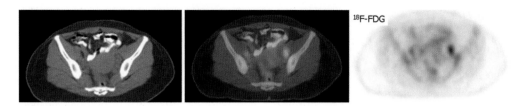

Fig. II.8.3C

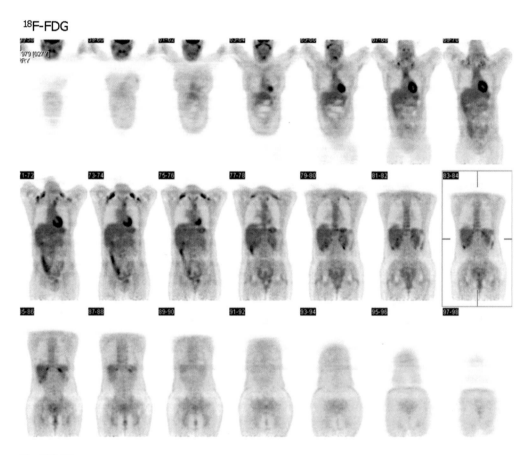

Fig. II.8.3D

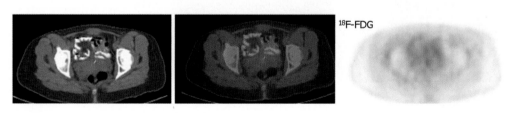

Fig. II.8.3E

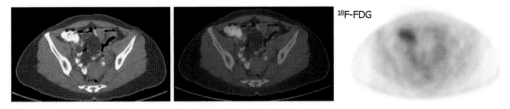

**Fig. II.8.3F**

### Findings

In the pretherapy PET/CT study, there is marked [18]F-FDG uptake within a large (approximately 50 × 50 mm) soft tissue mass originating in the cervix. Additional focally increased [18]F-FDG uptake is seen within external iliac lymph nodes bilaterally. The left external iliac lymph node measures 18 × 9 mm and the right measures 14 × 5 mm (Fig. II.8.3A–C).

The post-therapy PET/CT study performed approximately 3 months after completion of chemoradiation demonstrates minimal diffusely increased tracer uptake in the cervix, most probably related to post-radiation changes. There is a marked decrease in the size of the cervix as compared to the baseline study. There is also interval resolution of the [18]F-FDG uptake in the external iliac lymph nodes. There is decreased tracer activity in the lumbar spine and pelvic bones, due to the intervening radiation. Increased physiologic tracer activity is seen in the brown adipose tissue in the lower neck (Fig. II.8.3D–F).

### Discussion

Three-month post-therapy [18]F-FDG PET/CT demonstrates complete resolution of abnormal tracer uptake within the cervical mass and the pelvic lymph nodes. This is highly predictive of good prognosis.

Grigsby and colleagues[17] demonstrated that [18]F-FDG PET performed 3 months after completion of therapy is highly accurate in predicting long-term survival in patients with advanced cervical cancer treated with chemoradiation. A normal [18]F-FDG PET 3 months after therapy was indicative of an excellent prognosis, with a 5-year survival rate of 90% in patients with cervical cancer. In contrast, 5-year survival was only 45% in patients with persistent tracer uptake in the primary tumor or the nodal metastases seen before therapy. If the post-therapy PET study demonstrated new metastatic lesions, prognosis of the patients was poor with a 15% 5-year survival. These results were recently validated prospectively in 92 patients with cervical carcinoma treated with external irradiation, brachytherapy, and concurrent chemotherapy.[18] These patients underwent post-therapy PET 2–4 months after completion of therapy. [18]F-FDG PET showed a complete metabolic response in 71% of patients, partial metabolic response in 16%, and progressive disease in 13% of patients, with a significant difference in the 3-year progression-free survival of 78, 35, and 0%, respectively. The 3-year cause-specific survivals were 100, 51, and 0%, respectively. Multivariate analysis demonstrated that the post-therapy metabolic response was more predictive of survival than all known pretreatment prognostic factors. Thus, 3-month post-therapy [18]F-FDG uptake can be considered to represent a metabolic biomarker of tumor response and is a robust surrogate for prolonged follow-up to determine prognosis in cervical cancer.

### Diagnosis

1. Primary cervical squamous cell carcinoma.
2. Metastatic disease in external iliac lymph nodes bilaterally.
3. Metabolic response to chemoradiation.

## Case II.8.4 (DICOM Images on DVD)

### History

This 52-year-old woman with ovarian cancer was initially treated with total abdominal hysterectomy and bilateral salpingo-ophorectomy as well as omentectomy and chemotherapy. She presents with an elevated CA-125, and $^{18}$F-FDG PET/CT was performed for suspected recurrence (Fig. II.8.4A–F).

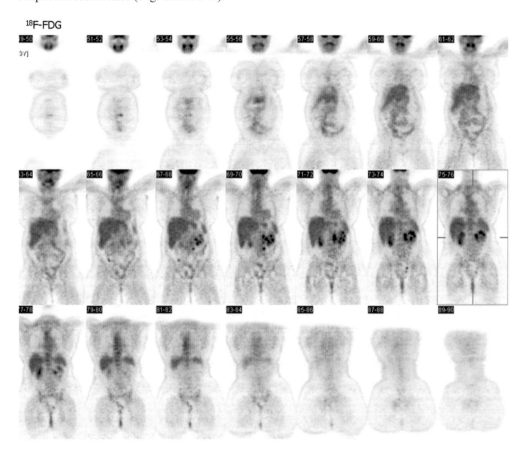

Fig. II.8.4A

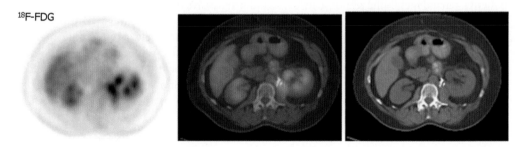

Fig. II.8.4B

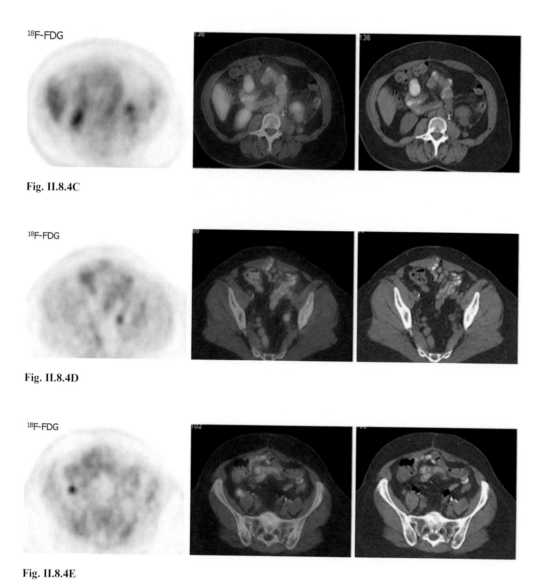

**Fig. II.8.4C**

**Fig. II.8.4D**

**Fig. II.8.4E**

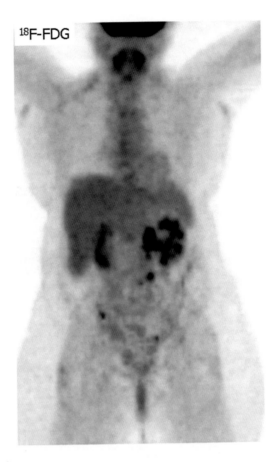

**Fig. II.8.4F (MIP image)**

### Findings

Intense ¹⁸F-FDG uptake is noted in multiple soft tissue nodules scattered throughout the abdomen and pelvis, consistent with recurrent disease (Fig. II.8.4A–F). There are multiple foci of markedly abnormal ¹⁸F-FDG uptake in the left para-aortic region adjacent to surgical clips (Fig. II.8.4A, B, F), and multiple soft tissue nodules in the left perinephric space demonstrating mildly increased tracer activity (Fig. II.8.4A, C, F). Additionally, there is increased ¹⁸F-FDG uptake within a 15 mm soft tissue nodule in the left pelvis, in a 9 mm nodule anterior to the right psoas muscle (Fig. II.8.4A, D–F), and in a small soft tissue nodule in the anterior abdomen in the region of the umbilicus (Fig. II.8.4A). Additional CT findings are seen on the DICOM images and described in the clinical report (see DVD).

### Discussion

The pattern of peritoneal involvement in this patient is typical for recurrent ovarian cancer. This pattern is associated with an unfavorable prognosis in comparison with recurrent disease presenting with discrete lesions.[37] Thus, early detection of localized recurrent disease may be beneficial. [18]F-FDG PET/CT has proven to be very useful in early detection of recurrent disease that is suitable for surgical resection.[27] Bristow and colleagues[27] demonstrated that in patients with rising CA-125 and negative or equivocal CT, [18]F-FDG PET has a sensitivity of 83% and PPV of 94% for detecting recurrent disease of at least 10 mm. Complete cytoreduction of the tumor was accomplished in 72% of patients with recurrent ovarian cancer larger than 10 mm. Some investigators have suggested that [18]F-FDG PET/CT is a sensitive post-therapy surveillance modality for detection of recurrent ovarian cancer. It assists in selecting the most appropriate treatment for individual patients. Chung and colleagues[28] studied 77 patients and demonstrated that the overall sensitivity, specificity, accuracy, PPV, and NPV of [18]F-FDG PET/CT were 93, 97, 95, 98, and 91%, respectively, for detection of recurrent ovarian cancer. PET/CT resulted in alteration of the management plan in 25% of patients by either avoiding previously planned diagnostic procedures or indicating the need for previously unplanned therapeutic procedures. Simcock and coworkers[29] demonstrated that [18]F-FDG PET/CT improves assessment of recurrent disease and provides prognostic information. In patients with rising CA-125, PET/CT results led to change in the distribution of known disease in 64% of patients and resulted in a major change in planned management in 58%. [18]F-FDG PET/CT identified a subgroup of women with apparently localized or no definite evidence of disease who had improved survival as compared with those patients with proven systemic disease.

**Diagnosis**

Recurrent ovarian cancer – diffuse abdominal carcinomatosis.

**Clinical Report: Body [18]F-FDG PET/CT (for DVD cases only)**

Indication

Localization of recurrent ovarian cancer.

History

This 52-year-old woman with ovarian cancer was initially treated with total abdominal hysterectomy, bilateral salpingo-ophorectomy and omentectomy, followed by chemotherapy. She also underwent bilateral pelvic lymphadenectomy. Approximately a year prior to current examination, she had recurrence in her left para-aortic region for which she underwent surgery and cisplatin washing. Subsequent [18]F-FDG PET/CT showed resolution of disease. She now presents with a suspicion of recurrence due to elevated CA-125.

Procedure

After oral administration of MD-Gastroview[TM] and intravenous administration of 555 MBq (15 mCi) [18]F-FDG, non-contrast CT images were obtained for attenuation correction and for fusion with PET images. PET was then obtained beginning approximately 87 min after injection of [18]F-FDG. The patient's fasting blood glucose level, measured before injection of [18]F-FDG, was 103 mg/dL. The area imaged spanned from the skull base to the upper thighs. The patient was positioned with arms up.

   Before administration of [18]F-FDG, intravenous access was established for patient hydration. In addition, a 16-French Foley catheter was inserted into the urinary bladder using standard aseptic technique. Furosemide, 20 mg, was administered by slow intravenous injection approximately 20 min after the injection of $^{18}$F-FDG. At the conclusion of the procedure, the intravenous line and Foley catheter were removed without incident. The patient tolerated the procedure well, without apparent complications.

## Findings

*Quality of the study*: The quality of this study is good.

*Head and neck*: There is physiologic distribution of the radiopharmaceutical in the cerebral cortex and lymphoid and glandular tissues of the neck.

*Chest*: The heart is normal. No pulmonary nodule is seen.

*Abdomen and pelvis*: There is increased $^{18}$F-FDG uptake in multiple soft tissue nodules scattered throughout the abdomen and pelvis, consistent with recurrent disease. There are multiple soft tissue nodules in the perinephric region of the left kidney, the larger nodules demonstrate increased $^{18}$F-FDG uptake, with the largest measuring 23 mm in maximum dimension. There are multiple left para-aortic soft tissue lymph nodes in the region of surgical clips demonstrating markedly abnormal tracer uptake. An additional soft tissue nodule is seen adjacent to the left diaphragmatic crus just above the origin of the renal arteries. There also is increased $^{18}$F-FDG uptake within a 15-mm soft tissue nodule in the left pelvis and a 9-mm nodule anterior to the right psoas muscle. There is a small umbilical hernia containing a portion of normal appearing bowel, with an adjacent $^{18}$F-FDG-avid soft tissue nodule.

The CT images demonstrate multiple soft tissue nodules scattered throughout the abdomen and pelvis. Multiple surgical clips are seen scattered throughout the abdomen and pelvis. There is mild anterior displacement of the left kidney secondary to posterior perinephric nodules. There is a small left extrarenal pelvis. The liver, pancreas, spleen, and bilateral adrenal glands are normal. There is a small hiatal hernia. The stomach and small and large bowels demonstrate normal wall thickness and caliber. A Foley catheter is seen within a decompressed urinary bladder. There are surgical clips adjacent to a small umbilical hernia containing a portion of normal appearing bowel.

*Musculoskeletal*: Evaluation of the osseous structures demonstrates no suspicious lytic or sclerotic lesions.

## Impression

Multifocal $^{18}$F-FDG uptake in the abdomen and pelvis, consistent with recurrent ovarian carcinoma.

## Case II.8.5

### History

This 56-year-old woman with endometrioid adenocarcinoma of the uterus initially treated with total abdominal hysterectomy and bilateral salpingo-ophorectomy as well as pelvic and abdominal lymphadenectomy presented to $^{18}$F-FDG PET/CT for further evaluation of a nodule in the anterior abdomen (Fig. II.8.5A–D).

$^{18}$F-FDG

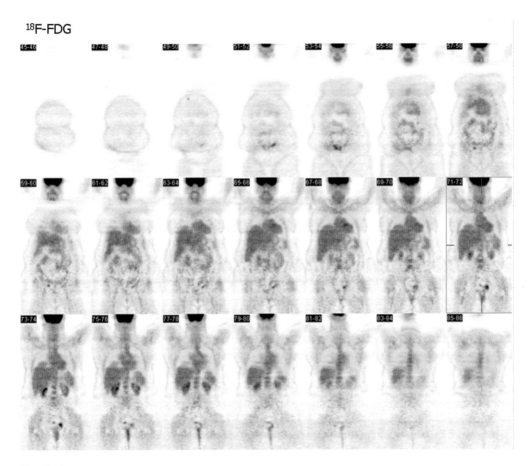

**Fig. II.8.5A**

$^{18}$F-FDG

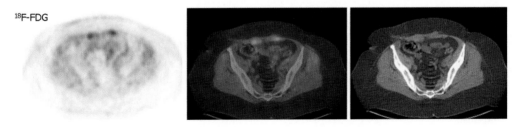

**Fig. II.8.5B**

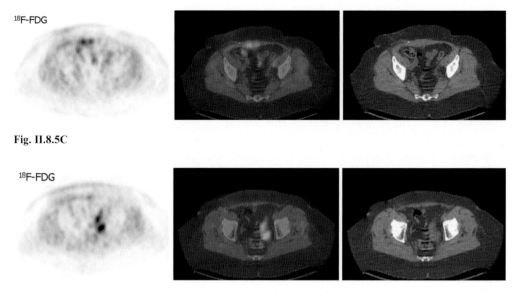

**Fig. II.8.5C**

**Fig. II.8.5D**

## Findings

There are multiple foci of increased [18]F-FDG activity along the anterior abdominal wall corresponding to slight thickening of the lower rectus muscle (Fig. II.8.5A–C). There is increased [18]F-FDG uptake within a soft tissue mass measuring 20 × 33 mm in the left pelvis, localized to the left iliac nodal chain (Fig. II.8.5D).

## Discussion

In patients with endometrial cancer, a significantly better prognosis has been noted when recurrences were detected during asymptomatic follow-up, supporting the benefit of surveillance programs in high-risk patients, whereas it seems to be of limited benefit for patients at low risk for recurrent disease.[38] Among patients with asymptomatic recurrent endometrial cancer, pelvic examination and conventional imaging can detect a large number of relapses.[38] Belhocine and colleagues[34] demonstrated that [18]F-FDG imaging has a sensitivity, specificity, diagnostic accuracy, PPV, and NPV of 96, 78, 90, 89, and 91%, respectively, for detection of residual or recurrent disease. PET confirmed recurrence initially suspected based on results of other tests in 88% of cases, but detected asymptomatic recurrences in an additional 12% of patients. In 35% of cases, PET significantly altered treatment decisions by detecting otherwise unsuspected distant metastases. Saga and colleagues[35] studied patients with endometrial cancer following therapy for detection of disease recurrence or to assess response to treatment. [18]F-FDG imaging had a sensitivity of 100%, specificity of 88%, and accuracy of 93% when evaluated in conjunction with CT/MRI. PET detected unsuspected metastatic disease in 19% of patients and changed the management of 33%. No false-negative result was noted for PET after a minimal follow-up of 5 months, thus suggesting a high NPV for this modality.

## Diagnosis

Recurrent endometrial cancer in abdominal wall and metastatic lymphadenopathy in pelvis.

# References

1. American Cancer Society. Cancer Facts & Figures 2009. Atlanta: American Cancer Society; 2009.
2. Lai CH, Yen TC, Chang TC. Positron emission tomography imaging for gynecologic malignancy. *Curr Opin Obstet Gynecol* 2007;19:37–41.
3. Havrilesky LJ, Kulasingam SL, Matchar DB, Myers ER. FDG-PET for management of cervical and ovarian cancer. *Gynecol Oncol* 2005;97:183–191.
4. Choi HJ, Roh JW, Seo SS, Lee S, Kim J-Y, Kim S-K, Kang KW, Lee JS, Jeong JY, Park S-Y. Comparison of the accuracy of magnetic resonance imaging and positron emission tomography/computed tomography in the presurgical detection of lymph node metastases in patients with uterine cervical carcinoma: A prospective study. *Cancer* 2006;106:914–922.
5. Loft A, Berthelsen AK, Roed H, Ottosen C, Lundvall L, Knudsen J, Nedergaard L, Højgaard L Engelholm SA. The diagnostic value of PET/CT scanning in patients with cervical cancer: a prospective study. *Gynecol Oncol* 2007;106:29–34.
6. Wright JD, Dehdashti F, Herzog TJ, Mutch DG, Huettner PC, Rader JS, Gibb RK, Powell MA, Gao F, Siegel BA, Grigsby PW. Preoperative lymph node staging of early-stage cervical carcinoma by [18F]-fluoro-2-deoxy-D-glucose-positron emission tomography. *Cancer* 2005;104:2484–2491.
7. Chou HH, Chang TC, Yen TC, Ng K-K, Hsueh S, Ma S-Y, Chang C-J, Huang H-J, Chao A, Wu T-I, Jung S-M, Wu Y-C, Lin C-T, Huang K-G, Lai C-H. Low value of [18F]-fluoro-2-deoxy-D-glucose positron emission tomography in primary staging of early-stage cervical cancer before radical hysterectomy. *J Clin Oncol* 2005;24:123–128.
8. Sironi S, Buda A, Picchio M, Perego P, Moreni R, Pellegrino A, Colombo M, Mangioni C, Messa C, Fazio F. Lymph node metastasis in patients with clinical early-stage cervical cancer: detection with integrated FDG PET/CT. *Radiology* 2005;238:272–279.
9. Lin LL, Mutic S, Low DA, LaForest R, Vicic M, Zoberi I, Miller T, Grigsby P. Adaptive brachytherapy treatment planning for cervical cancer using FDG-PET. *Int J Radiat Oncol Biol Phys* 2007;67:91–96.
10. Sakuragi N. Up-to-date management of lymph node metastasis and the role of tailored lymphadenectomy in cervical cancer. *Int J Clin Oncol* 2007;12:165–175.
11. Panici PB, Cutillo G, Angioli R. Modulation of surgery in early invasive cervical cancer. *Crit Rev Oncol Hematol* 2003;48:263–270.
12. Miller TR, Grigsby PW. Measurement of tumor volume by PET to evaluate prognosis in patients with advanced cervical cancer treated by radiation therapy. *Int J Radiat Oncol Biol Phys* 2002;53:353–359.
13. Kidd EA, Siegel BA, Dehdashti F, Grigsby PW. The standardized uptake value for F-18 fluorodeoxyglucose is a sensitive predictive biomarker for cervical cancer treatment response and survival. *Cancer* 2007;110:1738–1744.
14. Grigsby PW, Siegel BA, Dehdashti F. Lymph node staging by positron emission tomography in patients with carcinoma of the cervix. *J Clin Oncol* 2001;19:3745–3749.
15. Chung HH, Jo H, Kang WJ, Kim JW, Park N-H, Song Y-S, Chung J-K, Kang S-B, Lee H-P. Clinical impact of integrated PET/CT on the management of suspected cervical cancer recurrence. *Gynecol Oncol* 2007;104:529–534.
16. Yen TC, Lai CH, Ma SY, Huang K-G, Huang H-J, Hong J-H, Hsueh S, Lin W-J, Ng K-K, Chang T-C. Comparative benefits and limitations of (18)F-FDG PET and CT-MRI in documented or suspected recurrent cervical cancer. *Eur J Nucl Med Mol Imaging* 2006;33:1399–1407.
17. Grigsby PW, Siegel BA, Dehdashti F, Rader J, Zoberi I. Posttherapy [18F] fluorodeoxyglucose positron emission tomography in carcinoma of the cervix: Response and outcome. *J Clin Oncol* 2004;22:2167–2171.
18. Schwarz JK, Siegel BA, Dehdashti F, Grigsby PW. Association of posttherapy positron emission tomography with tumor response and survival in cervical carcinoma. *JAMA* 2007;298:2289–2295.
19. Johnson RJ. Radiology in the management of ovarian cancer. *Clin Radiol* 1993;48:75–82.
20. Lerman H, Metser U, Grisaru D, Fishman A, Lievshitz G, Even-Sapir E. Normal and abnormal 18F-FDG endometrial and ovarian uptake in pre- and postmenopausal patients: Assessment by PET/CT. *J Nucl Med* 2004;45:266–271.
21. Grab D, Flock F, Stohr I, Nüssle K, Rieber A, Fenchel S, Brambs H-J, Reske SN, Kreienberg R. Classification of asymptomatic adnexal masses by ultrasound, magnetic resonance imaging, and positron emission tomography. *Gynecol Oncol* 2000;77:454–459.

22. Yoshida Y, Kurokawa T, Kawahara K, Tsuchida T, Okazawa H, Fujibayashi Y, Yonekura Y, Kotsuji F. Incremental benefits of FDG positron emission tomography over CT alone for the preoperative staging of ovarian cancer. *AJR Am J Roentgenol* 2004;182:227–233.

23. Castellucci P, Perrone AM, Picchio M, Ghi T, Farsad M, Nanni C, Messa C, Meriggiola M, Pelusi G, Al-Nahhas A, Rubello D, Fazio F, Fanti S. Diagnostic accuracy of 18F-FDG PET/CT in characterizing ovarian lesions and staging ovarian cancer: Correlation with transvaginal ultrasonography, computed tomography, and histology. *Nucl Med Commun* 2007;28:589–595.

24. Chan JK, Cheung MK, Husain A, Teng NN, West D, Whittemore AS, Berek JS, Osann K. Patterns and progress in ovarian cancer over 14 years. *Obstet Gynecol* 2006;108:521–528.

25. Chan YM, Ng TY, Ngan HY, Wong LC. Quality of life in women treated with neoadjuvant chemotherapy for advanced ovarian cancer: a prospective longitudinal study. *Gynecol Oncol* 2003;88:9–16.

26. Avril N, Sassen S, Schmalfeldt B, Naehrig J, Rutke S, Weber WA, Werner M, Graeff H, Schwaiger M, Kuhn W. Prediction of response to neoadjuvant chemotherapy by sequential F-18-Fluorodeoxyglucose positron emission tomography in patients with advanced-stage ovarian cancer. *J Clin Oncol* 2005;23:7445–7453.

27. Bristow RE, del Carmen MG, Pannu HK, Cohade C, Zahurak ML, Fishman E, Wahl RL, Montz FJ. Clinically occult recurrent ovarian cancer: Patient selection for secondary cytoreductive surgery using combined PET/CT. *Gynecol Oncol* 2003;90:519–528.

28. Chung HH, Kang WJ, Kim JW, Park N-H, Song Y-S, Chung J-K, Kang S-B, Lee H-P. Role of [18F]FDG PET/CT in the assessment of suspected recurrent ovarian cancer: correlation with clinical or histological findings. *Eur J Nucl Med Mol Imaging* 2007;34:480–486.

29. Simcock B, Neesham D, Quinn M, Drummond E, Milner A, Hicks RJ. The impact of PET/CT in the management of recurrent ovarian cancer. *Gynecol Oncol* 2006;103:271–276.

30. Zhuang H, Yamamoto AJ, Sinha P, Pourdehnad M, Liu Y, Alavi A. Similar pelvic abnormalities on FDG positron emission tomography of different origins. *Clin Nucl Med* 2001;26:515–517.

31. Lee WL, Liu RS, Yuan CC, Chao HT, Wang PH. Relationship between gonadotropin-releasing hormone agonist and myoma cellular activity: Preliminary findings on positron emission tomography. *Fertil Steril* 2001;75:638–639.

32. Horowitz NS, Dehdashti F, Herzog TJ, Rader JS, Powell MA, Gibb RK, Grigsby PW, Siegel BA, Mutch DG. Prospective evaluation of FDG-PET for detecting pelvic and para-aortic lymph node metastasis in uterine corpus cancer. *Gynecol Oncol* 2004;95:546–551.

33. Suzuki R, Miyagi E, Takahashi N, Sukegawa A, Suzuki A, Koike I, Sugiura K, Okamoto N, Inoue T, Hirahara F. Validity of positron emission tomography using fluoro-2-deoxyglucose for the preoperative evaluation of endometrial cancer. *Int J Gynecol Cancer* 2007;17:890–896.

34. Belhocine T, De Barsy C, Hustinx R, Willems-Foidart J. Usefulness of (18)F-FDG PET in the posttherapy surveillance of endometrial carcinoma. *Eur J Nucl Med Mol Imaging* 2002;29:1132–1139.

35. Saga T, Higashi T, Ishimori T, Marcelo M. Yuji N, Takahiro M, Toru F, Kaori T, Shigeo Y, Toshihiro H, Masato K, Shingo F, Junji K. Clinical value of FDG-PET in the follow up of post-operative patients with endometrial cancer. *Ann Nucl Med* 2003;17:197–203.

36. Podoloff DA, Ball DW, Ben-Josef E, Benson AB, Cohen SJ, Coleman RE, Delbeke D, Ho M, Ilson DH, Kalemkerian GP, Lee RJ, Loeffler JS, Macapinlac HA, Morgan RJ, Siegel BA, Singhal S, Tyler DS, Wong RJ. NCCN Task Force: Clinical Utility of PET in a Variety of Tumor Types Task Force. *J Natl Compr Canc Netw* 2009;7 Suppl 2:S1–S23. http://www.nccn.org/professionals/physician_gls/f_guidelines.asp

37. Ferrandina G, Legge F, Salutari V, Paglia A, Testa A, Scambia G. Impact of pattern of recurrence on clinical outcome of ovarian cancer patients: Clinical considerations. *Eur J Cancer* 2006;42:2296–2302.

38. Sartori E, Pasinetti B, Carrara L, Gambino A, Odicino F, Pecorelli S. Pattern of failure and value of follow-up procedures in endometrial and cervical cancer patients. *Gynecol Oncol* 2007;107:S241–247.

# Chapter II.9
# Hybrid Imaging in Malignancies of the Urinary Tract, Prostate, and Testicular Cancers

Martine Klein and Marina Orevi

## Introduction

The main urologic malignancies include renal, bladder, prostate, and testicular cancers. Although positron emission tomography (PET) and PET/computed tomography (CT) play an increasing role in diagnosis and staging of many primary and metastatic tumors, it has been slow to be implemented into oncologic urology. Most malignant tumors are characterized by enhanced glucose metabolism, resulting in increased [18]F-fluorodeoxyglucose ([18]F-FDG) uptake, which can be imaged by PET. In urology, [18]F-FDG is a suboptimal tracer due to its variable uptake in some urological tumors and due to its accumulation and excretion through the urinary tract, potentially masking kidney, bladder, and prostate tumors. Thus, other PET tracers are being investigated for urologic malignancies.

Although PET imaging using [11]C-choline or [11]C-acetate that have negligible urinary excretion has already proved to be a better tool in evaluation of bladder and prostate malignancies, it is still challenging. Uptake of [11]C-choline or [11]C-acetate can be relatively low in small sized (<10 mm) loco-regional lymph node metastases. PET/CT allows for a more accurate localization of small, mild foci of activity.

The advantages of hybrid PET/CT imaging, combining functional features with anatomical detail, also apply to single photon emission computed tomography (SPECT)/CT imaging. In this context, radioimmunoscintigraphy of prostate cancer by capromab pendetide conjugated to [111]Indium (ProstaScint®) has significantly benefited from improved camera technology and the use of co-registration. In the management of testicular cancer, [18]F-FDG PET retains its relevance in particular in patients with residual or recurrent tumor and in monitoring treatment response.

## Renal Cancer

Renal cell carcinoma (RCC) is the most frequent neoplasm of the kidney in adults, accounting for 85% of renal malignancies.[1] Other renal tumors include transitional cell carcinoma (TCC), squamous cell carcinoma, lymphoma, and metastatic neoplasm (mainly from lung cancer and melanoma). The classic clinical presentation of RCC, described in

M. Klein (✉)

Department of Biophysics and Nuclear Medicine, Hadassah Hebrew University Medical Center, Jerusalem, Israel

e-mail: martine@hadassah.org.il

D. Delbeke, O. Israel (eds.), *Hybrid PET/CT and SPECT/CT Imaging*,
DOI 10.1007/978-0-387-92820-3_11, © Springer Science+Business Media, LLC 2010

only about 10% of patients, is a triad: hematuria, flank pain, and a palpable flank mass. In more than 50% of the patients, each of these triad terms can be the initial clinical manifestation of the tumor.

The role of imaging in RCC, and of PET in particular, is first to characterize the malignant nature of a renal mass and subsequently to detect loco-regional and distant metastases. The widespread use of ultrasonography (US) and CT has led to an increase in the number of incidentally discovered early stage RCCs in asymptomatic patients. An isolated RCC requires surgical excision of the tumor, usually radical nephrectomy. A renal mass is first evaluated by anatomic imaging modalities. A simple cyst is always benign and well characterized by contrast CT or US. A "complex" cyst can be a malignant tumor, while a solid mass represents cancer as a rule. Solid renal masses greater than 30 mm in diameter are generally resected and there is little role for additional imaging. Curative resection is feasible for localized disease. The sensitivity and specificity of helical CT for diagnosing RCC is 100% and 88–95%, respectively.[2] The sensitivity of CT for the detection of retro-peritoneal lymph node metastases is high, 95%, but it is associated with a rate of false-positive findings ranging from 3 to 43% when a nodal size of 10 mm or more is the criterion for malignancy. Thus, there is a need for more accurate imaging techniques for diagnosis and staging of RCC.

## PET/CT Imaging for Diagnosis and Staging of RCC

Only a small number of studies have investigated the role of $^{18}$F-FDG PET in evaluation of renal masses, reflecting the limitations related to the urinary excretory route of this tracer, which generates renal activity that needs to be differentiated from a malignant mass. There is general agreement that $^{18}$F-FDG PET has a limited role in the initial diagnosis of renal tumors compared to standard imaging modalities. Given the limitations of $^{18}$F-FDG as a tracer for renal tumors, other tracers are being investigated. $^{11}$C-acetate is retained by RCC, is cleared rapidly from normal parenchyma, and has no urinary excretion. Lawrentschuk and colleagues[3] reported a difficult case of RCC diagnosed by $^{18}$F-fluorothymidine (FLT), a radiolabeled compound based on the nucleic acid thymidine, and studied the role of $^{18}$F-misonidazole (MISO) in detecting hypoxia in RCC. However, detecting RCC in complex renal masses requires consistently high tracer uptake, which has not been shown by these tracers.

Approximately one-third of patients with RCC presents with metastatic disease and has a poor median survival of 10 months. Aide and colleagues[4] showed that the accuracy of $^{18}$F-FDG PET in detecting distant metastases of RCC was 94% versus 89% for CT. Overall, PET has a moderate sensitivity of 71–75% but a high positive predictive value (PPV) of 92–94% for detecting recurrent and metastatic RCC. Although a negative study cannot rule out metastatic disease, a positive PET should be considered as highly suspicious for local recurrence or metastases.[4-6] Currently, CT and bone scintigraphy are still the most commonly used imaging modalities for the evaluation of metastatic disease.

## PET/CT Imaging During Follow-Up and Recurrent RCC

$^{18}$F-FDG PET has been successful in monitoring the progression of RCC.[5] Because of the limited anatomic information, PET alone cannot replace CT in the follow-up of patients with RCC. However, PET/CT takes advantage of the high specificity of PET and the high sensitivity of CT in detecting metastatic RCC and can be useful in monitoring treatment response.

## Conclusions

[18]F-FDG imaging does not play a role in the primary diagnosis of RCC because of the significant renal excretion of the tracer. It has, however, a role in assessing metastatic spread and in detecting recurrent visceral, lymph node, and skeletal disease.

## Bladder Cancer

Bladder and related urothelial cancers represent about 4% of malignancies. In the United States, bladder cancer is the fourth most commonly diagnosed malignancy.[1] The mucosal surfaces of the collecting tubules, calyces, renal pelvis, ureter, bladder, and urethra have the same embryologic origin, and the term "urothelium" designates the lining surface epithelium. The ratio of tumors of the bladder compared to renal pelvis and to tumors of the ureter is 51 to 3 to 1, TCC being the most common urothelial neoplasm.

Bladder tumors are diagnosed mainly by direct visualization with cystoscopy and subsequent biopsy or resection. Most newly diagnosed malignancies are noninvasive, low-grade tumors that recur frequently, and rarely progress to muscle invasion or metastatic disease. [18]F-FDG imaging is unlikely to contribute to the evaluation of these limited tumors. However, high-grade or invasive bladder cancer is characterized by progressive local invasion, extension to adjacent organs, and development of regional and distant metastases. While organ-confined bladder cancer can be treated by radical cystectomy only, with a cure rate of more than 70%, pelvic lymphadenectomy is added in the case of invasive disease to the pelvis.[7] The risk of developing lymph node metastases in a patient with muscle-invasive bladder cancer is about 20%. The presence of regional node metastases increases the incidence of recurrence and distant disease with a 5-year survival of 20–25%. An accurate imaging modality identifying these patients could contribute to their management, since patients with positive lymph nodes benefit from chemotherapy more than from radical surgery. [18]F-FDG PET, based on metabolic changes has a potential advantage in detecting metastases in small lymph nodes compared to conventional imaging modalities.

## [18]F-FDG Imaging of Bladder Cancer

The spatial resolution of PET using [18]F-FDG for visualizing bladder cancer and pelvic lymph nodes is significantly limited by the urinary excretion of the radiotracer including pooling in the ureters and the bladder, and the variable bowel uptake. Different techniques have been recommended to reduce the amount of [18]F-FDG in the urinary bladder, such as forced diuresis or bladder catheter with continuous irrigation, but these are uncomfortable for the patient and have shown disappointing results. [18]F-FDG PET is therefore not being used in routine clinical practice for the detection and staging of bladder cancer. On the other hand, [18]F-FDG PET has a role in identifying distant metastases, in detecting recurrent pelvic tumor, and in differentiating between local recurrence and post-treatment fibrosis or necrosis. Sensitivity, specificity, and accuracy of [18]F-FDG PET for detecting nodal and distant metastasis were 60, 88, and 78%, respectively, in 55 patients with bladder cancer.[8] In another study, Kosuda and coworkers[9] identified all patients with distant metastatic disease involving the lungs, bone, and lymph nodes. Attempts have been made to increase the sensitivity of PET imaging for diagnosis and staging of bladder cancer using other tracers with negligible or no urine excretion.

## [11]C-Choline Imaging of Bladder Cancer

Choline acts as a precursor in the biosynthesis of phosphatidylcholine, a major phospholipid component in normal mammalian cell membranes.[10] Phosphorylation of choline is catalyzed by the enzyme cholinekinase. Cancer cells show increased choline uptake due to upregulated activity of cholinekinase and elevated levels of phosphatidylcholine. [11]C-choline has a very rapid blood clearance of approximately 7 min, and most of the tracer remains trapped within the cells, providing images of good diagnostic quality.

[11]C has a short half-life of 20 min and poses a logistic challenge in many institutions. [18]F-labeled choline derivates with a half-life of 110 min that have been synthetized[11] and show rapid clearance from the blood pool, but appear in the urinary bladder 3–5 min after injection, in contrast to [11]C-choline. This limitation can be overcome by dynamic pelvic acquisition since pathologic uptake begins 1 min post-injection, before urinary excretion and bladder filling.

With [11]C-choline minimal urinary excretion is still possible, and PET images are therefore acquired starting from the pelvis 3–5 min post-injection in order to avoid excretion into the ureters and bladder. Pitfalls due to the normal biodistribution and the minimal urinary excretion of [11]C-choline are the reason for the higher accuracy of [11]C-choline PET/CT as compared to PET stand-alone. In a pre-operative study of 19 tumors in 18 patients, [11]C-choline uptake was found in all primary TCCs, including 3 carcinomas in situ, 14 muscle-invasive bladder cancer, and 2 concomitant extensive TCCs of the ureter and renal pelvis, with an average standard uptake value (SUV) of $7.3 \pm 3.2$.[12] In addition, skeletal metastases were visualized on the [11]C-choline PET component in bones with normal architecture on the CT part that were confirmed by follow-up imaging studies. In early [11]C-choline PET only studies, tumors in situ were not visualized, and reported values were lower.[13] Hybrid imaging allows for the detection of small lymph node metastases and the resolution of challenges stemming from the normal biodistribution of labeled choline.

## [11]C-Acetate and [11]C-Methionine Imaging of Bladder Cancer

Shreve and colleagues[14] showed [11]C-acetate to be a potential PET tracer for various malignancies. As with choline, acetate uptake in tumor cells is related to cell membrane lipid synthesis. In addition, acetate has no urinary excretion and can be therefore useful for imaging of TCC. Preliminary results of a study comparing [11]C-choline and [11]C-acetate PET/CT imaging for the detection of TCC show lower SUV values for [11]C-acetate than for [11]C-choline (Klein and colleagues, unpublished results).

[11]C-Methionine is taken up proportional to the amino-acid transport and is primarily metabolized in the liver and pancreas with no significant renal excretion. The sensitivity of

[11]C-methionine PET for the detection of bladder cancer, although superior to [18]F-FDG PET, was found to be only of 78%.[15]

## Conclusions

[11]C-choline PET/CT seems to be the most promising imaging modality for the detection and staging of TCC. [18]F-FDG imaging is useful in the evaluation of loco-regional recurrence and of distant metastases.

## Prostate Cancer

Prostate cancer is the most common cancer and the second cause of death in men. More than 230,000 new cases are diagnosed each year, and the mortality rate in the United States exceeds 30,000 men per year.[1] The tumor may spread locally either through direct extension into the periprostatic fat or via ejaculatory ducts into the seminal vesicles, to regional lymph nodes through lymphatic channels, and hematogenously to the skeleton. Treatment of prostate cancer includes radical prostatectomy, radiotherapy, hormonal therapy, and, in cases of failure of the later, chemotherapy. Diagnosis of primary or recurrent prostate cancer is based on digital rectal examination, elevated serum levels of prostate specific antigen (PSA), and biopsy. The widespread use of the PSA serum assay has led to early diagnosis of prostate cancer, with more than 70% of tumors being organ-confined at diagnosis.[16] Staging is performed by transrectal ultrasound (TRUS), CT, or magnetic resonance imaging (MRI). Measurements of PSA serum values have made a significant change in management of prostate cancer both at screening and for detection of recurrent or persistent tumor. Detection of loco-regional disease versus distant metastases implies a change in management and prognosis of prostate cancer. In this respect, metabolic rather than anatomic imaging may play a role.

## PET/CT and SPECT/CT of Primary Prostate Cancer

There is general agreement that [18]F-FDG PET is not useful in the diagnosis or staging of primary prostate cancer, mainly because of low metabolic glucose activity of these malignant cells (due to their relatively slow cell replication) and of the accumulation of tracer activity in the bladder, which may mask the prostate bed.[12]

While radiolabeled choline (with either [11]C or [18]F) has the potential to be a promising tool for PET imaging of prostate cancer, its value is currently still debated. Sensitivity and specificity of [11]C-choline PET for detecting malignancy in patients with known prostate cancer range between 81–86% and 62–87%, respectively.[17,18] Although radiolabeled choline has been shown to have a higher lesion-based uptake than [18]F-FDG, no correlation between SUV of [11]C-choline and tumor grade or Gleason score has been found. In a study evaluating [11]C-choline PET/CT to identify malignant foci in the prostate, Farsad and colleagues[19] reported a sensitivity of 66%, specificity 81%, accuracy 71%, PPV 87%, and negative predictive value (NPV) of 55%. Martorana and coworkers[20] reported a sensitivity of 83% for detection of malignant nodules greater than 5 mm in size. However, PET/CT appeared to be only slightly more sensitive (66% versus 61%) and less specific (84% versus 97%) as compared to TRUS biopsy. The limited sensitivity of PET/CT is most likely due to several factors. Prostate cancer is frequently multifocal, [11]C-choline uptake may be relatively low (with an SUV ranging between 2.2 and 4.6), and the spatial resolution of PET/CT of approximately 5 mm may obviate visualization of smaller foci that can be detected at histopathology after radical prostatectomy. Moreover, false-positive findings occur due to [11]C-choline uptake in benign processes such as acute or chronic prostatitis, benign prostatic hypertrophy (BPH), prostatic intraepithelial neoplasia, as well as malignant lesions of different histologies.[18]

In addition to PET, endorectal coil MRI supplemented by spectroscopy is also based on choline metabolism. The sensitivity of PET/CT to assess extraprostatic extension, such as extra-capsular growth and seminal vesicle invasion, is low when compared to MRI (22% versus 63%).[20] Testa and colleagues[21] reported a comparable specificity for localizing cancer within the prostate with either 3D magnetic resonance (MR) spectroscopy and MRI, or PET/CT. However, PET/CT had a lower sensitivity of 55% versus 81% for 3D MR spectroscopy alone or combined with MRI. The advantage of whole body [11]C-choline PET/CT over other imaging modalities is its ability to detect distant metastases. This is of limited value following diagnosis of mainly low-stage disease due to widely used PSA screening. The prevalence of lymph node metastases at the time of diagnosis decreased from 23% in 1984 to 2% in 1995.[16]

Cellular uptake of [11]C-acetate in tumor cells is proportional to lipid synthesis. Prostate cancer is characterized by an increase in fatty acid synthesis and overexpression of the enzyme fatty acid synthase (FAS).[22] [11]C-acetate was found to be more sensitive than [18]F-FDG PET for detecting prostate cancer.[23] However, as with choline, the degree of uptake as measured by SUV may overlap for prostate cancer, BPH, and the normal prostate in patients 50 years or older.[24]

[111]In-capromab pentetide (ProstaScint®) is a murine antibody to an intracellular component of the prostatic specific membrane antigen (PSMA). Initial results demonstrated Prostascint scintigraphy® to have a sensitivity of 63% and a NPV of 92% for the detection of prostate cancer.[25] Prostascint® scintigraphy including both planar and SPECT has never been widely accepted for imaging of prostate cancer. A considerable amount of expertise is required to interpret these studies because of significant nonspecific binding and high blood pool activity leading to a low target-to-background ratio.

The use of SPECT/CT allows for better localization of foci of increased tracer uptake and subsequently enables a more confident interpretation of the images. In a study of 800 patients, Prostascint® SPECT/CT had a sensitivity of 79%, a specificity of 80%, and an overall accuracy of 80% for detection of prostate cancer.[26] Prostascint® SPECT/CT has been also utilized to guide focal brachytherapy in patients with prostate cancer. A 7-year follow-up of 239 patients demonstrated superior results in all risk categories compared with a 5-year meta-analysis of brachytherapy patients.[27] These data suggest that Prostascint® SPECT/CT can be used to deliver increased radiation doses to focal areas of increased tracer uptake inside the prostate.

## PET/CT and SPECT/CT of Metastatic Prostate Cancer

Only a small number of studies have used radiolabeled choline or acetate for primary staging of prostate cancer. PET imaging using [11]C-choline and [11]C-acetate have been proven to have a better performance than [18]F-FDG PET for diagnosis of nodal metastases. A limited number of studies using [11]C-methionine in primary staging of prostate cancer have also demonstrated that [11]C-methionine is superior to [18]F-FDG in detecting primary and metastatic lesions in prostate cancer.[28]

The skeleton is the most common site for distant metastases in prostate cancer. There are conflicting reports with respect to the accuracy of [18]F-FDG PET for detection of skeletal metastases. [18]F-FDG PET is considered to be more sensitive for the detection of skeletal metastases than for local or nodal disease. Shreve and colleagues [14] reported a sensitivity of 65% and PPV of 98% in 202 skeletal metastases. Yeh and coworkers [29] showed, however, that only 18% of lesions seen on bone scintigraphy showed [18]F-FDG uptake. Nunez and colleagues [28] described higher detectability rate of cervical spine metastases by [18]F-FDG PET as compared to bone scintigraphy. In a study by Morris and colleagues, [30] all lesions seen on [18]F-FDG PET were subsequently proven to be active disease.

Labeled choline, acetate, and methionine PET imaging have a better sensitivity than [18]F-FDG PET for diagnosis of skeletal metastases. The lesion-based sensitivity of [11]C-acetate PET and [18]F-FDG PET was 83 and 75%, respectively. [31] Nunez and cow-orkers [28] found that [11]C-methionine was more effective than [18]F-FDG for detecting skeletal metastases, with a sensitivity of 72 and 48% for [11]C-methionine and [18]F-FDG, respectively.

Even-Sapir and colleagues [32] compared planar skeletal scintigraphy with [99m]Tc-methylene-diphosphonate ([99m]Tc-MDP), bone SPECT, [18]F-fluoride PET, and PET/CT in 44 patients with high-risk prostate cancer. The sensitivity, specificity, PPV, and NPV of planar bone scintigraphy were 79, 57, 64, and 55%, respectively. The values for multiple field-of-view SPECT were 92, 82, 86, and 90%, respectively. For [18]F-fluoride PET, the values were 100, 62, 74, and 100%, respectively, whereas for [18]F-fluoride PET/CT, the values were 100% for all parameters.

## PET/CT and SPECT/CT in Recurrent Prostate Cancer

Recurrent prostate cancer is usually asymptomatic, and the diagnosis relies on rising PSA levels, with a reported incidence of PSA relapse ranging between 15 and 53%. [33] An increasing PSA profile after radiotherapy or after surgery is evidence of residual or recurrent disease. The treatment of local recurrence is either surgery or radiotherapy, whereas distant metas-tases are managed by systemic treatment. Both digital rectal examination and conventional imaging techniques detect local recurrence in only about 50% of cases since they are based on a minimum size of anatomical distortion, a criterion with obvious limitations particularly in post-therapy follow-up. The sensitivity of TRUS alone following radiation or surgery ranges between 25 and 54% for detection of local recurrence and is especially low at PSA values <1 ng/ml. The CT detection rate of local recurrence is only 36%, even in nodes larger than 20 mm, not suitable for early detection of relapse. [33] Endorectal MRI is highly efficient in detecting local recurrence, with a sensitivity of 95% and a specificity of 100%. [41] Although distant metastases are located mainly in the skeleton, the positive yield of [99m]Tc-MDP bone scintigraphy is less than 1–2% in patients with PSA levels below 10 ng/ml and significantly better when PSA levels are higher than 20 ng/ml. Ongoing studies are assessing the role of whole body PET to diagnose and localize recurrent prostate cancer in patients with biochem-ical relapse and whether there is a relationship between the performance of PET/CT and serum levels of PSA.

[18]F-FDG PET has a low tumor uptake in prostate cancer. The probability of a positive [18]F-FDG study increases with rising PSA. For PSA levels higher than 4 ng/ml, loco-regional recurrence is diagnosed in approximately 50% of cases. [18]F-FDG PET has not been found useful in patients with PSA values below 2.4 ng/ml. [15]

In a preliminary study assessing [11]C-choline PET, de Jong and colleagues [34] detected recurrent prostate cancer only in patients with a PSA level higher than 4 ng/ml. Similarly, in a study investigating 100 patients with prostate cancer and rising PSA levels, Cimitan and coworkers[35] recommended the use of $^{18}$F-choline PET/CT only in cases with a PSA higher than 4 ng/ml. More encouraging results were obtained when using state-of-the-art PET/CT techniques with oral and intravenous contrast enhancement for the CT component. PET/CT provides incremental information regarding the presence of nodal metastases, which is crucial to differentiate between local and regional recurrence and can lead to changes in patient management. The choice of the radiopharmaceutical for PET imaging of prostate cancer appears to be highly significant. $^{18}$F-choline has been reported to have a lower detectability rate even with the use of PET/CT. This is due to the early urinary excretion of $^{18}$F-choline compounds. Dynamic early and dual phase imaging has been recommended by some authors in order to overcome these limitations.

$^{11}$C-acetate PET is superior to $^{18}$F-FDG PET for diagnosis of loco-regional recurrence of prostate cancer. Omaya and colleagues[36] identified tumor recurrence in 27 of 46 patients with biochemical relapse and a mean PSA of 2.7 ng/ml. The sensitivity was, however, only 7% in patients with PSA values below 3 ng/ml. These results contrast with those of Albrecht and colleagues,[37] where $^{11}$C-acetate PET was positive in 9 of 15 patients with a median PSA of only 0.4 ng/ml. These better results were attributed to the use of image fusion of PET with CT. Image fusion of $^{11}$C-acetate PET with MRI using a software package also changed the characterization of equivocal lesions as either normal or abnormal in 10 and 18% of sites, respectively, and precisely defined the anatomical location of 73% of lesions.[38] In a study of 20 patients, $^{18}$F-choline and $^{11}$C-acetate PET/CT imaging detected local recurrent prostate cancer in half of the patients with PSA levels below 1 ng/ml.

A very limited number of studies report on the use of $^{11}$C-methionine in recurrent prostate cancer. Nunez and coworkers[28] compared the diagnostic yield of $^{18}$F-FDG and $^{11}$C-methionine in patients with progressing prostate cancer, defined as 50% increase in PSA levels and new or worsening skeletal metastases. The sensitivity for soft tissue and skeletal metastases was 70% each with $^{11}$C-methionine compared with 48 and 34%, respectively, for $^{18}$F-FDG.

As in staging of prostate cancer, SPECT/CT imaging has also optimized Prostascint® imaging in patients with recurrent disease. The use of Prostascint® has been expanded to include algorithms for patients with biochemical relapse, with preliminary encouraging results.

## Conclusions

Imaging of prostate cancer using PET and radioimmunoscintigraphy is still challenging. The yield of $^{18}$F-FDG PET for diagnosis and staging prostate cancer is low. Significant progress has been achieved with the use of radiolabeled choline compounds and $^{11}$C-acetate. $^{18}$F-fluoride PET/CT seems to be the best imaging technique for identifying skeletal metastases. Hybrid SPECT/CT imaging with Prostascint® as well as PET/CT are strongly advocated in order to improve the accuracy of these noninvasive imaging modalities.

## Testicular Cancer

Testicular tumors represent 1–2% of malignancies in men, with the highest incidence between the ages of 20 and 34 years. Primary testicular cancer occurs in approximately 7,000 men in the United States and causes 300 deaths per year,[1] with 95% being germ cell neoplasms and 5% Sertoli's or Leydig's cell tumors, most of them benign. Germ cell tumors are further divided into seminoma and nonseminoma germ cell tumors (NSGCT).

These malignancies generally present as a testicular mass, sometimes painful and tender. Few patients have gynecomastia, and up to 10% have distant metastases at presentation. Germ cell and NSGCT tumors differ in their biological behavior and metastasizing potential and therefore also in treatment. Seminoma is very radiosensitive. After orchiectomy and local radiotherapy, the cure rate exceeds 90%. NSGCT tend to spread early to retroperitoneal nodes and lungs. They are treated by surgery, radiation, and chemotherapy. Because of advances in chemotherapy, cure is now achieved in the majority of patients with minimal metastatic disease.

Diagnosis and staging of testicular tumors are currently based on clinical examination, tumor marker measurements, such as β-human chorionic gonadotropin (HCG), alpha-fetoprotein (AFP), and lactate dehydrogenase (LDH), imaging tests (US, CT of chest and abdomen), and histology of specimens obtained at surgery. Classification into low- and high-risk tumors is done by staging and the presence of prognostic factors, including blood vessel invasion by the primary tumor, the percentage of embryonal cancer in the tumor, and rising tumor markers.

Early after initiation of treatment, imaging studies can avoid further unnecessary treatment. They can also allow for planning treatment for cure when residual disease is detected. Conventional imaging modalities have a limited accuracy in staging of testicular cancers, with an overall 50% of patients being understaged and 25% overstaged by available techniques.[12] [18]F-FDG imaging may contribute its metabolic edge to the pretreatment assessment and for evaluating early response to treatment in testicular tumors.

## [18]F-FDG Imaging for Staging of Testicular Tumors

[18]F-FDG PET had a sensitivity of 70% and specificity of 100% in patients with stage I and II testicular tumors as compared to 40 and 78%, respectively, for CT.[39] [18]F-FDG imaging demonstrated a high sensitivity of 87%, specificity 94%, PPV 94%, and NPV 94% in staging of both seminoma and NSGT.[40,41] It could further identify 70% of patients with metastatic NSGCT who subsequently relapsed. In a study assessing patients with clinical stage I NSGCT, [18]F-FDG PET identified up to 21% patients with presumed disease who were not detected on CT, but relapse occurred in 47% patients with no tracer uptake for a median follow-up of 12 months. [18]F-FDG imaging is thus not highly sensitive to detect micrometastases.[42]

## [18]F-FDG Imaging of Residual and Recurrent Testicular Tumors

Most patients with bulky nodal disease have residual masses following treatment. The mass will often contain necrotic or fibrous tissue, requiring no further treatment. In patients with NSGCT, these masses may contain differentiated mature teratoma (MTD), a benign tumor at risk of future malignancy, which therefore needs to be removed. Serum tumor marker measurements and CT are the standard monitoring tools in these patients. However, CT cannot determine if the residual mass contains active tumor, and serum tumor markers are not sensitive or specific enough to diagnose the presence of active malignancy and cannot furthermore define the location of the tumor. [18]F-FDG PET can differentiate viable tumor from fibrosis, necrosis, or MTD without being able to differentiate between these non-malignant lesions.

In patients with advanced clinical stage seminoma (greater than IIB), CT or MRI detect residual masses in up to 80% of patients at 1 month after the end of chemotherapy. There is a risk of up to 30% of residual viable tumor in a lesion exceeding 30 mm in size and surgical resection is recommended.[43] In order to avoid unnecessary surgery, a better diagnostic tool is needed to select the patients who will benefit from resection of the residual mass. Negative [18]F-FDG in pure seminoma without teratomatous elements can reliably exclude residual disease following chemotherapy, regardless of tumor size, and thus spare unnecessary surgery.

## [18]F-FDG Imaging in Follow-up of NSGCT

Metastases of NSCGT occur primarily in retroperitoneal lymph nodes, followed by the lungs and mediastinal lymph nodes. Kollmansberger and colleagues[44] compared [18]F-FDG imaging with CT and serum marker changes after chemotherapy in patients with metastatic NSCGT. Sensitivity and specificity for prediction of residual mass viability were 59 and 92%, respectively, for PET, 55 and 86% for CT, and 42 and 100% for serum marker changes. Since this indicates that no method in itself appears sufficiently accurate to predict the viability of residual masses, it can be assumed that PET/CT will have in future an added value over separate PET and CT. The PPV and NPV of PET were 91 and 62%, respectively. While a positive PET image is a strong predictor for the presence of viable carcinoma or teratoma, 37% of all [18]F-FDG-negative PET masses at the end of treatment progressed during 6 months of follow-up or revealed MTD on histologic examination. Mature teratoma was the most frequent cause of false-negative PET in NSGCT.[41] [18]F-FDG imaging also adds important information in patients with multiple residual masses. In patients who underwent resection of one necrotic lesion in the presence of additional lesions that were all [18]F-FDG-negative, the probability of necrosis at the remaining nonresected lesions is higher than 90%.

## Conclusions

Although the sensitivity of [18]F-FDG imaging to detect testicular cancer is high, it does not identify micrometastases and cannot be totally relied on for accurate staging. It is most valuable in patients with residual or recurrent tumor leading to changes in patient management, with a high sensitivity and NPV in seminoma and high PPV in NSGCT.

## Guidelines and Recommendations for the use of [18]F-FDG PET and PET/CT

The National Comprehensive Cancer Network (NCCN) has incorporated [18]F-FDG PET and PET/CT in the practice guidelines and management algorithm of a variety of malignancies including genitourinary cancers. The use of [18]F-FDG PET (PET/CT where available) should only be considered as adjunct to conventional imaging technique for detection of distant metastases in: 1) Castration-resistant metastatic prostate cancer and; 2) in renal and muscle-invasive bladder carcinoma.[45]

## Case Presentations

## *Case II.9.1*

### History

A 64-year-old man had a hyperechogenic mass in the upper pole of the left kidney discovered on an abdominal US performed for evaluation of prostatism. Simple parenchymal cysts were seen in the lower pole of this kidney. CT showed contrast enhancement in the upper posterior renal mass (17 mm) and biopsy diagnosed RCC. The patient was referred to $^{18}$F-FDG PET/CT imaging for evaluation of a 10 mm pulmonary nodule observed in the left lower lobe (Fig. II.9.1A, B).

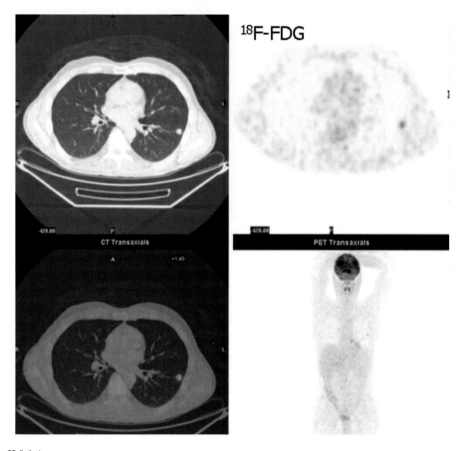

**Fig. II.9.1.A**

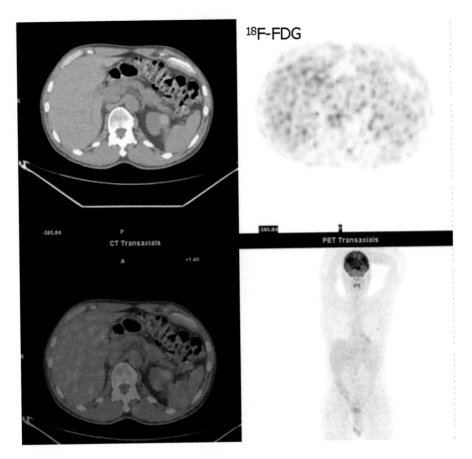

**Fig. II.9.1.B**

### Findings

A focus of moderately increased [18]F-FDG uptake (SUV 4.6) corresponding to a 10 mm nodule is seen in the lower lobe of the left lung (Fig. II.9.1A). There is no [18]F-FDG uptake in primary RCC in the upper pole of the left kidney seen on CT (Fig. II.9.1B) and there are no other abnormal PET findings.

### Discussion

Urinary [18]F-FDG accumulation often masks uptake in a renal tumor. In the present case, there is no significant [18]F-FDG uptake either in the simple cysts identified by US (not shown) or in the left renal mass. The absence of tracer uptake in a renal mass does not rule out malignancy. Uptake in the 10 mm left lung nodule is suspicious for a malignant lesion and may indicate either a metastasis or a primary lung tumor. At surgery, the left pulmonary nodule was resected and a RCC metastasis was diagnosed.

Ramdave and colleagues[5] identified a primary RCC in 15 of 17 patients with suspicious renal masses and reported that the accuracy of [18]F-FDG PET and CT were identical at 94%. However, in the largest series to date, sensitivity and specificity of [18]F-FDG PET for detection of primary RCC were 60 and 100% compared to 91.7 and 100% for CT, respectively.[46] Maijhail and coworkers[47] reported an overall sensitivity of 63.6%, specificity of 100%, and PPV of 100% for detection of RCC metastases with $^{18}$F-FDG PET. The average size of metastatic lesions identified by PET was larger than that of false-negative findings (22 mm versus 10 mm).$^{18}$F-FDG PET detected 64% of soft tissue metastases and 78% of skeletal metastases in patients with RCC. CT was more sensitive than $^{18}$F-FDG PET (91% versus 75%) for detection of pulmonary metastases.[46]

**Diagnosis**

1. Renal cell carcinoma.
2. Left pulmonary metastasis.

## Case II.9.2 (DICOM Images on DVD)

### History

A 60-year-old man underwent abdominal US, which identified a lesion in the left kidney, proven to be RCC by biopsy. Two years after left nephrectomy, a metastatic lytic lesion in the left acetabulum was diagnosed on CT and was treated by embolization and radiation, followed by metastasectomy 2 years later. $^{18}$F-FDG PET/CT performed at 9 months after surgery (Fig. II.9.2A) shows a focus of increasing $^{18}$F-FDG uptake in the left acetabulum next to the metallic hardware. The patient underwent major orthopedic surgery and was referred for follow-up PET/CT imaging 3 and 7 months after surgery (Fig. II.9.2B, C).

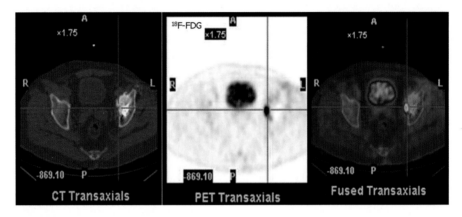

Fig. II.9.2.A

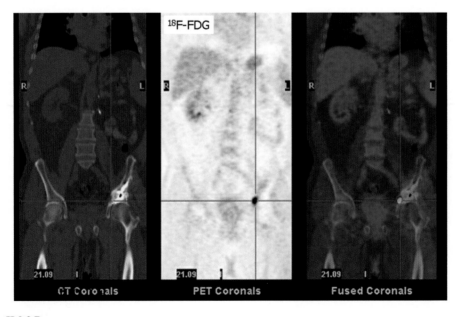

Fig. II.9.2.B

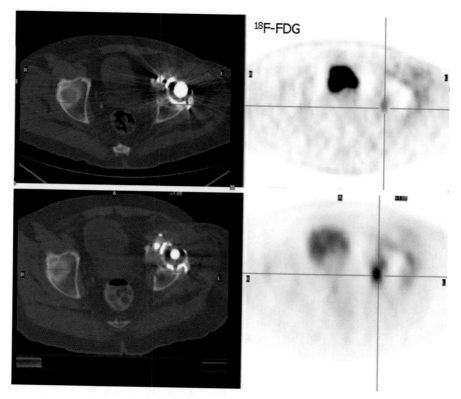

$^{18}$F-FDG

**Fig. II.9.2C**

## Findings

In Fig. II.9.2A, a focus of intense increased $^{18}$F-FDG uptake is seen in the left acetabulum medially and close to the metallic hardware. The intensity of the $^{18}$F-FDG uptake has increased significantly as compared to the findings on a PET/CT study performed 5 months earlier (not shown), with an increase in SUV from 7 to 20. Three months after extensive surgery, follow-up PET/CT (coronal slices Fig. II.9.2B and transaxial slices Fig. II.9.2C top row) shows mild increased activity around the left hip and a small focus of moderately increased uptake (SUV 4.8) at the posterior margin of the surgical excision in the left acetabulum. Four months later (Fig. II.9.2C, bottom row), the lesion has progressed and is more intense (SUV 12).

## Discussion

The findings are consistent with recurrent skeletal metastasis of RCC in the left acetabulum. The patient was referred to repeat $^{18}$F-FDG PET/CT studies since biopsy of the acetabular lesion could not be performed because of the previously implanted hardware and CT or MRI were not useful for the same reason. Post-surgical $^{18}$F-FDG-avid inflammatory changes can be observed at 2–3 months after surgery. However, the increase in intensity of the focal uptake observed on the sequence of the two PET/CT studies is worrisome for metastatic disease. On the basis of these PET/CT findings, the patient was treated with high-dose radiation focused to the findings on fused images.

Patients with advanced metastatic disease have a 0–2% survival rate, whereas solitary metastases can be resected surgically with a 5-year survival rate of approximately 30%.[8] [18]F-FDG PET has a sensitivity and accuracy for detecting skeletal metastases of 100%, while for skeletal scintigraphy the sensitivity and accuracy were 70.5 and 59.6%, respectively.[4] A different study reported, however, that [18]F-FDG PET had a sensitivity of only 77% and specificity of 87.2% as compared to 93.8 and 87.2%, respectively, for combined CT and skeletal scintigraphy.[48]

[18]F-FDG PET had a high accuracy of 100% as compared to 88% for CT for diagnosis of local recurrence and distant metastases in patients with RCC.[5]

## Diagnosis

RCC with recurrent skeletal metastasis.

## Follow-up

The left acetabular metastasis was treated by high-dose radiation focused on the PET/CT findings. Follow-up PET/CT studies performed 3 and 8 months after treatment showed a decrease in the intensity of tracer uptake in the left acetabulum (SUV of 5.6 and 3, respectively).

## Clinical Report: Body [18]F-FDG PET/CT (for DVD cases only; Corresponds to Fig. II.9.2C)

Indication

Restaging of metastatic renal cell carcinoma.

History

A 60-year-old man with a history of left nephrectomy for RCC presented 2 years later with a metastatic lytic lesion in the left acetabulum and was treated by embolization and radiotherapy. A second relapse in the left acetabulum occurred 2 years later and metastasectomy was performed. On follow-up [18]F-FDG PET/CT performed at 4 and 9 months after surgery, the intensity of a focus of [18]F-FDG uptake seen in the left acetabulum next to metallic hardware increased. Major orthopedic surgery was then performed with excision of the anterior left acetabulum, replacement by bone graft, fixation with metallic hardware, and total hip replacement. The patient was referred for follow-up PET/CT after surgery.

Procedure

The patient was fasted for more than 4 h and had a normal blood glucose level prior to [18]F-FDG injection. The PET acquisition was performed using a PET/CT system with CT (300 mA; 120 keV) being used for anatomical correlation and attenuation correction. Oral contrast (2 ml/kg) was administered during the uptake interval. PET emission images were acquired from the upper thighs to the top of the skull approximately 60 min after intravenous (IV) injection of 370 MBq (10 mCi) of [18]F-FDG.

Findings

> *Quality of the study*: The quality of this study is good.
>
> *Head and neck*: There is physiological distribution of $^{18}$F-FDG in the gray matter of the brain and in the lymphoid and glandular tissue of the neck.
>
> *Chest*: There is physiologic tracer uptake in the myocardium. On CT, a subcentimeter nodule is identified in the upper lobe of the right lung and in the medial segment of the left lingula, below the PET resolution, showing a slight increase in diameter when compared to previous CT studies. A pacemaker is seen in the left upper chest wall.
>
> *Abdomen*: The left kidney is absent (status post left nephrectomy).
>
> *Pelvis*: The patient is status post resection of the left acetabulum. As compared to the previous PET/CT study 4 months earlier, there is a focus of increased $^{18}$F-FDG uptake (SUV 12) in the left acetabulum, at the posterior margin of the surgical excision.

Impression

1. Recurrent RCC left acetabular metastasis, status post resection of the left acetabulum.
2. Two subcentimeter nodules in the right upper lung and in the left lingula, below the PET resolution, equivocal for metastases.

## Case II.9.3

### History

A 67-year-old man presented with macrohematuria. Cystoscopy revealed thickening of the right posterior bladder wall, and biopsy demonstrated a T2 TCC. CT was negative for metastases. The patient was referred for staging with $^{11}$C-choline PET/CT imaging prior to radical cystectomy (Fig. II.9.3A, B).

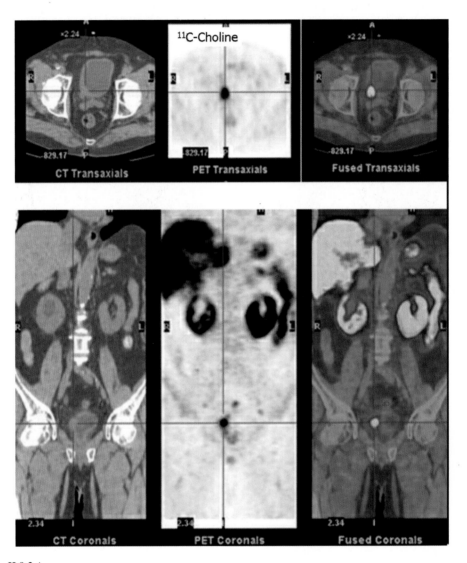

Fig. II.9.3.A

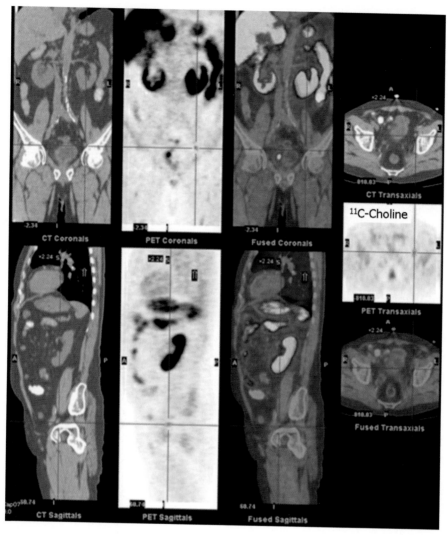

**Fig. II.9.3.B**

### Findings

A focal area of intense [11]C-choline uptake (SUV 5.6) is identified corresponding to the tumor in the right posterior wall of the bladder (Fig. II.9.3A). An additional focus of mildly increased tracer uptake (SUV 2) corresponding to a 6 mm lymph node is demonstrated in the left obturator area (Fig. II.9.3B). There is physiologic tracer uptake in the liver, spleen, kidneys, stomach, pancreas, small bowel, salivary glands, bone marrow, and of low intensity in the myocardium.

### Discussion

The findings are consistent with the known bladder TCC and with a small left obturator lymph node metastasis. With [11]C-choline it is imperative that imaging of the pelvic area starts no later than 3–4 min post-injection to avoid any physiologic tracer uptake in the bladder and ureters. This acquisition protocol allows detection of potential malignant involvement of the ureters. Intense physiologic accumulation of [11]C-choline in the renal cortex is seen as early as 5 min after tracer injection. This patient underwent radical cystectomy and a dissection of the pelvic lymphatics diagnosed a TCC metastasis in a left obturator lymph node.

CT and MRI are widely used for preoperative staging of bladder cancer with muscle invasion with an accuracy of 50 and 75%, respectively.[49] Both modalities rely on lymph node size criteria for diagnosis of metastases and disregard, as a rule, nodes smaller than 10 mm in diameter. Paik and colleagues[50] reported that CT visualized involved lymph nodes in 6 of 82 patients with invasive bladder cancer, with only 4 of them pathologically confirmed. In additional 13 patients, nodal metastases were not identified by CT. No SUV cutoff has been established for [11]C-choline uptake to differentiate between benign and malignant lesions. In a study performed in patient with TCC prior to surgery, loco-regional lymph nodes with a diameter of 5–18 mm had measured SUVs of 3.8 ± 1.4, including only one false-positive reactive node on histology.[49] Mild [11]C-choline uptake in a small lymph node is suspicious for malignant disease.

### Diagnosis

1. Muscle-invasive TCC of the urinary bladder.
2. Metastasis in a left obturator lymph node.

## Case II.9.4 (DICOM Images on DVD)

### History

This 64-year-old man presented with a vesical mass discovered on abdominal US performed for follow-up of RCC. Biopsy diagnosed muscle-invasive TCC of the left anterior bladder wall. CT was negative for metastases. The patient was assessed as part of a research protocol comparing $^{11}$C-choline and $^{11}$C-acetate PET/CT for diagnosis and staging of TCC of the bladder. (Fig. II.9.4A–C).

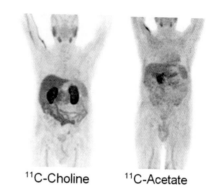

**Fig. II.9.4.A**

$^{11}$C-Choline        $^{11}$C-Acetate

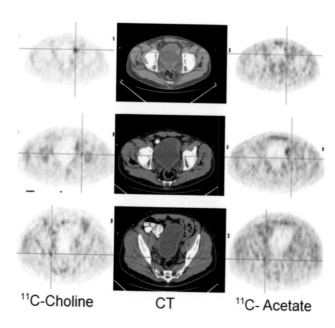

**Fig. II.9.4.B**       $^{11}$C-Choline        CT        $^{11}$C- Acetate

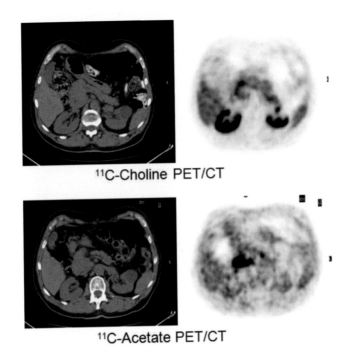

¹¹C-Choline PET/CT

¹¹C-Acetate PET/CT

**Fig. II.9.4.C**

## Findings

Both studies (Fig. II.9.4, A: maximum intensity projection (MIP) images, B: transaxial PET and CT slices) show a focus of increased tracer uptake corresponding to a thickenning in the left anterior wall of the bladder on CT and an additional focal uptake corresponding to a 6.7 mm right posterior pelvic lymph node. SUV in the bladder tumor is 5.2 and 2.9 for ¹¹C-choline and ¹¹C-acetate, respectively, and 3.4 for the right pelvic node for both tracers. A focus of mildly increased uptake (SUV 3) is seen only on ¹¹C-choline PET/CT corresponding to a 4.2 mm left obturator node. Additional foci of increased uptake are observed in bilateral inguinal lymph nodes on both studies. With ¹¹C-acetate, there is physiological uptake in the liver, spleen, kidneys, stomach, pancreas, small bowel, salivary glands, bone marrow, and myocardium (Fig. II.9.4A). Uptake is higher in the pancreas and lower in the kidneys with ¹¹C-acetate than with ¹¹C-choline (Fig. II.9.4C). There is a cyst in the left kidney seen on CT.

## Discussion

The findings are consistent with the known bladder TCC and with metastases involving bilateral pelvic and inguinal lymph nodes. The patient underwent radical cystectomy and dissection of the pelvic lymphatics. Metastases of TCC were found in right and left pelvic lymph nodes.

Although PET imaging demonstrates an increasing role in assessment of cancer patients it has been slow to develop in urologic malignancies, mainly because of the urinary excretion of ¹⁸F-FDG. ¹¹C-choline and ¹¹C-acetate are more favorable PET tracers for imaging of tumors of the urinary bladder. In a small number of cases comparing both tracers, the authors have noted that [11]C-choline imaging seems to provide studies with higher resolution than [11]C-acetate. Mildly increased tracer uptake is seen in small metastatic lymph nodes in present case using both tracers, thus emphasizing the importance of correlation with anatomical contrast-enhanced CT images and the contribution of hybrid PET/CT systems.

**Diagnosis**

1. Muscle-invasive TCC of the bladder.
2. Bilateral metastatic pelvic lymph nodes.

**Follow-up**

The patient underwent radical cystectomy and dissection of pelvic lymphatics. Nodal metastases of TCC were found in the right posterior and bilateral obturator lymph nodes. One 4.2 mm metastatic left obturator node was not identified by [11]C-acetate PET/CT. No dissection or biopsy of the inguinal lymph nodes was performed.

**Clinical Report: Body [11]C-choline PET/CT and [11]C-acetate PET/CT (for DVD cases only)**

Indication

Staging of a T2 TCC of the bladder.

History

This 64-year-old man presented with a urinary bladder mass discovered on routine abdominal US performed for follow-up of RCC. Biopsy diagnosed muscle-invasive TCC of the bladder (T2). CT was negative for metastases. The patient was included in a research protocol comparing the value of [11]C-choline and [11]C-acetate PET/CT for diagnosis and staging of advanced TCC of the bladder.

Procedure for [11]C-choline PET/CT

The patient was fasted for 4 h. Oral contrast (2 ml/kg) was administered during the hour before imaging. PET/CT was performed with CT being used for anatomical correlation and attenuation correction. CT (300 mA; 120 keV) acquisition was performed first. PET images acquisition started immediately after the IV injection of 370 MBq (10 mCi) [11]C-choline beginning with a FOV below the pelvis up and continuing to the top of the skull. The acquisition time for each FOV was 3.5 min, and image acquisition of the pelvic area was not delayed beyond 3.5 min after injection of [11]C-choline.

Findings for [11]C-choline PET/CT

*Quality of the study*: The quality of this study is good.
*Head and neck*: There is no [11]C-choline uptake in the normal brain. There is physiologic distribution in the lymphoid tissues of the neck.
*Chest*: There is low intensity physiologic uptake in the myocardium.

*Abdomen*: There is physiologic [11]C-choline uptake in the liver, more than in the spleen, pancreas (SUV 7), renal cortex (SUV 13), and the small bowel (SUV up to 6). A 25 mm simple cyst is identified in the anterior left kidney on CT. There is a 25 × 20 mm low density lesion in the right adrenal gland suggestive of a myelolipoma.

*Pelvis*: There is no increased tracer activity in the bladder.

There is a focus of increased tracer uptake in the left anterior wall of the bladder (SUV 5.2) corresponding to thickening of the wall on CT. Additional foci of increased [11]C-choline uptake correspond to a 6.7 mm right posterior pelvic lymph node (SUV 3.4), to a 4.2 mm left obturator and to a subcentimeter right obturator node (SUV 3 in both lesions). Other subcentimeter bilateral pelvic lymph nodes are identified on CT with no corresponding [11]C-choline uptake. Bilateral 10 mm inguinal nodes show mildly increased tracer uptake (SUV up to 2.5).

*Musculoskeletal*: Mildly increased bone marrow uptake

## Procedure for [11]C-acetate PET/CT (Performed the day after the [11]C-choline PET/CT)

The patient was fasted for 4 h. Oral contrast (2 ml/kg) was administered during the hour before imaging. PET/CT was performed with CT being used for anatomical correlation and attenuation correction. The CT (300 mA; 120 keV) acquisition was performed first, followed by IV injection of 370 MBq (10 mCi) of [11]C-acetate and immediate PET images acquisition starting from the field of view (FOV) below the pelvis up to the base of the skull. The duration of acquisition for each FOV was 3.5 min so that image acquisition of the pelvic area did not start later than 3.5 min after injection of [11]C-acetate.

## Findings for [11]C-acetate PET/CT

*Quality of the study*: The quality of this study is good.

*Neck*: There is physiologic [11]C-acetate distribution in the lymphoid tissues of the neck.

*Chest*: There is physiologic uptake in the myocardium.

*Abdomen*: There is physiologic [11]C-acetate uptake in the liver and of equal intensity in the spleen, intense uptake in the pancreas (SUV 9), and mild activity in the kidneys (SUV up to 4.8) and small bowel (SUV up to 4). On CT, there is also a 24.5 mm simple cyst in the anterior aspect of the left kidney and a 25 × 20 mm low density lesion in the right adrenal gland, suggestive of a myelolipoma.

*Pelvis*: There is no [11]C-acetate activity in the urinary bladder.

There is a focus of increased tracer uptake in the left anterior wall of the bladder (SUV 3.8) corresponding to thickening of the wall on CT, and focal uptake corresponding to a 6.7 mm right posterior pelvic lymph node (SUV 3.4). An additional focus of mildly increased [11]C-acetate uptake (SUV 3) corresponds to a subcentimeter right obturator node (SUV 3). Other subcentimeter bilateral pelvic lymph nodes including the 4.2 mm left obturator node avid on [11]C-choline PET/CT are identified on CT with no corresponding acetate uptake. Bilateral 10 mm inguinal nodes show increased acetate uptake (SUV up to 2.1).

*Musculoskeletal*: No abnormal finding.

Overall [11]C-acetate PET/CT demonstrates lower uptake than [11]C-choline-avid findings.

## Impression for [11]C-choline and [11]C-acetate PET/CT

1. TCC of the left anterior wall of the bladder.

2. Foci of increased $^{11}$C-acetate uptake in small subcentimeter right posterior and right obturator lymph nodes, suspicious for metastatic involvement. Other subcentimeter pelvic lymph nodes showing no abnormal tracer uptake are most likely not metastatic.
3. Suspicion of involvement of bilateral inguinal lymph nodes.
4. Left renal cyst.
5. Right adrenal lesion, most probable myelolipoma.

## *Case II.9.5*

### History

A 64-year-old man with elevated PSA levels was diagnosed with prostate cancer and referred to CT for staging. A 10 mm left iliac retroperitoneal lymph node at the level of L1 was described as suspicious for metastatic disease. Radiotherapy of the prostatic bed and involved lymph nodes was planned. ¹¹C-choline PET/CT was performed for restaging and to determine the extent of the radiotherapy field (Fig. II.9.5).

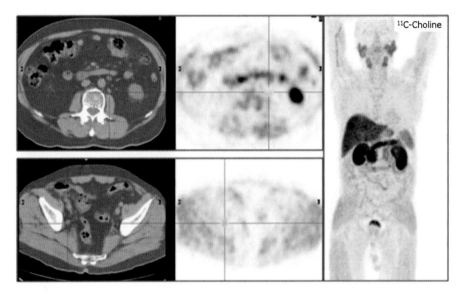

**Fig. II.9.5**

### Findings

Increased ¹¹C-choline uptake was seen in the prostatic bed corresponding to the known tumor (Fig. II.9.5 MIP). No abnormal ¹¹C-choline uptake is seen in the left retroperitoneal node identified on CT at the level of L1 (Fig. II.9.5 left, top row). A focus of mildly increased uptake is observed in the right pelvis (SUV 2) corresponding to a 13 mm right obturator lymph node (Fig. II.9.5 left, bottom row). In addition, there is physiological ¹¹C-choline uptake in bowel loops and pancreas.

### Discussion

The findings are consistent with primary prostate cancer and involve a right obturator lymph node. The absence of ¹¹C-choline uptake in the higher left retroperitoneal lymph node does not support the presence of tumor in this specific site. The patient received radiotherapy limited to the prostatic bed and to the pelvic area. Serum PSA levels decreased and the patient has no evidence of disease for a 2-year follow-up.

CT is of limited clinical utility in the evaluation of nodal staging using 10 mm size criteria. In a study by Lervan and colleagues,[51] only 1.5% of 861 high-risk patients with a

PSA of more than 20 ng/ml had suspicious lymph nodes on CT. De Jong and coworkers[52] compared the results of [11]C-choline PET with histological findings in pelvic lymph nodes and follow-up in 67 patients with prostate cancer assessed at staging and showed a sensitivity of 80%, specificity of 96%, and accuracy of 93%. PET/CT has the potential of being the most accurate imaging modality for detection of nodal involvement since [11]C-choline PET is more sensitive than CT and, on the other hand, CT improves the diagnostic accuracy of PET by improved differentiation of malignant lymph nodes from adjacent bowel activity. [11]C-choline PET/CT can be also used for radiation treatment planning.

**Diagnosis**

1. Primary prostate cancer.
2. Metastatic right obturator node.

## *Case II.9.6*

### History

A 59-year-old man presented 2 years after radical prostatectomy with a PSA of 3.5 ng/ml. Digital rectal examination, TRUS, and CT were negative for local recurrence or distant metastases. Skeletal scintigraphy and CT showed a typical pattern of Paget's disease in the right pelvis. The patient was referred to [11]C-choline PET/CT for restaging (Fig. II.9.6A, B).

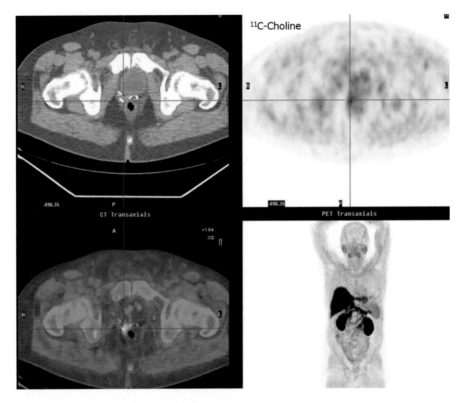

Fig. II.9.6.A

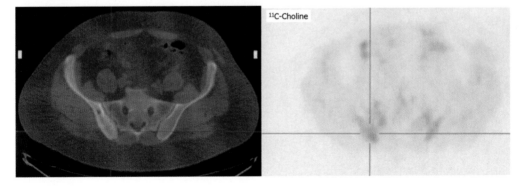

Fig. II.9.6.B

## Findings

A focus of increased $^{11}$C-choline uptake (SUV 2.7) corresponds to a slight soft tissue asymmetry on CT, in the area of the surgical bed (Fig. II.9.6A). An area of faintly increased choline uptake corresponds to a dense right iliac bone (Fig. II.9.6B). In addition, there is mild physiologic tracer activity in the urinary bladder, bone marrow, and small bowel loops.

## Discussion

The findings are consistent with local recurrence of prostate cancer at the site of resection and Paget's disease of the right iliac bone. PSA decreased after local secondary radiotherapy. Interpretation of $^{11}$C-choline PET is challenging. SUV can be as low as 1.5 in proven malignancy of both naïve and recurrent prostate cancer and at metastatic sites, and, with PET alone, identification and localization of a focus of increased $^{11}$C-choline uptake is often difficult. $^{11}$C-choline PET/CT is very helpful by precise localization of the focus of increased tracer uptake. CT allows to differentiate $^{11}$C-choline uptake in benign skeletal disease such as degenerative changes, osteophytes, facet joint disease, or incidental Paget's disease (Fig. II.9.6B) from skeletal metastases.

A rising PSA profile following radiotherapy or a value of 0.2 ng/ml after radical prostatectomy are evidence of recurrent tumor but cannot distinguish between local, regional, or distant relapse. In a group of 49 patients with suspected occult relapse due to a mean PSA level of 2.0 ng/ml, $^{11}$C-choline PET/CT had a sensitivity of 73%, PPV 88%, NPV 92%, and accuracy of 78% for diagnosis of local relapse. PET/CT was true positive in 23 of 33 patients and true negative in 12 of 13 cases.[53] In addition, 70% of patients with a favorable biochemical response to local radiotherapy were identified by PET/CT. In another study of 63 patients with biochemical recurrence, Krause and colleagues[54] demonstrated a relationship between the $^{11}$C-choline detection rate and serum PSA levels, from 36% for patients with PSA below 1 ng/ml, 43% for PSA value between 1 and 2 ng/ml, 62% for PSA between 2 and 4 ng/ml, respectively.

## Diagnosis

1. Local recurrence of prostate cancer.
2. Paget's disease in the right iliac bone.

## Case II.9.7

### History

This 26-year-old man presented with ongoing pain in an enlarged right testis. A stage II B/ C seminoma was diagnosed, and the patient underwent orchiectomy. CT showed a 50 mm right retroperitoneal mass and two additional small suspicious lesions. LDH values were elevated (1049 IU/l; normal range 48–115 IU/l). Additional markers were within the normal range. The patient was referred to $^{18}$F-FDG PET/CT for restaging and follow-up after chemotherapy (Fig. II.9.7A, B).

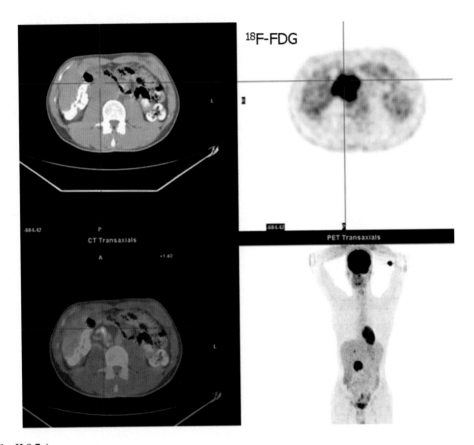

Fig. II.9.7.A

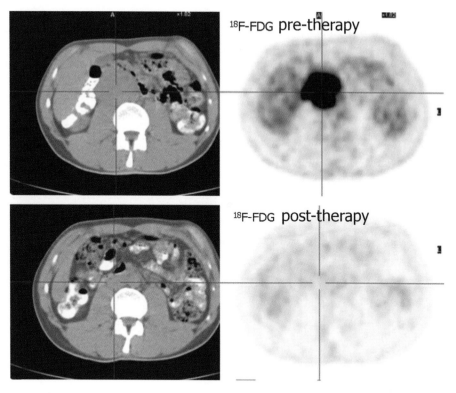

$^{18}$F-FDG pre-therapy

$^{18}$F-FDG post-therapy

**Fig. II.9.7.B**

**Findings**

A large area of intense $^{18}$F-FDG uptake corresponds to the 50 mm right retroperitoneal mass seen on CT (Fig. II.9.7A). The focus seen on the MIP image in the right upper abdomen represents physiological uptake in the right kidney. No other abnormal sites of increased tracer uptake are seen. Follow-up $^{18}$F-FDG PET/CT performed after three cycles of chemotherapy shows a dramatic decrease in size (to 15 mm) and disappearance of $^{18}$F-FDG uptake (Fig. II.9.7B, upper row pre-therapy, lower row post-therapy images).

**Discussion**

The findings are consistent with bulky metastatic seminoma and good response to treatment. LDH values decreased to normal. One year after treatment, the patient is in complete remission.

$^{18}$F-FDG imaging results were compared to histopathological diagnosis in 20 residual masses following chemotherapy for advanced disease.[55] The PPV was low, 25%, but the NPV was 100%, similar to additional prospective studies that reported a NPV of 96 and 100% in cohorts of 51 and 29 patients, respectively.[56,57] Histopathology of false-positive $^{18}$F-FDG-avid residual tumors revealed sarcoidosis, inflammation, and fibrosis or necrosis. In contrast, a PPV of 100% was found in a study of 51 patients with seminoma evaluated after chemotherapy.[56] Patients with seminoma present with pronounced desmoplastic inflammatory reactions in the early phase following chemotherapy. It is thus recommended to delay follow-up [18]F-FDG imaging by at least 2 months after completion of chemotherapy.

Considering its excellent NPV, [18]F-FDG PET has been proposed by the European Germ Cell Cancer Consensus Group as a good option for follow-up of residual masses, leading to a decrease in the number of unnecessary surgical interventions.[58]

**Diagnosis**

Metastatic seminoma achieving complete remission.

# References

1. Jemal A, Siegel R, Ward E, Murray T, Xu J, Thun MJ. Cancer statistics, 2007. *CA Cancer J Clin* 2007;57:43.
2. Kopka I, Fischer U, Zoeller G, Schmidt C, Ringert RH, Grabbe E. Dual-phased helical CT of the kidney. Value of the corticomedullary and nephrographic phase for evaluation of renal lesions and preoperative staging of renal cell carcinoma. *AJR Am J Roentgenol* 1997;169:1573–1578.
3. Lawrentschuk N, Poon AM, Scott AM. Fluorine-18 fluoro-thymidine: a new positron emission radio-isotope for renal tumors. *Clin Nucl Med* 2006;31:788–789.
4. Aide N, Cappele O, Bottet P, Bensadoun H, Regeasse A, Comoz F, Sobrio F, Bouvard G, Agostini D. Efficiency of [(18)F]FDG PET in characterizing renal cancer and detecting distant metastases: a comparison with CT. *Eur J Nucl Med Mol Imaging* 2003;30:1236–1245.
5. Ramdave S, Thomas GW, Berlangieri SU, Bolton DM, Davis I, Danguy HT, Macgregor D, Scott AM. Clinical role of F18-fluorodeoxyglucose positron emission tomography for detection and management of renal cell carcinoma. *J Urol* 2001;166:825–830.
6. Wu H, Yen R, Shen Y, Kao CH, Lin CC, Lee CC. Comparing whole body 18F-2-deoxyglucose positron emission tomography and technetium-99m methylene diphosphate bone scan to detect bone metastases in patients with renal cell carcinomas – a preliminary report. *J Cancer Res Clin Oncol* 2002;128:503–506.
7. Frank I, Cheville JC, Blute ML, Lohse CM, Nehra A, Weaver AL, Karnes RJ, Zincke H. Transitional cell carcinoma of the urinary bladder with regional lymph node involvement treated by cystectomy: Clinicopathologic features associated with outcome. *Cancer* 2003;97:2425–2431.
8. Drieskens O, Oyen R, Van Poppel H, Vankan Y, Flamen P, Mortelmans L. FDG-PET for preoperative staging of bladder cancer. *Eur J Nuc Med Mol Imaging* 2005;32:1412–1417.
9. Kosuda S, Kison PV, Greenough, Grossman HB, Wahl RL. Preliminary assessment of fluorine-18 fluorodeoxyglucose positron emission tomography in patients with bladder cancer. *Eur J Nuc Med* 1997;24:615–620.
10. Jana S, Blaufox MD. Nuclear medicine studies of the prostate, testes, and bladder. *Semin Nucl Med* 2006;36:51–72.
11. DeGrado TR, Baldwin SW, Wang S, Orr MD, Liao RP, Friedman HS, Reiman R, Price DT, Coleman RE. Synthesis and evaluation of $^{18}$F-labeled choline analogs as oncologic PET tracers. *J Nucl Med* 2001;42:1805–1814.
12. Gofrit ON, Mishani E, Orevi M, Klein M, Freedman N, Pode D, Shapiro A, Katz R, Libson E, Chisin R. Contribution of $^{11}$C-choline positron emission tomography/computerized tomography to preoperative staging of advanced transitional cell carcinoma. *J Urol* 2006;176:940–944.
13. de Jong IJ, Pruim J, Slsinga PH, Jongen MM, Mensink HJ, Vaalburg W. Visualization of bladder cancer using (11)C-choline PET: first clinical experience. *Eur J Nuc Med Mol Imaging* 2002; 29:1283–1288.
14. Shreve P, Chiao P-C, Humes HD, Schwaiger M, Gross MD. Carbon-11 acetate PET imaging of renal disease. *J Nucl Med* 1995;36:1595–1601.
15. Ahlstrom H, Malmstrom P-U, Letocha H, Andersson J, Langstrom B, Nilsson S. Positron emission tomography in the diagnosis and staging of urinary bladder cancer. *Acta Radiologica* 1996;37: 1870–1875.
16. Hankey BF, Feuer EJ, Clegg LX, Hayes GB, Legler JM, Prorok PC, Ries LA, Merrill RM, Kaplan RS. Cancer surveillance series: interpreting trends in prostate cancer – part I: Evidence of the effects of screening in recent prostate cancer incidence, mortality, and survival rates. *J Natl Cancer Inst* 1999;91:1017–1024.
17. Reske SN, Blumstein NM, Neumaier B, Gottfried H-W, Finsterbusch F, Kocot D, Möller P, Glatting G, Perner S. Imaging prostate cancer with 11C-choline PET/CT. *J Nucl Med* 2006;47:1249–1254.
18. Scher B, Seitz M, Albinger W, Tiling R, Scherr M, Becker H-C, Souvatzogluou M, Gildehaus F-J, Wester H-J, Dresel S. Value of 11C-choline PET and PET/CT in patients with suspected prostate cancer. *Eur J Nucl Med Mol Imaging* 2007;34:45–53.
19. Farsad M, Schiavina R, Castellucci P, Nanni C, Corti B, Martorana G, Canini R, Grigioni W, Boschi S, Marengo M, Pettinato C, Salizzoni E, Monetti N, Franchi R, Fanti S. Detection and localization of prostate cancer: correlation of (11)C-choline PET/CT with histopathologic step-section analysis. *J Nucl Med* 2005;46:1642–1649.

20. Martorana G, Schiavina R, Corti B, Farsad M, Salizzoni E, Brunocilla E, Bertaccini A, Manferrari F, Castellucci P, Fanti S. 11C-choline positron emission tomography/computerized tomography for tumor localization of primary prostate cancer in comparison with 12-core biopsy. *J Urol* 2006; 176:954–960.
21. Testa C, Schiavina R, Lodi R, Salizzoni E, Corti B, Farsad M, Kurhanewicz J, Manferrari F, Brunocilla E, Tonon C, Monetti N, Castellucci P, Fanti S, Coe M, Grigioni WF, Martorana G, Canini R, Barbiroli B. Prostate cancer: Sextant localization with MR imaging, MR spectroscopy, and 11C-choline PET/CT. *Radiology* 2007;244:797–806.
22. Swinnen JV, Verhoeven G. Androgens and the control of lipid metabolism in human prostate cancer cells. *J Steroid Biochem Mol Biol* 1998;65:191–198.
23. Oyama N, Akino H, Kanamaru H, Suzuki Y, Muramoto S, Yonekura Y, Sadato N, Yamamoto K, Okada K. 11C-acetate PET imaging of prostate cancer. *J Nucl Med* 2002;43:181–186.
24. Kato T, Tsukamoto E, Kuge Y, Takei T, Shiga T, Shinohara N, Katoh C, Nakada K, Tamaki N. Accumulation of [11C]acetate in normal prostate and benign prostatic hyperplasia: Comparison with prostate cancer. *Eur J Nucl Med Mol Imaging* 2002;29:1492–1495.
25. Manyak MJ, Hinkle GH, Olsen JO, Chiaccherini RP, Partin AW, Piantadosi S, Burgers JK, Texter JH, Neal CE, Libertino JA, Wright GL Jr, Maguire RT. Immunoscintigraphy with indium-111-capromab pendetide: Evaluation before definitive therapy in patients with prostate cancer. *Urology* 1999;54:1058–1063.
26. Wong TZ, Turkington TG, Polascik TJ, Coleman RE. ProstaScint (capromab pendetide) imaging using hybrid gamma camera-CT technology. *AJR Am J Roentgenol* 2005;184:676–680.
27. Ellis RJ, Kim EY, Zhou H, et al: Seven-Year biochemical disease-free survival rates following permanent prostate brachytherapy with dose escalation to biological tumor volumes (BTVs) identifies with SPECT/CT image fusion [abstract]. *Brachytherapy* 2005;4:107.
28. Nuñez R, Macapinlac HA, Yeung HW, Akhurst T, Cai S, Osman I, Gonen M, Riedel E, Scher HI, Larson SM. Combined 18F-FDG and 11C-methionine PET scans in patients with newly progressive metastatic prostate cancer. *J Nucl Med* 2002;43:46–55.
29. Yeh SD, Imbriaco M, Larson SM, Garza D, Zhang JJ, Kalaigian H, Finn RD, Reddy D, Horowitz SM, Goldsmith SJ, Scher HI. Detection of bony metastases of androgen-independent prostate cancer by PET-FDG. *Nucl Med Biol* 1996;23:693–697.
30. Morris MJ, Akhurst T, Osman I, Nunez R, Macapinlac H, Siedlecki K, Verbel D, Schwartz L, Larson SM, Scher HI. Fluorinated deoxyglucose positron emission tomography imaging in progressive metastatic prostate cancer. *Urology* 2002;59:913–918.
31. Fricke E, Machtens S, Hofmann M, Van den Hoff J, Bergh S, Brunkhorst T, Meyer GJ, Karstens JH, Knapp WH, Boerner AR. Positron emission tomography with 11C-acetate and 18F-FDG in prostate cancer patients. *Eur J Nucl Med Mol Imaging* 2003;30:607–611.
32. Even-Sapir E, Metser U, Mishani E, Lievshitz G, Lerman H Leibovitch I. The detection of bone metastases in patients with high-risk prostate cancer: 99mTc-MDP Planar bone scintigraphy, single- and multi-field-of-view SPECT, 18F-fluoride PET, and 18F-fluoride PET/CT. *J Nucl Med* 2006; 47:287–297.
33. Scher B, Seitz M. PET/CT imaging of recurrent prostate cancer. *Eur J Nucl Med Mol Imaging* 2008;35:5–8.
34. de Jong IJ, Pruim J, Elsinga PH, Vaalburg W, Mensink HJ. 11C-choline positron emission tomography for the evaluation after treatment of localized prostate cancer. *Eur Urol* 2003;44:32–38.
35. Cimitan M, Bortolus R, Morassut S, Canzonieri V, Garbeglio A, Baresic T, Borsatti E, Drigo A, Trovò MG. [(18)F]fluorocholine PET/CT imaging for the detection of recurrent prostate cancer at PSA relapse: experience in 100 consecutive patients. *Eur J Nucl Med Mol Imaging* 2006;33:1387–1398.
36. Oyama N, Miller TR, Dehdashti F, Siegel BA, Fischer KC, Michalski JM, Kibel AS, Andriole GL, Picus J, Welch MJ. 11C-acetate PET imaging of prostate cancer: detection of recurrent disease at PSA relapse. *J Nucl Med* 2003;44:549–555.
37. Albrecht S, Buchegger F, Soloviev D, Zaidi H, Vees H, Khan H, Keller A, Bischof Delaloye A, Ratib O, Miralbell R. 11C-acetate PET in the early evaluation of prostate cancer recurrence. *Eur J Nucl Med Mol Imaging* 2007;34:185–196.
38. Wachter S, Tomek S, Kurtaran A, Wachter-Gerstner N, Djavan B, Becherer A, Mitterhauser M, Dobrozemsky G, Li S, Pötter R, Dudczak R, Kletter K. 11C-acetate positron emission tomography imaging and image fusion with computed tomography and magnetic resonance imaging in patients with recurrent prostate cancer. *J Clin Oncol* 2006;24:2513–2519.
39. Albers P, Bender H, Yilmaz H, Schoeneich G, Biersack HJ, Mueller SC. Positron emission tomography in the clinical staging of patients with Stage I and II testicular germ cell tumors. *Urology* 1999;53:808–811.

40. Hain SF, O'Doherty MJ, Timothy AR, Leslie MD, Partridge SE, Huddart RA. Fluorodeoxyglucose PET in the initial staging of germ cell tumours. *Eur J Nucl Med* 2000;27:590–594.

41. Cremerius U, Wildberger JE, Borchers H, Zimny M, Jakse G, Günther RW, Buell W. Does positron emission tomography using 18-fluoro-2-deoxyglucose improve clinical staging of testicular cancer? Results of a study in 50 patients. *Urology* 1999;54:900–904.

42. Huddart RA, O'Doherty MJ, Padhani A, Rustin GJS, Mead JM, Joffe JK, Vasey P, Harland SJ, Logue J, Daugaard G, Hain SF, Kirk SJ, MacKewn JE, Stenning SP. 18fluorodeoxyglucose positron emission tomography in the prediction of relapse in patients with high-risk, clinical stage I nonseminomatous germ cell tumors: Preliminary report of MRC Trial TE22 – the NCRI Testis Tumour Clinical Study Group. *J Clin Oncol* 2007;25:3090–3095.

43. Flechon A, Bompas E, Biron P, Droz JP. Management of post-chemotherapy residual masses in advanced seminoma. *J Urol* 2002;168:1975–1979.

44. Kollmannsberger C, Oechsle K, Dohmen BM, Pfannenberg A, Bares R, Claussen CD, Kanz L, Bokemeyer C. Prospective comparison of [18F]fluorodeoxyglucose positron emission tomography with conventional assessment by computed tomography scans and serum tumor markers for the evaluation of residual masses in patients with nonseminomatous germ cell carcinoma. *Cancer* 2002; 94:2353–2356.

45. Podoloff DA, Ball DW, Ben-Josef E, Benson AB, Cohen SJ, Coleman RE, Delbeke D, Ho M, Ilson DH, Kalemkerian GP, Lee RJ, Loeffler JS, Macapinlac HA, Morgan RJ, Siegel BA, Singhal S, Tyler DS, Wong RJ. NCCN Task Force: Clinical Utility of PET in a Variety of Tumor Types Task Force. *J Natl Compr Canc Netw* 2009;7 Suppl 2:S1–S23. www.nccn.org/professionals/physician_gls/f_guidelines.asp

46. Kang DE, White RL Jr, Zuger JH, Sasser HC, Teigland CM. Clinical use of fluorodeoxyglucose F18 positron emission tomography for detection of renal cell carcinoma. *J Urol* 2004;171:1806–1809.

47. Maijhail NS, Urbain JL, Albani JM, Kanvinde MH, Rice TW, Novick AC, Mekhail TM, Olencki TE, Elson P, Bukowski RM. F-18 fluorodeoxyglucose positron emission tomography in the evaluation of distant metastases from renal cell carcinoma. *J Clin Oncol* 2003;21:3995–4000.

48. Ficarra V, Righetti R, Pilloni S, D'amico A, Maffei N, Novella G, Zanolla L, Malossini G, Mobilio G. Prognostic factors in patients with renal cell carcinoma : Retrospective analysis of 675 cases. *Eur Urol* 2002;41:190–198.

49. Kim B, Semelka RC, Ascher S, Chalpin DB, Carroll PR, Hricak H. Bladder tumor staging: comparison of contrast-enhanced CT, T1- and T2-weighted MR imaging, dynamic gadolinium-enhanced imaging, and late gadolinium-enhanced imaging. *Radiology* 1994;193:239–245.

50. Paik ML, Scolieri MJ, Brown SL, Spirnak JP, Resnick ML. Limitations of computerized tomography in staging invasive bladder cancer before radical cystectomy. *J Urol* 2000; 163:1693–1696.

51. Levran Z, Gonzalez JA, Diokno AC, Jafri SZ, Steinert BW. Are pelvic computed tomography, bone scan and pelvic lumphadenectomy necessary in the staging of prostate cancer? *Br J Urol* 1995;75:778–781.

52. de Jong IJ, Pruim J, Elsinga PH, Vaalburg W, Mensink HJ. Preoperative staging of pelvic lymph nodes in prostate cancer by 11C-choline PET. *J Nucl Med* 2003;44:331–335.

53. Reske SN, Blumstein NM, Glatting G. [(11)C]choline PET/CT imaging in occult local relapse of prostate cancer after radical prostatectomy. *Eur J Nucl Med Mol Imaging* 2008;35:9–17.

54. Krause BJ, Souvatzoglou M, Tuncel M, Herrmann K, Buck AK, Praus C, Schuster T, Geinitz H, Treiber U, Schwaiger M. The detection rate of [(11)C]Choline-PET/CT depends on the serum PSA-value in patients with biochemical recurrence of prostate cancer. *Eur J Nucl Med Mol Imaging* 2008; 35:18–23.

55. Hinz S, Schrader M, Kempkensteffen C, Bares R, Brenner W, Krege S, Franzius C, Kliesch S, Heicappel R, Miller K. The role of positron emission tomography in the evaluation of residual masses after chemotherapy for advanced stage seminoma. *J Urol* 2008;179:936–940.

56. De Santis M, Becherer A, Bokemeyer C, Stoiber F, Oechsle K, Sellner F, Lang A, Kletter K, Dohmen BM, Dittrich C, Pont J. 2-18Fluoro-deoxy-D-glucose positron emission tomography is a reliable predictor for viable tumor in postchemotherapy seminoma: an update of the prospective multicentric SEMPET trial. *J Clin Oncol* 2004; 22:1034–1039.

57. Ganjoo KN, Chan RJ, Sharma M, Einhorn LH. Positron emission tomography scans in the evaluation of postchemotherapy residual masses in patients with seminoma. *J Clin Oncol* 1999;17:3457–3460.

58. Krege S, Beyer J, Souchon R, Albers P, Albrecht W, Algaba F, Bamberg M, Bodrogi I, Bokemeyer C, Cavallin-Ståhl E. European consensus conference on diagnosis and treatment of germ cell cancer: A report of the second meeting of the European Germ Cell Cancer Consensus group (EGCCCG): part II. *Eur Urol* 2008 53:497–513.

# Chapter II.10
# Thyroid Cancer

Heather A. Jacene, Sibyll Goetze, and Richard L. Wahl

## Introduction

Thyroid cancer is a relatively rare disease, with an annual incidence of 1–4 per 100,000 and is more common in females. The incidence of thyroid cancer has increased in recent years, related to some extent to the earlier detection of sub-clinical disease, especially with the increased used of ultrasound (US). Many patients with thyroid cancer present with an incidentally discovered thyroid nodule on physical examination, at times self-examination, or diagnostic imaging. Some patients seek attention because of local symptoms such as dysphagia, dysphonia, hoarseness, or symptoms related to metastatic disease (cervical lymphadenopathy, pathologic fracture). Initial histological diagnosis is usually established by US and fine needle aspiration (FNA).[1]

The majority of thyroid malignancies are differentiated tumors. The most common thyroid cancer histology is papillary carcinoma (50–60%), followed by follicular carcinoma (20–30%). Subtypes of papillary carcinoma include the follicular, tall cell, columnar, and diffuse sclerosis variants. Although treatment is similar, follicular variant of papillary cancer and follicular cancer must be distinguished because the former behaves like papillary cancer. Medullary carcinoma, anaplastic carcinoma, thyroid lymphoma, and metastases originating in other tumors comprise the remaining thyroid malignancies and, considered separately, each is very rare. Survival rates are highly dependent on the type of thyroid cancer, but overall are excellent for patients with differentiated thyroid cancer. While 10-year survival rates for papillary and follicular carcinoma are 98 and 92%, respectively, this decreases to only 13% for patients with anaplastic carcinoma.[1]

Surgery is the treatment of choice for patients with localized thyroid carcinoma. Post-operative surveillance is performed with cervical US and serum tumor markers. Elevated or rising serum tumor markers suggest the presence of residual or recurrent disease. The role of hybrid single photon emission computed tomography (SPECT)/computed tomography (CT) and positron emission tomography (PET)/CT imaging in patients with thyroid carcinoma is primarily for localization of residual or recurrent disease once suspected.

H.A. Jacene (✉)
Division of Nuclear Medicine / PET, Russell H. Morgan Department of Radiology and Radiological Science, Johns Hopkins University School of Medicine, Baltimore, MD, USA
e-mail: hjacene1@jhmi.edu

D. Delbeke, O. Israel (eds.), *Hybrid PET/CT and SPECT/CT Imaging*,
DOI 10.1007/978-0-387-92820-3_12, © Springer Science+Business Media, LLC 2010

## Differentiated Thyroid Cancer

Cervical US and radioiodine imaging (diagnostic and post-therapy scans) are the main imaging procedures for evaluating patients with papillary and follicular thyroid cancer. Chest CT is also used to assess for and follow-up of pulmonary metastases. The role of CT and magnetic resonance imaging (MRI) (especially if [131]I therapy is planned) in loco-regional disease and restaging is evolving.

### *Radioiodine Whole-Body Scintigraphy with SPECT/CT*

Whole-body scintigraphy (WBS) performed after radioiodine ablation or therapy has the ability to detect new or additional metastases in 10–25% of cases, alter staging in 10%, and affect further management in 9–15% of patients.[2] Selected patients may also benefit from diagnostic WBS using [123]I or [131]I performed prior to therapy or during follow-up.

Although for decades WBS included mainly planar imaging, radioiodine-avid lesions may be difficult to localize on static scintigraphy alone. The high specificity of radioactive iodine for thyroid tissue results in poor definition of the body contours, and normal organs and iodine SPECT studies are therefore not helpful for further lesion localization and definition.

Precise characterization of radioiodine-avid foci is obtained through correct localization and is important for further patient management.[3] Radioiodine-avid metastases can be small and may occur in regions with distorted anatomy after surgery. SPECT/CT will improve the ability for their correct localization. On post-therapeutic WBS, the high activity contained in residual thyroid tissue often hampers cervical N-staging, a limitation that is overcome with SPECT/CT. Although radioiodine uptake is specific for tissue originating from the thyroid, false-positive findings can occur on planar WBS, related to benign processes, physiological radioiodine excretion, or artefacts due to contamination of the skin. By precise localization of radioiodine uptake, SPECT/CT is expected to improve the diagnostic accuracy of WBS and therefore to have a significant effect on patient management.

A small number of studies assessing the value of integrated SPECT/CT with radioiodine suggest that it has advantages over planar imaging and SPECT imaging alone.[4,5] The majority of radioiodine-avid foci were correctly classified as benign or malignant by hybrid imaging, further confirmed by clinical follow-up and US, CT, or MRI. In the patient-based analysis, SPECT/CT was found to change the therapeutic procedure in 25% of patients. In the future, the use of SPECT/CT to derive dosimetric estimates of radioiodine doses for treatment may constitute the breakthrough for rationally planned radionuclide therapy in patients with thyroid cancer.

### *[18]F-FDG PET/CT*

There is currently no well-established role for [18]F-fluorodeoxyglucose (FDG) PET/CT for routine diagnosis and follow-up of patients with differentiated thyroid carcinoma.

[18]F-FDG PET/CT is currently recommended for patients with differentiated thyroid cancer who have elevated thyroglobulin levels and negative radioiodine WBS post-therapy. A recent review of 21 studies performed between 1997 and 2006 that evaluated [18]F-FDG PET and PET/CT and included more than 10 patients per study concluded that these are useful imaging modalities in patients with thyroid cancer, with sensitivities in the range of 45–100% and specificity of 90–100% for diagnosis of recurrence.[6] The wide range of the reported sensitivity is related in part to the variability in parameters of the study protocols such as differences in patient selection, tumor characteristics, imaging devices, image analysis, and the gold standard used. [18]F-FDG imaging sensitivity is also related to serum thyroglobulin levels and to the site of the recurrent disease.[6]

The optimal [18]F-FDG imaging protocol in patients with differentiated thyroid cancer is still debated. A few studies have shown that thyrotropin-stimulating hormone (TSH) stimulation achieved by thyroid hormone withdrawal increases the sensitivity of [18]F-FDG imaging.[7,8] This increase in sensitivity must be weighed against the side effects of hypothyroidism. The results of studies evaluating recombinant humanized TSH (rhTSH) stimulation prior to [18]F-FDG scanning show conflicting data. Some authors have found an increased detection rate of [18]F-FDG-avid lesions with rhTSH stimulation,[9,10] while others did not.[11,12] No studies have performed a direct comparison of endogenous versus exogenous TSH stimulation. A recent study on 63 patients demonstrated that TSH stimulation moderately increases the sensitivity for [18]F-FDG positive lesions.[13]

Patients with [18]F-FDG-avid disease have been shown to have a worse prognosis as compared to patients with negative studies.[14,15] The glycolytic rate expressed by SUVmax levels, number of lesions, and [18]F-FDG-avid disease volume may all be significant predictors of mortality.[14,15] In patients with aggressive differentiated thyroid cancer variants, [18]F-FDG imaging therefore should be performed before aggressive treatment is started.[6]

## Hürthle Cell Carcinoma

Hürthle cell carcinoma (also called oncocytic or oxyphilic carcinoma) comprises approximately 3–6% of all thyroid malignancies. Hürthle cells are histologically distinct variants of follicular cells and can be also found in benign thyroid lesions. Diagnosis of malignancy is based on the presence of angioinvasion, capsular invasion, and/or metastases. Hürthle cell carcinomas have a higher rate of distant metastases than papillary or follicular carcinomas and only rarely accumulate radioiodine, thus precluding the routine use of radiodine WBS. Thyroglobulin levels may be normal or elevated.[1]

A meta-analysis of [18]F-FDG imaging in this patient population, including data from a multi-center study, reported an overall sensitivity of 92%, specificity 80%, positive predictive value (PPV) 92%, negative predictive value (NPV) 80%, and accuracy of 89% for detection of Hürthle cell carcinoma.[16] A more recent study reported higher performance indices with a sensitivity of 96% and a specificity of 95%.[17] [18]F-FDG imaging detected more sites of disease and has a higher PPV than CT[16,17] and demonstrated more sites of disease in 3 of 6 patients with both positive [18]F-FDG and WBS studies, as well as 10 patients with negative WBS who had positive [18]F-FDG imaging studies.[17]

## Anaplastic Thyroid Cancer

Anaplastic thyroid cancer (ATC) represents less than 2% of all thyroid malignancies and affects mainly the elderly population. The tumors grow very rapidly, and patients present with symptoms and signs of upper aero-digestive tract obstruction or invasion (i.e., dysphagia, dyspnea, hoarseness, pain, stridor). The major differential diagnosis is thyroid lymphoma. The two entities cannot be distinguished by imaging, and diagnosis is made by tissue biopsy with immunohistochemistry.[1]

Treatment options for patients with ATC are limited, and median survival at diagnosis is 8 months.[1] Consequently, there is no real role for timely and sophisticated imaging procedures for follow-up of patients with ATC because results do not usually change outcomes. [18]F-FDG imaging has not been methodologically studied in patients with ATC, yet several case reports have shown that it is a very [18]F-FDG avid malignancy because of its poor differentiation.[18–20]

## Medullary Thyroid Cancer

Medullary thyroid cancer (MTC) is a neuroendocrine malignancy that arises from parafollicular C-cells in the thyroid gland. The parafollicular C cells secrete calcitonin, a hormone that is involved in bone mineral metabolism, vitamin D regulation, and satiety. MTC accounts for 3–10% of all thyroid neoplasms, and, in most cases, approximately 75% are sporadic. The other 25% are familial cases, either as part of multiple endocrine neoplasias or isolated familial MTC. MTC is insensitive to chemotherapy and radiation therapy. Complete surgical excision including lymph node dissection provides the best chance for cure and the best prognosis. After surgery, serum calcitonin and carcinoembryonic antigen (CEA) levels are used for surveillance.

Imaging studies are performed when results of these tests raise the suspicion of recurrence or in the presence of new symptoms, and when potential treatment options are considered.[21] The most frequently used imaging modalities to stage and re-stage MTC are US and CT. Various radiopharmaceuticals have been also evaluated including [131]I- or [123]I-meta-iodo-benzyl-guanidine (MIBG) and somatostatin receptor scintigraphy (SRS) with[111]In-pentetreotide, with moderate and variable results. The sensitivity of MIBG for the detection of recurrent, residual, or metastatic MTC is around 30%,[22] and the sensitivity of SRS ranges from 25 to 71%.[23,24] Specificity of MIBG and SRS for detection of MTC is higher. Other radiopharmaceuticals such as [201]Tl-chloride, [99m]Tc-sestamibi, and radio-labeled anti-CEA antibodies have also been evaluated but have shown disappointing results. Pentavalent [99m]Tc-dimercaptosuccinic acid appears to perform better than MIBG and SRS.[25]

The role of [18]F-FDG imaging in patients with MTC was recently reviewed.[26] A wide range of sensitivities, between 41–88%, and specificities, 33–79%, have been reported, with conflicting results even in more recent studies.[27,28] Some of the differences in performance may be explained by differences in the completeness of initial surgery or the clinical indications for performing the study, such as rising calcitonin levels and negative anatomical imaging studies[28] versus rising calcitonin levels alone.[27] The sensitivity of [18]F-FDG imaging is related to the serum calcitonin levels, with best results being reported at serum levels higher than 1,000 pg/mL.[29,30]

MTC is generally a slow growing tumor with no overexpression of glucose transporters.[31] An additional disadvantage of [18]F-FDG imaging is the detection of small volume disease in cervical lymph nodes and miliary hepatic metastases. Despite these limitations, [18]F-FDG performs better than other scintigraphic techniques for the detection of MTC and is more sensitive than CT or MRI, but not US, for detecting cervical or mediastinal metastases, and than bone scintigraphy for diagnosis of skeletal metastases.[29] More than a single sensitive method may be required for the diagnosis of recurrent or metastatic MTC, and [18]F-FDG imaging may be particularly useful when other imaging modalities are negative.

## Thyroid Incidentalomas on [18]F-FDG PET/CT

[18]F-FDG PET/CT is not specifically used for diagnosis of thyroid cancer. However, focal [18]F-FDG uptake can be incidentally found in the thyroid gland. In patients with no prior history of thyroid disease, such an incidental focus has a high probability of malignancy, and further workup is required, usually US with biopsy.[32] The NPV for the detection of malignancy in a thyroid nodule visualized on the CT portion of the PET/CT study has not been established. These lesions will most likely go undetected, and less follow-up is therefore available. Diffuse thyroid tracer uptake has been found in up to 3% of patients undergoing [18]F-FDG imaging and can be associated with lymphocytic thyroiditis among other causes.[33]

## Guidelines and Recommendations for the Use of [18]F-FDG PET and PET/CT

The National Comprehensive Cancer Network (NCCN) has incorporated [18]F-FDG PET and PET/CT in the evaluation and management algorithm of a variety of malignancies including thyroid cancer.[34] The use of [18]F-FDG PET (PET/CT where available) should be considered in the evaluation of suspected recurrence of papillary, follicular, and Hurthle cell carcinoma if radioiodine scan is negative and thyroglobulin levels are > 10 ng/mL. The role of [18]F-FDG PET is limited in MTC.

A multidisciplinary panel of experts assessed meta-analyses and systematic reviews published in the [18]F-FDG PET literature before March 2006 and made recommendations for the use of FDG PET in oncology.[35] The panel concluded that [18]F-FDG PET should routinely be performed on patients previously treated for well-differentiated (follicular or papillary) thyroid cancer when the findings of [131]I WBS are negative and the thyroglobulin serum levels are >10 ng/mL.

## Case Presentations

### Case II.10.1 (DICOM Images on DVD)

#### History

A 32-year-old female with a history of papillary thyroid carcinoma presented with lower neck lymphadenopathy suspicious for recurrent disease. Previous treatment included thyroidectomy and administration of 370 MBq (100 mCi) of [131]I for remnant thyroid ablation. The patient received rhTSH, and with a TSH level of 105 uIU/mL, her thyroglobulin was 57.4 ng/mL. She was referred for a [123]I WBS to detect and localize recurrent papillary thyroid carcinoma. Images were obtained 24 h after oral administration of 55 MBq (1.5 mCi) of [123]I (Fig. II.10.1A-C).

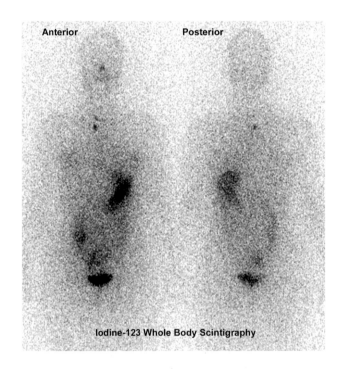

Fig. II.10.1A

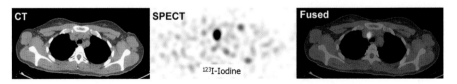

Fig. II.10.1B

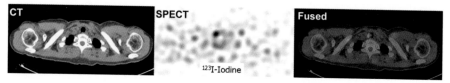

Fig. II.10.1C

## Findings

On WBS, there are two focal areas of [123]I uptake in the right lower neck and upper mediastinum highly suspicious for recurrent thyroid cancer (Fig. II.10.1A). SPECT/CT of the neck and upper thorax was obtained for better localization of these foci. The prominent, inferior focus fuses to a 12 mm right upper paratracheal lymph node located behind the right sternoclavicular joint, anterior and right of the trachea (Fig. II.10.1B). The second, more subtle focus of uptake fuses to a 5 mm right upper paratracheal soft tissue density (Fig. II.10.1C).

## Discussion

The findings are consistent with recurrent, radioiodine-avid papillary thyroid carcinoma. No additional foci of abnormal tracer activity are seen outside the neck and superior mediastinum region to suggest the presence of distant metastases.

The standard technique for radioiodine metastatic surveys in patients with differentiated thyroid cancer is WBS, a highly specific study that lacks, however, anatomic details. SPECT/CT overcomes this limitation. Ruf and colleagues[36] evaluated 25 patients after radioiodine therapy with inconclusive foci on WBS. They found that SPECT/CT changed image interpretation, as compared to planar and SPECT alone, that resulted in a change in therapy in 25% of patients. Tharp and coworkers[5] demonstrated similar results. SPECT/CT had incremental diagnostic value in 57% of 71 patients undergoing conventional WBS for follow-up of thyroid carcinoma. It allowed more precise lesion localization and, therefore, characterization of findings, and the authors concluded that SPECT/CT influenced the referring physician's approach to therapeutic administration of radioiodine, surgery, external beam radiation, and medical treatment.

Traditionally, patients have been prepared for follow-up WBS by withdrawal of thyroid hormone replacement, which is ceased for 4–6 weeks, or, alternatively, patients are switched to triiodothyronine ($T_3$) for 2 weeks prior to complete hormone withdrawal to decrease symptomatic hypothyroidism. A TSH level of 30 uIU/L or higher improves the sensitivity of WBS. A decade ago, rhTSH was approved for stimulation prior to thyroglobulin testing with or without WBS.[37] RhTSH is given as two 0.9 mg intramuscular injections on consecutive days, followed by radioiodine administration the next day. WBS is performed at standard time points after radioiodine administration. Clinical studies have shown that the sensitivity of WBS with rhTSH stimulation is similar to hormone withdrawal,[35] and the absence of even short-term hypothyroidism positively affects the quality of life of patients.[38]

## Diagnosis

Recurrent, papillary thyroid carcinoma in right upper paratracheal lymph nodes.

## Clinical Report: $^{123}$I Metastatic Survey with SPECT/CT (for DVD cases only)

Indication

Suspected recurrent thyroid carcinoma.

History

A 32-year-old female with a history of 50 mm papillary thyroid carcinoma, status post-thyroidectomy, and 370 MBq (100 mCi) of $^{131}$I remnant thyroid ablation. Approximately 6 months later, a follow-up CT study revealed residual lower neck adenopathy. The patient presented for $^{123}$I WBS to evaluate for residual or recurrent thyroid cancer.

Procedure

The patient received rhTSH in preparation for this study. At the time of this study, the TSH level was 105 uIU/mL and thyroglobulin of 57.4 ng/mL. Serum beta human chorionic gonadotrophin (HCG) was negative.

$^{123}$I (55 MBq = 1.5 mCi) was administered orally, and 24 h delayed WBS and spot views of the head and neck were acquired in the anterior and posterior projections. SPECT/CT of the thorax was obtained with the patient's arms raised.

Findings

*Quality of the study*: The quality of this study is good.
*Whole-body planar images*: There is a focus of intense $^{123}$I accumulation in the lower neck or superior mediastinum, to the right of midline. Above this lesion, there is a second, more subtle focus of $^{123}$I accumulation. Physiologic $^{123}$I accumulation is visualized in the nasopharynx, oropharynx, stomach, bowel, bladder, and both breasts.
*SPECT/CT*: The inferior and more intense focus of $^{123}$I activity corresponds to a 12 mm right upper paratracheal lymph node, behind the right sternoclavicular joint. The second, more subtle area of uptake fuses to a 5 mm right upper paratracheal soft tissue density.
No other abnormalities are visualized on CT.

Impression

1. Right upper paratracheal lymph node, 12 mm in diameter, with intense $^{123}$I activity, most consistent with iodine-avid thyroid cancer metastasis.
2. Right upper paratracheal soft tissue mass, 5 mm in diameter, with increased $^{123}$I activity, highly suspicious for a second iodine-avid metastatic focus of thyroid cancer.

## Case II.10.2 (DICOM Images on DVD)

### History

This 34-year-old female with a history of a 17 mm papillary carcinoma in the right lobe of the thyroid gland, was found at surgery (sub-total thyroidectomy) to have metastatic disease in several central neck lymph nodes. The patient received 2,812 MBq (76 mCi) of [131]I for remnant thyroid ablation. A post-treatment WBS did not reveal disease outside the thyroid bed. Ten months later, the patient presented with an elevated stimulated thyroglobulin levels (490 ng/mL) and received 5,550 MBq (150 mCi) of [131]I. Post-treatment WBS revealed [131]I uptake in the region of the thyroid bed extending substernally. She underwent completion thyroidectomy and resection of recurrent disease in a 20 mm right paratracheal mass. Elevated stimulated thyroglobulin level persisted after surgery. [123]I WBS raised the possibility of residual mediastinal disease, and the patient received 7,400 MBq (200 mCi) of [131]I. Stimulated WBS 9 months later was negative, while thyroglobulin levels were lower, but still elevated (10 ng/mL). US of the neck revealed a suspicious left level VI lymph node, diagnosed as metastatic papillary thyroid cancer on FNA. The patient was referred for [18]F-FDG PET/CT to assess the whole extent of disease (Fig. II.10.2A–C).

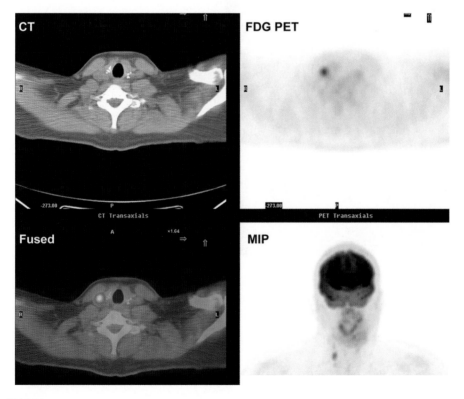

Fig. II.10.2A

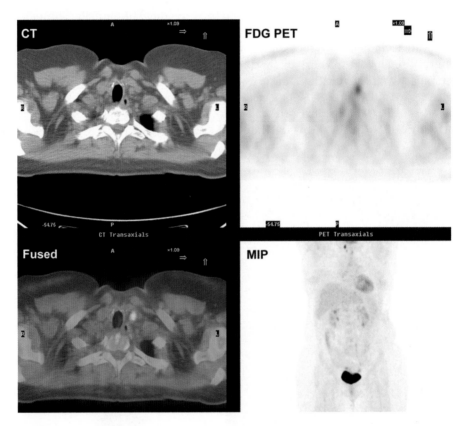

Fig. II.10.2B

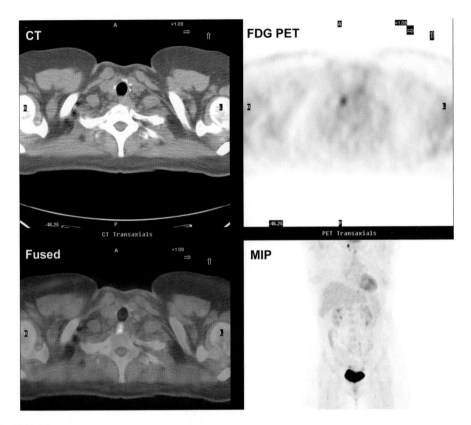

**Fig. II.10.2C**

## Findings

Three foci of increased $^{18}$F-FDG activity are seen in the head and neck region. A focus of intense $^{18}$F-FDG activity fuses to a soft tissue density on CT posterior to the right sternocleidomastoid muscle, probably a right level IV cervical lymph node (Fig. II.10.2A). There is a 7 mm left level VI lymph node with moderate $^{18}$F-FDG activity corresponding to the biopsy proven recurrence (Fig. II.10.2B), and a 5 mm $^{18}$F-FDG-avid right central neck lymph node posterior to the trachea, right lateral to the esophagus (Fig. II.10.2C).

## Discussion

The findings in the left neck are consistent with the biopsy proven recurrence in the left level VI lymph node and a right central neck lymph node metastasis posterior to the trachea. The more intense $^{18}$F-FDG uptake in the 7 mm right level IV cervical lymph node was also suspicious for malignancy and confirmed by US-guided FNA, which revealed metastatic papillary carcinoma.

   The additional positive right level IV lymph node detected on $^{18}$F-FDG PET/CT has significant implications for further clinical management in this case. Disease in this node indicates that metastases have spread outside the central neck compartment, and right lateral neck dissection is necessary. In a review of the lymph node anatomy,[39] the central neck is shown to include all lymph nodes medial to the carotid arteries from the inferior body of the hyoid bone to the level of the brachiocephalic vein (levels VI and VII). Central and lateral neck dissections require different surgical approaches.

The largest study evaluating the use of [18]F-FDG imaging in differentiated thyroid cancer was a multi-center retrospective analysis that included 222 patients. The overall sensitivity and specificity of [18]F-FDG for the detection of disease was 75 and 90%, respectively.[11] In the subgroup of 166 patients with negative WBS, the sensitivity was 85%. [18]F-FDG PET was more sensitive but not more specific than WBS.

The diagnostic accuracy for detection of differentiated thyroid cancer is higher for PET/CT, 93%, as compared to 78% for PET alone.[40] PET/CT also had an incremental value when compared to the side-by-side interpretation of PET and CT in 74% of patients.

[18]F-FDG PET/CT has been reported to alter therapy in 9–54% of patients with differentiated thyroid cancer.[6,38] In patients with known disease in the neck, previously planned surgery may be more extensive, and aggressive local treatment may be cancelled if distant metastases are found on [18]F-FDG PET/CT.

## Diagnosis

Papillary thyroid cancer with bilateral central and right lateral neck lymph node metastases.

## Clinical Report: Body [18]F-FDG PET/CT (for DVD cases only)

Indication

To evaluate the extent of disease in a patient with radioiodine-negative thyroid cancer and persistently elevated thyroglobulin levels.

History

A 34-year-old female with a history of a 17 mm papillary carcinoma in the right lobe of the thyroid gland, status post sub-total thyroidectomy and remnant thyroid ablation with 2,812 MBq (76 mCi) of [131]I. At surgery, metastatic disease was found in several central neck lymph nodes. Ten months later, the patient received 5,550 MBq (150 mCi) of [131]I for elevated stimulated thyroglobulin level (490 ng/mL). Post-treatment WBS revealed [131]I activity in the region of the thyroid bed extending substernally. The patient underwent completion of thyroidectomy and resection of recurrent disease in a 20 mm right paratracheal mass. Elevated stimulated thyroglobulin level persisted post-operatively and the [123]I WBS raised the possibility of residual mediastinal disease. The patient received 7,400 MBq (200 mCi) [131]I. Nine months later, stimulated WBS was negative with lower, but still elevated, thyroglobulin levels (10 ng/mL). US of the neck revealed a suspicious left level VI lymph node that was metastatic papillary thyroid cancer on FNA. The patient was referred for [18]F-FDG PET/CT in search for additional sites of disease.

Procedure

The fasting blood glucose level was 83 mg/dl. [18]F-FDG (873 MBq = 23.6 mCi) was administered intravenously. Oral contrast was administered. After an [18]F-FDG uptake period of approximately 60 min, CT without intravenous contrast and PET images were acquired from the vertex of the skull to the mid-femurs. The CT scan without intravenous contrast was used for attenuation correction and localization.

Findings

*Quality of the study*: The quality of this study is good.

*Head and neck*: There is a focus of intense $^{18}$F-FDG activity, which fuses to a soft tissue density on CT posterior to the right sternocleidomastoid muscle, probably a right level IV cervical lymph node. There is a 7 mm left level VI lymph node with moderate $^{18}$F-FDG activity corresponding to the biopsy proven recurrence. There is a 5 mm right central neck lymph node posterior to the trachea, lateral to the esophagus. These findings are highly suspicious for metastatic thyroid carcinoma. Surgical clips are seen in the region of the thyroid bed consistent with history of thyroidectomy.

*Chest*: There is a focus of $^{18}$F-FDG activity corresponding to the distal esophagus. This may represent mild reflux esophagitis or may be within the physiologic normal range. There is a 3 mm right lower lobe lung nodule that is too small to be characterized by $^{18}$F-FDG PET/CT. Physiologic $^{18}$F-FDG activity is seen in the myocardium, blood pool, and bilateral breast tissue.

*Abdomen and pelvis*: There is a focus of moderate $^{18}$F-FDG activity corresponding to the uterus. There are 2 foci of $^{18}$F-FDG activity in the adnexal regions bilaterally, corresponding to both ovaries. These findings are most likely physiologic and related to the menstrual cycle in a patient of this age.

Impression

1. A 7 mm left level VI lymph node with moderate $^{18}$F-FDG activity, consistent with biopsy proven recurrence of thyroid carcinoma.
2. Focus of intense $^{18}$F-FDG activity, which fuses to a soft tissue density on CT posterior to the right sternocleidomastoid muscle, probably a right level IV cervical lymph node, highly suspicious for metastatic thyroid carcinoma.
3. A 5 mm right central neck lymph node posterior to the trachea and lateral to the esophagus with increased $^{18}$F-FDG activity, highly suspicious for metastatic thyroid carcinoma.
4. A 3 mm right lower lobe lung nodule that is too small to be characterized by $^{18}$F-FDG PET/CT. In a patient with a history of cancer, recommend follow-up dedicated thoracic CT in 12 months to evaluate the stability of this nodule over time.
5. $^{18}$F-FDG activity fusing to the endometrial cavity and bilateral ovaries, most likely physiologic, related to the menstrual cycle in a patient of this age group.
6. Focus of $^{18}$F-FDG activity in the distal esophagus, which may represent mild reflux esophagitis or may be within the physiologic normal range.

## Case II.10.3

### History

This 46-year-old male with a history of a 35 mm Hürthle cell carcinoma presented initially with back pain, mainly while sitting. CT revealed a mass involving the left ilium and sacrum. Biopsy revealed a thyroid neoplasm. He received external beam radiation to the left pelvic lesion and ultimately underwent total thyroidectomy. [123]I WBS indicated that the pelvic lesion was radioiodine-avid, and the patient received a therapeutic dose of [131]I. Post-treatment WBS demonstrated the presence of remnant tissue in the thyroid bed and multiple skeletal metastases. The patient continued to complain of pain and therefore underwent embolization and radiofrequency ablation of the ilio-sacral mass. His stimulated thyroglobulin levels declined initially from 66,000 to 6,110 ng/mL but subsequently increased to 25,000 ng/mL. A therapeutic dose of 20,535 MBq (555 mCi) [131]I was administered. He presented for post-treatment WBS (Fig. II.10.3A, B).

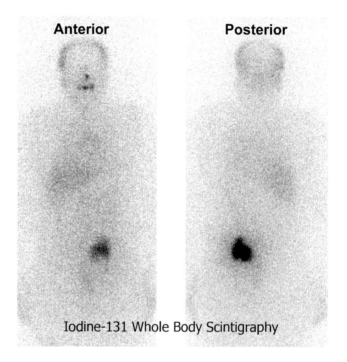

**Anterior**          **Posterior**

Iodine-131 Whole Body Scintigraphy

**Fig. II.10.3A**

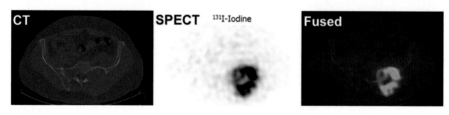

**Fig. II.10.3B**

**Findings**

On WBS, there is a intense focus of [131]I accumulation in the left pelvic region (Fig. II.10.3A). SPECT/CT demonstrates that the focus of activity fuses to a left ilio-sacral lytic lesion (Fig. II.10.3B). The periphery of the mass demonstrates the most intense activity while the center is photopenic. CT shows partial destruction of the iliac bone and the sacrum and posterior extension of the mass into the left gluteal muscles.

**Discussion**

The findings on the post-treatment [131]I SPECT/CT are most consistent with active, iodine-avid Hürthle cell carcinoma in the left ilio-sacral mass. The central photopenic area suggests the presence of necrosis. This is probably related to prior treatment with embolization and radiofrequency ablation.

Only 10% of Hürthle cell carcinomas are radioiodine-avid, with WBS sensitivity ranging between 18 and 65%.[17,41] The rationale for the initial WBS in this patient was to determine if his metastases were indeed radioiodine-avid. After confirming that this was indeed the case, the patient was able to receive therapeutic doses of [131]I, which led initially to some decline of the thyroglobulin level.

Patients with Hürthle cell carcinoma have an intermediate prognosis, between differentiated and anaplastic carcinomas. Overall 20-year survival is 65% for Hürthle cell carcinoma versus 81–87% for papillary and follicular carcinomas.[1] Negative prognostic factors for Hürthle cell carcinoma include tumor size greater than 40 mm, extrathyroidal extension, and the presence of nodal and distant metastases.[42] The level of [18]F-FDG uptake in Hürthle cell carcinoma, expressed as SUVmax, provides prognostic information, with a significant difference in 5-year overall survival, 92% in patients with an SUVmax < 10, but only 64% in patients with a tumor SUVmax > 10.[17]

**Diagnosis**

Radioiodine-avid residual active Hürthle cell carcinoma in left ilio-sacral mass.

## Case II.10.4

### History

This 72-year-old male with a history of ATC initially presented with hoarseness. CT revealed a mass arising from the right lobe of the thyroid gland, extending from the level of the epiglottis to the right lung apex, and the patient received external beam radiation therapy and chemotherapy. He also has a long-standing history of lymphocytic thyroiditis treated with thyroid hormone replacement. The patient was referred for [18]F-FDG PET/CT to assess the extent of disease (Fig. II.10.4A, B).

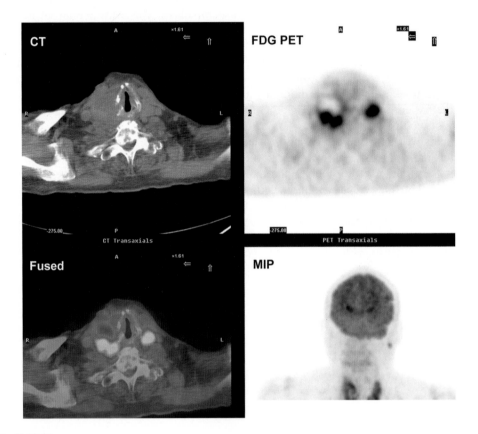

Fig. II.10.4A

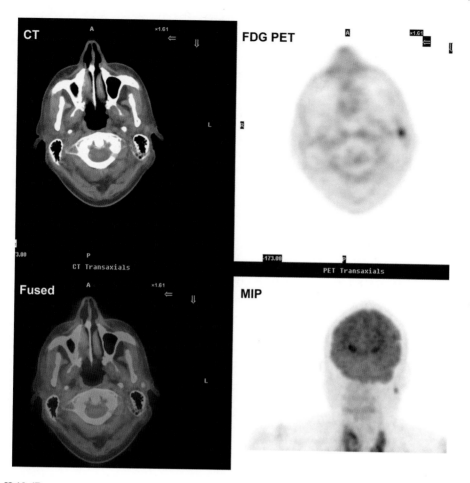

**Fig. II.10.4B**

### Findings

There is a 52 × 50 mm solid and cystic mass arising from the right lobe of the thyroid gland. The solid component of the mass demonstrates intense $^{18}$F-FDG activity while the cystic component is photopenic (Fig. II.10.4A). There is erosion of the right thyroid cartilage on the CT component, associated with moderate $^{18}$F-FDG activity. The left lobe of the thyroid gland is enlarged and demonstrates intense $^{18}$F-FDG activity (Fig. II.10.4A). There is an additional focus of intense $^{18}$F-FDG activity corresponding to a 7 × 6 mm left parotid lymph node (Fig. II.10.4B).

### Discussion

The right-sided thyroid mass and intense uptake in the left lobe of the thyroid gland are most consistent with diffuse infiltration of the thyroid gland with the known ATC. Although the patient has a history of lymphocytic thyroiditis, which can accumulate $^{18}$F-FDG, the size and intensity of the tracer uptake renders malignancy the more likely diagnosis. The [18]F-FDG-avid left parotid lymph node is suspicious for metastatic disease. In isolation, the differential diagnosis of increased [18]F-FDG uptake in a parotid nodule includes Warthin's tumor, pleomorphic adenoma, oncocytoma, and metastatic disease. On CT, the right thyroid cartilage appears eroded, with associated increased [18]F-FDG activity, suggesting tumor invasion. MRI or direct inspection at surgery is, however, the recommended technique to detect early bone and cartilage invasion by tumor due to their higher resolution as compared to [18]F-FDG PET.[43]

A small subset of patients with ATC have more favorable prognostic features, including tumors less than 40 mm in diameter and unilateral tumors without local invasion. With multi-modality therapy, long-term survival may be achieved in some of these patients. In this setting, [18]F-FDG imaging may play a role in monitoring therapy and for diagnosis of recurrent or metastatic disease.[19,20]

**Diagnosis**

1. ATC exhibiting a right mass and diffuse invasion of the thyroid gland.
2. Possible ATC metastasis in left parotid lymph node.

## Case II.10.5

### History

This 62-year-old male presented with abdominal pain, 25 pound weight loss and anorexia, and CT which demonstrated multiple hepatic lesions. Biopsy of one of these hepatic lesions revealed a well-differentiated neuroendocrine tumor, and he received multiple cycles of chemotherapy over the next year. Follow-up CT scan revealed miliary hepatic lesions, an enlarged multi-nodular left lobe of the thyroid, sub-centimeter mediastinal lymph nodes, and diffuse sclerotic lesions in the spine and pelvis suspicious for metastatic disease. He was referred for SRS with [111]In-pentetreotide (Fig. II.10.5A–C).

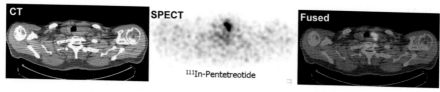

Fig. II.10.5A

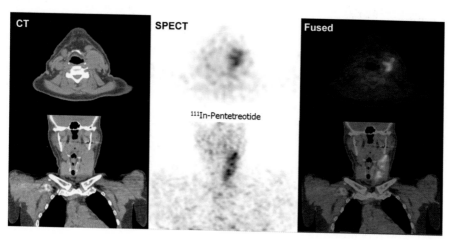

Fig. II.10.5B

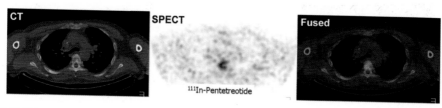

Fig. II.10.5C

## Findings

There is intense tracer uptake corresponding to an enlarged left lobe of the thyroid gland (Fig. II.10.5A). The right lobe of the thyroid gland does not show increased tracer uptake and appears normal on the CT component. Level II/III left cervical lymph nodes with intense tracer uptake are also demonstrated (Fig. II.10.5B). There is mild sclerosis of a mid-thoracic vertebral body on CT with intense [111]In-pentetreotide uptake. The sclerotic lesion in the posterior aspect of a right rib does not show increased [111]In-pentetreotide activity (Fig. II.10.5C). The hepatic lesions did not have significant abnormal [111]In-pentetreotide uptake (not shown).

## Discussion

The findings are most consistent with a somatostatin receptor positive neuroendocrine tumor in the left lobe of the thyroid gland, with metastatic disease in left cervical lymph nodes and a mid-thoracic vertebra.

While this patient had been diagnosed with metastatic well-differentiated neuroendocrine tumor, the primary malignancy was unknown. The findings on SRS raise the possibility of metastatic MTC. The differential diagnosis includes metastatic disease to thyroid, lymph nodes, and bone originating in other well-differentiated neuroendocrine tumors or other malignancies that express somatostatin receptors such as lymphoma, breast cancer, small cell lung cancer, and Merkel cell tumors. No focal abnormal tracer activity was seen in the lungs or breast tissue, however.

Subsequent to the SRS, the patient developed compressive symptoms due to the large mass in the neck and underwent left hemithyroidectomy with left central and levels 2–4 neck dissection. Pathology revealed a 70 mm MTC with metastatic disease in 21 of 34 lymph nodes. At the time of surgery, serum calcitonin levels were elevated at 7,582 pg/mL (normal range ≤ 10 pg/mL).

The sensitivity of SRS for detection of MTC ranges from 25 to 71%.[23,24] The reported variability in performance of SRS is considered to be related to a heterogeneous expression of somatostatin receptors.[44] SPECT/CT has been shown to have an added value over SPECT imaging alone in neuroendocrine tumors by providing complimentary anatomic and functional information. Most reports include also a small number of patients with MTC.[45,46] With SPECT/CT, lesion localization is precise, extent of disease is more accurately assessed, and tracer avidity of lesions visualized on CT can be identified and confirmed, with prognostic and therapeutic implications.

## Diagnosis

1. Medullary thyroid cancer.
2. Metastatic left neck lymphadenopathy.
3. Active and treated skeletal metastases.
4. Treated hepatic metastases.

## Case II.10.6

### History

This 55-year-old female with a history of multiple recurrences of MTC presented with indeterminate anatomic imaging findings and rising serum calcitonin and CEA levels. Her past therapies included total thyroidectomy, multiple surgical resections of sites of recurrent disease, and external beam radiation therapy. She was referred for $^{18}$F-FDG PET/CT with a suspicion of recurrence in order to detect and localize MTC (Fig. II.10.6A, B).

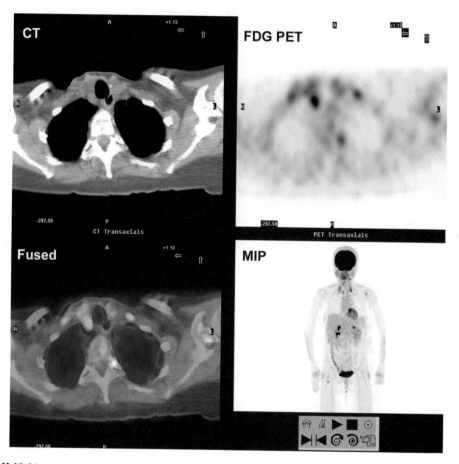

Fig. II.10.6A

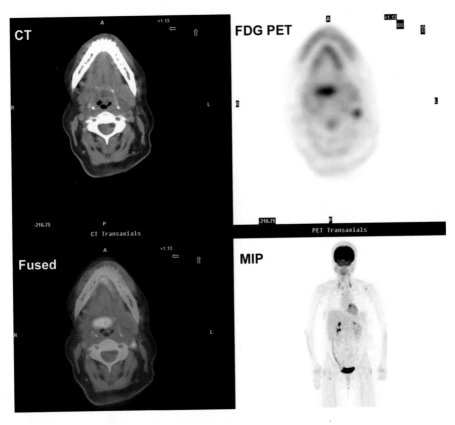

**Fig. II.10.6B**

## Findings

There is a $13 \times 8$ mm right paratracheal lymph node showing intense [18]F-FDG activity. There is an additional focus of intense [18]F-FDG activity in the left transverse process of an upper thoracic vertebra (Fig. II.10.6A). Focal, intense [18]F-FDG uptake is also shown in a $7 \times 5$ mm level II left cervical lymph node (Fig. II.10.6B). Additional foci of [18]F-FDG uptake are seen in the proximal left humerus and right femur (maximum intensity projection (MIP) images). Intense, linear [18]F-FDG activity is seen in the scalene muscles on both sides (MIP images). Physiologic [18]F-FDG activity is visualized in the soft palate (Fig. II.10.6B).

## Discussion

In a patient with a history of MTC and rising serum tumor markers, these findings are most consistent with recurrence in left cervical and right paratracheal lymph nodes and skeletal metastases. The level II left cervical lymph node does not meet CT size criteria (diameter greater than 15 mm) for malignancy. This is one of the limitations of conventional imaging. Although inflammatory lymph nodes in the neck can be false positive on [18]F-FDG imaging, the lesion in this case is asymmetric and has a high level of tracer intensity.

The symmetric $^{18}$F-FDG activity in the scalene muscles appears intense and focal on the transaxial images and might be confused with metastatic lymph nodes. Scalene muscle uptake of $^{18}$F-FDG is not uncommon, it occured in one series in 36% of 410 patients and is related mainly to muscle use (or strain). Uptake is most commonly bilateral, symmetric, and linear, and best appreciated on coronal or MIP images.[47]

**Diagnosis**

1. Recurrent MTC to right paratracheal and level II left cervical lymph nodes.
2. Skeletal metastases in right proximal femur, left scapula, and the left transverse process of an upper thoracic vertebra.
3. Physiologic scalene muscle and soft palate $^{18}$F-FDG uptake.

## Case II.10.7

### History

This 66-year-old female with a history of right nasal cavity mucosal melanoma treated with resection 5 years prior to current examination presented with a 2-week history of epistaxis. Endoscopic biopsy revealed local recurrence. The patient was referred for $^{18}$F-FDG PET/CT in search for loco-regional and distant metastases (Fig. II.10.7A, B).

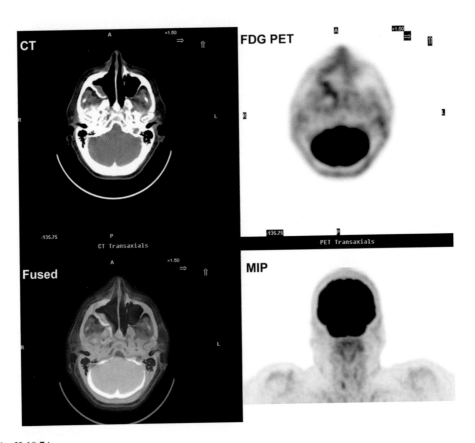

Fig. II.10.7A

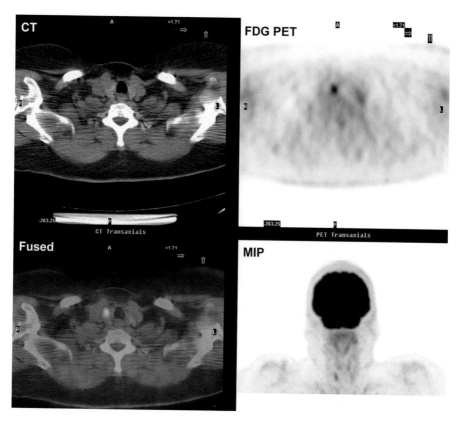

**Fig. II.10.7B**

### Findings

There is a focus of moderate [18]F-FDG activity corresponding to a soft tissue mass in the lateral aspect of the right nasal cavity (Fig. II.10.7A). A nodule in the right lower pole of the thyroid gland demonstrates moderate to intense [18]F-FDG activity (Fig. II.10.7B).

### Discussion

The lesion in the right nasal cavity is consistent with the biopsy-proven recurrent melanoma. The metabolically active thyroid nodule needs further evaluation. The primary differential diagnosis includes a primary thyroid malignancy versus a benign thyroid adenoma. However, there are uncommon reports of melanoma metastases to the thyroid gland.

Salvatori and colleagues[32] reviewed the literature between 1990 and 2006 regarding the incidental detection of focal [18]F-FDG uptake in the thyroid during whole-body PET scanning and found 15 reports. The frequency of abnormal [18]F-FDG uptake in the thyroid, some including diffuse tracer activity, ranged from 0.1 to 40%. The incidence of thyroid cancer in patients with focal abnormal [18]F-FDG activity within the thyroid gland ranged from 27 to 63%. False positives were due mainly to benign thyroid adenomas. In contrast to focal [18]F-FDG uptake, diffuse increased tracer activity in the thyroid gland appears to be associated mainly with thyroiditis.[33] In present case, the patient underwent FNA of the thyroid nodule, which revealed papillary thyroid carcinoma. Total thyroidectomy was performed, revealing a 6-mm lesion with no extrathyroidal or vascular invasion, and negative lymph nodes.

**Diagnosis**

1. Recurrent melanoma of the right nasal cavity mucosa.
2. Papillary thyroid carcinoma.

# References

1. Fraker D, Skarulis M, Livolsi V. Thyroid Tumors. In: DeVita V, Hellman S, Rosenberg SA, eds.: *Cancer: Principles and Practice of Oncology, 6th ed.* Philadelphia, PA: Lippincott Williams & Wilkens: 2001;1740–1762.
2. Cooper DS, Doherty GM, Haugen BR, Kloos RT, Lee SL, Mandel SJ, Mazzaferri EL, McIver B, Sherman SI, Tuttle RM. Management guidelines for patients with thyroid nodules and differentiated thyroid cancer. *Thyroid* 2006;16:109–142.
3. Shapiro B, Rufini V, Jarwan A, Geatti O, Kearfott KJ, Fig LM, Kirkwood ID, Gross MD. Artifacts, anatomical and physiological variants, and unrelated diseases that might cause false-positive whole-body 131-I scans in patients with thyroid cancer. *Semin Nucl Med* 2000;30:115–132.
4. Even-Sapir E, Keidar Z, Sachs J, Engel A, Bettman L, Gaitini D, Guralnik L, Werbin N, Iosilevsky G, Israel O. The new technology of combined transmission and emission tomography in evaluation of endocrine neoplasms. *J Nucl Med* 2001;42:998–1004.
5. Tharp K, Israel O, Hausmann J, Bettman L, Martin WH, Daitzchman M, Sandler MP, Delbeke D. Impact of 131I-SPECT/CT images obtained with an integrated system in the follow-up of patients with thyroid carcinoma. *Eur J Nucl Med Mol Imaging* 2004;31:1435–1442.
6. Leboulleux S, Schroeder PR, Schlumberger M, Ladenson PW. The role of PET in follow-up of patients treated for differentiated epithelial thyroid cancers. *Nat Clin Pract Endocrinol Metab* 2007;3:112–121.
7. Moog F, Linke R, Manthey N, Tiling R, Knesewitsch P, Tatsch K, Hahn K, Grünwald F, Biersack H-J. Influence of thyroid-stimulating hormone levels on uptake of FDG in recurrent and metastatic differentiated thyroid carcinoma. *J Nucl Med* 2000;41:1989–1995.
8. van Tol KM, Jager PL, Piers DA, Pruim J, de Vries EGE, Dullaart RPF, Links TP. Better yield of (18)fluorodeoxyglucose-positron emission tomography in patients with metastatic differentiated thyroid carcinoma during thyrotropin stimulation. *Thyroid* 2002;12:381–387.
9. Chin BB, Patel P, Cohade C, Ewertz M, Wahl R, Ladenson P. Recombinant human thyrotropin stimulation of fluoro-D-glucose positron emission tomography uptake in well-differentiated thyroid carcinoma. *J Clin Endocrinol Metab* 2004;89:91–95.
10. Petrich T, Borner AR, Otto D, Hofmann M, Knapp W. Influence of rhTSH on [(18)F]fluorodeoxyglucose uptake by differentiated thyroid carcinoma. *Eur J Nucl Med Mol Imaging* 2002;29:641–647.
11. Grunwald F, Kalicke T, Feine U, Lietzenmayer R, Scheidhauer K, Dietlein M, Schober O, Lerch H, Brandt-Mainz K, Burchert W, Hiltermann G, Cremerius U, Biersack HJ. Fluorine-18 fluorodeoxyglucose positron emission tomography in thyroid cancer: results of a multicentre study. *Eur J Nucl Med* 1999;26:1547–1552.
12. Wang W, Macapinlac H, Larson SM, Yeh SDJ, Akhurst T, Finn RD, Rosai J, Robbins RJ. [18F]-2-fluoro-2-deoxy-D-glucose positron emission tomography localizes residual thyroid cancer in patients with negative diagnostic (131) I whole body scans and elevated serum thyroglobulin levels. *J Clin Endocrinol Metab* 1999;84:2291–2302.
13. Leboulleux S, Schroeder PR, Busaidy NL, Auperin A, Corone C, Jacene HA, Ewertz ME, Bournaud C, Wahl RL, Sherman SI, Ladenson PW, Schlumberger M. Assessment of the incremental value of recombinant TSH stimulation before FDG PET/CT imaging to localize residual differentiated thyroid cancer. *J Clin Endocrinol Metab* 2009;94:1310–1316.
14. Robbins RJ, Wan Q, Grewal RK, Reibke R, Gonen M, Strauss HW, Tuttle RM, Drucker W, Larson SM. Real-time prognosis for metastatic thyroid carcinoma based on 2-[18F]fluoro-2-deoxy-D-glucose-positron emission tomography scanning. *J Clin Endocrinol Metab* 2006;91:498–505.
15. Wang W, Larson SM, Fazzari M, Tickoo SK, Kolbert K, Sgouros G, Yeung H, Macapinlac H, Rosai J, Robbins RJ. Prognostic value of [18F]fluorodeoxyglucose positron emission tomographic scanning in patients with thyroid cancer. *J Clin Endocrinol Metab* 2000;85:1107–1113.
16. Plotkin M, Hautzel H, Krause BJ, Schmidt D, Larisch R, Mottaghy FM, Boerner A-R, Herzog H, Vosberg H, Müller-Gärtner H-W. Implication of 2-18fluor-2-deoxyglucose positron emission tomography in the follow-up of Hurthle cell thyroid cancer. *Thyroid* 2002;12:155–161.
17. Pryma DA, Schoder H, Gonen M, Robbins RJ, Larson SM, Yeung HWD. Diagnostic accuracy and prognostic value of 18F-FDG PET in Hurthle cell thyroid cancer patients. *J Nucl Med* 2006;47:1260–1266.
18. Jadvar H, Fischman AJ. Evaluation of rare tumors with [F-18]Fluorodeoxyglucose positron emission tomography. *Clin Positron Imaging* 1999;2:153–158.
19. Nguyen BD, Ram PC. PET/CT staging and posttherapeutic monitoring of anaplastic thyroid carcinoma. *Clin Nucl Med* 2007;32:145–149.

20. Poppe K, Lahoutte T, Everaert H, Bossuyt A, Velkeniers B. The utility of multimodality imaging in anaplastic thyroid carcinoma. *Thyroid* 2004;14:981–982.
21. Donovan DT,Gagel RF. Medullary Thyroid Carcinoma and the Multiple Endocrine Neoplasms. In: Falk S, ed.: *Thyroid Disease: Endocrinology, Surgery, Nuclear Medicine, and Radiotherapy, 2nd ed.* Philadelphia, PA: Lippincott-Raven: 1997:619–644.
22. Rufini V, Salvatori M, Garganese MC, Di GD, Lodovica MM, Troncone L. Role of nuclear medicine in the diagnosis and therapy of medullary thyroid carcinoma. *Rays* 2000;25:273–282.
23. Baudin E, Lumbroso J, Schlumberger M, Leclere J, Giammarile F, Gardet P, Roche A, Travagli JP, Parmentier C. Comparison of octreotide scintigraphy and conventional imaging in medullary thyroid carcinoma. *J Nucl Med* 1996;37:912–916.
24. Frank-Raue K, Bihl H, Dorr U, Buhr H, Ziegler R, Raue F. Somatostatin receptor imaging in persistent medullary thyroid carcinoma. *Clin Endocrinol (Oxf)* 1995;42:31–37.
25. Clarke SE, Lazarus CR, Wraight P, Sampson C, Maisey MN. Pentavalent [99mTc]DMSA, [131I]MIBG, and [99mTc]MDP – an evaluation of three imaging techniques in patients with medullary carcinoma of the thyroid. *J Nucl Med* 1988;29:33–38.
26. Khan N, Oriuchi N, Higuchi T, Endo K. Review of fluorine-18-2-fluoro-2-deoxy-D-glucose positron emission tomography (FDG-PET) in the follow-up of medullary and anaplastic thyroid carcinomas. *Cancer Control* 2005;12:254–260.
27. Giraudet AL, Vanel D, Leboulleux S, Aupérin A, Dromain C, Chami L, Tovo NN, Lumbroso J, Lassau N, Bonniaud G, Hartl D, Travagli J-P, Baudin E, Schlumberger M. Imaging medullary thyroid carcinoma with persistent elevated calcitonin levels. *J Clin Endocrinol Meta* 2007;92:4185–4190.
28. Iagaru A, Masamed R, Singer PA, Conti PS. Detection of occult medullary thyroid cancer recurrence with 2-deoxy-2-[F-18]fluoro-D-glucose-PET and PET/CT. *Mol Imaging Biol* 2007;9:72–77.
29. de Groot JW, Links TP, Jager PL, Kahraman T, Plukker JT. Impact of 18F-fluoro-2-deoxy-D-glucose positron emission tomography (FDG-PET) in patients with biochemical evidence of recurrent or residual medullary thyroid cancer. *Ann Surg Oncol* 2004;11:786–794.
30. Ong SC, Schoder H, Patel SG, Tabangay-Lim IM, Doddamane I, Gönen M, Shaha AR, Tuttle RM, Shah JP, Larson SM. Diagnostic accuracy of 18F-FDG PET in restaging patients with medullary thyroid carcinoma and elevated calcitonin levels. *J Nucl Med* 2007;48:501–507.
31. Musholt TJ, Musholt PB, Dehdashti F, Moley JF. Evaluation of fluorodeoxyglucose-positron emission tomographic scanning and its association with glucose transporter expression in medullary thyroid carcinoma and pheochromocytoma: a clinical and molecular study. *Surgery*1997;122:1049–1060.
32. Salvatori M, Melis L, Castaldi P, Maussier ML, Rufini V, Perotti G, Rubello D. Clinical significance of focal and diffuse thyroid diseases identified by (18)F-fluorodeoxyglucose positron emission tomography. *Biomed Pharmacother* 2007;61:488–493.
33. Karantanis D, Bogsrud TV, Wiseman GA, Mullan BP, Subramaniam RM, Nathan MA, Peller PJ, Bahn RS, Lowe VJ. Clinical significance of diffusely increased 18F-FDG uptake in the thyroid gland. *J Nucl Med* 2007;48:896–901.
34. Podoloff DA, Ball DW, Ben-Josef E, Benson AB, Cohen SJ, Coleman RE, Delbeke D, Ho M, Ilson DH, Kalemkerian GP, Lee RJ, Loeffler JS, Macapinlac HA, Morgan RJ, Siegel BA, Singhal S, Tyler DS, Wong RJ. NCCN Task Force: Clinical Utility of PET in a Variety of Tumor Types Task Force. *J Natl Compr Canc Netw* 2009;7 Suppl 2:S1–S23. http://www.nccn.org/professionals/physician_gls/f_guidelines.asp
35. Fletcher JW, Djulbegovic B, Soares HP, Siegel BA, Lowe VJ, Lyman GH, Coleman E, Wahl R, Paschold JC, Avril N , Einhorn LH, Suh WW, Samson D, Delbeke D, Gorman M, Shields AF. Recommendations for the use of FDG(fluorine-18, (2-[18F]Fluoro-2-deoxy-D-glucose) Positron emission tomography in oncology. *J Nucl Med* 2008;49:480–508.
36. Ruf J, Lehmkuhl L, Bertram H, Sandrock D, Amthauer H, Humplik B, Ludwig Munz D, Felix R. Impact of SPECT and integrated low-dose CT after radioiodine therapy on the management of patients with thyroid carcinoma. *Nucl Med Commun* 2004;25:1177–1182.
37. Ladenson PW. Recombinant thyrotropin versus thyroid hormone withdrawal in evaluating patients with thyroid carcinoma. *Semin Nucl Med* 2000;30:98–106.
38. Schroeder PR, Haugen BR, Pacini F, Reiners C, Schlumberger M, Sherman SI, Cooper DS, Schuff CG, Braverman LE, Skarulis MC, Davies TF, Mazzaferri EL, Daniels GH, Ross DS, Luster M, Samuels MH, Weintraub BD, Ridgway EC, Ladenson PW. A comparison of short-term changes in health-related quality of life in thyroid carcinoma patients undergoing diagnostic evaluation with recombinant human thyrotropin compared with thyroid hormone withdrawal. *J Clin Endocrinol Metab* 2006;91:878–884.

39. Som PM, Curtin HD, Mancuso AA. An imaging-based classification for the cervical nodes designed as an adjunct to recent clinically based nodal classifications. *Arch Otolaryngol Head Neck Surg* 1999;125:388–396.

40. Palmedo H, Bucerius J, Joe A, Strunk H, Hortling N, Meyka S, Roedel R, Wolff M, Wardelmann E, Biersack H-J, Jaeger U. Integrated PET/CT in differentiated thyroid cancer: diagnostic accuracy and impact on patient management. *J Nucl Med* 2006;47:616–624.

41. Yen TC, Lin HD, Lee CH, Chang SL, Yeh SH. The role of technetium-99m sestamibi whole-body scans in diagnosing metastatic Hurthle cell carcinoma of the thyroid gland after total thyroidectomy: A comparison with iodine-131 and thallium-201 whole-body scans. *Eur J Nucl Med* 1994;21:980–983.

42. Stojadinovic A, Hoos A, Ghossein RA, Urist MJ, Leung DHY, Spiro RH, Shah HP, Brennan MF, Singh B, Shaha AR. Hurthle cell carcinoma: A 60-year experience. *Ann Surg Oncol* 2002;9:197–203.

43. Lowe VJ, Kim H, Boyd JH, Eisenbeis JF, Dunphy FR, Fletcher JW. Primary and recurrent early stage laryngeal cancer: preliminary results of 2-[fluorine 18]fluoro-2-deoxy-D-glucose PET imaging. *Radiology* 1999;212:799–802.

44. Papotti M, Kumar U, Volante M, Pecchioni C, Patel YC. Immunohistochemical detection of somatostatin receptor types 1–5 in medullary carcinoma of the thyroid. *Clin Endocrinol(Oxf)* 2001;54:641–649.

45. Krausz Y, Keidar Z, Kogan I, Even-Sapir E, Bar-Shalom R, Engel A, Rubinstein R, Sachs J, Bocher M, Agranovicz S, Chisin R, Israel O. SPECT/CT hybrid imaging with 111In-pentetreotide in assessment of neuroendocrine tumours. *Clin Endocrinol(Oxf)* 2003;59:565–573.

46. Pfannenberg AC, Eschmann SM, Horger M, Lamberts R, Vonthein R, Claussen CD, Bares R. Benefit of anatomical-functional image fusion in the diagnostic work-up of neuroendocrine neoplasms. *Eur J Nucl Med Mol Imaging* 2003;30:835–843.

47. Jacene HA, Goudarzi B, Wahl RL. Scalene muscle uptake: a potential pitfall in head and neck PET/CT. *Eur J Nucl Med Mol Imaging* 2008;35:89–94.

# Chapter II.11
# Endocrine Tumors

Yodphat Krausz

## Introduction

Endocrine tumors constitute a heterogeneous group of neoplasms that originate in the pituitary, thyroid, and parathyroid glands, the endocrine pancreatic islets, and the neuroendocrine (NE) cells in the adrenal glands or dispersed in the digestive and respiratory tracts.

Management of patients with endocrine tumors depends on their early detection since surgery is the mainstay of treatment. Localization and staging are based on conventional anatomical modalities including computed tomography (CT), ultrasound (US), or magnetic resonance imaging (MRI), and on scintigraphic functional techniques characterized by unique uptake and transport mechanisms in the presence of high density of membrane receptors. Conventional imaging is the major diagnostic tool for localization of morphological abnormalities. Functional and metabolic imaging using single-photon emission computed tomography (SPECT) or positron emission tomography (PET) and various tumor-avid radiopharmaceuticals may, however, detect a tumor prior to its visualization on CT, or may express the functional significance of anatomical findings, with impact on treatment strategy. The functional techniques are limited in the presence of small lesion size, low resolution and relatively low contrast, and scarcity of anatomical delineation. Furthermore, concurrent foci may reflect the bio-distribution of the radiotracer or processes unrelated to the underlying disease.

Hybrid functional and anatomical imaging systems have led to a major breakthrough in diagnosis, staging, and follow-up of patients with endocrine tumors. Fusion images clarify the nature of the abnormality, and optimize diagnosis and staging of the disease processes. The anatomical maps provide precise localization of SPECT or PET findings and allow for exclusion of disease in sites of physiological tracer uptake. In addition, hybrid imaging systems equipped with a low-dose CT may be used as a bridge to diagnostic high-resolution, contrast-enhanced CT or MRI of a specific area of interest.

This chapter evaluates the contribution of hybrid SPECT/CT and PET/CT to image analysis and to management of patients with gastroenteropancreatic (GEP) and neural crest tumors, and parathyroid adenoma.

Y. Krausz (✉)
Department of Medical Biophysics and Nuclear Medicine, Hadassah Hebrew University Medical Center, Jerusalem, Israel
e-mail: yodphat@hadassah.org.il

D. Delbeke, O. Israel (eds.), *Hybrid PET/CT and SPECT/CT Imaging*,
DOI 10.1007/978-0-387-92820-3_13, © Springer Science+Business Media, LLC 2010

## Imaging Protocols

Hybrid imaging systems allow for sequential acquisition of anatomic transmission (CT) and functional emission (either PET or SPECT) data during a single session by using a single imaging device.

In our experience the routinely used SPECT/low-dose CT imaging devices combine a dual-head, variable gamma camera with a low-dose or diagnostic CT mounted on the same gantry.[1-4] The study is performed after tracer administration, following planar imaging. CT acquisition is performed according the manufacturer's guidelines for the specific device, and SPECT is acquired using tracer-adapted protocols. For $^{99m}$Tc- and $^{123}$I-labeled radio-pharmaceuticals, high-resolution, low-energy collimators are used, and 360° SPECT images are obtained in a matrix size of 128 × 128, with a 3° angle step, at 20 s per frame for $^{111}$In, a 6° angle step at 30 s per frame study is acquired using medium-energy collimators. Reconstruction is performed iteratively, with the ordered subsets expectation maximization (OSEM) technique. The resultant transaxial, sagittal, and coronal emission data are registered with the transmission data to generate hybrid images fusing, superimposed anatomical (CT), and functional (SPECT) images.

Hybrid PET/CT systems provide high-quality images of both PET and CT, precise alignment of the two data sets, as well as CT attenuation correction of PET images. PET/CT has significant advantages over PET stand-alone, including the more accurate localization of foci of abnormal tracer uptake, differentiation of pathologic from physiologic activity, and enhancement in guiding and monitoring the efficacy of therapy.

For $^{18}$F-fluorodeoxyglucose (FDG) imaging, patients fast at least 4 h prior to tracer injection, and a PET/CT study is acquired from vertex to mid-thigh, after a 60–90 min uptake period. $^{18}$F-FDG, while being a widely accepted radiopharmaceutical in clinical oncology, has, however, a limited role in assessment of endocrine tumors. Amine precursors and somatostatin analogs have been labeled with positron emitters, such as $^{11}$C (T1/2 = 20 min), $^{18}$F (T1/2 = 110 min), and $^{68}$Ga (T1/2 = 68 min), as an alternative for $^{18}$F-FDG imaging in NE tumors. For CT acquisition, which is usually the first step of the study, oral contrast agents and intravenous (IV) contrast can be administered. PET images are subsequently acquired for 2–5 min per bed position according to the type of system and acquisition protocol. PET data are reconstructed with and without attenuation correction and are fused with the corresponding CT slices. Transaxial, coronal, and sagittal PET, CT, and PET/CT images, as well as a maximum intensity projection (MIP) in three-dimensional cine mode of the PET data are presented for review.

## SPECT/CT and PET/CT Tracers for Imaging of NE Tumors

NE tumors constitute a rare class of well-differentiated solid tumors characterized by membrane-bound dense-core secretory granules, marker proteins, and neuropeptide cell type-specific hormonal products. Functioning tumors may secrete biologically active substances. Non-functioning tumors may only exhibit immunopositivity for markers, with no distinct clinical syndrome.

NE tumors include GEP tumors, neural crest tumors, and medullary thyroid cancer (MTC, discussed in Chapter II.10). Some of these tumors have a low proliferation rate, go undetected for years, and benefit only from complete surgical removal prior to spread. Once metastases are present, tumor debulking may prolong survival and provide significant symptomatic relief. When the disease is non-resectable, unnecessary surgery may be spared, and tumor-targeted treatment with labeled ligands is suggested. Accurate staging has therefore a significant impact on planning the treatment strategy.

NE tumors may be difficult to localize because of their small size, multiplicity, and presence in hollow organs, and thus can benefit from integration of anatomical and functional imaging techniques. The main anatomical modalities used in diagnosis and staging of NE tumors include conventional, intra-operative, and endoscopic US, CT, MRI, and selective arteriography. These techniques fail to disclose tumor sites that are either too small to have caused morphological alterations, too numerous to permit clear characterization, or obscured by structural changes related to previous surgery.

Functional imaging modalities can detect the presence of metastatic disease throughout the body and identify small tumor sites prior to conventional imaging. These techniques are based on detection of high-density membrane receptors using somatostatin receptor scintigraphy (SRS), on the unique uptake of analogs of hormone precursors, expression of transporters, and synthesis as well as storage of hormones, using meta-iodo-benzyl-guanidine (MIBG) and amine precursors.

Overexpression of receptors, identified with somatostatin analogs labeled with [111]In and [68]Ga, using SPECT/CT and PET/CT, respectively, has led to a major breakthrough in the management of NE tumors. This involves mainly improved localization of an occult primary tumor, precise staging, early detection of recurrence, monitoring treatment effects, and determining receptor status for targeted therapy. These imaging modalities have thus become essential diagnostic tools assessing patients with NE tumors prior to initiation of treatment.[5]

The radiopharmaceutical of choice for SRS is [111]In-diethylene triamine pentaacetic acid (DTPA)-Octreotide ([111]In-pentetreotide), which binds preferentially to somatostatin receptor (SSTR) subtypes II and V, with a reported sensitivity of 82–95%. SRS lacks structural details for anatomical delineation. Specificity is also hampered by the tracer bio-distribution related to receptor status of various organs as well as to the elimination route via the kidneys and the gastrointestinal tract (GIT). False-positive results may also derive from other concomitant disease processes and have been reported to adversely affect the clinical management in 2.7% of patients.[6] These limitations may be overcome by SPECT/CT. When the disease is confined to a single organ, such as the liver, a single mode of organ-specific therapy is suggested. When a soft tissue mass has invaded an adjacent bone, futile surgery is spared. In extensive, unresectable disease, systemic therapy is required. Hybrid imaging also facilitates quantification of the degree of uptake of radiolabeled ligands administered for therapeutic purposes following the visualization of tumor sites on diagnostic scans.

False-negative SRS using [111]In-pentetreotide is mostly encountered in the presence of low density of SSTRs with resulting lack of tumor uptake. The relatively poor spatial resolution of planar and SPECT studies is also one of the reasons for the poor tumor detectability rate, particularly for small tumors.

Somatostatin analogs have been synthesized and radiolabeled for diagnosis and therapy, following structural modifications, with the use of alternative chelators and radiometals resulting in considerable changes in SSTR affinity profiles. DOTA-Tyr3-octreotide (DOTATOC) with improved binding affinity, internalization rate, and selectivity for SSTR2 and DOTA-1-NaI3-octreotide (DOTANOC) with a broader SSTR subtype profile have been labeled with [111]In, [68]Ga, and [86]Y for diagnostic and therapeutic applications. The newer somatostatin analogs, DOTATOC and DOTANOC, have improved pharmacokinetics, faster tumor uptake, and more rapid clearance, and the increased tumor-to-background contrast improves tumor visualization. Labeling with a positron-emitting radioisotope adds the advantages of high-resolution imaging, which enhances lesion detectability, and the ability to quantitate tracer uptake for planning and monitoring peptide receptor radionuclide therapy. [68]Ga-DOTATOC had higher detection rates of NE tumors as compared with CT, [111]In-DOTATOC, and [111]In-DTPA-octreotide-SPECT.[7,8] The newer [68]Ga-DOTANOC analog further increases image quality and has been suggested for routine receptor PET/CT studies.[9,10]

Additional functional modalities are based on uptake of amine precursors and MIBG into the NE cell. MIBG is a guanidine derivative that exploits the specific type 1 amine uptake mechanism at the cell membrane and from the cytoplasm and is stored within intracellular vesicles. MIBG can be labeled with the single-photon emitters [123]I and [131]I, and used for diagnostic and therapeutic purposes, respectively.

NE cells are also characterized by their unique capacity to take up and decarboxylate aromatic amine precursors such as 5-hydroxytryptophan (HTP) and dihydroxyphenylala-nine (DOPA). Following decarboxylation, these precursors are converted into the corresponding amines serotonin and dopamine, stored in intracellular vesicles. Tracers such as [11]C-5-HTP, [11]C-DOPA, or [18]F-DOPA have been developed for localization of carcinoid and endocrine pancreatic tumors, and 6-[18]F-fluorodopamine for pheochromocytoma.

Overall, [11]C-5-HTP-PET has the potential to detect more tumor sites than SRS and CT, visualizing the primary tumor in 84% compared with 47 and 42% of patients for SRS and CT, respectively.[11] [18]F-DOPA PET has also been suggested to play a complementary role in the evaluation of NE tumors, mainly when MIBG, SRS, CT, or MRI have failed to identify the tumor, but not as a substitute for these other modalities.[12,13]

[18]F-FDG, the most widely used PET tracer for diagnosis, staging, and treatment monitoring in clinical oncology, fails to detect well-differentiated tumors associated with a low proliferative rate and has only been suggested in less-differentiated GEP tumors with high proliferative activity and in metastatic MTC associated with rapidly increasing carcinoembryonic antigen (CEA) levels.[14]

## SPECT/CT and PET/CT of GEP Tumors

According to recent World Health Organization criteria, GEP tumors (carcinoid and islet cell tumors), have been subdivided into well-differentiated endocrine tumors, well-differentiated and poorly differentiated endocrine carcinoma. In the past, carcinoid tumors were classified according to the site of origin, with the GIT and lung being the main locations for the primary tumor. The tumors can originate from the foregut (respiratory tract, thymus, stomach, duodenum, and pancreas), midgut (small intestine, appendix, right colon), or the hindgut (transverse colon, sigmoid, and rectum), with accordingly different metastatic spread and different symptomatology.

The primary GIT carcinoid requires surgical removal to prevent complications,[15] but is difficult to diagnose at an early stage because of small size, multiplicity of lesions, and intramural location in hollow organs. CT and MRI detect larger primary tumors (10–30 mm), liver and lymph node metastases, mesenteric invasion, and vascular encasement, and colonoscopy identifies tumors in the distal ileum, ileocecal valve, or the ascending colon.[16–18] SRS has a sensitivity ranging between 80 and 90% for diagnosis of the primary carcinoid, regional lymph nodes, and distant metastases, superior to that of CT and MRI.

Endocrine pancreatic tumors, classified according to their hormonal secretion include gastrinomas, of which 90% are malignant, with metastases detected in 60–80% of patients at the time of diagnosis, glucagonomas and VIPomas, which also show metastases in 90 and 60% of cases, respectively, at presentation. Insulinoma is benign in 90% of patients. Endocrine pancreatic tumors and their metastases can be localized in about 50% of cases using US, CT, MRI, and/or angiography.[19–21] CT is the imaging modality of choice for detection of islet cell tumors, and MRI is used for detection of small functional tumors.[22] SRS has an overall sensitivity of 80–95% for GEP tumors.[19,23]

Several reports have shown the contribution of SPECT/CT as an adjunct to SRS in patients with GEP tumors, mainly by delineating soft tissue tumors, detecting invasion into adjacent bones, identifying previously unknown, or changing the location of tumor sites, with further impact on management of up to one third of the patient population.[24–27] When SRS is negative, SPECT/CT may confirm the absence of receptor density in a tumor visualized on CT.

Various PET tracers have been used in GEP tumors. The labeled precursor of serotonin, [11]C-5-HTP, has been found superior to SRS and CT in patients with carcinoid, with a potential role in treatment monitoring of these patients.[11,28] Pathological uptake of [18]F-DOPA has also been documented in GIT carcinoid, with an overall sensitivity of 65% compared with 29% for [18]F-FDG PET, 57% for SRS, and 73% for CT and MRI. Conventional imaging was reported to be the most sensitive tool for detection of visceral metastases, whereas [18]F-DOPA was superior in diagnosis of primary tumors and lymph node metastases.[29] [18]F-DOPA appears to be also highly accurate in detection of skeletal metastases and superior to SRS in all organs except for the liver.[30] [18]F-DOPA PET/CT changed the clinical management in 84% of patients with GEP tumors.[31]

Comparison of [18]F-FDG PET with SRS demonstrates the difference between metabolic activity and receptor expression in NE tumors, with FDG-avidity being demonstrated in less-differentiated GEP tumors where SRS failed to detect any lesion.[32,33]

In summary, SRS SPECT/CT using [111]In-pentetreotide or PET/CT using [68]Ga-labeled analogs are valuable tools for assessment of well-differentiated GEP tumors, with significant impact on patient management. PET using [68]Ga-DOTANOC contributes especially for diagnosis of small tumors bearing only a low density of SSTRs. [11]C-5-HTP is highly sensitive and exceeds both SRS and CT in tumor visualization, with the exception of poorly differentiated or non-functioning tumors.[18]F-FDG may be useful in distinguishing tumors characterized by rapid growth and aggressive behavior. Hybrid imaging defines the localization and functional status of the tumor, optimizes the surgical approach in patients with resectable tumors, and helps tailor the optimal treatment strategy for advanced disease.

## SPECT/CT and PET/CT of Neural Crest Tumors

Pheochromocytoma, a tumor originating in the adrenergic nervous system, resides mainly in the adrenal gland, and is best visualized by CT or MRI, with an overall sensitivity of 93–100%. The prevalence of malignancy ranges from 13 to 26%. The diagnostic modality of choice for metastatic disease is scintigraphy using [123]I-MIBG, with an overall sensitivity of 86–88% and specificity of 96–99%. Expression of tumor-specific catecholamine transport and storage mechanisms by pheochromocytoma tumor cells provides the basis for scintigraphy, mainly using [123]I-MIBG. Spatial resolution of [123]I-MIBG scans remains limited even with SPECT, and [123]I-MIBG-avid foci may require anatomical correlation, using SPECT/CT.

Hybrid images may contribute to diagnosis when unilateral, asymmetric, low-intensity uptake occurs in one of the adrenal glands, characterizing areas of normal [123]I-MIBG biodistribution or excretion, and also facilitates detection of recurrent or metastatic disease in the vicinity of normal structures with high tracer uptake such as the myocardium and liver.[34] Furthermore, SPECT/CT can differentiate between [123]I-MIBG-avid retroperitoneal recurrence and adrenal gland hyperplasia following contralateral adrenalectomy and optimize characterization of equivocal findings on CT.[35]

It has been suggested that when an MIBG scan is negative, [18]F-FDG-PET and SRS may provide additional information, although not specific for pheochromocytoma. The sensitivity of [18]F-FDG for solitary benign or malignant pheochromocytoma is of approximately 70%, detecting and localizing dedifferentiated and/or rapidly growing tumors. SRS has also been suggested for evaluation of non-MIBG-avid tumors, mainly when malignant or metastatic, with sensitivity of approximately 90%, but has not been recommended for initial diagnostic work-up.

Other PET radiopharmaceuticals, including [18]F-DOPA and [11]C-hydroxyephedrine have been suggested for patients with negative [123]I-MIBG scintigraphy.[36] [18]F-DOPA has been reported to have both a sensitivity and specificity of 100% in patients with adrenal pheochromocytoma as compared to a sensitivity of 71% for [123]I-MIBG.[37] [18]F-DOPA had, however, a lower lesion-based detectability rate when compared to CT or MRI.[38] An additional somatostatin analog, DOTA-D-Phen1-Tyr3-Thr8-octreotide labeled with [68]Ga ([68]Ga-DOTATATE) showed more lesions with higher uptake and better resolution compared to [123]I-MIBG in patients with malignant pheochromocytoma, with potential impact on therapy with [90]Y-labeled DOTATATE.[39]

Neuroblastoma (NB) is one of the most common solid extracranial malignancy in children and will be discussed in more details in Chapter II.15. [123]I-MIBG scintigraphy is used for diagnosis of a primary lesion that is inaccessible to biopsy, staging, determining prognosis, radio-guided surgery, and response to therapy, and for defining the need for targeted radiotherapy. SPECT/CT improves the delineation of physiologic, diffuse intra-luminal bowel activity, localization of tumor sites, and detection of bone and bone marrow involvement. Similar to pheochromocytoma, SPECT/CT may characterize tumor recurrence adjacent to organs with physiologic [123]I-MIBG activity. In this group of pediatric patients, SPECT/CT may also clarify the nature of the diffuse heterogeneous physiologic uptake in the right heart, sometimes misinterpreted as malignant paramedian mediastinal, sternal, or vertebral sites of tumor involvement.[40] SPECT/CT can also differentiate between bilateral symmetric upper thoracic activity, probably related to physiologic muscular or brown fat uptake, and malignant lesions such as skeletal metastases in the scapulae or ribs, or malignant supraclavicular lymphadenopathy.[35] SPECT/CT has been advocated as a tool for quantification of radiation dose delivered during [131]I-MIBG therapy, using CT-based measurements of tumor volume-of-interest.[41] Most neuroblastomas accumulate [18]F-FDG, and PET has been found to be equal or superior to MIBG scans for identifying soft tissue and extracranial skeletal metastases, for revealing small lesions, and for delineating the extent and localizing sites of disease.[42,43]

In summary, SPECT/CT is an important tool for localization of MIBG-avid sites and for characterization of their benign or malignant significance, with subsequent impact on treatment with [131]I-MIBG. Additional radiopharmaceuticals, including [18]F-FDG and more specific PET tracers, have been suggested for diagnosis and staging of pheochromo-cytoma in patients with a negative MIBG scan at presentation.

## SPECT/CT of Parathyroid Adenoma

The most appropriate therapeutic approach for parathyroid adenoma, which accounts for 85% of primary hyperparathyroidism, is surgery. The classic surgical procedure of bilateral neck exploration has been gradually replaced by minimally invasive surgical procedures that are associated with a low risk of hypoparathyroidism or recurrent laryngeal nerve injury and also allow for shortening of the time of surgery and hospitalization. These new approaches include unilateral neck exploration, minimally invasive parathyroidectomy, endoscopic surgery, and video-assisted thoracic surgery.

The new surgical approaches to hyperparathyroidism have become feasible due to the improved preoperative localization using diagnostic modalities such as scintigra-phy with $^{99m}$Tc-sestamibi scintigraphy. A meta-analysis covering 10 years in the English literature reported that $^{99m}$Tc-sestamibi scintigraphy had an average sensitiv-ity and specificity of 91 and 99%, respectively.[44] An additional non-statistical sys-tematic meta-analysis including 52 studies reported sensitivity ranging between 39 and above 90%, with surgical findings serving as gold standard.[45]

About 80–85% of parathyroid adenomas are located adjacent to the thyroid gland. The combined use of $^{99m}$Tc-sestamibi and US is considered the imaging strategy of choice for localization of a cervical parathyroid adenoma. In case of an ectopic parathyroid adenoma, which can occur in 8–11% of patients, CT is superior to US for localization to the retrotracheal, retroesophageal and mediastinal space. Most authors now favor a wide application of $^{99m}$Tc-sestamibi SPECT in addition to planar scintigraphy prior to initial surgery, either at the early or delayed phase, because of its increase in sensitivity from 74–87% to 91–96% when compared with planar scinti-graphy.[45–49] $^{99m}$Tc-sestamibi SPECT does not provide, however, detailed anatomical information. It lacks landmarks for precise tomographic orientation in the mediast-inal compartment.

Several reports have documented the role of $^{99m}$Tc-sestamibi SPECT/CT in visua-lization of a parathyroid adenoma. SPECT/CT precisely localizes the majority of adenomas prior to surgery, including the ectopic lesions, with a localization rate of 88% as compared to 53% for both planar $^{99m}$Tc-sestamibi scintigraphy and cervical US.[50] SPECT/CT had a sensitivity of 91%, specificity 95%, PPV 82%, and NPV of 97%, as compared to 85, 93, 76, and 95%, respectively, for SPECT stand-alone and 68, 90, 65, and 91%, respectively, for CT.[51] SPECT/CT had a major impact, pre-dominantly in ectopic parathyroid adenomas, as documented in several studies includ-ing patients with primary hyperparathyroidism who subsequently underwent neck or mediastinal exploration.[24,52,53] In addition to the benefits of SPECT/CT for precise localization of lesions, CT attenuation correction of the SPECT data increases image contrast, but has no impact on detection rate.[54] SPECT/CT can lead to a modifica-tion of the surgical approach in patients with an uncommon location of the para-thyroid glands to the retrotracheal space.[55] In an extensive study of 833 patients with primary hyperparathyroidism who underwent scintigraphic evaluation of parathyroid adenomas using various protocols, SPECT/CT, performed in 180 patients, did not contribute to a reduction of the false positive rate. However, SPECT/CT after negative planar scintigraphy identified a solitary focus in six patients, with verification at surgery in five of them.[56] Early SPECT/CT in combination with delayed imaging was statistically significantly superior to any single or dual phase planar or SPECT studies, suggesting that dual phase imaging with early SPECT/CT should be part of the preoperative evaluation of patients with primary hyperparathyroidism in the era of minimally invasive parathyroidectomy.[57]

In summary, planar [99m]Tc-sestamibi scintigraphy diagnoses a parathyroid adenoma in the neck in the majority of patients with primary hyperparathyroidism, mainly with the thyroid serving as an anatomical landmark in the early phase of the study. SPECT/CT, however, contributes to localization of ectopic adenomas and may facilitate the surgical intervention in patients with multinodular goiter and/or distorted anatomy after neck surgery or radioiodine ablation of the thyroid for unrelated diseases.

## Summary

A thorough understanding of the physiology, pathophysiology, and clinical context of SSTRs and metabolic processes, with careful analysis of fused functional–anatomic images, facilitates the interpretation of studies and the subsequent management of patients with endocrine tumors. Best results are obtained with a combination of functional imaging tests, such as SRS with SPECT/CT or PET/CT and high-resolution morphological imaging, such as contrast-enhanced CT and/or MRI. SSTRs are expressed on most NE tumors, therefore the high efficacy of labeled somatostatin analogs for imaging and therapy. [18]F-FDG appears to be of value mainly in poorly differentiated NE tumors. Positron emitters such as [11]C-5HTP and [11]C- or [18]F-DOPA have been found superior to CT and SRS in detection of NE tumors, predominantly of small foci of disease. Functional imaging with PET using these compounds is now being employed to complement rather than to replace other imaging modalities.

SPECT/CT and PET/CT play an increasing role in imaging of endocrine tumors, for functional characterization and staging of disease during initial work-up and for early detection of tumor recurrence after treatment, especially in the presence of inconclusive anatomical studies, as well as for dosimetric estimation for targeted radionuclide therapy. Hybrid imaging provides better definition of tumors that are radiotracer-avid and of their relationship with adjacent structures, defines the functional significance of lesions on CT, and improves the specificity of SPECT and/or PET data by excluding disease at sites of physiological uptake or excretion.

## Case Presentations

### *Case II.11.1 (DICOM Images on DVD)*

**History**

This 50-year-old man was referred for SRS following the incidental diagnosis of a well-differentiated NE tumor in a mesenteric mass. The patient had been previously followed with CT after diagnosis of Hodgkin's disease involving the mediastinum 9 years prior to current examination. A recent CT demonstrated a solitary 34 × 25 mm mass in the mesentery, above the level of aortic bifurcation, with moderate $^{18}$F-FDG-avidity on PET/CT (Fig. II.11.1A), but no mediastinal recurrence. Fine needle aspiration (FNA) suggested the diagnosis of a primary or metastatic well-differentiated NE tumor (carcinoid). $^{111}$In-pentetreotide SPECT/CT was performed in search of a primary tumor, for staging and determination of receptor status (Fig. II.11.1B–D).

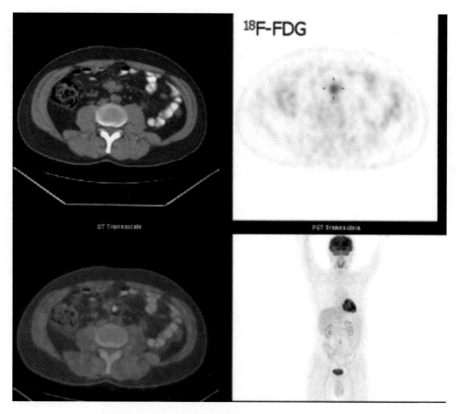

**Fig. II.11.1A**

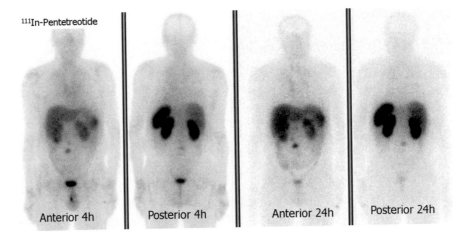

Fig. II.11.1B

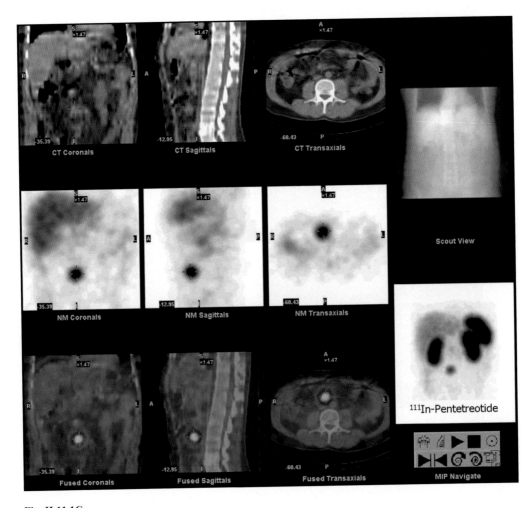

Fig. II.11.1C

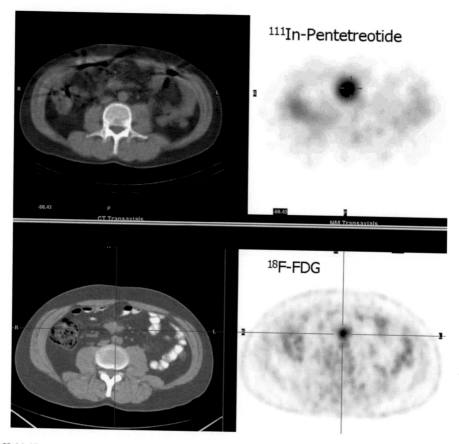

**Fig. II.11.1D**

**Findings**

Whole-body (WB) SRS shows a focus with high density of receptors in the mid-abdomen
(Fig. II.11.1B) corresponding to a 36 × 27 mm mesenteric mass on the CT component of the
SPECT/CT (Fig. II.11.1C, D, upper row) and PET/CT (Fig. II.11A, D, lower row) and to
the [18]F-FDG-avid tumor site (Fig. II.11A, D, lower row). Additional low-intensity foci are
visualized on the WB study at the level of the third part of the duodenum and in the right
paramediastinal area, with no corresponding CT abnormality (Fig. II.11.1B).

**Discussion**

The patient, with Hodgkin's disease in complete remission, was diagnosed with an
[18]F-FDG-avid NE tumor in the mesentery, which expressed high density of SSTRs.
The primary tumor was not detected on CT or colonoscopy.

Primary carcinoid of the GIT is difficult to diagnose at an early stage because of its small
size and location in the walls of hollow organs.[17] Receptor expression in the primary tumor
and metastatic foci is found in mainly well-differentiated tumors, whereas [18]F-FDG-avidity
is documented in carcinoid with high Ki-67 expression, poor differentiation, and a high
proliferation rate.[33] The mesenteric mass in this patient showed both receptor expression

and [18]F-FDG-avidity, but all techniques failed to identify the primary tumor, including colonoscopy, which was also negative. Capsule endoscopy, however, identified an ileal polypoid lesion, consistent with carcinoid.

### Diagnosis

Well-differentiated NE carcinoma in small intestine with mesenteric metastasis.

### Follow-up

At surgery, the primary well-differentiated neuroendocrine carcinoma was identified in the small bowel, 120 cm proximal to the ileocecal valve, 10 mm in diameter, with invasion of the muscularis, and a proliferation index of less than 1%. The tumor was removed along with a solitary metastatic lymph node (30 mm) among nine nodes examined. Follow up CT of the abdomen at 10 months after surgery was within normal limits.

### Clinical Report: Body [18]F-FDG PET/CT, and [111]In-Pentetreotide SPECT/CT (for DVD cases only)

Indication

Staging of well-differentiated NE tumor.

History

This 50-year-old man presented with a $34 \times 25$ mm mesenteric tumor mass detected on CT performed for follow-up of Hodgkin's disease. [18]F-FDG-avidity was documented on PET in the tumor mass. On FNA, a well-differentiated NE tumor was diagnosed, and the patient was referred for further evaluation with [111]In-pentetreotide imaging.

Procedure: PET/CT

The patient was instructed to fast for 5 h and had a normal blood glucose level prior to [18]F-FDG injection. PET/CT with low-dose CT for anatomical correlation and attenuation correction of PET emission images was initiated 65 min after the IV injection of 381 MBq (10.3 mCi) of [18]F-FDG and covered the area from vertex to mid-thighs.

Procedure: [111]In-Pentetreotide SRS

Planar images were acquired from vertex to mid-thighs at 4 h and 24 h after IV injection of 222 MBq (6 mCi) of [111]In-pentetreotide, with SPECT/CT of the chest, abdomen, and pelvis performed at 24 h after tracer injection.

Findings: PET/CT

> *Quality of study*: The quality of the study is good. There is physiologic distribution of the radiopharmaceutical in the brain, myocardium, bowel, liver, and renal collecting system.
> *Brain*: Within normal range.
> *Head and neck*: No definite abnormality.

*Chest*: On the CT portion of the PET/CT, there are bronchiectases seen in the right upper lobe.

*Abdomen*: Moderate $^{18}$F-FDG uptake is identified in a mesenteric $36 \times 27$ mm mass below the level of the aortic bifurcation.

*Pelvis*: On the CT portion of the PET/CT, two renal calculi are identified in the left kidney.

Findings: $^{111}$In-Pentetreotide SRS

*Quality of study*: The quality of the study is adequate. There is physiologic distribution of the radiopharmaceutical to the liver, spleen, and kidneys.

*Skull*: Within normal range

*Head and neck*: No definite abnormality

*Chest*: Faint uptake in the paramediastinal area, with no corresponding abnormality on the CT component of the SPECT/CT.

*Abdomen*: Moderate tracer uptake is demonstrated in the mesenteric mass. Faint focal uptake is also visualized cranially to this mass, but with no corresponding CT abnormality.

*Pelvis*: No focal increased density of receptors was identified.

Impression

Moderate $^{18}$F-FDG and $^{111}$In-pentetreotide uptake in a mesenteric mass diagnosed as a well-differentiated NE tumor on FNA. No other foci of abnormal $^{18}$F-FDG uptake or $^{111}$In-pentetreotide were identified. Surgery was recommended.

## *Case II.11.2*

### History

This 86-year-old man presented with excessive diarrhea and weight loss for 18 months. A mass was detected on CT in the body of the pancreas, and the patient was referred to [111]In-pentetreotide SPECT/CT for assessment of the SSTR status (Fig. II.11.2A, B).

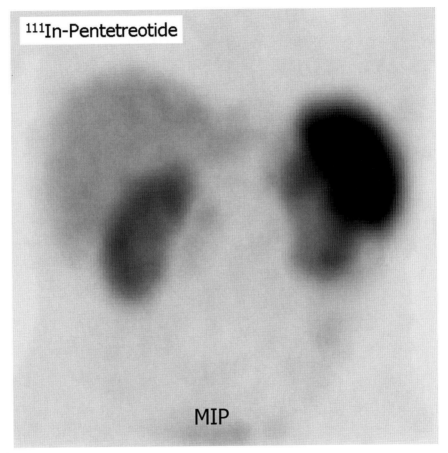

**Fig. II.11.2A**

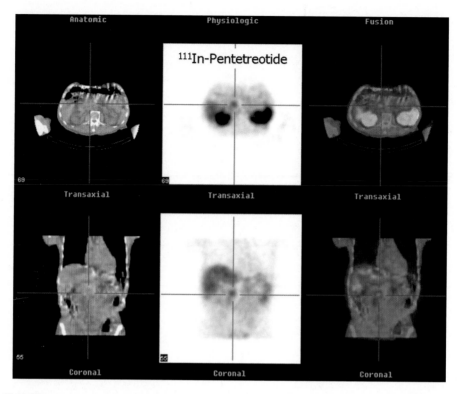

**Fig. II.11.2B**

### Findings

Planar (not shown) and 3D MIP SPECT images show a faint focus of low intensity tracer uptake in the vicinity of the right kidney that does not indicate the presence of any significant receptor density (Fig. II.11.2A). Attenuation-corrected transaxial (upper row) and coronal (lower row) SPECT/CT images show a focus of slightly increased tracer activity in an area anterior, superior, and medial to the upper pole of the right kidney, corresponding to the tumor visualized on the CT component in the body of the pancreas (Fig. II.11.2B). Given the patient's history and clinical symptoms, this was considered to represent a VIPoma within the body of the pancreas. No pathological tumor sites suggestive of metastatic disease were visualized.

### Discussion

VIPoma is a rare tumor of the endocrine pancreas associated with secretory diarrhea. Pancreatic VIPomas are usually solitary, more than 30 mm in diameter. In most cases, because of the size of the tumor, CT can readily detect the primary tumor.[19] Approximately 60–70% of VIPomas are metastatic at the time of diagnosis. SRS has been used for the detection of both the primary tumor and its metastases.[20] Whereas in this case no VIP plasma measurements were available, symptoms and CT finding in the region of the pancreas, associated with a relatively high density of SSTRs detected on SRS, suggested the presence of a VIPoma. The presence of these receptors in the

primary tumor indicated that octreotide may represent a therapeutic option for relief of symptoms. The patient was not due to undergo surgical resection of the pancreatic tumor.

**Diagnosis**

VIPoma in body of the pancreas.

## Case II.11.3

**History**

This 55-year-old female was referred for re-staging of an endocrine carcinoma of the pancreas. The patient had undergone Whipple operation 5 years prior to the current examination, with removal of a tumor (30 mm in diameter) with a high mitotic rate and staining positive for chromogranin and synaptophysin. Follow-up CT revealed the presence of enlarged retroperitoneal lymph nodes. The patient was referred for re-staging and assessment of receptor status using [111]In-pentetreotide SRS (Fig. II.11.3A, B).

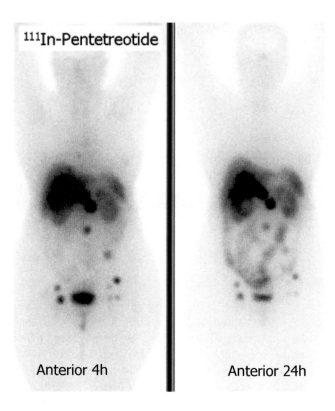

**Fig. II.11.3A**

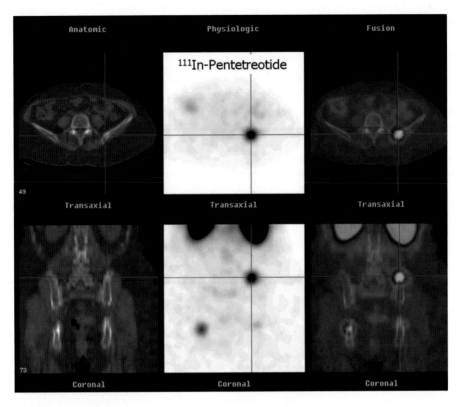

**Fig. II.11.3B**

## Findings

Anterior WB [111]In-pentetreotide scintigraphy at 4 and 24 h after injection of the radiotracer (Fig. II.11.3A) shows multiple sites of abnormal uptake in the abdomen, predominant in the liver, and additional pathological foci in the pelvis and the mid-chest. SPECT/CT (Fig. II.11.3B, transaxial – upper row, coronal slices – lower row) at the level of the pelvis demonstrates the presence of a focus of abnormal uptake localized to an osteoblastic lesion in the left iliac bone seen on the CT component of the SPECT/CT. An additional pathological focus is localized in the right ischium.

The findings were consistent with metastatic disease to liver and bones expressing high density of SSTRs. The patient was referred for peptide radio-receptor therapy, using the labeled somatostatin analog [177]Lu-octreotate. Major regression of hepatic and skeletal metastases was seen on follow-up CT and SRS. The patient reported a symptomatic improvement for 22 months after therapy.

## Discussion

Overexpression of receptors that can be identified with SRS has led to a major breakthrough in the management of NE tumors. SPECT/CT improves the ability to identify and localize occult primary tumors, staging, and early detection of recurrence, as well as defining the receptor status for targeted therapy. SRS with SPECT/CT has become an essential diagnostic modality prior to management of patients with NE tumors.[5]

### Diagnosis

Pancreatic NE carcinoma with disseminated hepatic and skeletal metastases expressing high density of SSTRs.

## Case II.11.4

### History

This 54-year-old woman was referred for $^{123}$I-MIBG SPECT/CT during follow-up of a left adrenal pheochromocytoma (200 × 150 × 100 mm), which had been surgically removed 3 years prior to current examination. There was no clinical or biochemical evidence of recurrence (Fig. II.11.4A, B).

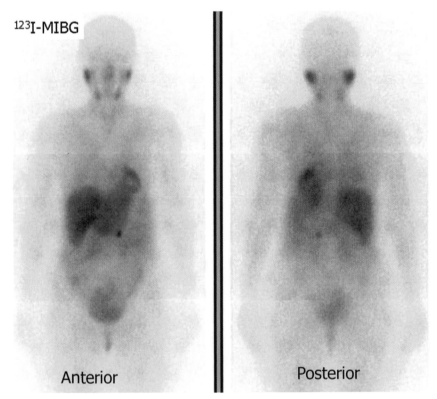

Fig. II.11.4A

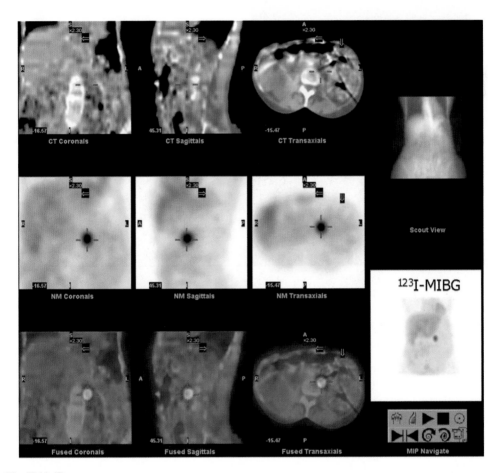

**Fig. II.11.4B**

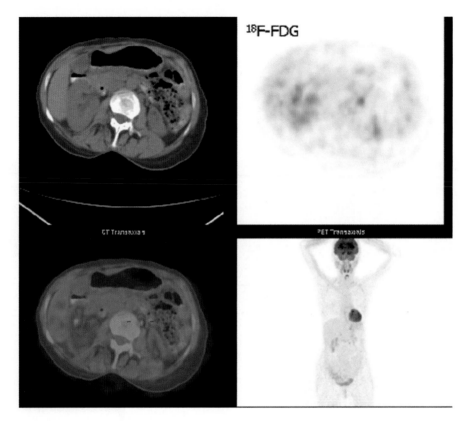

**Fig. II.11.4C**

## Findings

Anterior and posterior WB [123]I-MIBG scintigraphy, 24 h after tracer injection, shows a focus of increased activity in the left upper abdomen (Fig. II.11.4A). SPECT/CT in coronal (left), sagittal (center), and transaxial slices (right) at the level of the abdomino-pelvic region localizes this focus of increased activity to the left paravertebral area of L-3 with no well-defined abnormality detected on the CT component (Fig. II.11.4B).[18]F-FDG PET/CT acquired prior to surgical exploration of a possible tumor recurrence shows an [18]F-FDG-avid focus of moderate intensity in the same area as seen on [123]I-MIBG SPECT/CT (Fig. II.11.4C).

## Discussion

[123]I-MIBG scintigraphy is currently the first-choice functional modality for assessment of patients with pheochromocytoma, with improved sensitivity following the use of [123]I for labeling.[36] Recurrence is suspected when [123]I-MIBG uptake is more intense than that of the liver, as documented in this patient. SPECT/CT improved the localization of the [123]I-MIBG-avid focus but failed to identify a corresponding morphological abnormality.

[18]F-FDG PET, with a sensitivity in the range of 70%, is indicated mainly when the [123]I-MIBG study fails to disclose tumor recurrence.[32] In this particular patient,[18]F-FDG PET/CT was acquired despite the documented [123]I-MIBG avidity, because of the lack of biochemical evidence of recurrence and the lack of any CT abnormalities on the very low dose CT component of the SPECT/CT system used.

## Diagnosis

Suspected recurrence of pheochromocytoma in left adrenal bed.

## Case II.11.5

### History

This 37-year-old man was referred to $^{123}$I-MIBG SPECT/CT, following resection of a huge right adrenal pheochromocytoma (220 × 160 × 130 mm), for further characterization of lung lesions visualized on the CT study performed prior to surgery (Fig. II.11.5A–D).

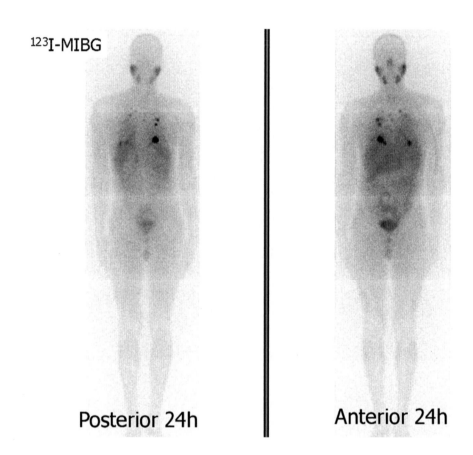

Fig. II.11.5A

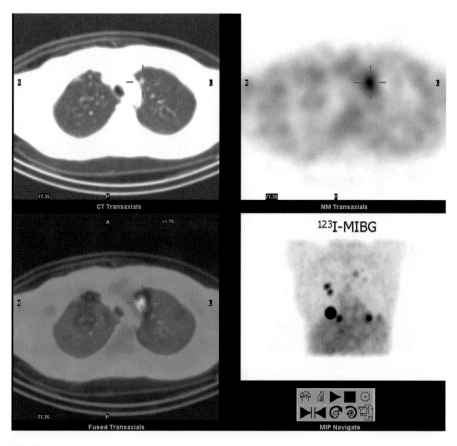

**Fig. II.11.5B**

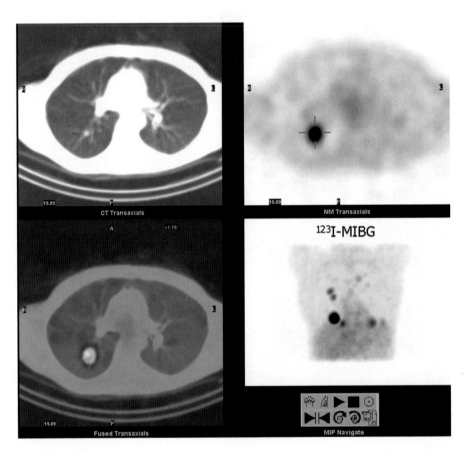

Fig. II.11.5C

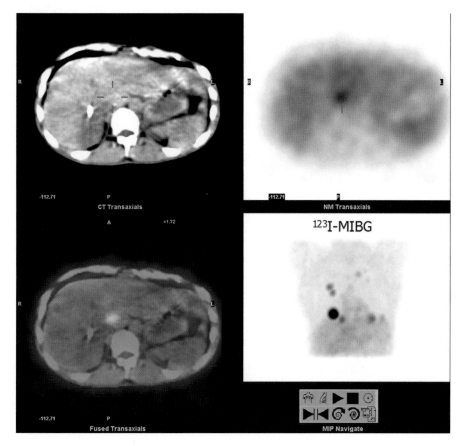

**Fig. II.11.5D**

## Findings

Anterior and posterior WB [123]I-MIBG scintigraphy (Fig. II.11.5A) performed at 24 h after tracer injection shows several lesions in the chest and probable involvement of the upper abdomen. The sites of intense focal [123]I-MIBG activity correspond to several nodules in both lungs seen on the CT component of the SPECT/CT study of the thorax (Fig. II.11.5B, C). An additional [123]I-MIBG-avid focus was localized by SPECT/CT to the liver, with no corresponding abnormality on the low-dose CT component of the study (Fig. II.11.5D). Findings were consistent with [123]I-MIBG-avid pheochromocytoma metastatic to the lungs and liver. The patient was referred for treatment with [131] I-MIBG.

## Discussion

The patient presented with an 18 cm tumor mass in the right abdomen on CT that was initially thought to involve the liver and/or the right adrenal gland. Furthermore, multiple lung lesions were documented. The initial cytological and biopsy diagnosis suggested the presence of adrenocortical carcinoma. However, following surgical resection of the tumor, pheochromocytoma with multiple foci of vascular invasion was diagnosed. [123]I-MIBG scintigraphy showed several [123]I-MIBG-avid lesions in the lungs and an additional solitary lesion in the liver. The patient was then referred for [131]I-MIBG treatment. Chromogranin in the plasma decreased from 22,620 ng/mL prior to surgery to 332 ng/mL (normal: 19–98 ng/mL) after the initial dose of [131]I-MIBG therapy.

## Diagnosis

[123]I-MIBG-avid pheochromocytoma, metastatic to lungs and liver.

## *Case II.11.6*

### History

This 64-year-old woman was referred for preoperative localization of a parathyroid adenoma prior to re-exploration. She has a history of $^{131}$I treatment for toxic multinodular goiter 6 years prior to current examination and presented with persistent primary hyperparathyroidism including calcium serum level of 11.3 mg/dL and parathormone (PTH) serum level of 12.6 pmol/L (normal <6.8 pmol/L), following failed initial neck exploration. (Fig. II.11.6A–C).

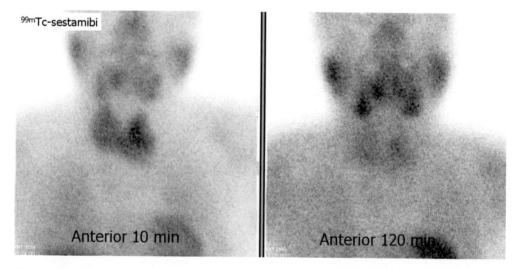

**Fig. II.11.6A**

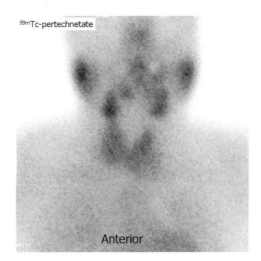

**Fig. II.11.6B**

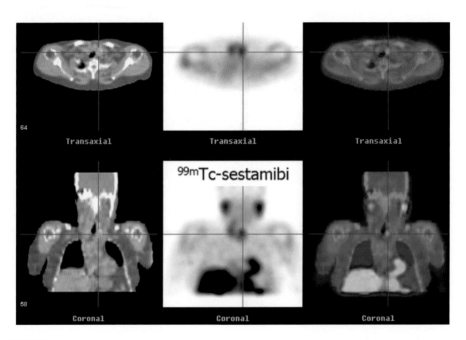

**Fig. II.11.6C**

**Findings**

Anterior planar images of the neck and chest were acquired for 15 min at 10 and 120 min after injection of $^{99m}$Tc-sestamibi and show heterogenous tracer uptake with mild predominance and retention in the upper half of the left thyroid lobe (Fig. II.11.6A). Planar thyroid scintigraphy, which can be also used for visual subtraction with the early $^{99m}$Tc-sestamibi images, is obtained following injection of $^{99m}$Tc-pertechnetate and demonstrates heterogenous uptake in both lobes of the gland (Fig. II.11.6B). SPECT/CT images of the neck and chest were acquired following the early planar study (Fig. II.11.6C) and demonstrate the presence of a parathyroid adenoma precisely localized in the left posterior paratracheal space. These findings guided the surgical re-exploration, and a 12 × 6 × 3 mm, 0.5 g parathyroid adenoma located between the trachea and the esophagus was excised. Following surgery, serum calcium decreased to 8.7 mg/dL.

**Discussion**

SPECT/CT facilitated the surgical exploration and excision of the cervical parathyroid adenoma after failed initial surgery in a patient previously treated with $^{131}$I for toxic multinodular goiter. All the above circumstances presented a challenge for the diagnosis and localization of the adenoma to the surgical team, which was solved by SPECT/CT. This modality facilitates image interpretation and planning of the surgical procedure. SPECT/CT improves significantly the success rate of minimally invasive parathyroidectomy when the adenoma is located in ectopic sites such as deep in the neck or in the mediastinum.[50,53]

**Diagnosis**

Left upper parathyroid adenoma located posteriorly between the trachea and the esophagus.

## *Case II.11.7*

### History

This 49-year-old female presented with primary hyperparathyroidism, with serum calcium level of 11.1 mg/dL and PTH serum level of 8.24 pmol/L (normal < 6.8 pmol/L), and was referred for preoperative localization of a parathyroid adenoma with $^{99m}$Tc-sestamibi SPECT/CT (Fig. II.11.7A, B).

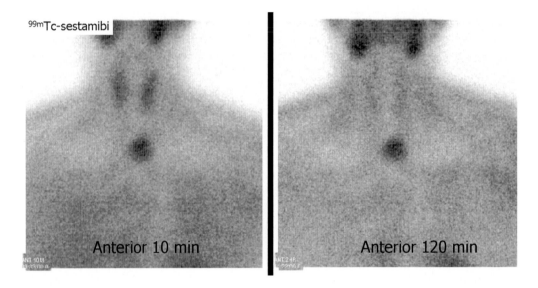

**Fig. II.11.7A**

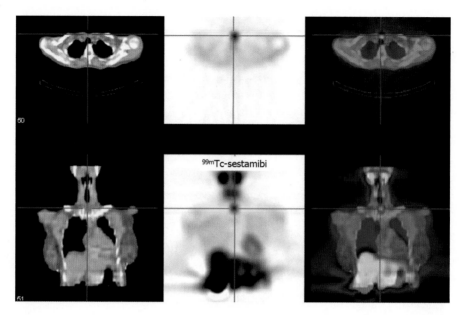

Fig. II.11.7B

## Findings

Early and delayed planar scintigraphy demonstrates the presence of a focus of increased sestamibi activity, interpreted as confined to the superior mediastinum (Fig. II.11.7A). Non-attenuation-corrected transaxial (upper row) and coronal (lower row) SPECT/CT images localize the focus of increased tracer activity to the mid-neck, above the suprasternal notch, anterior to the trachea. These findings guided the surgical exploration, and a 28 × 14 × 5 mm, 1.0 g parathyroid adenoma was excised. After surgery, the serum calcium decreased to 8.2 mg/dL.

## Discussion

Planar images suggested the presence of an ectopic parathyroid adenoma in the superior mediastinum. SPECT/CT, however, localized the adenoma to the mid-lower neck, above the manubrium, in the pre-tracheal space, thus sparing a median sternotomy. The CT data of the SPECT/CT procedure provide detailed anatomical information and allow precise localization of the foci of uptake especially in the lower neck and mediastinal compartment.

## Diagnosis

Ectopic parathyroid adenoma in the mid-anterior lower neck.

## Case II.11.8

### History

This patient with a history of well-differentiated NE carcinoma of the terminal ileum (typical carcinoid) presented with rising serum chromogranine levels. He was referred to $^{68}$Ga-DOTATOC PET/CT for staging (Fig. II.11.8).

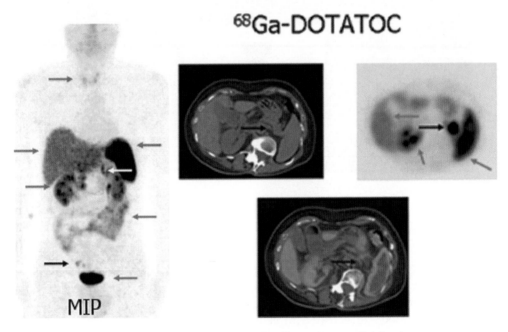

**Fig. II.11.8** (Images courtesy of F. Mottaghy and L. Mortelmans, Leuven, Belgium.)

### Findings

MIP image of the $^{68}$Ga-DOTATOC study (Fig. II.11.8-left) demonstrates the presence of SSTR positive intraperitoneal metastasis in a right pelvis lymph node (black arrow) and an additional suspicious focus of unclear location in the left upper abdomen (white arrow). There is physiological tracer uptake in the thyroid, spleen, liver, kidneys, diffuse in the bowel and the urinary bladder (blue arrows). Transaxial slices of the $^{68}$Ga-DOTATOC-PET/CT (Fig. II.11.8-right) located the suspicious lesion in the left upper abdomen to a mass in the tail of the pancreas (black arrow). There is intense physiological $^{68}$Ga-DOTATOC uptake in the spleen, and of lower intensity in the liver and right kidney (blue arrows).

### Diagnosis

NE tumor in tail of pancreas.

### Follow-up

The tracer-avid lesion in the tail of the pancreas was histologically confirmed as a well-differentiated NE carcinoma of the pancreas.

# References

1. Bocher M, Balan A, Krausz Y, Shrem Y, Lonn A, Wilk M, Chisin R. Gamma camera-mounted anatomical X-ray tomography: technology, system characteristics and first images. *Eur J Nucl Med* 2000;27:619–627.
2. Krausz Y, Israel O. Single-photon emission computed tomography/computed tomography in endocrinology. *Semin Nucl Med* 2006;36:267–274.
3. Keidar Z, Israel O, Krausz Y. SPECT/CT in tumor imaging: technical aspects and clinical applications. *Semin Nucl Med* 2003;33:205–218.
4. Schillaci O. Hybrid SPECT/CT: A new era for SPECT imaging? *Eur J Nucl Med Mol Imaging* 2005;32:521–524.
5. Gibril F, Jensen RT. Diagnostic uses of radiolabelled somatostatin receptor analogues in gastroenteropancreatic endocrine tumours. *Dig Liver Dis* 2004;36 Suppl 1:S106–120.
6. Gibril F, Reynolds JC, Chen CC, Yu F, Goebel SU, Serrano J, Doppman JL, Jensen RT. Specificity of somatostatin receptor scintigraphy: A prospective study and effects of false-positive localizations on management in patients with gastrinomas. *J Nucl Med* 1999;40:539–553.
7. Gabriel M, Decristoforo C, Kendler D, Dobrozemsky G, Heute D, Uprimny C, Kovacs P, Von Guggenberg E, Bale R, Virgolini IJ. [68]Ga-DOTA-Tyr3-octreotide PET in neuroendocrine tumors: comparison with somatostatin receptor scintigraphy and CT. *J Nucl Med* 2007;48: 508–518.
8. Buchmann I, Henze M, Engelbrecht S, Eisenhut M, Runz A, Schäfer M, Schilling T, Haufe S, Herrmann T, Haberkorn U. Comparison of [68]Ga-DOTATOC PET and [111]In-DTPAOC (Octreoscan) SPECT in patients with neuroendocrine tumours. *Eur J Nucl Med Mol Imaging* 2007;34:1617–1626.
9. Baum R, Niesen A, Leonhardi J, Wortmann R, Mueller D, Roesch F. Receptor PET/CT imaging of neuroendocrine tumours using the Ga-68 labelled, high affinity somatostatin analogue DOTA-1-Nal3 octreotide (DOTA-NOC): Clinical results in 327 patients. *Eur J Nucl Med Mol Imaging* 2005;32 Suppl 1:S54–55.
10. Prasad V, Fetscher S, Baum RP. Changing role of somatostatin receptor targeted drugs in NET: Nuclear Medicine's view. *J Pharm Pharm Sci* 2007;10:321s–337s.
11. Orlefors H, Sundin A, Garske U, Juhlin C, Oberg K Skogseid B, Langstrom B, Bergstrom M, Eriksson B. Whole-body (11)C-5-hydroxytryptophan positron emission tomography as a universal imaging technique for neuroendocrine tumors: comparison with somatostatin receptor scintigraphy and computed tomography. *J Clin Endocrinol Metab* 2005;90:3392–3400.
12. Nanni C, Fanti S, Rubello D. 18F-DOPA PET and PET/CT. *J Nucl Med* 2007;48:1577–1579.
13. Krausz Y, Freedman N, Orevi M, Mishani E, Barak D, Glser B, Rubinstein R, Klein M, Gross DJ, Chisin R. FDOPA-PET in neuroendocrine tumors: An open question? *J Nucl Med* 2007;48 (Suppl 2):127P.
14. Junik R, Drobik P, Malkowski B, Kobus-Blachnio K. The role of positron emission tomography (PET) in diagnostics of gastroenteropancreatic neuroendocrine tumours (GEP NET). *Adv Med Sci* 2006; 51:66–68.
15. de Herder WW, Lamberts SW. Gut endocrine tumours. *Best Pract Res Clin Endocrinol Metab* 2004; 18:477–495.
16. Gore RM, Berlin JW, Mehta UK, Newmark GM, Yaghmai V. GI carcinoid tumors: appearance of the primary and detecting metastases. *Best Pract Res Clin Endocrinol Metab* 2005;19:245–263.
17. Plöckinger U, Rindi G, Arnold R, Eriksson B, Krenning EP, de Herder WW, Goede A, Caplin M, Öberg K, Reubi JC, Nilsson O, Delle Fave G, Ruszniewski P, Ahlman H, Wiedenmann B. guidelines for the diagnosis and treatment of neuroendocrine gastrointestinal tumours. A consensus statement on behalf of the European neuroendocrine tumour society (ENETS). *Neuroendocrinology* 2004;80:394–424.
18. Nikou GC, Lygidakis NJ, Toubanakis C, Pavlatos S, Tseleni-Balafouta S, Giannatou E, Mallas E, Safioleas M. Current diagnosis and treatment of gastrointestinal carcinoids in a series of 101 patients: The significance of serum chromogranin-A, somatostatin receptor scintigraphy and somatostatin analogues. *Hepatogastroenterology* 2005;52:731–741.
19. Virgolini I, Traub-Weidinger T, Decristoforo C. Nuclear medicine in the detection and management of pancreatic islet-cell tumours. *Best Pract Res Clin Endocrinol Metab* 2005;19:213–227.
20. McLean AM, Fairclough PD. Endoscopic ultrasound in the localisation of pancreatic islet cell tumours. *Best Pract Res Clin Endocrinol Metab* 2005;19:177–193.

21. Gouya H, Vignaux O, Augui J, Dousset B, Palazzo L, Louvel A, Chaussade S, Legmann P. CT, endoscopic sonography, and a combined protocol for preoperative evaluation of pancreatic insulinomas. *AJR Am J Roentgenol* 2003;181:987–992.

22. Noone TC, Hosey J, Firat Z, Semelka R. Imaging and localization of islet-cell tumours of the pancreas on CT and MRI. *Best Pract Res Clin Endocrinol Metab* 2005;19:195–211.

23. Gibril F, Reynolds JC, Doppman JL, Chen CC, Venzon DJ, Termanini B, Weber HC, Stewart CA, Jensen RT. Somatostatin receptor scintigraphy: its sensitivity compared with that of other imaging methods in detecting primary and metastatic gastrinomas. A prospective study. *Ann Intern Med* 1996;125:26–34.

24. Even-Sapir E, Keidar Z, Sachs J, Engel A, Bettman L, Gaitini D, Guralnik L, Werbin N, Iosilevsky G, Israel O. The new technology of combined transmission and emission tomography in evaluation of endocrine neoplasms. *J Nucl Med* 2001;42:998–1004.

25. Krausz Y, Keidar Z, Kogan I, Even-Sapir E, Bar-Shalom R, Engel A, Rubinstein R, Sachs J, Bocher M, Agranovicz S, Chisin R, Israel O. SPECT/CT hybrid imaging with In[111]-Pentetreotide in assessment of neuroendocrine tumors. *Clin Endocrinol* 2003;59:565–573.

26. Pfannenberg AC, Eschmann SM, Horger M, Lamberts R, Vonthein R, Claussen CD, Bares R. Benefit of anatomical-functional image fusion in the diagnostic work-up of neuroendocrine neoplasms. *Eur J Nucl Med Mol Imaging* 2003;30:835–843.

27. Hillel PG, van Beek EJ, Taylor C, Lorenz E, Bax N, Prakash V, Tindale WB. The clinical impact of a combined gamma camera/CT imaging system on somatostatin receptor imaging of neuroendocrine tumors. *Clin Radiol* 2006;61:579–587.

28. Oberg K, Eriksson B. Nuclear medicine in the detection, staging and treatment of gastrointestinal carcinoid tumours. *Best Pract Res Clin Endocrinol Metab* 2005;19:265–276.

29. Hoegerle S, Altehoefer C, Ghanem N, Koehler G, Waller CF, Scheruebl H, Moser E, Nitzsche E. Whole-body 18F-DOPA PET for detection of gastrointestinal carcinoid tumours. *Radiology* 2001;220:373–380.

30. Becherer A, Szabo M, Karanikas G, Wunderbaldinger P, Angelberger P, Raderer M, Kurtaran A, Dudczak R, Kletter K. Imaging of advanced neuroendocrine tumors with (18)F-FDOPA PET. *J Nucl Med* 2004;45:1161–1167.

31. Ambrosini V, Tomassetti P, Rubello D, Campana D, Nanni C, Castellucci P, Farsad M, Montini G, Al-Nahhas A, Franchi R, Fanti S. Role of 18F-dopa PET/CT imaging in the management of patients with [111]In-pentetreotide negative GEP tumors. *Nucl Med Commun* 2007;28:473–477.

32. Adams S, Baum R, Rink T, Schumm-Dräger PM, Usadel K-H, Hör G. Limited value of fluorine-18 fluorodeoxyglucose positron emission tomography for the imaging of neuroendocrine tumors. *Eur J Nucl Med* 1998;25:79–83.

33. Belhocine T, Foidart J, Rigo P, Najjar F, Thiry A, Quatresooz P, Hustinx R. Fluorodeoxyglucose positron emission tomography and somatostatin receptor scintigraphy for diagnosing and staging carcinoid tumours: Correlations with the pathological indexes p53 and Ki-67. *Nucl Med Commun* 2002;23:727–734.

34. Bar-Shalom R, Keidar Z, Krausz Y. Prospective Image Fusion: The Role of SPECT/CT and PET/CT Iin Henkin RE, Bova D, Dillehay GL (eds): *Nuclear Medicine, 2nd Ed.* St. Louis, MO: C.V. Mosby, 2006.

35. Rozovsky K, Koplewitz BZ, Krausz Y, Revel-Wilk S, Weintraub M, Chisin R, Klein M. The added value of SPECT/CT for the correlation of MIBG scan and diagnostic CT in neuroblastoma and pheochromocytoma. *AJR Am J Roentgenol* 2008;190:1085–1090.

36. Ilias I, Pacak K. Diagnosis and management of tumors of the adrenal medulla. *Horm Metab Res* 2005;37:717–721.

37. Hoegerle S, Nitsche E, Altehoefer C, Ghanem N, Manz T, Brink I, Reincke M, Moser E, Neumann HP. Pheochromocytomas: detection with 18F DOPA whole body PET – initial results. *Radiology* 2002;222:507–512.

38. Timmers HJ, Hadi M, Carrasquillo JA, Chen CC, Martiniova L, Whatley M, Ling A, Eisenhofer G, Adams KT, Pacak K. The effects of carbidopa on uptake of 6-18F-Fluoro-L-DOPA in PET of pheochromocytoma and extraadrenal abdominal paraganglioma. *J Nucl Med* 2007;48:1599–1606.

39. Win Z, Al-Nahhas A, Towey D, Todd J, Rubello D, Lewington V, Gishen P. 68 Ga-DOTATATE PET in neuroectodermal tumors: first experience. *Nucl Med Commun* 2007;28:359–363.

40. Ozer S, Dobrozemsky G, Kienast O, Beheshti M, Becherer A, Niederle B, Kainberger F, Dudczak R, Kurtaran A.Value of combined XCT/SPECT technology for avoiding false positive planar [123]I-MIBG scintigraphy. *Nuklearmedizin* 2004;43:164–170.

41. Tang HR, Da Silva AJ, Matthay KK, Price DC, Huberty JP, Hawkins RA, Hasegawa BH. Neuroblastoma imaging using a combined CT scanner-scintillation camera and 131I-MIBG. *J Nucl Med* 2001;42:237–247.

42. Shulkin BL, Hutchinson RJ, Castle VP, Yanik GA, Shapiro B, Sisson JC. Neuroblastoma: positron emission tomography with 2-[fluorine-18]-fluoro-2-deoxy-D-glucose compared with metaiodobenzylguanidine scintigraphy. *Radiology* 1996;199:743–750.

43. Kushner BH, Yeung HW, Larson SM, Kramer K, Cheung NK. Extending positron emission tomography scan utility to high-risk neuroblastoma: fluorine-18 fluorodeoxyglucose positron emission tomography as sole imaging modality in follow-up of patients. *J Clin Oncol* 2001;19:3397–3405.

44. Denham DW, Norman J. Cost-effectiveness of preoperative sestamibi scan for primary hyperparathyroidism is dependent solely upon the surgeon's choice of operative procedure. *J Am Coll Surg* 1998;186:293–305.

45. Gotthardt M, Lohmann B, Behr TM, Bauhofer A, Franzius C, Schipper ML, Wagner M, Höffken H, Sitter H, Rothmund M, Joseph K, Nies C. Clinical value of parathyroid scintigraphy with technetium-99m methoxyisobutylisonitrile: discrepancies in clinical data and a systematic metaanalysis of the literature. *World J Surg* 2004;28:100–107.

46. Arici C, Cheah WK, Ituarte PH, Morita E, Lynch TC, Siperstein AE, Duh Q-Y, Clark OH. Can localization studies be used to direct focused parathyroid operations? *Surgery* 2001;129:720–729.

47. Moka D, Voth E, Dietlein M, Larena-Avellaneda A, Schicha H. Technetium 99m-MIBI-SPECT: A highly sensitive diagnostic tool for localization of parathyroid adenomas. *Surgery* 2000;128:29–35.

48. Lorberboym M, Minski I, Macadziob S, Nikolov G, Schachter P. Incremental diagnostic value of preoperative 99mTc-MIBI SPECT in patients with a parathyroid adenoma. *J Nucl Med* 2003;44:904–908.

49. Schachter PP, Issa N, Shimonov M, Czerniak A, Lorberboym M. Early, postinjection MIBI-SPECT as the only preoperative localizing study for minimally invasive parathyroidectomy. *Arch Surg* 2004;139:433–437.

50. Buhl T, Mollerup C, Mortensen J. Precise preoperative localization of parathyroid adenomas with combined 99mTc-MIBI SPECT/Hawkeye (low-dose CT) scanning [abstr]. *J Nucl Med* 2004;45(suppl):16.

51. Martin P, Alcan I, Berges L, Fuss M, Jortay A, Paternot J, Bergmann P. Contribution of 99mTc-MIBI SPECT/CT fusion imaging in hyperparathyroidism: first experience with the new hybrid SPECT/CT GE Hawkeye [abstr]. *Eur J Nucl Med Mol Imaging* 2004;31(suppl 2):246.

52. Kaczirek K, Prager G, Kienast O, Dobrozemsky G, Dudczak R, Niederle B, Kurtaran A. Combined transmission and 99mTc-sestamibi emission tomography for localization of mediastinal parathyroid glands. *Nuklearmedizin* 2003;42:220–223.

53. Krausz Y, Bettman L, Guralnik L, Yosilevsky G, Keidar Z, Bar-Shalom R, Even-Sapir E, Chisin R, Israel O. Tc99m-MIBI SPECT/CT in primary hyperparathyroidism. *World J Surgery* 2006; 30:76–83.

54. Ruf J, Seehofer D, Denecke T, Stelter L, Rayes N, Felix R, Amthauer H. Impact of image fusion and attenuation correction by SPECT-CT on the scintigraphic detection of parathyroid adenomas. *Nuklearmedizin* 2007;46:15–21.

55. Serra A, Bolasco P, Satta L, Nicolosi A, Uccheddu A, Piga M. Role of SPECT/CT in the preoperative assessment of hyperparathyroid patients. *Radiol Med* 2006;111:999–1008.

56. Sharma J, Mazzaglia P, Milas M, Berber E, Schuster D, Halkar R, Siperstein A, Weber C. Radionuclide imaging for hyperparathyroidism (HPT): Which is the best technetium-99m sestamibi modality? *Surgery* 2006;140:856–863.

57. Lavely WC, Goetze S, Friedman KP, Leal JP, Zhang Z, Garret-Mayer E, Dackiw AP, Tufano RP, Zeiger MA, Ziessman HA. Comparison of SPECT/CT, SPECT, and planar imaging with single- and dual-phase (99m)Tc-sestamibi parathyroid scintigraphy. *J Nucl Med* 2007;48:1084–1089.

# Chapter II.12
# Lymphoma

Michal Weiler-Sagie and Ora Israel

## Introduction

Lymphoma is a malignancy that originates in the lymphocytes. There are many types of lymphoma, and overall they are divided into two large groups: non-Hodgkin's lymphoma (NHL), representing the majority (approximately 85%) of these tumors, and Hodgkin's disease (HD). Lymphomas account for about 5% of all cases of cancer in the United States, and their incidence is rising.[1] A significant portion of lymphomas are curable with appropriate treatment.

## Non-Hodgkin's Lymphoma

Among the many subtypes of NHL, the most common are diffuse large B-cell lymphoma (DLCL) and follicular lymphoma (FL), which account for 30 and 20% of all NHLs, respectively.[2] The median age of patients at diagnosis is the sixth decade of life (except for lymphoblastic and Burkitt NHL, which affect children and young adults). Patients usually present with painless peripheral adenopathy. Symptoms may vary depending on the pathological subtype and the site of disease. Most cases present with advanced stage disease, and B symptoms such as fever, night sweats, or weight loss occur in about 20% of these patients. Mediastinal involvement is less common. Extranodal disease is encountered in 15–20% of patients with DLCL, involving mainly the bone marrow and the gastrointestinal tract (GIT) but has been described in almost every organ [reviewed in Adult Non-Hodgkin Lymphoma Treatment[3]].

Tissue diagnosis is essential at presentation in all patients with NHL. Based on histological diagnosis, several NHL classifications have been recommended. The most recent one, the World Health Organization (WHO) classification (2001), identifies distinct clinico-pathologic NHL entities based on immunophenotypic and genetic features. It divides NHLs into more than 30 B-cell, T-cell, and natural killer (NK)-cell neoplasms, many of which have a unique natural history. NHLs are characterized by the histologic pattern of growth, cell size, rate of proliferation, and level of differentiation. Tumors that grow in a nodular pattern, which vaguely resemble normal B-cell lymphoid follicular structures, are generally less aggressive than lymphomas proliferating in a diffuse pattern. Lymphomas of small lymphocytes have, as a rule, a more indolent course than those of large lymphocytes.

M. Weiler-Sagie (✉)
Department of Nuclear Medicine, Rambam Health Care Campus, Haifa, Israel
e-mail: m_weiler@rambam.health.gov.il

D. Delbeke, O. Israel (eds.), *Hybrid PET/CT and SPECT/CT Imaging*,
DOI 10.1007/978-0-387-92820-3_14, © Springer Science+Business Media, LLC 2010

513

Excisional lymph node or surgical biopsy of an extranodal site is the most accurate diagnostic method. Immuno-histochemistry has become a routine procedure, necessary for accurate sub-classification. Flow cytometry and genetic analysis can help in cases with inconclusive histological and immuno-histochemistry review. Additional workup includes detailed patient history determining the presence of B symptoms, physical examination with documentation of adenopathy, hepato-splenomegaly and defining performance status, laboratory tests, imaging studies, and bone marrow biopsy.

Staging is based on the Ann Arbor staging system, initially developed for HD. Stage I disease is characterized by the involvement of a single lymph node region, stage II involves two or more lymph node regions on the same side of the diaphragm, stage III involves lymph nodes on both sides of the diaphragm, and stage IV is characterized by multifocal involvement of one or more extralymphatic organs. The international prognostic index (IPI), used to identify patients with aggressive NHL that are most likely to relapse, defines five significant risk factors: age, serum lactic dehydrogenase (LDH), performance status, stage, and extranodal involvement. Patients with two or more risk factors have a less than 50% chance of 5-year relapse-free and overall survival (OS). The FL International Prognostic Index (FLIPI) identified five significant risk factors in patients with FL: age, serum LDH, stage, hemoglobin levels, and number of nodal areas. Patients with a single risk factor have a 10-year OS rate of 85%, as compared to 40% in the presence of three or more risk factors. Patients at high risk of relapse may benefit from more aggressive therapies.

In relationship to clinical behavior, NHLs are divided into two prognostic groups: indolent and aggressive lymphoma. Indolent NHL has a relatively good prognosis with a median survival of 10 years. It is usually not curable in advanced clinical stages. Most indolent types are nodular (or follicular) lymphoma with FLs representing about 70% of cases. Less common subtypes also classified as indolent are marginal zone lymphoma (nodal, splenic, and mucosa-associated lymphatic tissue; MALT), small lymphocytic lymphoma (SLL), lymphoplasmacytic, mycosis fungoides, primary cutaneous anaplastic large cell, and Hairy cell leukemia. B symptoms are unusual but bone marrow involvement is common (50–80%). Spontaneous regression occurs in up to 20% of patients. Disease may "wax and wane" for years without therapy or progress rapidly and require treatment. Therapeutic options vary from a "watch and wait" policy to autologous hematopoietic cell transplantation (AHCT). Early stage I and II indolent NHL can be effectively treated with radiation therapy alone.[4]

Treatment options for advanced stage disease include rituximab, a chimeric human-murine monoclonal antibody (anti-CD-20), chemotherapy, radiation therapy, or a combination of all above-mentioned options.

While aggressive NHL has a shorter natural history, a significant number of patients in this group can be cured. Subtypes classified as aggressive NHL include DLCL, mantle cell lymphoma (MCL), anaplastic large cell, peripheral and angioimmunoblastic T-cell, and extranodal T-/NK-cell lymphoma. Burkitt and lymphoblastic lymphoma are considered highly aggressive disease. Treatment consists of intensive combination chemotherapy regimens, with the addition of rituximab further improving chance of survival. Five year OS of aggressive NHL ranges between 50–60%, and 30–60% of patients can be cured. Most relapses occur in the first 2 years after completion of therapy. Salvage treatment with high-dose chemotherapy followed by AHCT leads to cure of 10–20% of relapsing patients.

# Hodgkin's Disease

Most cases of HD are classified as "classic" HD [reviewed in Adult Hodgkin Lymphoma Treatment[5]]. Cell histology of classic HD is less important than in NHL. Treatment options and prognosis depend on stage of disease rather than the histologic subtype. HD has a bimodal incidence curve; the first peak occurs in young adulthood, at the age of 15–35, and the second at the age of over 55. HD usually presents as painless adenopathy in the supraclavicular and/or cervical regions and has a contiguous pattern of spread. Mediastinal involvement is common, occurring in more than 85% of patients. B symptoms are found in 30–40% of patients with stage III or IV disease, but only in less than 10% with stage I or II disease. Bone marrow involvement occurs in 5% of patients, and bone marrow biopsy is performed in the presence of B symptoms or low blood count.

The WHO classifies HD as classical with four subtypes (nodular sclerosis, mixed cellularity, lymphocyte-depleted, lymphocyte rich) and nodular lymphocyte-predominant HD (LPHD), the latter representing about 5% of all cases. The distinction between classic HD and LPHD is clinically significant because of their different natural histories, prognosis, and treatment options. LPHD is usually diagnosed in asymptomatic young males with cervical or inguinal lymph nodes but no mediastinal involvement and is characterized by earlier-stage disease, longer survival, and less treatment failure.

Diagnosis of HD is made as a rule by excisional lymph node biopsy and requires the presence of Hodgkin or Reed-Steinberg cells with a background of inflammatory cells. The current Ann Arbor staging classification for HD was adopted in 1971 and modified 18 years later at the Cotswolds meeting. Imaging plays an important role in staging of HD. On chest X-rays and computed tomography (CT), "bulky" disease with a mediastinal-to-mass ratio (MMR) of 33% or more, or adenopathy measuring 10 cm or more in its greatest dimension, are associated with worse prognosis.

Over 75% of patients with HD can be cured with combination chemotherapy and/or radiation therapy. Patients can be divided into major prognostic groups, further used for defining the appropriate treatment strategy:

   early favorable – stage I or II without any risk factors is treated with chemotherapy and involved-field radiation (IF-XRT) or chemotherapy alone;
   early unfavorable – stage I or II with at least one of the following risk factors: large mediastinal mass, extranodal involvement, elevated erythrocyte sedimentation rate (ESR), >3 involved lymph node areas, B symptoms, is treated with chemotherapy and IF-XRT or chemotherapy alone;
   advanced disease – stage III or IV, divided into advanced favorable and unfavorable HD according to the IPI score calculated from seven factors: albumin levels, hemoglobin levels, gender, age, stage, white blood cell (WBC) count, and absolute lymphocytic count.

Patients with less than three adverse risk factors have advanced favorable HD, with 60–80% 5-year freedom-from-progression (FFP) with first-line chemotherapy. Patients with 4–7 adverse factors are considered as advanced unfavorable disease with 42–51% 5-year FFP.

Salvage therapy and AHCT are administered to patients who relapse, with high response rates of 73–88%, but even non-responders benefit from AHCT with long-term remissions achieved in 20–30% of patients.

## $^{18}$F-FDG Imaging for Diagnosis of NHL and HD

In patients presenting with adenopathy or mediastinal masses, with or without B symptoms, the differential diagnosis includes lymphoma as well as inflammatory or infectious
conditions, granulomatous processes, other lymphoproliferative diseases, and metastatic
adenopathy. All of the above can take up $^{18}$F-fluorodeoxyglucose ($^{18}$F-FDG), which is a
non-specific indicator of metabolic activity. Diagnosis of lymphoma is made by tissue
sampling. $^{18}$F-FDG positron emission tomography (PET)/CT is an appropriate test in
certain clinical settings when lymphoma is suspected, such as finding the most appropriate
site for biopsy in patients without obviously accessible nodal sites or with exclusively
extranodal disease. In patients with peripheral adenopathy in which needle biopsy rather
than excisional biopsy is considered, $^{18}$F-FDG imaging can improve the yield of biopsy
guiding toward the lesion, which is not only most accessible but also has the highest and
most homogenous tracer uptake. This may help circumvent sampling errors in large lymph
nodes with necrotic tissue or small but benign lymph nodes.

## $^{18}$F-FDG Imaging at Initial Staging of Lymphoma

### $^{18}$F-FDG Avidity of HD and NHL

Sensitivity and specificity of $^{18}$F-FDG imaging are high for HD and for most histological
subtypes of NHL. The degree of uptake is variable and does not correlate with a specific
histologic subtype or grade of lymphoma, with the exception of SLL, which has a known
lower intensity uptake. $^{18}$F-FDG PET detected disease in at least one site in 161/172
patients with lymphoma, with a detection rate of 98% in HD, 100% in DLCL, 98% in
FL, and 100% in MCL. Lower detection rates were reported for marginal zone, 67%, and
peripheral T-cell lymphoma, 40%.[6] On a site-based analysis involving 255 lymphoma
patients, over 97% of HD and aggressive or highly aggressive NHL were $^{18}$F-FDG-avid
as compared to somewhat lower uptake rates in indolent NHL, specifically 91% for FL,
82% in extranodal marginal zone B-cell MALT, and approximately 50% for SLL and
splenic marginal zone lymphoma (SMZL).[7]

### Comparative Performance of $^{18}$F-FDG Imaging and CT

$^{18}$F-FDG is the metabolic tracer of choice for imaging of lymphoma. It is highly sensitive
and superior to CT in detecting nodal and extranodal involvement in most histologic
subtypes of lymphoma [reviewed in the literature by Seam et al.[8]]. In discordant cases,
$^{18}$F-FDG PET resulted in upstaging by detection of additional lymphoma sites, such as
lymph nodes of 1 cm or smaller, or splenic and hepatic infiltration.[9–11] $^{18}$F-FDG PET/
CT provides more sensitive and specific imaging data than either modality alone.[12]
PET/CT performed without intravenous contrast and a low-dose (40–80 mA) CT
component is more sensitive and specific than contrast-enhanced full-dose stand-alone
CT for evaluation of nodal and extranodal lymphoma involvement.[13–15] Tatsumi and
colleagues[15] evaluated the status of 1,537 anatomic sites in 20 patients with HD and 33
patients with NHL on unenhanced low-dose PET/CT studies. Concordant PET and CT
findings were found in 1,489 sites. Among the 48 discordant sites, PET correctly
characterized 31 true positive and 9 true negative lesions further confirmed by biopsy

or follow-up. In a meta-analysis of the role of $^{18}$F-FDG PET in staging of lymphoma including mostly DLCL-NHL and HD, as well as few FL[13] the pooled sensitivity for patient-based data from 14 studies was 91%, with a false-positive rate of 10%. The maximum joint sensitivity and specificity was 88%.

## Diagnosis of Bone Marrow Involvement

$^{18}$F-FDG imaging can detect focal or multifocal bone and/or bone marrow involvement in patients with lymphoma with a negative iliac crest bone marrow biopsy, subsequently confirmed by histopathology or magnetic resonance imaging (MRI).[16] $^{18}$F-FDG PET cannot replace bone marrow aspiration because of false-negative studies, more common when there is involvement of only 10–20% of the medullary space. Based on a recent meta-analysis, estimates of $^{18}$F-FDG PET sensitivity for detecting marrow infiltration in NHL and HD were 43 and 76%, respectively.[17]

## $^{18}$F-FDG Staging Criteria in HD and NHL

According to the International Harmonization Project (IHP), $^{18}$F-FDG imaging is strongly recommended for staging of patients with $^{18}$F-FDG-avid, potentially curable lymphoma such as DLCL and HD to better define the whole extent of disease.[18] In HD, staging is the dominant factor in determining the treatment strategy and prognosis of patients, while for NHL histological classification has the highest significance. For incurable, $^{18}$F-FDG-avid, indolent, and aggressive NHL (e.g., FL, MCL) and for variably $^{18}$F-FDG-avid NHL, a study needs to be performed at staging if response to treatment will also be evaluated by $^{18}$F-FDG PET, since the baseline test will determine the presence of $^{18}$F-FDG avidity and assist in interpreting mid- and end-of-treatment studies.[18,19] Worldwide, $^{18}$F-FDG PET/CT is used routinely for staging and subsequently for assessing response to treatment and follow-up of patients with lymphoma.

Radiotherapy is a major therapeutic tool in treatment of lymphomas. IF-XRT is a first-line treatment option for early favorable HD and for low-stage indolent NHLs. Radiation treatment is also used, in combination with chemotherapy, in some advanced stage lymphomas. Conventionally, radiation field planning has been based on anatomical imaging. The additional metabolic information provided by $^{18}$F-FDG imaging can potentially decrease radiation volume and dose, thus reducing radiation toxicity, important mainly in children and adolescents.[20]

## $^{18}$F-FDG Imaging for Monitoring Therapy Response in Lymphoma

### Definition of Response

The Cotswold meeting and the National Cancer Institute (NCI) international working group defined the criteria for response to treatment in HD and NHL in 1999.[21,22] Revised criteria incorporating $^{18}$F-FDG imaging have been recommended by the International Harmonization Project (IHP) in 2007.[18,19] Complete response (CR) is defined as disappearance of all detectable clinical evidence of disease. This definition which has been previously based on the extent of anatomical shrinkage of masses on CT includes at present also a residual mass of an $^{18}$F-FDG-avid lymphoma on CT with none or minimal $^{18}$F-FDG uptake, irrelevant of the size of the mass. For lymphomas with variable $^{18}$F-FDG avidity, regression to normal size on CT determines CR. Partial response (PR) indicates a >50% decrease in size of lymphoma lesions and of the degree of $^{18}$F-FDG uptake in one or more previously involved sites. Stable disease (SD) relates to $^{18}$F-FDG uptake in prior sites of disease with no new sites on either PET or CT. Tumor progression (TP) defines a patient in PR or SD who shows > 50% increase in size with $^{18}$F-FDG uptake of a previous lymphoma site, or a new, $^{18}$F-FDG-avid lymph node, >1.5 cm in diameter. Relapse is defined if the criteria noted above for TP are met in a patient who had previously achieved CR.

## Timing of $^{18}$F-FDG Imaging in Assessing Response to Treatment in Lymphoma

Effective radio- and chemotherapy kill cancer cells by first-order kinetics, meaning that a given treatment dose will kill the same fraction, but not necessarily the same number of cancer cells regardless of the size of the tumor. A therapy dose that kills 90% (1-log unit) of the cells will have to be repeated at least 10 times to eliminate a newly diagnosed cancer. Cure of lymphoma with the standard six cycles of therapy, assuming no interval re-growth, requires at least 1.5 log units of tumor cell killing per cycle, or a 99.9% reduction in the number of viable cancer cells after two cycles.[23] The resolution of $^{18}$F-FDG PET for detecting lymphoma is 0.5 cm, which translates to a tumor size of approximately 0.1–1.0 g, or $10^8$–$10^9$ cells. After the first 2–3 log units of tumor cell killing, depending on the initial size of the tumor, it is likely that the residual viable tumor cell mass will be below the PET detection threshold. Therefore, while a negative $^{18}$F-FDG PET study after two cycles of therapy implies that the rate of tumor cell killing for this lymphoma is sufficient to produce cure, a negative test at the end of treatment is expected to have less predictive value because it does not differentiate between patients with high and low tumor killing rates. A positive $^{18}$F-FDG PET study after two cycles of therapy suggests that fewer than 2 or 3 log units of tumor cells have been eliminated and it is therefore unlikely that the 10 or 11 log units needed for cure will be reached by six to eight cycles. A positive test at the end of six cycles of therapy indicates with high probability that the lymphoma is resistant to treatment.

## During and End-of-Treatment $^{18}$F-FDG Imaging in Lymphoma

For assessing response during treatment a PET/CT study is performed after one to four cycles of chemotherapy. The IHP recommends the study be performed at least 3 weeks after the previous cycle of treatment to allow time for the chemotherapeutic effect to take hold and to avoid transient fluctuations in $^{18}$F-FDG uptake that can occur early after treatment due to tumor "stunning."[19] A significant decrease in tumor uptake is expected to occur after one to two cycles of treatment in both NHL and HD. A negative $^{18}$F-FDG PET/CT study during treatment suggests that the patient has achieved CR, keeping in mind, however, that PET cannot detect microscopic disease. At the completion of treatment, studies are also performed at least 3 weeks after the last cycle of chemotherapy.

They are delayed for 6–12 weeks after radiotherapy to reduce the chances for increased [18]F-FDG uptake related to inflammatory reactions initiated by radiation.[18,19] Numerous studies have assessed the role of [18]F-FDG PET performed after one to four cycles of chemotherapy to predict outcome.[24–27] Haioun and colleagues[24] treated 90 patients with aggressive NHL and prospectively assessed [18]F-FDG PET after two cycles. Significantly more [18]F-FDG-negative patients (83%) achieved CR compared with only 58% of [18]F-FDG-positive patients, with a 2-year estimated OS of 90 and 61%, respectively. [18]F-FDG PET was a prognostic factor independent of the IPI score. Schot and cow-orkers,[27] in a study of 101 patients with aggressive lymphoma, found that the IPI score in conjunction with [18]F-FDG PET response after two cycles provides more accurate prog-nosis for outcome of second-line treatment in recurrent NHL. Hutchings and colleagues[25] evaluated 77 patients with HD after two cycles of chemotherapy and found that [18]F-FDG PET was of similar accuracy after two cycles as in later studies and stronger than estab-lished prognostic factors. Juweid and coworkers[28] evaluated 54 patients with aggressive NHL who underwent [18]F-FDG PET at 1–16 weeks after completion of chemotherapy. Progression-free survival was significantly shorter in patients with a positive as compared to those with a negative study.

## *[18]F-FDG Imaging of a Residual Mass*

During or at the end of treatment anatomical imaging modalities cannot distinguish between a residual mass composed of fibrotic or necrotic tissue and residual active disease. This is accurately achieved by [18]F-FDG imaging, which can differentiate between residual lymphoma and non-viable tissue. Patients showing [18]F-FDG uptake in a shrinking mass in the mid- or end-of-treatment study are more likely to have TP or relapse, thus suggesting the need for a change in treatment. In a study of 58 patients with HD and NHL who had residual masses on CT after treatment, a positive [18]F-FDG PET study correlated with a significantly poorer progression-free survival, with a negative predictive value (NPV) of 100% for HD and with a positive predictive value (PPV) of 100% for NHL.[29] In a study of 28 patients with a residual mass, the NPV and PPV of [18]F-FDG PET at 1 year were 95 and 60%, respectively, and the disease-free survival for PET-negative and positive patients was 95 and 40%, respectively. These results suggest that a patient with HD with a [18]F-FDG-negative residual mediastinal mass is unlikely to relapse, while, on the other hand, a positive study carries a significantly higher risk of relapse and demands further diagnostic procedures and a closer follow-up.[30]

## *Pitfalls in Interpretation*

[18]F-FDG-avid sites detected in patients with lymphoma evaluated during or after treatment need to be interpreted with caution in view of potential, mainly treatment-related false-positive results.[31,32] Physiologic uptake of [18]F-FDG in brown fat can mimic nodal involve-ment. Following granulocyte colony stimulating factor (G-CSF) treatment, there is diffuse uptake in the skeleton (and spleen), which should not be misinterpreted as lymphomatous bone marrow involvement. [18]F-FDG uptake in a hyperplasic thymus needs to be differen-tiated from recurring disease in the mediastinum. After radiation therapy to the mediastinum, paramediastinal [18]F-FDG lung uptake may be due to post-radiation pneumonitis or, alter-natively, to a concurrent infectious process, mainly in patients with no pulmonary

involvement at presentation. New [18]F-FDG uptake in lymph nodes that were involved at presentation is more suspicious for recurrence than new uptake in new sites, which can also represent reactive nodes to a concurrent local process unrelated to the primary diagnosis. This represents the most common cause for false-positive nodal uptake, occurring more often in the cervical, axillary, and inguinal regions.[33]

## [18]F-FDG Imaging for Diagnosis and Restaging of Lymphoma Recurrence

Relapse occurs in about 20–30% of the patient with HD, usually in the first 3 years after treatment.[34] Intensive follow-up of patients with lymphoma subtypes that have low cure rates is of questionable value because early detection of relapse is unlikely to result in a significant change in patient management. In contrast, salvage therapies for recurrent HD are associated with a high response rate, which therefore justifies close follow-up. Early detection of relapse enables initiation of treatment when the tumor load is low and the patient is symptom-free. Relapse of HD is usually identified as a result of the investigation of symptoms rather than by routine screening of asymptomatic patients.[34] Follow-up of HD using the recommendations issued by the Cotswold Committee in 1989 should be done every 3 months for the first 2 years, every 4 months in the third year, every 6 months in years 4 and 5, and once a year thereafter.[22] Evidence-based data on the value of follow-up of patients with HD who have achieved a CR are lacking. Investigations are indicated when there are new symptoms or signs suspicious of possible disease recurrence.[34,35] In a study assessing [18]F-FDG PET in diagnosis of preclinical relapse in HD,[36] 36 patients were examined at the end of treatment and every 4–6 months for 2–3 years thereafter. [18]F-FDG abnormalities preceded CT findings and correctly identified all four patients who relapsed, including two who were symptom-free. [18]F-FDG PET appears therefore as a good tool to identify a relapse even in asymptomatic patients.[34,35] However, in the same study, there was a high rate of false-positive [18]F-FDG PET, which incorrectly suggested relapse in six patients.

Aggressive NHL has high cure rates and salvage therapy is effective. There are no clear recommendations for routine imaging follow-up in asymptomatic NHL after treatment. Scarce literature data indicate that CT diagnosed 13%[37] and 6%[38] of preclinical relapses in intermediate or aggressive NHL.

Patients with indolent NHL are followed up with [18]F-FDG PET in order to decide when to start treatment, such as after appearance of clinical symptoms, in the presence of significant TP, or when an indolent lymphoma transforms to an aggressive type of disease. [18]F-FDG imaging can help in identifying some of these scenarios and may be therefore more successful than CT.[39] An increase in [18]F-FDG uptake intensity in sites of lymphoma is suggestive of histologic transformation and PET/CT can be used to direct confirming biopsy to these sites.[40]

## Summary

The vast majority of lymphoma subtypes are [18]F-FDG avid, and PET is therefore a valuable tool for evaluation of these subtypes. [18]F-FDG PET/CT is better than either modality alone in evaluating patients with lymphoma, mainly by accurately defining sites of increased tracer uptake unrelated to lymphoma, thus reducing the false-positive rate.

[18]F-FDG imaging is useful in staging of lymphoma, with better diagnosis of splenic, hepatic, and bone marrow involvement as compared to CT. [18]F-FDG PET/CT performed early during treatment can detect non-responding patients and suggest a change in the therapeutic strategy. Positive [18]F-FDG PET/CT studies during or at the end of treatment are associated with worse prognosis. [18]F-FDG PET/CT can distinguish between a residual mass consisting of necrotic and fibrotic tissue and residual active lymphoma, can detect relapse during follow-up, and can identify transformation of low- to high-grade lymphoma. [18]F-FDG PET/CT studies provide a metabolic guiding tool and thus optimize the process of selecting a site for biopsy with a subsequent decrease tissue sampling errors.

## Guidelines and Recommendations for the Use of [18]F-FDG-PET and PET/CT

The National Comprehensive Cancer Network (NCCN) has incorporated [18]F-FDG PET in the practice guidelines and management algorithm of most Hodgkin's lymphoma (HL) and NHL.[41,42] The use of [18]F-FDG PET (PET/CT where available) is recommended in the following clinical scenarios:

1) Baseline for lymphoma that are potentially curative (HD, DLCL);
2) Baseline to exclude systemic disease in clinically localized lymphoma (HD, DLCL, FL, Mantle cell, AIDS-related B cell, nodal and splenic marginal zone, peripheral T cell, MALT);
3) To evaluate residual masses;
4) To monitor therapy of aggressive lymphoma (HD, DLCL).

[18]F-FDG PET is not indicated

1) To monitor therapy if CT is normal.
2) For surveillance.

A multidisciplinary panel of experts reviewed meta-analyses and systematic reviews published in the [18]F-FDG PET literature before March 2006 and made recommendations for the use of [18]F-FDG PET in oncology.[43] The panel concluded that:

1) [18]F-FDG PET should routinely be obtained in addition to the conventional workup in the pretreatment staging of lymphoma;
2) [18]F-FDG PET may be added to bone marrow biopsy for staging and restaging lymphoma;
3) [18]F-FDG PET should routinely be added to the conventional workup for restaging or detecting recurrence in patients to whom curative treatment was administered. However, if the [18]F-FDG PET findings are positive, further confirmation by biopsy is mandatory. [18]F-FDG PET is not recommended for detecting relapse in asymptomatic patients.

Consensus recommendations regarding the use of [18]F-FDG PET for assessment response have been published by the imaging subcommittee of the IHP[19]:

1) Pre-therapy [18]F-FDG PET imaging is strongly encouraged but not mandatory for aggressive lymphoma (HL, DLCL, MCL, and FL) because they are routinely [18]F-FDG avid. However, pre-therapy [18]F-FDG PET imaging is mandatory for lymphomas that are not typically [18]F-FDG avid if response treatment will also be evaluated with [18]F-FDG PET.

2) The timing of $^{18}$F-FDG PET is critical to avoid equivocal interpretations. $^{18}$F-FDG PET should be performed at least 3 weeks and preferably 6–8 weeks after completion of chemotherapy and 8–12 weeks after radiation therapy. For evaluation during therapy, $^{18}$F-FDG PET imaging should be performed as close as possible before the next cycle of therapy.

3) Visual assessment alone is adequate for interpreting PET findings as positive or negative. Mediastinal blood pool activity is used as a reference for assessment of residual masses greater than 2 cm.

4) Specific criteria for defining PET positivity in liver, spleen, lung, and bone marrow are described in the review article.

5) Treatment monitoring during the course of therapy should only be done in the setting of clinical trials.

In the revised response criteria for lymphoma based on PET and CT article, Cheson and colleagues[18] recommend performance of a baseline $^{18}$F-FDG PET/CT in routinely $^{18}$F-FDG-avid lymphoma only (HL, DLCL) and in these patients after completion of therapy. In lymphoma with indolent NHL (FL and MCL) and other NHL with variable tracer avidity, baseline $^{18}$F-FDG PET is recommended only if overall response rate (ORR) or complete remission are end-point, and $^{18}$F-FDG PET is recommended after completion of therapy if positive at baseline. At mid-treatment, $^{18}$F-FDG PET is recommended only in clinical trials.

## Case Presentations

### *Case II.12.1 (DICOM Images on DVD)*

#### History

This 47-year-old female had elevated serum LDH levels on routine blood sample. Abdominal ultrasonography and whole-body CT showed an enlarged spleen with hypoechogenic areas. The patient was referred to $^{18}$F-FDG PET/CT with the suspicion of lymphoma (Fig. II.12.1A–D).

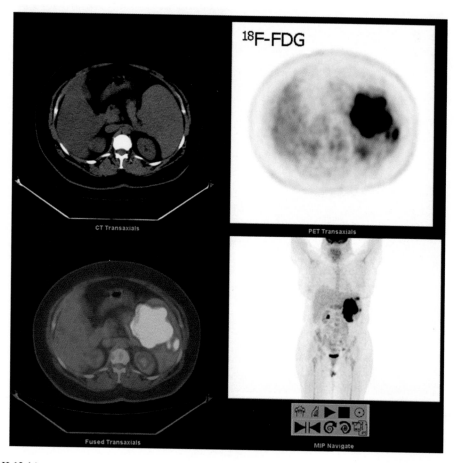

**Fig. II.12.1A**

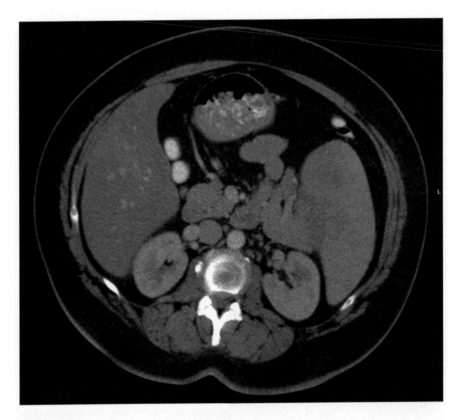

**Fig. II.12.1B**

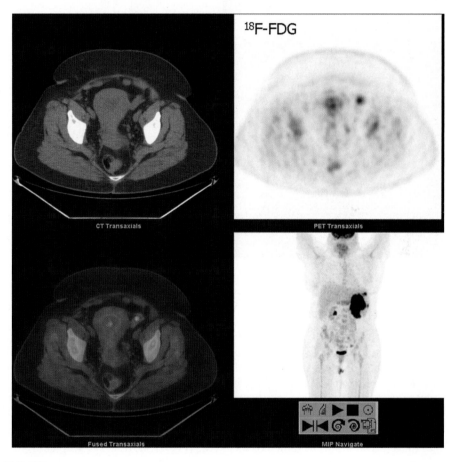

**Fig. II.12.1C**

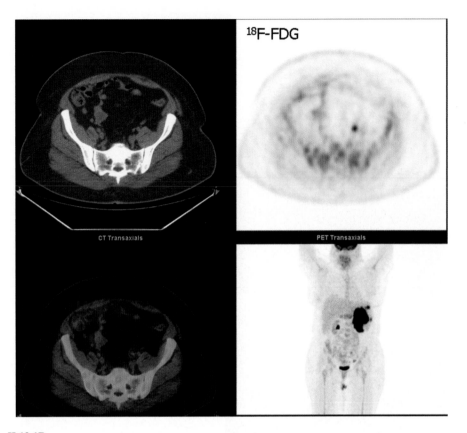

**Fig. II.12.1D**

### Findings

On whole-body [18]F-FDG PET/CT, the spleen is enlarged to 15 cm in the largest axial dimension and contains a large area of intense pathological [18]F-FDG uptake also involving lymph nodes in the adjacent hilum and tail of the pancreas. There are several additional small [18]F-FDG-avid foci corresponding to hypodense splenic lesions on the CT with contrast (Fig. II.12.1A,B). On maximal intensity projection (MIP) images, there are additional focal sites of increased [18]F-FDG activity in the mid- and left pelvis. The suspicious foci in the anterior aspect of the lower mid- and left pelvis are localized by fused PET/CT images to the left ovary and the lumen of the uterus (Fig. II.12.1C). The suspicious focus in the left upper posterior pelvis is localized by fused images to the left ureter (Fig. II.12.1D). There is also mild bone marrow uptake. Additional CT findings are seen on the Digital Imaging and Communications in Medicine (DICOM) images and described in the clinical report (see DVD).

### Discussion

This patient presented with laboratory and imaging data suspicious for lymphoma. Diagnosis is based on tissue sampling and biopsy should be performed in the easiest to approach region in order to minimize morbidity associated with the procedure. A peripheral lymph node is the best option. In this case, bone marrow biopsy was normal. CT pointed to the spleen as the single site of disease and did not identify a peripheral suspicious lesion as a potential site for biopsy. Before proceeding to splenic biopsy or diagnostic splenectomy, $^{18}$F-FDG PET/CT can aid in the search of better sites to biopsy. This test cannot be used to diagnose lymphoma since $^{18}$F-FDG uptake is non-specific. In this patient, no additional sites of disease were identified, and diagnostic splenectomy was preformed.

PET/CT studies including a low-dose non-enhanced CT has a higher sensitivity and specificity than stand-alone contrast-enhanced CT for evaluation of nodal and extranodal lymphoma.[13–15] In current example, the diagnostic contrast-enhanced CT was of additional value in delineating the loco-regional extent of the process involving both lymph nodes in the splenic hilum and the tail of the pancreas as proven by the pathology specimen. PET/CT, however, excluded the presence of additional distant sites of disease suspected by the focal $^{18}$F-FDG-avid lesions in the pelvis by localizing the increased tracer activity to sites of physiologic biodistribution such as the ovary and uterus during menstruation, and urinary excretion of $^{18}$F-FDG in the ureter.

## Diagnosis

DLCL of the spleen with local invasion to a LN at the splenic hilum and to the tail of the pancreas.

## Follow-Up

The patient underwent splenectomy, and DLCL of the spleen with local invasion to LN at the splenic hilum and the tail of the pancreas was diagnosed. She received six courses of chemotherapy with a protocol consisting of CHOP and Rituximab, achieved CR, and has no evidence of disease for a follow-up of 4 years.

## Clinical Report: Body $^{18}$F-FDG PET/CT (for DVD cases only)

Indication

Suspected lymphoma of spleen, detection of peripheral site to biopsy.

History

This 47-year-old female had elevated serum LDH levels on routine blood sample. Abdominal ultrasonography and whole-body CT showed an enlarged spleen with hypoecogenic areas.

Procedure

The patient was fasted for more than 4 h and had a normal blood glucose level prior to $^{18}$F-FDG injection. PET acquisition was performed with a PET/CT scanner with a low-dose CT being used for anatomical correlation and attenuation correction. PET emission images were started 110 min after IV injection of 555 MBq (15 mCi) of $^{18}$F-FDG and covered the area from the base of the skull through the upper thighs.

Findings

> *Quality of study*: The quality of the study is good. Motion of the head is notable (mis-registration between PET and CT images). There is tracer activity according to the physiologic distribution of the radiopharmaceutical including the brain, myocardium, bowel, liver, and renal collecting system.
>
> *Head and neck*: within normal range.
>
> *Chest*: within normal range.
>
> *Abdomen and pelvis*: The spleen is enlarged to 15 cm in largest axial dimension and contains an area of intense pathological $^{18}$F-FDG uptake involving lymph nodes of up to $15 \times 8$ mm in the adjacent hilum and tail of the pancreas. (There are several additional small $^{18}$F-FDG-avid foci corresponding to hypodense splenic lesions on the CT with contrast.) There is a small focus of $^{18}$F-FDG uptake medial to the iliac vessels at the level of S1 localized by fused images to the ureter. Foci of increased tracer uptake are seen in the anterior aspect of the left pelvis at the level of the acetabulum and at the same level in the mid-pelvis, corresponding to the left ovary and the lumen of the uterus, respectively. On CT numerous very small (below 5 mm) mesenteric and left para-aortic, bilateral pelvic, and inguinal lymph nodes are visible, with no corresponding $^{18}$F-FDG uptake. Steatosis of the liver is demonstrated.
>
> *Musculoskeletal*: There is mild bone marrow hyperplasia.

Impression

1. Abnormal $^{18}$F-FDG uptake in a large hypodense lesion in the spleen with direct extension to splenic hilum lymph nodes, and additional foci of increased tracer activity in hypodense lesions in the spleen, consistent with malignancy.
2. Very small, <5 mm in diameter, mesenteric, para-aortic, pelvic, and inguinal non-avid lymph nodes seen on CT.
3. Fatty liver.
4. Focal increased $^{18}$F-FDG uptake in the left ureter on PET, representing physiologic urinary tracer excretion.
5. Physiologic $^{18}$F-FDG uptake on PET in the left ovary and lumen of uterus during menstruation.

## Case II.12.2

### History

This 37-year-old male presented with abdominal pain and weight loss. On physical examination, an enlarged spleen and left axillary adenopathy were noted. CT showed left axillary and mediastinal adenopathy, an enlarged spleen with hypodense areas, massive adenopathy in the hepatic hilum, and enlarged mesenteric and retroperitoneal lymph nodes. An excisional lymph node biopsy from the left axilla was diagnostic for DLCL. Bone marrow biopsy showed no evidence of lymphoma. [18]F-FDG PET/CT was performed for staging (Fig. II.12.2A), after two cycles and at the end of chemotherapy (Fig. II.12.2B).

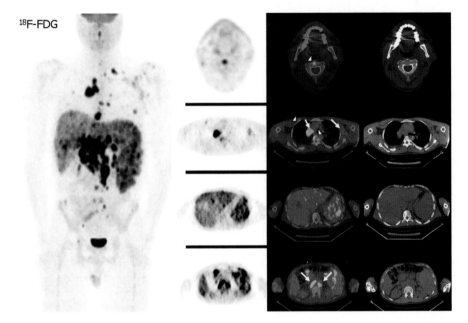

**Fig. II.12.2A**

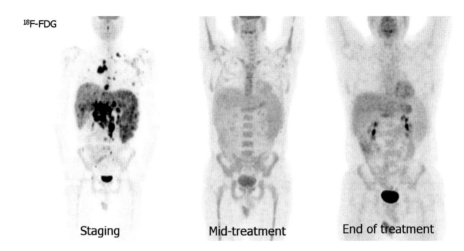

Fig. II.12.2B

## Findings

Baseline PET/CT (Fig. II.12.2A) demonstrates foci of abnormal $^{18}$F-FDG uptake in multiple enlarged lymph nodes, up to $30 \times 30$ mm in diameter above the diaphragm, in a mesenteric mass $100 \times 60$ mm in size and in additional enlarged lymph nodes up to $30 \times 25$ mm below the diaphragm (arrows), as well as diffuse heterogenic increased tracer uptake in the liver and in an enlarged spleen, and multiple abnormal tracer uptake foci in the skeleton (arrowheads) including cervical, thoracic, and lumbar vertebrae, the left scapula and clavicle, sternum, multiple ribs, the right ilium, and the left sacroiliac region, with no corresponding abnormalities on the CT scan.

PET/CT performed after two cycles of chemotherapy (Fig. II.12.2B, MIP-center image) shows diffuse increased skeletal and splenic tracer uptake most probably related to G-CSF treatment. PET/CT performed at the end of treatment (Fig. II.12.2B, MIP-right image) shows no sites of abnormal $^{18}$F-FDG activity and no evidence of active disease.

## Discussion

NHL has frequently an extranodal presentation, mainly to the GIT, but almost any organ can be involved. $^{18}$F-FDG imaging is superior to CT in detecting extranodal disease in the spleen, liver, and potentially the bone marrow.[15,16] In this patient, there are multiple foci of $^{18}$F-FDG uptake in the skeleton with no concurrent findings on CT. Bone marrow biopsy, based on sampling of the iliac bone, was falsely negative in this case. In patients with multifocal bone marrow involvement such as this one, PET performs better as compared to patients with diffuse involvement.[17]

PET/CT performed during treatment demonstrates diffuse $^{18}$F-FDG uptake throughout the skeleton and in the spleen. Since there had been initial bone marrow and splenic involvement, this uptake may be related to persistent disease but with a lower likelihood considering the dramatic response in all other sites and also because of the diffuse pattern of uptake, which is different from the multiple focal lesions on the baseline study. Interview of the patient confirmed recent administration of G-CSF, which affects the biodistribution of $^{18}$F-FDG.[32]

Aggressive NHL responds well to chemotherapy as demonstrated in this case by the mid- and end-of-treatment studies, which show no evidence of active lymphoma. Negative $^{18}$F-FDG studies at mid- and end-of-treatment are associated with good prognosis.[24–28] The patient achieved CR and has no evidence of disease for a follow-up of 3 years.

**Diagnosis**

1. DLCL, stage IV.
2. Good response to treatment.

## Case II.12.3 (DICOM Images on DVD)

### History

This 56-year-old male was diagnosed with anemia on routine blood tests. Chest X-rays done as part of the workup showed a mediastinal mass. CT revealed a large mediastinal mass and cervical lymphadenopathy. Abdominal ultrasound was normal. CT-guided biopsy of the mediastinal mass diagnosed classical HD. Bone marrow biopsy was normal. The patient was referred to [18]F-FDG PET/CT for staging (Fig. II.12.3A, B) and after two cycles of chemotherapy (Fig. II.12.3C).

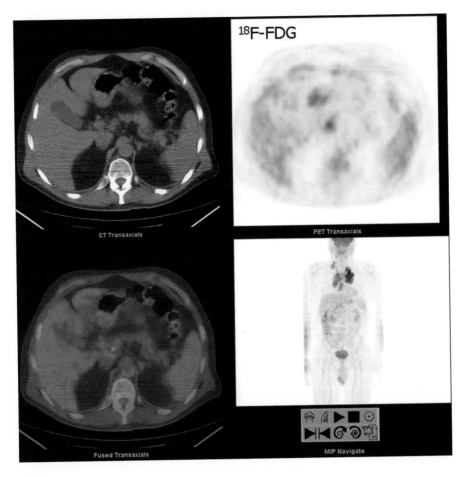

**Fig. II.12.3A**

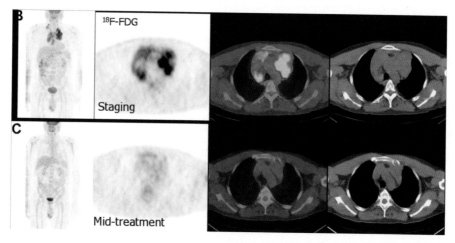

**Fig. II.12.3 B, C**

## Findings

A large area of heterogeneous abnormal $^{18}$F-FDG uptake is seen in a 125 × 50 mm mediastinal mass with additional foci of pathological uptake in the lower neck, the right pulmonary hilum, subcarinal region, and lower posterior mediastinum as demonstrated in the MIP image (Fig. II.12.3A, B). An additional small $^{18}$F-FDG focus corresponding to a 13 × 9 mm celiac lymph node is noted below the diaphragm (Fig. II.12.3A). PET/CT acquired after two courses of chemotherapy demonstrates a residual mediastinal mass with no abnormal $^{18}$F-FDG activity (Fig. II.12.3C).

## Discussion

This is a typical case of HD diagnosed by CT with a painless mediastinal mass and supradiaphragmatic lymphadenopathy. $^{18}$F-FDG PET/CT identified all sites of disease diagnosed by CT and detected an additional nodal site below the diaphragm in a slightly enlarged celiac chain lymph node that was overlooked on CT. This resulted in upstaging of the patient from stage II to stage III disease. PET/CT is more sensitive than CT or PET alone in staging of HD and aggressive NHL with a sensitivity of about 90%.[13] In a previous report $^{18}$F-FDG PET/CT resulted in upstaging of up to 20% of cases showing discordance with CT and had an impact on patient management in up to 30% of cases.[8,9]

PET/CT acquired after two courses of chemotherapy showed no sites of abnormal $^{18}$F-FDG activity (Fig. II.12.3C). High-stage HD has good prognosis with 5-year survival of about 50%. PET/CT performed during treatment is a valuable tool for risk stratification in HD.[25] The CT component of the study performed during treatment demonstrates the presence of a residual mediastinal mass (Fig. II.12.3C). Anatomical imaging cannot distinguish between residual viable lymphoma and a residual mass of necrotic and fibrotic tissue. $^{18}$F-FDG provides important metabolic information and thus enables differentiation between responders to chemotherapy and non-responders early during treatment.

The patient continued to receive treatment and is scheduled for a post-treatment $^{18}$F-FDG PET/CT study.

**Diagnosis**

1. Classical HD of the nodular sclerosis type, stage III.
2. Good metabolic response to treatment demonstrated on PET/CT during treatment.


**Clinical Report: Body $^{18}$F-FDG PET/CT (for DVD cases only)**

Indication

Staging of HD diagnosed by core biopsy of a mediastinal mass.


History

This 56-year-old male was diagnosed with anemia on routine blood test. Chest X-rays done as part of the workup showed a mediastinal mass. CT revealed a large mediastinal mass and cervical lymphadenopathy. Abdominal ultrasound was normal. Bone marrow biopsy was normal.


Procedure

Oral contrast was administered prior to the procedure. The patient was fasted for more than 4 h and had normal blood glucose levels prior to $^{18}$F-FDG injection. Acquisition was performed with a PET/CT scanner with a low-dose CT being used for anatomical correlation and attenuation correction. PET emission images were started 90 min after IV injection of 518 MBq (14 mCi) of $^{18}$F-FDG and covered the area from the base of the skull through the upper thighs.


Findings

  *Quality of study*: The quality of the study is good. There is physiologic distribution of the radiopharmaceutical in the brain, bowel, liver, and renal collection system.
  *Head and neck*: Abnormal uptake in the right lower neck localized to several lymph nodes of varying size, the largest one measuring 23 × 10 mm.
  *Chest*: Heterogeneous abnormal $^{18}$F-FDG uptake is seen in a lymph node aggregate in the left thoracic inlet forming a confluence with a large anterior mediastinal mass involving both sides and measuring 125 × 50 mm in its greatest dimensions. There are additional foci of abnormal uptake in enlarged mediastinal lymph nodes in the subcarinal region and in mild-to-moderate right hilar adenopathy. There are moderate calcifications in the left anterior descending coronary artery.
  *Abdomen and pelvis*: Focal pathological uptake is seen in a slightly enlarged, 13 × 9 mm, lymph node in the celiac chain. On CT there is a very small cortical cyst in the right kidney, a small umbilical hernia containing fat only and an enlarged prostate.
  *Musculoskeletal*: within normal range.

Impression

1. Abnormal $^{18}$F-FDG uptake in a mediastinal mass, in multiple enlarged lymph nodes above the diaphragm, and in a single lymph node below the diaphragm, consistent with HD involvement.
2. Very small right renal cortical cyst.
3. Small umbilical hernia containing fat.
4. Enlarged prostate.

## Case II.12.4

### History

This 55-year-old female was diagnosed and treated for SLL in the right groin and achieved CR 1 year prior to current examination. She was hospitalized due to progressive weakness that developed over 2 months. She was referred for $^{18}$F-FDG PET/CT with the suspicion of recurrence (Fig. II.12.4A–C).

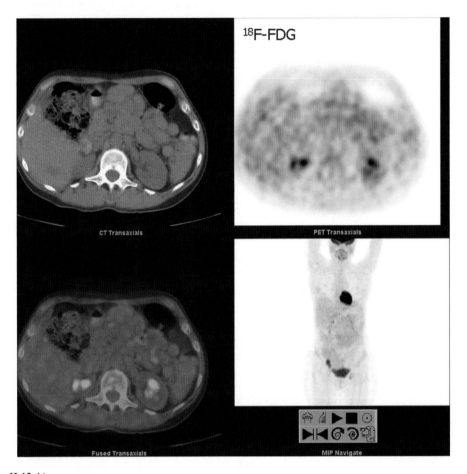

**Fig. II.12.4A**

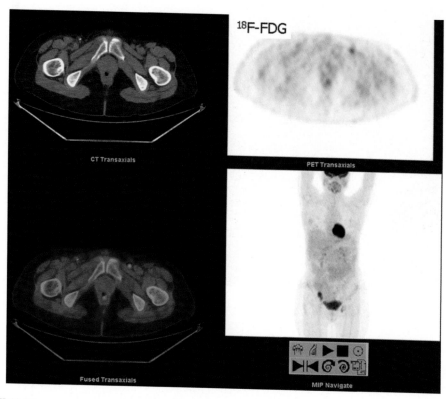

**Fig. II.12.4B**

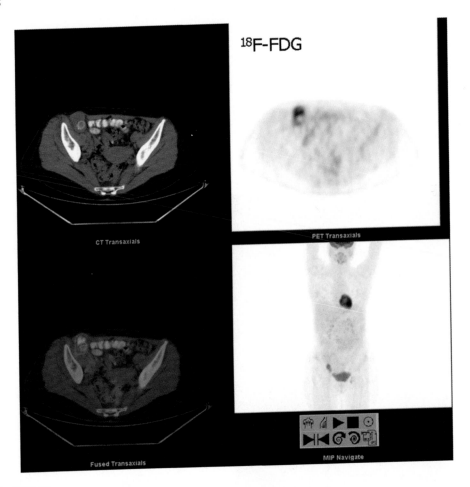

**Fig. II.12.4C**

## Findings

[18]F-FDG PET/CT demonstrates low-intensity [18]F-FDG uptake in a mesenteric mass 110 × 70 mm in largest axial dimensions extending from the level of the upper poles of the kidneys to the level of L5 (Fig. II.12.4A). Additional [18]F-FDG-avid foci are localized in both inguinal regions corresponding on the left to an enlarged 15 × 9 mm inguinal lymph node (Fig. II.12.4B) and on the right to a hypodense fluid collection 30 × 45 mm in size (Fig. II.12.4C). Sampling of the left inguinal node diagnosed recurrent SLL. The right inguinal lesion was diagnosed as an infectious process at the site of previous surgery.

## Discussion

[18]F-FDG PET has a high sensitivity and specificity for most histological subtypes of lymphoma. The intensity of uptake varies and does not correlate with the histological subtype or grade of lymphoma, with the exception of SLL, a low-grade lymphoma with known low-intensity uptake.[7,39] In Fig. II.12.4A, the faint, diffuse uptake in the anterior

aspect of the abdomen would have been difficult to interpret as disease if the mesenteric lymph nodes would have not been seen on CT. In a study that compared $^{18}$F-FDG and CT for detection of lymphoma, PET was not superior to CT below the diaphragm.[7] The site of recurrence in the left inguinal lymph node is easier to define due to the focal nature of the uptake and the low background in the groin. In the abdomen, however, uptake in liver, spleen, bowel loops, and blood vessels are responsible for relatively high background activity that can mask low-intensity uptake in involved lymph nodes. The low-intensity uptake in sites of SLL contrasts with the high-intensity uptake focus in the right groin, which is related to an infectious process at a site of previous surgery and radiation. $^{18}$F-FDG uptake is not specific to lymphoma and indicates the presence of a metabolically active process that utilizes glucose and may be due to infection, inflammation, or neoplasm. The intensity of uptake is also not indicative of the underlying process. Correlation with patient history and complaints, physical examination, and laboratory studies is essential.

**Diagnosis**

1. Recurrent SLL.
2. Post-surgical infection in right groin.

## Case II.12.5

### History

This 12-year-old female was diagnosed with HD by excisional biopsy of a cervical lymph node. She was referred to [18]F-FDG PET/CT for staging prior to treatment and had repeat studies after three and five courses of chemotherapy (Fig. II.12.5A–C).

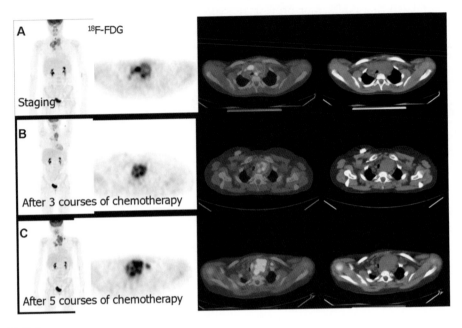

**Fig. II.12.5**

### Findings

[18]F-FDG PET/CT at presentation (Fig. II.12.5A) shows heterogeneous uptake in a mass extending from the anterior aspect of the base of the neck through the anterior mediastinum bilaterally (95 × 40 mm in the largest axial dimensions) and along the retrocaval–pretracheal region to the right suprahilar level. The mid-treatment study (Fig. II.12.5B) performed after three courses of chemotherapy shows some improvement with a decrease in size and intensity of the mediastinal [18]F-FDG uptake with corresponding anatomical shrinkage of the tumor on the CT component (90 × 35 mm in the largest axial dimensions). There is, however, significant residual abnormal uptake in the mediastinal mass. [18]F-FDG PET/CT performed after five courses of chemotherapy (Fig. II.12.5C) shows TP with abnormal [18]F-FDG activity that has increased in extent and intensity in a mediastinal mass that has enlarged on CT to 100 × 50 mm in the largest axial dimensions and now displaces the trachea to the right. In additional, there is a new focus of uptake in an enlarged left supraclavicular lymph node, 17 × 14 mm in size.

## Discussion

This patient had stage II HD. After three courses of chemotherapy, [18]F-FDG PET/CT demonstrated the presence of residual active disease. [18]F-FDG PET/CT is used to monitor response to therapy in both HD and NHL. Patients with residual uptake during treatment have a worse prognosis than patients with a negative study.[24–27] PET/CT performed during treatment can separate early responders to chemotherapy from non-responders. In most lymphoma patients, chemotherapy is highly effective, and no [18]F-FDG uptake can be found as early as 1 day after onset of therapy.[23] PET is limited in detecting disease below a certain tumor volume. In this particular patient, the chemotherapy regimen was intensified after mid-treatment PET/CT results that showed an unsatisfactory response. TP further detected by PET/CT led to induction of salvage chemotherapy and AHCT after which the patient achieved CR and has no evidence of disease for a follow-up of 3 years.

## Diagnosis

1. HD, refractory to first-line chemotherapy.
2. CR after salvage therapy and AHCT.

## Case II.12.6

### History

This 66-year-old female was diagnosed with grade II FL by diagnostic biopsy from a lymph node in the right groin, the only site of disease by CT. Bone marrow biopsy showed no evidence of disease. The patient was considered to have stage I disease and was treated with local radiotherapy. She was referred for [18]F-FDG PET/CT to assess response to radiation therapy and for periodical studies thereafter to monitor the status of the disease and as an aid in further treatment decisions (Fig. II.12.6A-G, *time after initial diagnosis, # treatment initiated after scan).

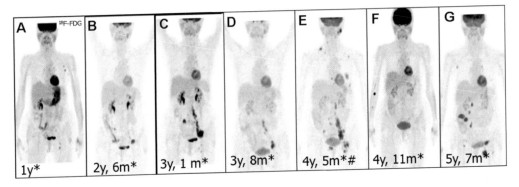

Fig. II.12.6A–G

### Findings

MIP images of serial [18]F-FDG PET/CT studies are presented. The first study (Fig. II.12.6A) demonstrates the presence of abnormal [18]F-FDG uptake in lymph nodes in the left axilla and left groin, consistent with sites of active disease. Diffuse increased uptake in the stomach was further diagnosed as chronic gastritis by endoscopic biopsy. Chemotherapy was initiated. A study performed 1 year after completion of chemotherapy (Fig. II.12.6B) demonstrates a new focus of increased [18]F-FDG uptake in lymph nodes in the left groin and the right internal iliac chain. The caring physician recommended a watchful waiting policy. The next study was performed 6 months later (Fig. II.12.6C) and shows TP in nodal sites below the diaphragm, along the iliac vessels and in the left groin. The watchful waiting policy was continued. An additional study was performed 7 months later (Fig. II.12.6D) and demonstrates disease regression with a decrease in number and intensity of foci of abnormal uptake in lymph nodes along the left iliac vessels and in the left groin. No uptake is seen in the right internal iliac region. An additional study was performed 9 months later following new patient complaints of swelling in the left submandibular region (Fig. II.12.6E). It demonstrates TP with multiple new foci of abnormal [18]F-FDG uptake in sclerotic and lytic lesions in the skeleton involving the right pubis, bilateral sacroiliac regions, T9 and T11 vertebrae, the lower ribs, and a soft tissue mass also involving a rib in the posterior aspect of the left lower chest wall. There were also additional new foci of increased tracer activity in lymph nodes above the diaphragm including the left submandibular region. The previously demonstrated lesions below the diaphragm increased in number and in intensity of uptake. Following this study, second-line chemotherapy combined with Rituximab was initiated, and complete remission was demonstrated by PET/CT at the end of treatment (Fig. II.12.6F). An additional study was performed after 8 months (Fig. II.12.6G) due to new swelling of the left groin and demonstrated recurrence in multiple nodal sites above and below the diaphragm.

## Discussion

FL is the most common indolent lymphoma subtype representing about 70% of all patients. Indolent NHL has a relatively good prognosis with median survival of up to 10 years, but is, as a rule, not curable in advanced clinical stages.[2] In this patient, chemotherapy was effective for only a short period with relapses documented in the second and last studies (Fig. II.12.6B, G). Spontaneous regression occurs in up to 20% of FL, and waxing and waning adenopathy has been described, similar to that documented between the second and third study, followed by spontaneous regression of disease (between the third and fourth study), and then repeat progression (between the fourth and fifth study). In present case, $^{18}$F-FDG PET/CT was performed as an aid to guide the decision-making process on when and how to treat. Treatment was initiated based on the fact that the patient became symptomatic and on PET/CT, which demonstrated progression of disease. Another role for $^{18}$F-FDG imaging in patients with indolent NHL is to detect transformation to aggressive disease as may be suggested by an increase in $^{18}$F-FDG intensity in a previously low-uptake site.[40]

In the first study (Fig. II.12.6A), diffuse gastric uptake is notable. This could represent an extranodal site of lymphoma, physiologic tracer uptake, or gastritis. $^{18}$F-FDG uptake is non-specific and cannot differentiate between the different etiologies. The GIT is the most common site of extranodal involvement, with the stomach being the most common site within the GIT. Lymphomatous involvement seems therefore a reasonable option, while, on the other hand, gastritis is a common disease. In this case, endoscopic examination and tissue sampling diagnosed gastritis.

## Diagnosis

1. Recurrent grade II FL.
2. Gastritis.

## Case II.12.7

### History

This 35-year-old male complained of weight loss. CT performed as part of his work-up demonstrated the presence of a mediastinal mass. Biopsy diagnosed HD. Bone marrow biopsy was normal. The patient was referred to $^{18}$F-FDG PET/CT for staging prior to treatment (Fig. II.12.7A) and following repeat studies during and at the end of treatment, 6 months after completion of treatment for routine follow-up (Fig. II.12.7B).

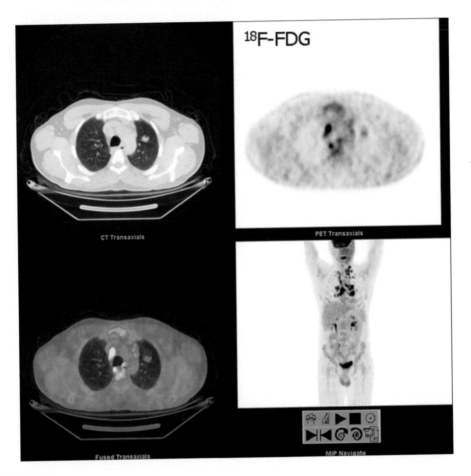

**Fig. II.12.7A**

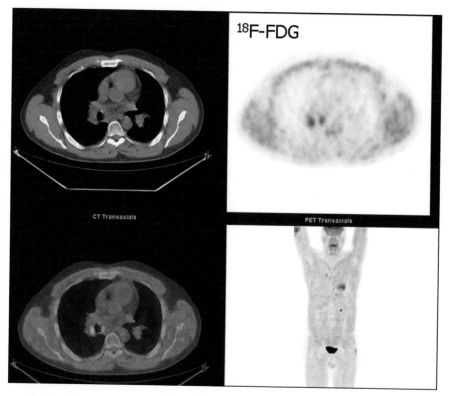

**Fig. II.12.7B**

## Findings

$^{18}$F-FDG PET/CT at staging (Fig. II.12.7A) demonstrates abnormal foci of tracer uptake in lymph nodes along the left side of the neck, in the supra- and infraclavicular region bilaterally, and in multiple mediastinal locations. Abnormal foci of tracer uptake of lesser intensity were noted in lesions in both lungs. Mid- and end-of-treatment studies were negative. A PET/CT study performed for routine follow-up 6 months later (Fig. II.12.7B) demonstrates new sites of increased $^{18}$F-FDG activity in the right pulmonary hilum and in an enlarged subcarinal lymph node (23 × 16 mm), which are areas of HD involvement at presentation. These new findings were interpreted as suspicious for recurrent disease. Bronchoscopic biopsy from the lesion in the right pulmonary hilum confirmed the diagnosis. There is diffuse tracer uptake in skeletal muscles.

## Discussion

The staging PET/CT study showed multiple $^{18}$F-FDG-avid foci in lung nodules (Fig. II.12.7A), raising the suspicion for pulmonary lymphomatous involvement. The differential diagnosis includes concurrent inflammatory, infectious, or granulomatous lung disease. The patient's history and the CT features of the pulmonary findings can help in making the correct diagnosis. The presence of a single focus of abnormal $^{18}$F-FDG uptake, especially in advanced-age smokers, should raise the possibility of a synchronous primary lung malignancy. In this young, previously healthy non-smoker, the most likely diagnosis is HD involvement, which indicates stage IV disease. Appearance of new lung uptake foci in studies performed after initiation of treatment is more problematic since the prevalence of benign lung lesions, such as opportunistic infections, chemotherapy-induced. or post-radiation pneumonitis, rises. It has been therefore suggested that new [18]F-FDG-avid lung nodules in studies performed during or after treatment in patients without established pulmonary lymphoma at staging, in conjunction with evidence of CR in all other disease sites, should be considered unrelated to lymphoma.[19]

The mid- and end-of-treatment studies show no evidence of disease. The patient returned for a routine follow-up study 6 months later (Fig. II.12.7B), and recurrence in previously involved mediastinal lymph nodes was diagnosed.

Diffuse uptake in skeletal muscles (Fig. II.12.7B) indicates a change in the pattern of the biodistribution of [18]F-FDG and can be related to intense physical activity the day prior to the study, to elevated insulin levels, most frequently due to noncompliance to fasting instructions.

## Diagnosis

Early relapse of HD.

## Case II.12.8

### History

This 60-year-old male with a history of FL presented with marked adenopathy in the right axilla. CT demonstrated extensive lymphadenopathy above and below the diaphragm, most prominent in the right axilla and the left para-aortic region, suggestive of recurrent lymphoma. A biopsy from the right axilla was non-diagnostic, consisting of necrotic tissue. $^{18}$F-FDG PET/CT scan was performed (Fig. II.12.8A, B) for guiding repeat biopsy to a metabolically active site.

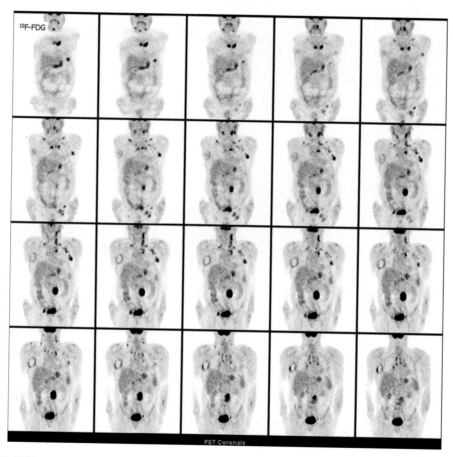

Fig. II.12.8A

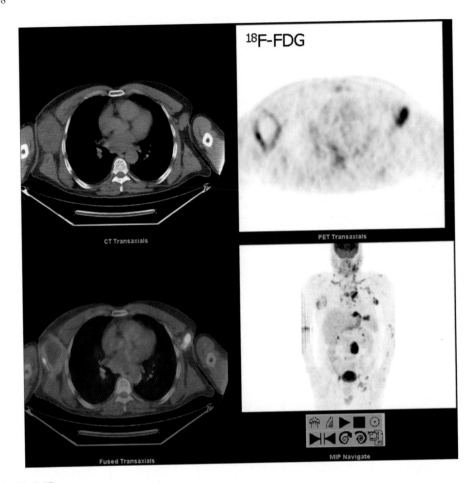

**Fig. II.12.8B**

### Findings

Multiple foci of increased tracer activity of variable intensity are demonstrated in enlarged lymph nodes above and below the diaphragm (Fig. II.12.8A, B). There are also multiple sites of abnormal [18]F-FDG uptake in the skeleton including both clavicles, the left acromion, T8, T9, L3 vertebrae, and the iliac bones. There is only moderate [18]F-FDG activity at the borders of the large, mainly hypodense right axillary lymph node, which has been the site of the previous biopsy (Fig. II.12.8B)

### Discussion

[18]F-FDG PET/CT was performed in search of the most suitable site for repeat biopsy after the first procedure had been non-diagnostic. In a study involving 56 patients with known lymphoma, ultrasound biopsy guided by [18]F-FDG PET/CT findings was found to be a safe and effective tool to diagnose recurrence.[41] In present case, PET/CT indicated the potential cause for previously unsuccessful tissue sampling. The large photopenic area in the center of the mass, also hypodense on CT, surrounded by a thin border of low-intensity FDG activity

(Fig. II.12.8B), suggests that most of this large lesion is necrotic. Furthermore, PET/CT findings guide toward appropriate sites for repeat tissue sampling in enlarged peripheral lymph nodes with high-intensity, homogenous $^{18}$F-FDG uptake, as demonstrated in the left axilla and the right groin. In patients with recurrent FL, it is particularly important to direct biopsy to the site with most intense uptake, since FL is prone to transformation to aggressive forms of lymphoma, which may display more intense uptake.[44] Biopsy from the left axilla was performed and established the diagnosis of recurrent FL, the same histology as at initial presentation.

The study also identified multiple focal sites of increased $^{18}$F-FDG uptake throughout the skeleton with no corresponding findings on CT. Bone marrow involvement was confirmed by biopsy.

**Diagnosis**

Recurrent grade II FL.

## Case II.12.9

### History

This 36-year-old female was diagnosed with HD by mediastinal biopsy. The staging PET/CT study showed abnormal $^{18}$F-FDG uptake in multiple nodal sites above the diaphragm. A mid-treatment study after two courses of chemotherapy showed CR, confirmed at the end of chemotherapy and after completion of radiation treatment to the mediastinal mass. The patient performed periodic follow-up PET/CT (Fig. II.12.9A–C, *time after initial diagnosis).

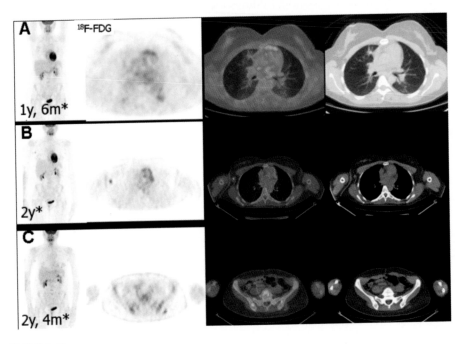

**Fig. II.12.9 A–C**

### Findings

During follow-up, there are new low-intensity foci of increased $^{18}$F-FDG activity in para-mediastinal lesions in the upper zones of the lungs (Fig. II.12.9A). The next follow-up study performed 6 months later (Fig. II.12.9B) demonstrates a new focus of increased $^{18}$F-FDG activity in a right axillary lymph node (10 × 10 mm) and disappearance of the paramediastinal findings. An additional study performed 4 months later (Fig. II.12.9C) demonstrates the presence of a new, low-intensity focus of increased $^{18}$F-FDG activity in a subcutaneous granuloma in the left buttock.

### Discussion

Lymphoma has an overall cure rate of up to 80%. Therefore, most follow-up $^{18}$F-FDG PET/CT studies show no evidence of disease. $^{18}$F-FDG is, however, not lymphoma-specific and is taken up by various active metabolic processes unrelated to the primary disease, of various malignant, infectious, or inflammatory etiologies.[31,32] A study including 1,120 post-treatment studies in 848 lymphoma patients reported a false-positive rate of 5% under strict interpretation criteria. [18]F-FDG-avid foci were considered positive for lymphoma only when uptake occurred at sites of previous disease, in asymmetric lymph nodes, or in nodal stations unlikely to be affected by inflammation. [18]F-FDG-avid foci were considered benign in regions of physiological uptake (urinary tract, GIT, muscles), symmetrical nodal uptake, lesions unrelated to lymphoma already identified by other imaging modalities, and very low or non-focal uptake.[33]

In the present case, the first follow-up study showed new low-intensity, paramediastinal [18]F-FDG activity in upper lung lesions (Fig. II.12.9A). In this specific clinical setting, these findings were attributed to post-radiation pneumonitis, which indeed resolved on the next study (Fig. II.12.9B). Subsequently, a moderately intense focus of tracer uptake was demonstrated in an axillary nodal site. The intensity of uptake was not high, this site had not been involved initially, and reactive axillary lymphadenopathy is common. This was stated in the report issued for this study, and the findings resolved on follow-up (Fig. II.12.9C). The new low-intensity lesion seen on the next study (Fig. II.12.9C) was a subcutaneous granuloma in the left buttock.

## Diagnosis

1. No evidence of HD on follow-up studies.
2. Transient foci of increased [18]F-FDG activity due to inflammatory processes.

# References

1. Jemal A, Siegel R, Ward E, Murray T, Xu J, Thun MJ.Cancer statistics, 2007. *CA Cancer J Clin* 2007;57:43–66.
2. Armitage JO, Weisenburger DD. New approach to classifying non-Hodgkin's lymphomas: Clinical features of the major histologic subtypes. Non-Hodgkin's Lymphoma classification project. *J Clin Oncol* 1998;16:2780–2795.
3. Adult Non-Hodgkin Lymphoma Treatment, National Cancer Institute, U.S. National Institutes of Health, last updated on 12/17/2007 (Accessed December 20th 2007, at http://www.cancer.gov/cancer topics/pdq/treatment/adult-non-hodgkins/healthprofessional).
4. Ardeshna KM, Smith P, Norton A, Hancock BW, Hoskin PJ, MacLennan KA, Marcus RE, Jelliffe A, Hudson GV, Linch DC. Long-term effect of a watch and wait policy versus immediate systemic treatment for asymptomatic advanced-stage non-Hodgkin lymphoma: A randomised controlled trial. *Lancet* 2003;362:516–522.
5. Adult Hodgkin Lymphoma Treatment, National Cancer Institute, U.S. National Institutes of Health, last updated on 7/17/2007 (Accessed December 20th 2007, at http://www.cancer.gov/cancertopics/pdq/treatment/adulthodgkins/healthprofessional).
6. Elstrom R, Guan L, Baker G, Nakhoda K, Vergilio JA, Zhuang H, Pitsilos S, Bagg A, Downs L, Mehrotra A. Utility of FDG-PET scanning in lymphoma by WHO classification. *Blood* 2003;101:3875–3876.
7. Tsukamoto N, Kojima M, Hasegawa M, Oriuchi N, Matsushima T, Yokohama A, Saitoh T, Handa H, Endo K, Murakami H. The usefulness of 18F-fluorodeoxyglucose positron emission tomography (18F-FDG-PET) and a comparison of 18F-FDG-PET with 67Gallium scintigraphy in the evaluation of lymphoma: Relation to histologic subtypes based on the World Health Organization classification. *Cancer* 2007;110:652–659.
8. Seam P, Juweid ME, Cheson BD. The role of FDG-PET scans in patients with lymphoma. *Blood* 2007;110:3509–3516.
9. Buchmann I, Reinhardt M, Elsner K, Bunjes D, Altehoefer C, Finke J, Moser E, Glatting G, Kotzerke J, Guhlmann CA, Schirrmeister H, Reske SN. 2-(fluorine-18)fluoro-2-deoxy-D-glucose positron emission tomography in the detection and staging of malignant lymphoma. A bicenter trial. *Cancer* 2001;91:889–899.
10. Moog F, Bangerter M, Diederichs CG, Guhlmann. A, Kotzerke J, Merkle E, Kolokythas O, Herrmann. F, Reske SN. Lymphoma: role of whole-body 2-deoxy-2-[F-18]fluoro-D-glucose (FDG) PET in nodal staging. *Radiology* 1997;203:795–800.
11. Moog F, Bangerter M, Diederichs CG, Guhlmann A, Merkle E, Frickhofen N, Reske SN. Extranodal malignant lymphoma: detection with FDG PET versus CT. *Radiology* 1998;206:475–481.
12. Raanani P, Shasha Y, Perry C, Metser U, Naparstek E, Apter S, Nagler A, Polliack A, Ben-Bassat I, Even-Sapir E. Is CT scan still necessary for staging in Hodgkin and non-Hodgkin lymphoma patients in the PET/CT era? *Ann Oncol* 2006;17:117–122.
13. Isasi CR, Lu P, Blaufox MD. A metaanalysis of 18F-2-deoxy-2-fluoro-D-glucose positron emission tomography in the staging and restaging of patients with lymphoma. *Cancer* 2005;104:1066–1074.
14. Schaefer NG, Hany TF, Taverna C, Seifert B, Stumpe KD, von Schulthess GK, Goerres GW. Non-Hodgkin lymphoma and Hodgkin disease: Coregistered FDG PET and CT at staging and restaging – do we need contrast-enhanced CT? *Radiology* 2004;232:823–829.
15. Tatsumi M, Cohade C, Nakamoto Y, Fishman EK,Wahl RL. Direct comparison of FDG PET and CT findings in patients with lymphoma: initial experience. *Radiology* 2005;237:1038–1045.
16. Moog F, Bangerter M, Kotzerke J, Guhlmann A, Frickhofen N, Reske SN. 18-F-fluorodeoxyglucose-positron emission tomography as a new approach to detect lymphomatous bone marrow. *J Clin Oncol* 1998;16:603–609.
17. Pakos EE, Fotopoulos AD, Ioannidis JP. 18F-FDG PET for evaluation of bone marrow infiltration in staging of lymphoma: A meta-analysis. *J Nucl Med* 2005;46:958–963.
18. Cheson BD, Pfistner B, Juweid ME, Gascoyne RD, Specht L, Horning SJ, Coiffier B, Fisher RI, Hagenbeek A, Zucca E, Rosen ST, Stroobants S, Lister TA, Hoppe RT, Dreyling M, Tobinai K, Vose JM, Connors JM, Federico M, Diehl V. Revised response criteria for malignant lymphoma. *J Clin Oncol.* 2007;25:579–586.
19. Juweid ME, Stroobants S, Hoekstra OS, Mottaghy FM, Dietlein M, Guermazi A, Wiseman GA, Kostakoglu L, Scheidhauer K, Buck A, Naumann R, Spaepen K, Hicks RJ, Weber WA, Reske SN,

Schwaiger M, Schwartz LH, Zijlstra JM, Siegel BA, Cheson BD. Use of positron emission tomography for response assessment of lymphoma: consensus of the Imaging Subcommittee of International Harmonization project in Lymphoma: *J Clin Oncol* 2007;25:571–578.

20. Hudson MM, Krasin MJ, Kaste SC. PET imaging in pediatric Hodgkin's lymphoma. *Pediatr Radiol* 2004;34:190–198.

21. Cheson BD, Horning SJ, Coiffier B, Shipp MA, Fisher RI, Connors JM, Lister TA, Vose J, Grillo-López A, Hagenbeek A, Cabanillas F, Klippensten D, Hiddemann W, Castellino R, Harris NL, Armitage JO, Carter W, Hoppe R, Canellos GP. Report of an international workshop to standardize response criteria for non-Hodgkin's lymphomas. NCI sponsored international working group. *J Clin Oncol* 1999;17:1244.

22. Lister TA, Crowther D, Sutcliffe SB, Glatstein E, Canellos GP, Young RC, Rosenberg SA, Coltman CA, Tubiana M. Report of a committee convened to discuss the evaluation and staging of patients with Hodgkin's disease: Cotswolds meeting. *J Clin Oncol* 1989;7:1630–1636.

23. Kasamon YL, Jones RJ, Wahl RL. Integrating PET and PET/CT into the risk-adapted therapy of lymphoma. *J Nucl Med* 2007;48 Suppl 1:19S–27S.

24. Haioun C, Itti E, Rahmouni A, Brice P, Rain J-D, Belhadj K, Gaulard P, Garderet L, Lepage E, Reyes F, Meignan M. [18F]fluoro-2-deoxy-D-glucose positron emission tomography (FDG-PET) in aggressive lymphoma: an early prognostic tool for predicting patient outcome. *Blood* 2005;106:1376–1381.

25. Hutchings M, Loft A, Hansen M, Pedersen LM, Buhl T, Jurlander J, Buus S, Keiding S, D'Amore F, Boesen A-M, Berthelsen AK, Specht L. FDG-PET after two cycles of chemotherapy predicts treatment failure and progression-free survival in Hodgkin lymphoma. *Blood* 2006;107:52–59.

26. Avril NE, Weber WA. Monitoring response to treatment in patients utilizing PET. *Radiol Clin North Am* 2005;43:189–204.

27. Schot BW, Zijlstra JM, Sluiter WJ, van Imhoff GW, Pruim J, Vaalburg W, Vellenga E. Early FDG-PET assessment in combination with clinical risk scores determines prognosis in recurring lymphoma. *Blood* 2007;109:486–491.

28. Juweid ME, Wiseman GA, Vose JM, Ritchie JM, Menda Y, Wooldridge JE, Mottaghy FM, Rohren EM, Blumstein NM, Stolpen A, Link BK, Reske SN, Graham MM, Cheson BD. Response assessment of aggressive non-Hodgkin's lymphoma by integrated International Workshop Criteria and fluorine-18-fluorodeoxyglucose positron emission tomography. *J Clin Oncol* 2005;23:4652–4661.

29. Naumann R, Vaic A, Beuthien-Baumann B, Bredow J, Kropp J, Kittner T, Franke W-G, Ehninger G. Prognostic value of positron emission tomography in the evaluation of post-treatment residual mass in patients with Hodgkin's disease and non-Hodgkin's lymphoma. *Br J Haematol* 2001;115:793–800.

30. Weihrauch MR, Re D, Scheidhauer K, Ansén S, Dietlein M, Bischoff S, Bohlen H, Wolf J, Schicha H, Diehl V, Tesch H. Thoracic positron emission tomography using 18F-fluorodeoxyglucose for the evaluation of residual mediastinal Hodgkin disease. *Blood* 2001;98:2930–2934.

31. Bar-Shalom R. Normal and abnormal patterns of 18F-fluorodeoxyglucose PET/CT in lymphoma. *Radiol Clin North Am* 2007;45:677–688, vi–vii.

32. Kazama T, Faria SC, Varavithya V, Phongkitkarun S, Ito H, Macapinlac HA. FDG PET in the evaluation of treatment for lymphoma: clinical usefulness and pitfalls. *Radiographics* 2005;25:191–207.

33. Castellucci P, Zinzani P, Pourdehnad M, Alinari L, Nanni C, Farsad M, Battista G, Tani M, Stefoni V, Canini R, Monetti N, Rubello D, Alavi A, Franchi R, Fanti S. 18F-FDG PET in malignant lymphoma: significance of positive findings. *Eur J Nucl Med Mol Imaging* 2005;32:749–756.

34. Radford JA, Eardley A, Woodman C, Crowther D. Follow up policy after treatment for Hodgkin's disease: too many clinic visits and routine tests? A review of hospital records. *BMJ* 997;314:343–346.

35. Torrey MJ, Poen JC, Hoppe RT. Detection of relapse in early-stage Hodgkin's disease: Role of routine follow-up studies. *J Clin Oncol* 1997;15:1123–1130.

36. Jerusalem G, Beguin Y, Fassotte MF, Belhocine T, Hustinx R, Rigo P, Fillet G. Early detection of relapse by whole-body positron emission tomography in the follow-up of patients with Hodgkin's disease. *Ann Oncol* 2003;14:123–130.

37. Elis A, Blickstein D, Klein O, Eliav-Ronen R, Manor Y, Lishner M. Detection of relapse in non-Hodgkin's lymphoma: Role of routine follow-up studies. *Am J Hematol* 2002;69:41–44.

38. Guppy AE, Tebbutt NC, Norman A, Cunningham D. The role of surveillance CT scans in patients with diffuse large B-cell non-Hodgkin's lymphoma. *Leuk Lymphoma* 2003;44:123–125.

39. Karam M, Novak L, Cyriac J, Ali A, Nazeer T, Nugent F. Role of fluorine-18 fluoro-deoxyglucose positron emission tomography scan in the evaluation and follow-up of patients with low-grade lymphomas. *Cancer* 2006;107:175–183.

40. Schoder H, Noy A, Gonen M, Weng L, Green D, Erdi YE, Larson SM, Yeung HW. Intensity of 18fluorodeoxyglucose uptake in positron emission tomography distinguishes between indolent and aggressive non-Hodgkin's lymphoma. *J Clin Oncol* 2005;23:4643–4651.
41. Podoloff DA, Advani RH, Allred C, Benson AB, Brown E, Burstein HJ, Carlson RW, Coleman RE, Czuczman MS, Delbeke D, Edge SB, Ettinger DS, Grannis FW, Hillner BE, Hoffman JM, Keil K, Komaki R, Larson SM, Mankoff DA, Rozenzweig KE, Skibber JM, Yahalom J, Yu JM, Zelenetz AD. NCCN Task Force Report: Positron Emission Tomography (PET/Computed tomography (CT) scanning in cancer. *J Natl Compr Canc Netw* 2007;5 Suppl 1:S1–S22.
42. http://www.nccn.org/professionals/physiciangls/fguidelines.asp.
43. Fletcher JW, Djulbegovic B, Soares HP, Siegel BA, Lowe VJ, Lyman GH, Coleman E, Wahl R, Paschold JC, Avril N, Einhorn LH, Suh WW, Samson D, Delbeke D, Gorman M, Shields AF. Recommendations for the use of FDG (fluorine-18, (2-[18 F]Fluoro-2-deoxy-D-glucose) positron emission tomography in oncology. *J Nucl Med* 2008;49:480–508.
44. Soudack M, Bar-Shalom R, Israel O, Ben-Arie Y, Levy Z, Gaitini D. Utility of sonographically guided biopsy in metabolically suspected recurrent lymphoma. *J Ultrasound Med* 2008;27:225–231.

# Chapter II.13
# Melanoma

**Ronald C. Walker, Laurie B. Jones-Jackson, Aaron C. Jessop, and Dominique Delbeke**

## Introduction

The National Cancer Institute Surveillance, Epidemiology, and End Results (SEER) database has demonstrated an increase in the annual incidence of cutaneous melanoma of 619% and an increase in annual mortality of 165% from 1950 to 2000. In 2004 an estimated 55,000 Americans were newly diagnosed with cutaneous melanoma, and approximately 7,900 died from this disease. Of all cancers in the United States, cutaneous melanoma ranks fifth in incidence among men and seventh among women. It is the most common cancer in women aged 20–29 and the second leading cause of lost productive years. Efforts to reduce the incidence of cutaneous melanoma include identification and screening of persons at high risk and encouragement of the use of sun protection. A prior cutaneous melanoma confers 10 times greater risk of a second melanoma, with the highest incidence within the first 2 years of the initial diagnosis. Inherited mutations in the *CDKN2A* and *CDK4* genes, documented in some families with hereditary melanoma, confer a 60–90% lifetime risk of melanoma.[1]

## Cutaneous Melanoma

### Diagnosis

Diagnosis of cutaneous melanoma is based on physician and/or patient examinations followed by biopsy of suspicious lesions. High-risk factors for development of melanoma include a prior personal or a family history of the disease, fair skin, and multiple pigmented skin lesions including atypical moles or freckles. Prior severe sunburns, especially multiple and occurring during childhood, also increase the lifetime risk of cutaneous melanoma. Both skin and mucous membranes must be examined annually in high-risk patients. Biopsy is necessary to verify the diagnosis.[1]

R.C. Walker (✉)
Department of Radiology and Radiological Sciences, Vanderbilt University Medical Center, Nashville, TN, USA
e-mail: ronald.walker@vanderbilt.edu

D. Delbeke, O. Israel (eds.), *Hybrid PET/CT and SPECT/CT Imaging*,
DOI 10.1007/978-0-387-92820-3_15, © Springer Science+Business Media, LLC 2010

## *Staging*

### TNM Staging

After biopsy confirmation of a newly diagnosed cutaneous melanoma, pathologic staging is important to establish both the prognosis and the subsequent surgical management. The Breslow system, empirically derived by Alexander Breslow in 1970, has been replaced by the Tumor, Node, Metastasis (TNM) system of clinical and pathologic staging adopted in 2002 by the American Joint Commission on Cancer (AJCC) (Table II.13.1). TNM staging has demonstrated improved correlation with melanoma-specific outcome analysis and includes the impact on survival based on risk factors, which had not been incorporated in the older staging system, specifically the presence or the absence of ulceration over the majority of the primary lesion and the results of sentinel lymph node (SLN) biopsy as to the presence or the absence of micro- or macrometastases. Research to incorporate additional data, such as blood levels of S-100β or melanoma inhibitory proteins, serum alkaline phosphatase or tyrosinase/melanoma antigen recognized by T cells 1 (MART-1) reverse transcription-polymerase chain reaction (RT-PCR)

**Table II.13.1**  AJCC melanoma TNM classification

| T classification | Thickness | Ulceration status |
|---|---|---|
| T1 | ≤1.0 mm | a: Without ulceration and level II/III |
|  |  | b: With ulceration or level IV/V |
| T2 | 1.01–2.0 mm | a: Without ulceration |
|  |  | b: With ulceration |
| T3 | 2.01–4.0 mm | a: Without ulceration |
|  |  | b: With ulceration |
| T4 | >4.0 mm | a: Without ulceration |
|  |  | b: With ulceration |
| **N classification** | **No. of metastatic nodes** | **Nodal metastatic mass** |
| N1 | 1 node | a: Micrometastasis[a] |
|  |  | b: Macrometastasis† |
| N2 | 2–3 nodes | a: Micrometastasis[a] |
|  |  | b: Macrometastasis[b] |
|  |  | c: In transit met(s)/satellite(s) without metastatic nodes |
| N3 | >3 metastatic nodes, or matted nodes, or in transit met(s)/satellite(s) with metastatic node(s) |  |
| **M classification** | **Site** | **Serum lactate dehydrogenase (LDH)** |
| M1a | Distant skin, subcutaneous, or nodal metastases | Normal |
| M1b | Pulmonary metastases | Normal |
| M1c | All other visceral metastases | Normal |
|  | Any distant metastasis | Elevated |

[a] Micrometastases are diagnosed after sentinel or elective lymphadenectomy.
[b] Macrometastases are defined as clinically detectable nodal metastases confirmed by therapeutic lymphadenectomy or when nodal metastasis exhibits gross extracapsular extension.
(Reprinted with permission of American Society of Clinical Oncology from Balch CM, Buzaid AC, Soong S, et al. Final Version of the American Joint Committee on Cancer Staging System for Cutaneous Melanoma. *J Clin Oncol* 2001; 19: 3635–3648.)

analysis[2-4] and evaluation of genetic risk factors, is ongoing but with unclear specific value for routine clinical use at this time. Incorporation of molecular markers is likely to be introduced in future staging systems. The only blood test criterion incorporated in the current AJCC melanoma staging is the level of lactate dehydrogenase (LDH) in advanced disease, demonstrating an inverse correlation with survival.[5]

The presence of metastatic disease in the SLN defines stage III or higher, disease. Long-term outcome is inversely related to the number of metastatic lymph nodes discovered by sampling both the SLN and other locoregional nodes in the SLN group. Within stage III, subgroups IIIa–c are related to the number of metastatic nodes, the presence of microscopic versus macroscopic disease in any of the nodes, and the presence or the absence of ulceration on histopathological examination of the primary lesion. Ulceration is defined as tumor breakthrough of the epidermis on microscopic examination, with an actual macroscopic ulcer crater seldom present (Table II.13.2).[5] Long-term survival of patients with stage IIC disease, defined as ulceration positive but SLN negative, is as poor as that of patients in the stage III disease, which demonstrates the significance of the presence of

**Table II.13.2**   Correlation of AJCC TNM stage with pathologic stage for cutaneous melanoma

| Pathologic stage | TNM designation | Thickness of primary (mm) | Ulceration present | SLN metastasis[a] |
|---|---|---|---|---|
| 1A | T1a | 1 | No | – |
| 1B | T1b | 1 | Yes[b] | – |
| | T2a | 1.01–2.0 | No | – |
| IIA | T2b | 1.01–2.0 | Yes | – |
| | T3a | 2.01–4.0 | No | – |
| IIB | T3b | 2.01–4.0 | Yes | – |
| | T4a | >4.0 | No | – |
| IIC | T4b | >4.0 | Yes | – |
| IIIA | N1a | Any | No | 1 micro |
| | N2a | Any | No | 2–3 micro |
| IIIB | N1a | Any | Yes | 1 micro |
| | N1b | Any | No | 1 macro |
| IIIB | N2a | Any | Yes | 2–3 micro |
| | N2b | Any | No | 2–3 macro |
| IIIC | N1b | Any | Yes | 1 macro |
| | N2b | Any | Yes | 2–3 macro |
| | N3 | Any | Any | >3 Any |
| IV[c] | M1a / M1b / M1c | Any | Any | Any |

[a] SLN metastasis status refers to the absence (–) of metastatic disease, the single most powerful predictor of long-term recurrence/outcome; the number of metastatic nodes found at SLN sampling; regional lymphadenectomy; microscopic (micro) versus macroscopic (macro) metastatic disease – pathologic staging.

The presence or the absence of primary lesion ulceration on histopathological examination is second only to the SLN status as a predictor of outcome.

Clinical "microscopic" lymph node metastasis refers to nodal involvement discovered by pathologic examination that was not apparent on pre-surgical physical examination or imaging studies.

Clinical "macroscopic" lymph node involvement is defined as pre-surgical metastatic lymphadenopathy evident on either physical and/or radiologic examination.

[b] Level 1B can demonstrate either cytopathological ulcerations or Clark level IV or V invasion.

[c] The presence of distant metastatic disease defines stage IV cutaneous melanoma. M1a has the least poor outcome, with metastases limited to the skin, lymph nodes, and subcutaneous tissues. M1b (pulmonary metastasis) and M1c (metastasis not involving the regions defined by M1a or M1b or elevated serum LDH) have the poorest outcome, with survival at 1 year less than 50% as a rule.

(Derived with permission of The Massachusetts Medical Society from Tsao et al.[1])

ulceration thought to be a surrogate for the aggressiveness of the tumor. The presence of four or more metastatic lymph nodes, or three matted nodes, regardless of other considerations, defines stage IIIC. While increasing thickness of the primary tumor and the presence of ulceration are factors that each negatively affect prognosis, the presence or the absence of metastatic disease in the SLN confers the most powerful significance on long-term survival.[6]

### Early Stage Melanoma: Role of SPECT/CT for SLN Localization and Biopsy

In stage I and II disease, with tumor thickness $\leq 4$ mm and no clinical evidence of spread, up to 75–80% of patients do not show nodal metastases at lymphadenectomy, a procedure that thus could be spared, lowering the morbidity and surgery-related cost.

The sentinel node concept states that the first node(s) to receive lymphatic drainage from a tumor (the "sentinel node") will always contain malignant cells if lymphatic spread of the tumor has occurred. Histopathology of the SLN will therefore reflect the histopathology of the entire nodal bed. Lymphoscintigraphy is useful in identifying patients who are most likely to benefit from lymphadenectomy. Nodal basins identified by lymphoscintigraphy are discordant with the expected drainage pattern in over 60% of patients with head and neck melanoma and one-third of patients with truncal lesions. If elective lymph node dissection is based on clinical experience or classic anatomic patterns, the procedure will be misdirected in approximately 50% of cases. Mainly in the head and neck and shoulder regions, but also in an area within 10 cm of the midline, there is unpredictable lymphatic drainage, making lymphoscintigraphy essential for identification of the SLN(s). Trunk lesions can drain to multiple sites, including cervical, supraclavicular, and inguinal lymph nodes. Upper extremity lesions can drain to the epitrochlear and/or axillary lymph nodes, and lower extremity lesions can drain to popliteal and/or inguinal lymph nodes.

Using minimally invasive surgery the SLN is identified during lymphoscintigraphy via a small hand-held gamma probe, and subsequently excised. Wide excision of the primary site is performed during the same procedure. If the SLN is proven to be positive for melanoma by conventional hematoxylin and eosin (H&E) staining or by RT-PCR analysis, the patient subsequently undergoes regional lymphadenectomy.

The results of the Multicenter Selective Lymphadenectomy Trial (MSLT) suggest that patients staged with a SLN procedure have a significantly better 5-year disease-free survival when compared to patients staged without identification of the SLN, thus demonstrating the important role of SLN sampling for accurate staging.[7] The Society of Nuclear Medicine (SNM) has published procedure guidelines for SLN localization in management of patients with melanoma.[8] The scintigraphic procedure is used, as a rule, in conjunction with methylene blue dye injected in the operating room. Blue and radioactive nodes are excised and extensively assessed histopathologically. This technique has been well-validated in patients with melanoma, with a false negative rate of <1%. The status of the SLN histology is predictive of >99% of all recurrent lymph node metastases. In intermediate-level (stages I and II) melanoma, nodal "skip" metastases have not been reported.

While nuclear medicine professionals have performed localization of the SLN by lymphoscintigraphy for decades, a recent augmentation of this established procedure is to incorporate the use of single photon emission computed tomography (SPECT)/computed tomography (CT), with the CT component most commonly used for anatomic localization, and also for attenuation correction. Superior anatomic information that can be obtained in systems incorporating a diagnostic CT is of unclear clinical significance at present.

SPECT/CT is not always needed for accurate localization of the SLN, but it is useful in anatomically complex regions and/or in regions where lymphatic drainage can be variable, such as the head and neck or the trunk.[9]

In an early report of the incremental value of SPECT/CT for SLN localization in 34 consecutive patients, including 28 with melanoma, 50% of patients with melanoma of the trunk demonstrated multiple drainage basins by SPECT/CT, as did 33% of patients with tumors of the head and neck. In patients with head and neck or trunk melanoma, 43% of SLNs that were correctly identified on SPECT/CT were not visualized on planar scintigraphy. Limitations of planar images were due mainly to scatter artifacts near the injection site, failure to identify in-transit lymph nodes, and failure to recognize deep nodes associated with a drainage basin that could not be clearly appreciated on planar images. SPECT/CT was of no added value in localization of the SLN in patients with melanoma of the extremities or in a single patient with a penile primary. Recent investigations support the use of SPECT/CT for appropriate SLN localization in patients with melanoma of the head and neck or the trunk.[9,10]

The sensitivity of $^{18}$F-fluorodeoxyglucose ($^{18}$F-FDG) positron emission tomography (PET) for detection of metastases in stage I and II disease, with primary lesion thickness $\leq$ 4 mm, is extremely low compared to SLN biopsy if there is no clinically palpable lymphadenopathy because $^{18}$F-FDG PET cannot detect micrometastases. The sensitivity of $^{18}$F-FDG imaging is 14% for detection of nodal metastases when the tumor volume is less than 78 mm$^3$ and 90% when the tumor volume is greater than 78 mm$^3$.[11]

### High-Risk Melanoma: Role of $^{18}$F-FDG Imaging

Approximately 50–70% of patients with high-risk melanoma (thickness > 4 mm) have nodal metastases and more than 10% have distant metastases, with a 5-year survival of less than 50%. $^{18}$F-FDG PET is recommended in these patients, and multiple studies report sensitivity ranging between 84 and 97% for lesion detection.[12]

## Detection of Recurrence and Restaging with $^{18}$F-FDG PET and PET/CT

Recurrence is common in cutaneous melanoma (Chart II.13.1). Early detection of recurrence is difficult. There are no established blood markers for early detection of recurrent and/or residual disease.

Cutaneous melanoma remains an aggressive malignancy that is resistant to effective treatment in advanced stages. The most successful approach for long-term benefit remains prevention and early surgical treatment when appropriate. Significant mortality occurs even with stage II disease. The current AJCC staging criteria include only one serum test, the level of LDH, for staging and restaging of disease, with other blood tests considered to be investigational at present. Serum LDH level determination is of limited utility since it is only elevated in advanced, stage IV disease, with patient survival typically less than 1 year. A surveillance chest radiograph is of little value for detection of early recurrence. Likewise, while physical examination may demonstrate evidence of recurrent disease, it indicates the presence of high risk, "macroscopic" disease by the time it becomes evident. The SLN bed, a region with high likelihood for recurrence, is difficult to examine clinically due to the presence of surgical scar, especially if a regional dissection was performed. Accordingly, long-term follow-up of patients with cutaneous melanoma remains problematic.[1,5,13]

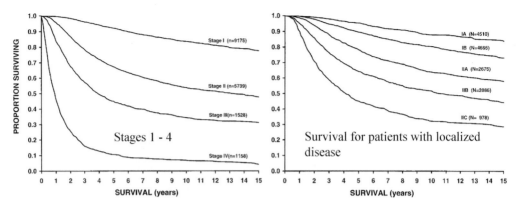

**Chart II.13.1** Melanoma-specific K-M survival statistics for newly diagnosed patients with stages I–IV cutaneous melanoma (*left*), with similar K-M survival statistics for patients with localized disease (stages I and II, *right*) at the time of diagnosis. Note that survival for stage IIC is lower than for stage III disease. Differences in survival between all stages are significant for both graphs (p < 0.0001). Numbers in parentheses refer to the number of patients in each staging group in the American Joint Committee on Cancer melanoma database. (Reprinted with permission of American Society of Clinical Oncology from Balch et al.[5])

A prospective evaluation of a proposed follow-up strategy for patients with melanoma showed that imaging was of no significant value in routine follow-up of patients with stage I and II melanoma. For stage III disease, however, following regional lymphadenectomy, imaging techniques should be used every 6 months for 10 years, specifically abdominal ultrasound, chest radiography, and CT.[14] In recent years, PET/CT has proven itself to be the whole-body imaging modality of choice for detection of recurrence.[15]

The use of imaging for effective whole-body melanoma surveillance requires the use of CT, brain magnetic resonance imaging (MRI), and/or [18]F-FDG PET/CT. Of these modalities, [18]F-FDG PET/CT is the imaging modality of choice for initial staging and restaging of stage III and IV melanoma. Because of frequent small focal densities seen on CT and/or focal regions of uptake of [18]F-FDG that do not represent tumor, baseline imaging can be very helpful, allowing for detailed comparison to follow-up examinations. [18]F-FDG PET/CT is superior to CT alone in evaluation of the abdomen and pelvis but inferior to breath-hold CT for evaluation of small pulmonary metastases and to MRI for evaluation of cerebral metastases.[9] A meta-analysis on the use of whole-body [18]F-FDG PET in management of patients with melanoma reported a sensitivity of 92%, specificity of 90%, and a change in management based on [18]F-FDG PET imaging in 22% of patients.[16]

Baseline[18]F-FDG PET/CT in stage III melanoma improves staging accuracy and can prevent unnecessary surgery for presumed limited disease or futile resection of a solitary metastasis when, in fact, other sites of disease are present. In a retrospective analysis of 257 patients, Bastiaannet and coworkers[17] found that [18]F-FDG PET/CT upstaged 22% of patients from stage III to stage IV disease, changed the treatment in 17% of patients, and found unrelated premalignant or malignant conditions, mainly colorectal tumors, in 4% of patients.

While many melanoma metastases are [18]F-FDG-avid, not all tumor sites accumulate the radiopharmaceutical. However, most metastases that do not accumulate [18]F-FDG will be visible on the CT portion of the PET/CT examination. In a prospective study of 124 patients with melanoma, Strobel and colleagues[18] demonstrated improved accuracy in staging or restaging patients when the CT component was interpreted separately and in addition to the PET/CT study because not all foci of tumor involvement were $^{18}$F-FDG-avid. $^{18}$F-FDG PET/CT demonstrated a sensitivity, specificity, and accuracy of 85, 96, and 91%, respectively, when only areas of increased uptake were considered as possibly representing tumor. When the CT performed for anatomic localization and attenuation correction was interpreted, both separately and together with the $^{18}$F-FDG PET images, sensitivity, specificity, and accuracy increased to 98, 94, and 96%, respectively (p = 0.016). Not surprisingly, most metastases detected only on CT were in the lungs, with other locations including a small subcutaneous nodule in the gluteal region, an iliac node and a muscle metastasis.

Similarly, in a retrospective study of 250 patients with metastatic cutaneous melanoma, Reinhardt and coworkers[19] reported separate overall N- and M-staging accuracy of $^{18}$F-FDG PET/CT of 97% as compared to the PET-only accuracy of 93% and CT-only accuracy of 79% (all differences were statistically significant). This study included patients in multiple clinical settings, specifically initial staging, treatment assessment, restaging, and follow-up.

## Choroidal Melanoma

Choroidal melanoma is the most common primary intraocular malignancy in adults, with an incidence of 4.3 cases/million annually in the United States, mostly occurring in patients of European (Caucasian) ancestry. In Japan, the incidence is much lower, at 0.25 cases/million annually. Choroidal (also called uveal) melanoma is well demonstrated on MRI in 70% of cases, with contrast-enhanced orbital CT and ultrasound also commonly used. While in this group of patients $^{18}$F-FDG PET/CT is useful in detection of whole-body metastases, it is not sensitive for detection of the primary lesion. $^{123}$I-iodoamphetamine ($^{123}$I-IMP) SPECT is superior to $^{18}$F-FDG PET/CT for visualization of the primary lesion and can also be useful for detection of the extent of disease and local recurrence in the head and neck region. The reported detectability rate of the primary tumor by $^{18}$F-FDG PET/CT is typically 0% for small (T1) tumors, 30–50% for T2 tumors, and 50–75% for T3 tumors. Distant metastases at the time of diagnosis are very rare in T1 or T2 lesions, and range between 2 and 4% with T3 primary tumors at initial presentation.[20–22]

The cause for the low sensitivity of $^{18}$F-FDG PET/CT in detection of orbital melanoma is unknown but has been hypothesized to be related to the relatively low metabolic rate in many primary melanomas of the eye compared to extraocular locations, the superficial, sheet-like configuration of many ocular tumors and the difficult visual discrimination of the tumor from the normal high uptake in brain and muscles of $^{18}$F-FDG. However, since orbital metastases of various malignancies are often visualized quite well compared to primary ocular melanoma, these explanations remain speculative. At this time MRI is the modality of choice for imaging of orbital tumors, with diagnostic, IV contrast-enhanced orbital CT, ultrasound, and 24-h post-injection $^{123}$I-IMP SPECT also useful.[23]

## Summary

Both cutaneous and ocular melanomas remain malignancies with poor prognosis that are resistant to treatment excluding resection for cure in cases of localized disease. For cutaneous melanoma, this requires complete surgical extirpation. The best options for patients are prevention followed by early detection and appropriate surgical treatment, including biopsy of the SLN. The use of SPECT/CT for localization of the SLN for primary tumors of the trunk or of the head and neck region is strongly supported. SPECT/CT has been used to allow more accurate identification of the draining lymph nodal bed(s) and to improve SLN identification. Imaging of any type is of little value for patients with localized (stage I or II) disease or for patients with microscopic disease in regional lymph nodes, beyond the imaging used for localization of the SLN.

For patients with stage III macroscopic disease or stage IV melanoma, whole-body $^{18}$F-FDG PET/CT (from vertex to feet) imaging is the best single imaging modality for staging or restaging patients, including localization of solitary metastasis considered for surgical resection, the only means of somewhat effective control of stage IV disease.

MRI remains superior to other imaging options for evaluation of cerebral metastases or choroidal tumors. A dedicated, breath-hold multidetector row CT (MDCT) is superior for detection of small pulmonary nodules that are easily missed on $^{18}$F-FDG PET/CT. A multiphasic MDCT is likewise superior for evaluation of small and/or metabolically quiescent metastases of the liver or spleen. All these imaging modalities should be considered for complete staging and restaging of the melanoma patient.

## Guidelines and Recommendations for the Use of $^{18}$F-FDG PET and PET/CT

The National Comprehensive Cancer Network (NCCN) has incorporated $^{18}$F-FDG PET and PET/CT in the practice guidelines and management algorithm of a variety of malignancies including melanoma.[24] The use of $^{18}$F-FDG PET (PET/CT where available) is recommended in the following clinical scenarios:

1. Initial evaluation of clinical stage III and IV.
2. Evaluation of recurrence and metastases.

A multidisciplinary panel of experts assessed meta-analyses and systematic reviews published in the $^{18}$F-FDG PET literature before March 2006 and made recommendations for the use of FDG PET in oncology.[25] The panel concluded that $^{18}$F-FDG PET should routinely be added to conventional imaging for staging and detecting recurrent melanoma.

## Case Presentations

## *Case II.13.1*

### History

A 72-year-old male with a primary cutaneous melanoma of the scalp treated with local resection was referred to ^18F-FDG PET/CT for initial staging after diagnostic biopsy (Fig. II.13.1A–E).

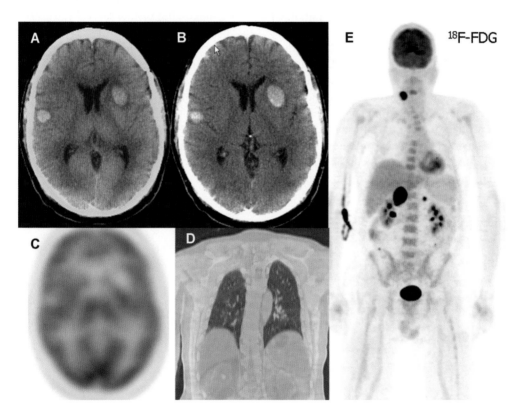

Fig. II.13.1A-E

### Findings

The CT component at the level of the brain demonstrates hemorrhagic cerebral metastases seen as areas of increased density compared to the cerebral tissue (Fig. II.13.1A, fused PET/CT, and Fig. II.13.1B, CT-only). On the PET portion these lesions show tracer uptake similar to the background or areas of relative photopenia (Fig. II.13.1C). A subcentimeter left pulmonary metastasis is seen on coronal PET/CT image of the lungs (Fig. II.13.1D), viewed at lung windows.

There is abnormal uptake on maximal intensity projection (MIP) image (Fig. II.13.1E) in the right neck involving a 30 mm level 2A nodal mass. There is also abnormal uptake in an enlarged right (40 mm) and a normal sized left (8 mm) adrenal gland, in a subcentimeter lesion in the upper margin of the right iliac wing and in a subtle [18]F-FDG-avid focus localized to a very small lesion in the soft tissues of the left lower abdominal quadrant.

Due to the presence of cerebral, nodal, adrenal, and pulmonary metastases, the patient was defined as stage IV disease with M1a, M1b, and M1c metastases.

## Discussion

The prognosis of this patient is poor, with the majority of stage IV patients surviving less than 1 year after diagnosis. Not apparent on the MIP images, but seen on the CT portion of the PET/CT, are hemorrhagic cerebral metastases. They demonstrate [18]F-FDG uptake equal to or less than that of the surrounding normal cerebral tissue. This case demonstrates that the CT portion of the PET/CT study must be evaluated as a stand-alone examination, in particular in patients with advanced stage melanoma. Strobel and colleagues[18] have demonstrated significant improvement in sensitivity, specificity, and accuracy in staging and restaging of melanoma with [18]F-FDG PET/CT when the CT component is interpreted independently and in addition to the PET component since not all malignant lesions are FDG-avid. This case also demonstrates that various regions of the body must be viewed with appropriately adjusted CT window-width and window-level settings (such as lung versus mediastinum or brain) to accurately appreciate the full extent of disease.

## Diagnosis

1. Melanoma metastatic to the neck, lung, adrenal glands, right iliac bone, and soft tissues seen on both PET and CT.
2. Hemorrhagic cerebral metastases seen on CT.

## *Case II.13.2*

### History

A 65-year-old male underwent wide excision of a melanoma of the right upper back with a positive SLN in the right axilla, followed by regional lymph node dissection (RLND) of the right axillary nodal basin. Several lymph nodes contained metastatic tumor. Despite the relatively recent surgery, the treating physicians requested $^{18}$F-FDG PET/CT for whole-body staging, suspecting stage IV disease (Fig. II.13.2).

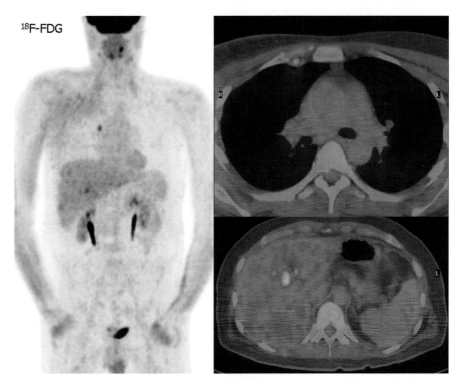

**Fig. II.13.2**

### Findings

There is mild, diffuse increased tracer uptake as a result of the recent right axillary RLND (MIP image, left). Focal areas of $^{18}$F-FDG uptake are seen in the right parasternal region corresponding to a 10 mm right internal mammary node (MIP, left, and upper right) and in several hepatic lesions, the largest 20 mm in diameter (MIP, left, and lower right).

There is mild diffuse whole-body soft tissue uptake, potentially due to recent eating, other causes of stimulation of endogenous insulin, or failure to restrict his physical activity as instructed the day prior to the PET/CT. Images of the lower extremities and of the brain were performed with no significant abnormalities (not shown).

**Discussion**

The MIP image demonstrates the expected surgically induced $^{18}$F-FDG uptake related to an inflammatory reaction after the recent right axillary RLND. $^{18}$F-FDG PET/CT images of the chest (upper right) and of the upper abdomen (lower right) demonstrate metastatic disease in a right internal mammary lymph node and in the liver, respectively. The patient was diagnosed as stage IV disease with distant nodal and visceral involvement.

This case demonstrates the power of whole-body $^{18}$F-FDG PET/CT for staging of cutaneous melanoma. While a region of recent surgery can demonstrate iatrogenically induced uptake of $^{18}$F-FDG for approximately 2–3 months following the procedure, regions outside the surgical bed can be evaluated without significant interference.

In patients with stage I–III disease, the SLN bed is a high-risk area for future recurrence, as are the regions either near the excised primary tumor bed or along the drainage routes from the primary site to the SLN group. Because of complex variability in lymphatic drainage routes in melanoma, especially in the trunk and in the head and neck, SLN mapping is essential for proper identification of the actual nodal station draining the primary lesion. SPECT/CT should also be considered for SLN localization, especially in the anatomically complex regions of the head and neck or trunk.[9,10]

**Diagnosis**

1. Metastases in a right internal mammary lymph node and the liver.
2. Inflammatory changes in the right axilla due to recent RLND.

## Case II.13.3 (DICOM Images on DVD)

### History

This 32-year-old male was diagnosed with melanoma of the neck 8 years ago. He was treated with surgical resection but did not receive chemo- or radiation therapy. The patient presented with increasing shortness of breath and pleuritic chest pain and was referred to $^{18}$F-FDG PET/CT for restaging (Fig. II.13.3A, B).

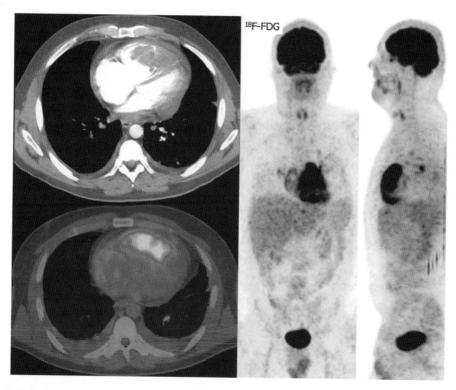

**Fig. II.13.3A**

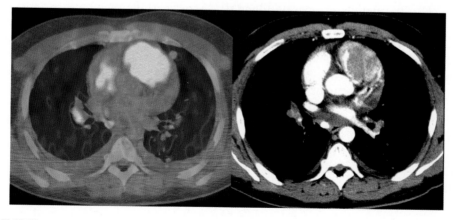

**Fig. II.13.3B**

## Findings

There is an $^{18}$F-FDG-avid 40 × 70 mm mass in the right ventricle of the heart seen on the anterior and lateral MIP images (Fig. II.13.3A, center and right) and the transaxial PET/CT image (Fig. II.13.3A, lower left). The contrast-enhanced CT (Fig. II.13.3A, upper left) clearly defines the cardiac mass. Several $^{18}$F-FDG-avid pulmonary nodules and hilar and mediastinal lymph nodes are demonstrated. There are also small bilateral pleural effusions.

## Discussion

Biopsy of the right ventricular mass revealed melanoma. The most common tumors to metastasize to the heart and/or pericardium are lung and breast cancer, lymphoma, and melanoma. While melanoma is the least common of these tumors in terms of total annual incidence, it is the malignancy that most often metastasizes to the heart on a percentage basis. Cardiac metastases are found in 46–71% of patients dying from melanoma at autopsy. Cardiac metastases can be located within the chambers, as in the present case, or within the myocardium. Involvement of the myocardium or pericardium is often associated with arrhythmia, which can be fatal. Whereas most cancers demonstrate a low signal on T1-weighted MRI images before IV contrast administration, melanin, which contains paramagnetic metals, appears bright.[26]

## Diagnosis

1. Melanoma metastatic to the right ventricle, mediastinal and hilar lymph nodes, and lungs.
2. Tumor or thromboemboli to the proximal pulmonary arteries apparent from comparing sites of obvious emboli seen on the contrast-enhanced CT (DICOM images provided on the DVD with the PET/CT DICOM images) with PET/CT.

## Follow-up

A few days after the $^{18}$F-FDG PET/CT study was performed, the patient underwent a contrast-enhanced CT examination of the chest and abdomen DICOM images provided on the DVD). By carefully comparing filling defects seen in the pulmonary arteries (Fig. II.13.3B, right), compatible with pulmonary emboli, with areas of uptake seen on the fused PET/CT images (Fig. II.13.3B, left), it is apparent that at least some of what appeared to be $^{18}$F-FDG-avid hilar lymph nodes are $^{18}$F-FDG-avid lesions in the proximal pulmonary artery branches, bilaterally. The differential diagnosis includes either bland or septic thromboemboli and/or tumor emboli.

## Clinical Report: Body $^{18}$F-FDG PET/CT (for DVD cases only)

Indication

Restaging of cutaneous melanoma.

History

This 32-year-old male with a history of melanoma of the neck diagnosed 8 years ago, treated with surgical resection only, presented with increasing shortness of breath and pleuritic chest pain.

Procedure

The fasting blood glucose level was 82 mg/dL. Sixty minutes after the IV administration of 481 MBq (13.0 mCi) of $^{18}$F-FDG, PET images were acquired from the vertex of the brain to the proximal femora in a single acquisition with the arms down. A separate acquisition was performed from the proximal femora through the feet. Whole-body low-dose CT without intravenous contrast was acquired to correct for attenuation and to provide anatomic localization.

Findings

*Quality of the study* : The overall quality of the study is good.

*Head and neck* : Tracer uptake in the head and neck region is physiologic.

*Chest* : There is intense $^{18}$F-FDG uptake in a right ventricular mass, measuring approximately 40 × 70 mm in maximal axial dimensions. The precise size of the mass is difficult to determine due to normal physiologic myocardial $^{18}$F-FDG uptake, cardiac and respiratory motion, and lack of significant attenuation differences on CT between the mass and the blood within the heart. In addition, there is intense $^{18}$F-FDG uptake corresponding to bilateral hilar lymphadenopathy and in the major pulmonary arteries. There are multiple nodules in both lungs, some of which demonstrate mild to moderate $^{18}$F-FDG avidity. Additional CT findings include small bilateral pleural effusions and calcified mediastinal lymph nodes.

*Abdomen and pelvis* : There is physiologic $^{18}$F-FDG activity in the bowel, liver and the renal collecting system.

*Musculoskeletal* : Degenerative changes of the thoracolumbar spine are noted.

Impression

1. Intense $^{18}$F-FDG uptake within the known right ventricular mass and bilateral hilar lymph nodes, consistent with metastatic disease.
2. Multiple bilateral pulmonary nodules, some showing mild to moderate $^{18}$F-FDG avidity, consistent with metastatic disease.
3. Additional CT findings include bilateral pleural effusions, calcified granulomatous nodal disease in the mediastinum, and degenerative changes in the thoracolumbar spine.
4. $^{18}$F-FDG uptake in the major pulmonary arteries, considered to represent additional metastatic sites.

## Case II.13.4

### History

This 33-year-old female presented for baseline staging of a choroidal melanoma. Because primary choroidal melanoma is unusual at this age, there was additional concern that the lesion was a metastasis from an unknown primary (Fig. II.13.4A, B).

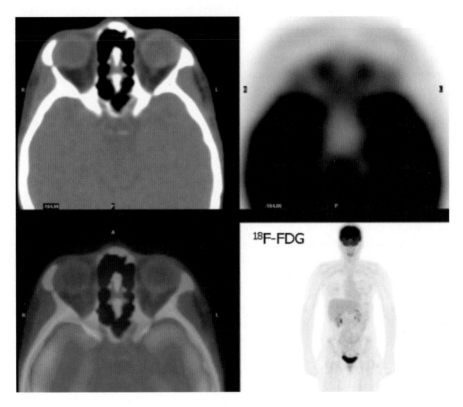

**Fig. II.13.4A**

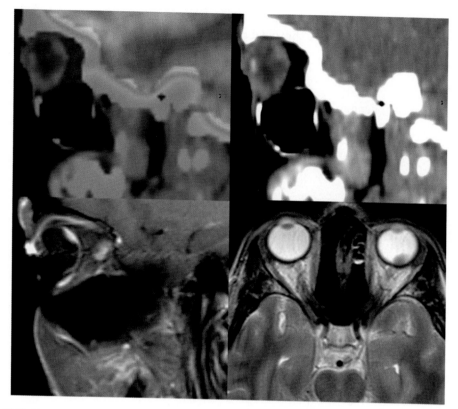

**Fig. II.13.4B**

## Findings

The whole-body [18]F-FDG PET/CT is normal excluding a 9 mm soft tissue density involving the choroidal region of the left eye seen on CT with no [18]F-FDG uptake (Fig. II.13.4A). Software fusion of the sagittal [18]F-FDG PET/CT and accompanying CT with post-gadolinium enhanced T1-weighted sagittal (Fig. II.13.4B, left column) and T2-weighted axial (Fig. II.13.4B, right column) MRI images show the "en plaque" left eye choroidal melanoma.

## Discussion

While unusual for her age, theses findings suggested a primary choroidal melanoma with no evidence of additional lesions. [18]F-FDG imaging has a poor sensitivity for choroidal melanoma, probably for a combination of reasons including the proximity of the tumor to the uptake in the brain and extraocular muscles, blurring associated with eye movement during imaging, a relatively low metabolic rate compared to cutaneous melanoma, as well as the small size and the often flat or "en plaque" shape of the lesion.[23]

MRI is the imaging modality of choice in choroidal melanoma, providing excellent evaluation of the primary tumor (Fig. II.13.4B) and of possible extraocular extension.[20–22] [18]F-FDG PET/CT is the preferred modality for whole-body imaging, and, with the use of breath-hold CT acquisition protocols, the procedure of choice to diagnose or exclude small pulmonary nodules. The negative whole-body PET/CT study of this patient was accepted for final diagnosis of a primary choroidal tumor rather than a metastatic lesion.

## Diagnosis

Choroidal melanoma not [18]F-FDG-avid, better characterized by MRI than CT.

## Case II.13.5

### History

This 28-year-old male with stage IIIB melanoma of the right upper back diagnosed 2 years previously, treated with wide excision and both axillary and cervical lymph node dissection, was referred to $^{18}$F-FDG PET/CT for restaging (Fig. II.13.5).

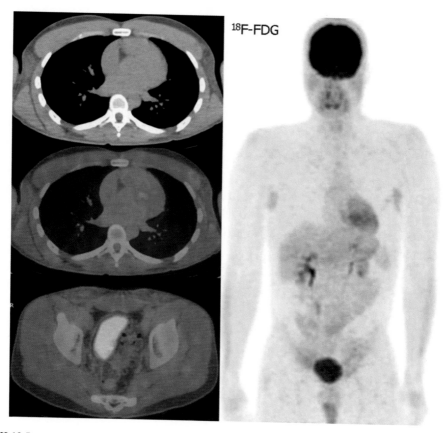

**Fig. II.13.5**

## Findings

The transaxial CT (top left), fused PET/CT (center and bottom, left), and MIP (right) image of this $^{18}$F-FDG PET/CT examination (lower limbs not shown) demonstrate a normal, physiologic tracer uptake pattern as well as subcutaneous symmetric uptake of $^{18}$F-FDG in the axillary and inguinal regions corresponding to stranding on the CT and PET/CT transaxial images.

## Discussion

While melanoma can produce an area of poorly defined subcutaneous increased density and $^{18}$F-FDG uptake on PET/CT, bilateral symmetric uptake limited to the axillary and inguinal regions would be unusual for hypermetabolic tumor lesions. Indeed, this pattern of uptake is commonly seen at sites of tumor vaccine injections and must be recognized as such on $^{18}$F-FDG PET/CT studies performed for staging or restaging of melanoma. This patient had indeed received numerous tumor vaccine injections in these regions and had no evidence of recurrent disease.

## Diagnosis

1. No evidence of recurrent melanoma.
2. $^{18}$F-FDG uptake in subcutaneous tissue at sites of vaccine injection, due to inflammatory changes.

## Case II.13.6 (DICOM Images on DVD)

### History

A 58-year-old male with a history of melanoma of the face was previously treated with wide excision, right parotid and right neck dissection, followed by radiation therapy. A prior $^{18}$F-FDG PET/CT (not shown) 1 year after treatment showed no evidence of residual tumor. The patient presented 2 years after initial treatment with suspected recurrence on physical examination and was referred for $^{18}$F-FDG PET/CT for restaging (Fig. II.13.6A–C).

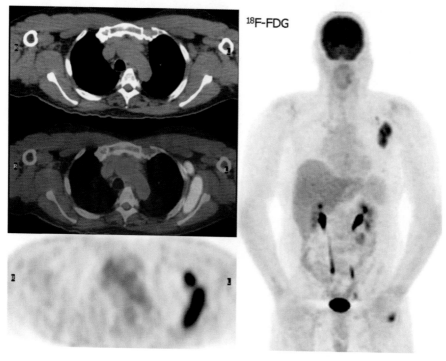

**Fig. II.13.6A**

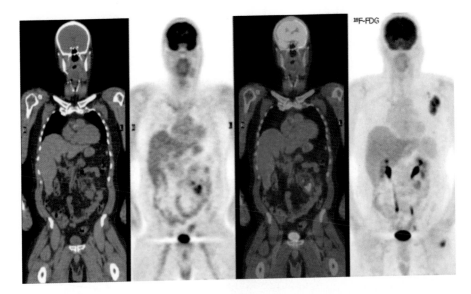

Fig. II.13.6B

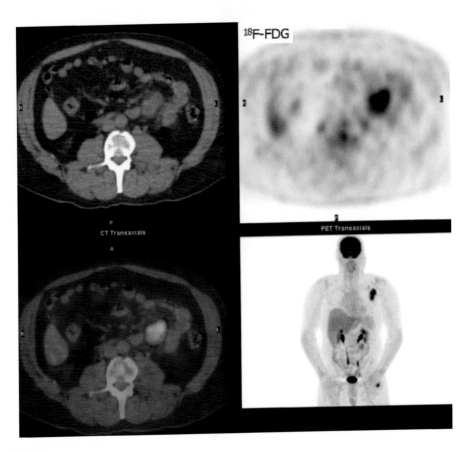

Fig. II.13.6C

## Findings

There is evidence of recurrence in the left axillary lymph nodes and the left subscapularis muscle (Fig. II.13.6A). There is also increased tracer uptake in the left mid-abdominal region corresponding to mesenteric adenopathy and in the left hand (not to be misinterpreted as the injection site which was the right arm) (Fig. II.13.6B, C).

## Discussion

This case demonstrates the power of whole-body imaging with $^{18}$F-FDG PET/CT to demonstrate the full extent of disease in a single examination. If clinically important for further patient management, an MRI examination of the brain, breath-hold CT of the lungs, and multi-phasic contrast-enhanced CT of the liver and spleen can demonstrate metastatic disease not seen with $^{18}$F-FDG PET/CT. However, the presence of additional metastatic foci that could be potentially demonstrated by these later examinations would not change the restaging status and further approach in this patient. Unless additional imaging will affect management of patients with disseminated disease, whole-body $^{18}$F-FDG PET/CT is the only imaging examination needed.[9,15,16]

## Diagnosis

Widely metastatic melanoma.

## Clinical Report: Body $^{18}$F-FDG PET/CT (for DVD cases only)

Indication

Restaging of melanoma.

History

This 58-year-old male with a history of melanoma of the right face was treated with wide local excision, right parotid and right neck dissection 2 years previously and completed radiation therapy 1 year ago. A $^{18}$F-FDG PET/CT scan following treatment demonstrated no evidence of residual disease. He presents now for restaging, 2 years from initial diagnosis, with clinical evidence of recurrence.

Procedure

The fasting blood glucose was 106 mg/dL. $^{18}$F-FDG 403 MBq (10.9 mCi) was administered intravenously in a right hand vein. After a 55-min distribution time, low dose non-contrast-enhanced CT was acquired to correct for attenuation and for anatomic localization. PET was acquired over the brain, neck, thorax, abdomen, and pelvis. The arms are positioned along the sides. Similar imaging sequences were then acquired for the entire lower extremities.

Findings

*Quality of the study*: The overall quality of the study is good.

*Head and neck*: Physiologic uptake of $^{18}$F-FDG is seen in the brain and the glandular and lymphoid tissue of the neck. On CT, there are findings consistent with the known extensive surgical procedures in the right neck including right parotid and neck dissection. No abnormal $^{18}$F-FDG activity is seen in this area.

*Chest*: Mild physiologic uptake of $^{18}$F-FDG is seen in the myocardium. Intense $^{18}$F-FDG uptake is seen in multiple left axillary lymph nodes, the largest of which measures 28 mm in greatest axial diameter. An additional site of intense $^{18}$F-FDG uptake involves most of an enlarged left subscapularis muscle seen on CT. No abnormalities are seen in the lungs except for a single calcified granuloma at the right apex, with no $^{18}$F-FDG uptake. The mediastinum is unremarkable.

*Abdomen and pelvis*: Physiologic $^{18}$F-FDG uptake is seen in the genitourinary and gastrointestinal tract. Intense $^{18}$F-FDG activity is seen in the 46 mm left mid-abdominal mesenteric mass, consistent with metastasis. Intense $^{18}$F-FDG uptake is also seen in an 18 mm mesenteric nodule in the left mid-quadrant, superior to this large mass at the level of the inferior pole of the left kidney. On CT the liver appears within normal limits. The spleen appears within normal limits, except for splenic granulomas. The kidneys and adrenal glands demonstrate a normal non-contrasted appearance. There is diverticulosis without diverticulitis.

*Musculoskeletal*: There is intense $^{18}$F-FDG activity corresponding to a 25 mm nodule within the dorsal aspect of the left hand, consistent with a metastasis and in the enlarged left subscapularis muscle previously mentioned.


Impression

1. Intense $^{18}$F-FDG uptake in left axillary lymphadenopathy, the largest lymph node measures 28 mm in greatest axial diameter, consistent with metastasis.
2. Intense $^{18}$F-FDG activity corresponding to a large area within the left subscapularis muscle, consistent with soft tissue metastasis.
3. Intense $^{18}$F-FDG uptake in a 46 mm mesenteric mass and an 18 mm mesenteric nodule superior to the larger mass, consistent with metastases.
4. Intense $^{18}$F-FDG uptake in a 25 mm nodule in the dorsal aspect of the left hand, consistent with metastasis.
5. Extensive surgical changes in the right face and neck, with no corresponding abnormal $^{18}$F-FDG activity.
6. Additional incidental findings on CT are delineated above.

## Case II.13.7

### History

This 42-year-old male with a 2-year history of right parietal scalp nevus recently diagnosed as melanoma following a punch biopsy (Breslow thickness of 0.672 mm, Clark level 4) was referred for lymphoscintigraphy with SLN localization (Fig. II.13.7A–D).

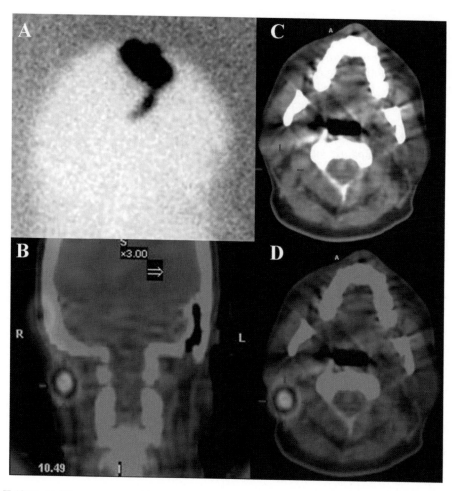

**Fig. II.13.7A–D** (Case courtesy of Peeyush Bhargava, MD, Michael E. DeBakey VA Medical Center, Houston, TX.)

### Findings

Planar scintigraphy (Fig. II.13.7A) demonstrates the peri-tumoral injection site and early inferior drainage of the radioisotope. Additional planar views revealed foci of uptake posterior and inferior to the ear (not shown). However, there are several lymph nodes in this region, both deep and superficial, and planar studies failed to demonstrate which specific lymph node was the SLN. SPECT/CT imaging clearly demonstrates the SLN located in the posterior triangle representing a deep lymph node in the right occipital chain posterior to the mastoid (Fig. II.13.7B-coronal SPECT/CT, C-axial CT, and D-axial SPECT/CT).

Following this precise localization, the patient underwent wide local excision with 2 cm margins and biopsy of the SLN. Dissection directed by the SPECT/CT images and by the further use of an intra-operative gamma probe allowed clear identification of the SLN. Histopathological examination did not show malignant involvement in the SLN.

## Discussion

As discussed previously, the lymphatic drainage of the head and neck region and of the trunk is unpredictable. Because of the complex anatomy and variable routes of drainage, subtle activity in deep lymph nodes can be masked by overlying structures. In this case specifically, the SLN was not seen on planar imaging during lymphoscintigraphy. Without SPECT/CT, such deep SLNs can be missed and secondary lymph nodes can be misidentified as the SLN. Multiple drainage routes can also exist. In this setting, the associated complex relationships are best imaged with SPECT/CT, thereby allowing the correct identification of the SLN.[8–10]

## Diagnosis

Successful localization of the SLN via SPECT/CT.

# References

1. Tsao H, Atkins MB, Sober AJ. Management of cutaneous melanoma. *New Engl J Med* 2004;351:998–1012.
2. Domingo-Domenech J, Molina R, Castel T, Montagut C, Puig S, Conill C, Martí R, Vera M, Auge JM, Malvehy J, Grau JJ, Gascon P, Mellado B. Serum protein S-100 predicts clinical outcome in patients with melanoma treated with adjuvant interferon – comparison with tyrosinase re-PCR. *Oncology* 2005;68:341–349.
3. Garbe C, Leiter, U, Ellwanger U, Blaheta HJ, Meier F, Rassner G, Schittek B. Diagnostic value and prognostic significance of protein S-100β, melanoma-inhibitory activity, and tyrosinase/MART-1 reverse transcription-polymerase charin reaction in the follow-up of high-risk melanoma patients. *Cancer* 2003;97:1737–1745.
4. Wascher RA, Morton DL, Kuo C, Elashoff RM, Wang H-J, Gerami M, Hoon DSB. Molecular tumor markers in the blood: early prediction of disease outcome in melanoma patients treated with a melanoma vaccine. *J Clin Oncol* 2003;21:2558–2563.
5. Balch CM, Buzaid AC, Soong SJ, Atkins MB, Cascinelli N, Coit DG, Fleming ID, Gershenwald JE, Houghton Jr A, Kirkwood JM, McMasters KM, Mihm MF, Morton DL, Reintgen DS, Ross MI, Sober A, Thompson JA, Thompson JF. Final version of the American Joint Committee on Cancer staging system for cutaneous melanoma. *J Clin Oncol* 2001;19:3635–3648.
6. Gershenwald JE, Thompson W, Mansfield PF, Lee JE, Colome MI, Tseng C-H, Lee JJ, Balch CM, Reintgen DS, Ross MI. Multi-institutional melanoma lymphatic mapping experience: the prognostic value of sentinel lymph node status in 612 stage I or II melanoma patients. *J Clin Oncol* 1999;17:976–983.
7. Morton DL, Thompson JF, Cochran AJ, Mozzillo N, Elashoff R, Essner R, Nieweg OE, Roses DF, Hoekstra HJ, Karakousis CP, Reintgen DS, Coventry BJ, Glass EC, Wang H-J, for the MSLT Group. Sentinel-node biopsy or nodal observation in melanoma. *N Engl J Med* 2006;355:1307–1317. Erratum in: *N Engl J Med* 2006;355:1944.
8. Alazraki N, Glass EC, Castronovo F, Valdes Olmos RA, Podoloff D. Society of Nuclear Medicine procedure guideline for lymphoscintigraphy and the use of intraoperative gamma probe for sentinel lymph node localization in melanoma of intermediate thickness. *J Nucl Med* 2002;93:1414–1418.
9. Belhocine TZ, Scott AM, Evan-Sapir E, Urbain JL, Essner R. Role of nuclear medicine in the management of cutaneous malignant melanoma. *J Nucl Med* 2006;47:957–967.
10. Even-Sapir E, Lerman H, Lievshitz G, Khafif A, Fliss DM, Schwart A, Gur E, Skornick Y, Schneebaum S. Lymphoscintigraphy for sentinel node mapping using a hybrid SPECT/CT system. *J Nucl Med* 2003;44:1413–1420.
11. Wagner JD, Schauwecker DS, Davidson D, Wenck S, Jung SH, Hutchins G. FDG-PET sensitivity for melanoma lymph node metastases is dependent on tumor volume. *J Surg Oncol* 2001;77:237–242.
12. Friedman KP, Wahl RL. Clinical use of positron emission tomography in the management of cutaneous melanoma. *Semin Nucl Med* 2004;34:242–253.
13. Balch CM, Soong S, Gershenwald JE, Thompson JF, Reintgen DS, Cascinelli N, Urist M, McMasters KM, Ross MI, Kirkwood JM, Atkins MB, Thompson JA, Coit DG, Byrd D, Desmond R, Zhang Y, Liu P-Y, Lyman JH, Morabito A. Prognostic factors analysis of 17,600 melanoma patients: Validation of the American Joint Committee on Cancer melanoma staging system. *J Clin Oncol* 2001;19:3622–3634.
14. Garbe C, Paul A, Kohler-Späth H. Prospective evaluation of a follow-up schedule in cutaneous melanoma patients: Recommendations for an effective follow-up strategy. *J Clin Oncol* 2003;21:520–529.
15. Garbe C, Eigentler TK. Diagnosis and treatment of cutaneous melanoma: State of the art 2006. *Melanoma Res* 2007;17:117–127.
16. Schwimmer J, Essner R, Patel A, Jahan SA, Shepherd JE, Park K, Phelps ME, Czernin J, Gambhir SS. A review of the literature for whole-body FDG PET in the management of patients with melanoma. *Q J Nucl Med* 2000;44:153–167.
17. Bastiaannet E, Oyen WJG, Meijer S, Hoekstra OS, Wobbes T, Jager PL, Hoekstra HL. Impact of [$^{18}$F]fluorodeoxyglucose positron emission tomography on surgical management of melanoma patients. *Br J Surg* 2006;93:243–249.
18. Strobel K, Dummer R, Husarik D, Lago MP, Hany MF, Steinert HC. High-risk melanoma: Accuracy of FDG PET/CT with added CT morphologic information for detection of metastases. *Radiology* 2007;244:566–674.

19. Reinhardt MJ, Joe AY, Jaeger U, Huber A, Matthies A, Bucerius J, Roedel R, Strunk H, Bieber T, Biersack H-J, Tüting T. Diagnostic performance of whole body dual modality 18F-FDG PET/CT imaging for N- and M-staging of malignant melanoma: Experience with 250 consecutive patients. *J Clin Oncol* 2006;24:1178–1187.

20. Kato K, Kubota T, Ikeda M, Tadokoro M, Abe S, Nakano S, Nishino M, Kobayashi H, Ishigaki T. Low efficacy of [18]F-FDG PET for detection of uveal malignant melanoma compared with [123]I-IMP SPECT. *J Nucl Med* 2006;47:404–409.

21. Reddy S, Kurli M, Tena LB, Finger PT. PET/CT imaging: Detection of choroidal melanoma. *Br J Ophthalmol* 2005;89:1265–1269.

22. Finger PT, Kurli M, Reddy S, Tena LB, Pavlick AC. Whole body PET/CT for initial staging of choroidal melanoma. *Br J Ophthalmol* 2005;89:1270–1274.

23. Lane KA, Bilyk JR. Preliminary study of positron emission tomography in the detection and management of orbital malignancy. *Ophthal plast Reconstr Surg* 2006;22:361–365.

24. http://www.nccn.org/professionals/physician_gls/f_guidelines.asp.

25. Fletcher JW, Djulbegovic B, Soares HP, Siegel BA, Lowe VJ, Lyman GH, Coleman E, Wahl R, Paschold JC, Avril N, Einhorn LH, Suh WW, Samson D, Delbeke D, Gorman M, Shields AF. Recommendations for the Use of FDG(fluorine-18, (2-[[18]F]Fluoro-2-deoxy-D-glucose) positron emission tomography in oncology. *J Nucl Med* 2008;49:480–508.

26. Chiles C, Woodard PK, Gutierrez FR, Link KM. Metastatic involvement of the heart and pericardium: CT and MR imaging. *Radiographics* 2001;21:439–449.

# Chapter II.14
# Malignancy of the Bone: Primary Tumors, Lymphoma, and Skeletal Metastases

Einat Even-Sapir, Gideon Flusser, and Arye Blachar

## Skeletal Metastases, Bone Lymphoma, and Multiple Myeloma

Most malignant skeletal lesions initiate intramedullary. As the intramedullary malignant deposit enlarges, the surrounding bone undergoes osteoclastic and osteoblastic activity. Tumor cells may destroy bone directly or produce mediators that stimulate reabsorption by osteoclasts.[1] Based on the balance between the two processes, the radiographic appearance of a malignant skeletal lesion may be lytic, blastic, or mixed.[2] Detection of malignant skeletal involvement is based on either direct visualization of tumor cells or of the secondary reaction of the bone to the present malignant cells. $^{18}$F-Fluorodeoxyglucose ($^{18}$F-FDG) directly accumulates in tumor cells and may therefore identify malignant skeletal involvement at early stages when confined to the marrow, before the cortical skeletal reaction has occurred, while increased accumulation of $^{99m}$Tc-methylene diphosphonate ($^{99m}$Tc-MDP), used for skeletal scintigraphy (BS), or of $^{18}$F-fluoride, a positron emission tomography (PET) bone-seeking agent, depends on the presence of secondary reactive high bone turnover and osteoblastic changes.[3–5]

## $^{18}$F-FDG PET/CT for Diagnosis of Malignant Skeletal Lesions

$^{18}$F-FDG PET is superior to BS in detecting skeletal involvement in various malignant diseases.[6,7] The normal red marrow demonstrates only low-intensity $^{18}$F-FDG uptake. Therefore, increased intramedullary tracer uptake suggests the presence of early malignant bone marrow involvement prior to an identifiable bone reaction, thus preceding detection of early skeletal metastases by BS and computed tomography (CT).[8] $^{18}$F-FDG PET can detect all types of skeletal metastases including lytic, blastic, and mixed lesions. However, there are data suggesting that $^{18}$F-FDG PET is more sensitive in detecting lytic metastases as compared to blastic lesions, which are considered to be relatively less aggressive.[9]

In baseline $^{18}$F-FDG PET studies performed prior to therapy, a pattern of heterogeneous patchy or focal intramedullary uptake suggests the presence of early malignant involvement of the bone marrow.[10,11] Lymphomatous involvement is commonly marrow-based. Accumulating data indicate that $^{18}$F-FDG PET can identify early lymphomatous infiltration of the marrow.

E. Even-Sapir (✉)
Department of Nuclear Medicine, Tel-Aviv Sourasky Medical Center, Tel Aviv University, Tel Aviv, Israel
e-mail: evensap@tasmc.health.gov.il

D. Delbeke, O. Israel (eds.), *Hybrid PET/CT and SPECT/CT Imaging*,
DOI 10.1007/978-0-387-92820-3_16, © Springer Science+Business Media, LLC 2010

Involvement of the marrow by multiple myeloma (MM) precedes bone destruction. The use of $^{18}$F-FDG PET in imaging MM is evolving. It has the goals to provide correct staging of disease in order to avoid unnecessary treatment in patients with monoclonal gammopathy of undetermined significance (MGUS) and/or smoldering myeloma, treat patients with impending overt skeletal disease as early as possible, identify subgroups of patients with poor risk, and to accurately identify patients with nonsecretory myeloma.[12] Positive $^{18}$F-FDG PET reliably indicates the presence of active MM while a negative study suggests MGUS.[13]

## $^{18}$F-FDG PET/CT for Monitoring Response to Therapy

$^{18}$F-FDG PET/CT imaging allows accurate separation between active malignant skeletal involvement and bone repair. Successful treatment is reflected by decrease or even disappearance of uptake. A "burnt out" malignant skeletal lesion may remain abnormal on the CT component of the PET/CT study with no increased $^{18}$F-FDG accumulation.[14,15]

$^{18}$F-FDG uptake is affected by therapy. Timing of performance of PET/CT is therefore of major importance for accurate assessment of the response of malignant skeletal lesions to treatment. Early (less than 2 weeks) after chemotherapy, metabolic shutdown (stunning) of tumor cells can lead to a degradation in the performance of $^{18}$F-FDG PET/CT and subsequent false-negative results. Granulocyte colony-stimulating factors (G-CSF) therapy may alter the marrow distribution of the tracer, mimicking the pattern of extensive malignant marrow involvement. Follow-up PET/CT should therefore be performed long enough time after the G-CSF peak effect.[16] Bones included in the radiation field may show increased, normal, or reduced $^{18}$F-FDG uptake compared to the neighboring structures depending on the time interval from radiotherapy.

## Advantages of $^{18}$F-FDG PET/CT in Malignant Skeletal Involvement

Scintigraphically detected skeletal lesions often require further validation with a contemporaneous CT. This can be currently obtained in a single setting using hybrid single photon emission computed tomography (SPECT)/CT or PET/CT systems, which enable the characterization of each lesion with respect to its uptake and morphological appearance.

Hybrid imaging may overcome the inherent limitation of $^{18}$F-FDG PET stand-alone imaging caused by the fact that $^{18}$F-FDG accumulates in both soft tissue and skeletal metastases, through accurate localization of abnormal tracer uptake to the appropriate tissue. The presence of skeletal metastases in the vicinity of physiologic $^{18}$F-FDG uptake, such as in the skull for instance, may be difficult to assess.[17] $^{18}$F-FDG PET/CT imaging allows accurate localization of the precise level of an abnormality in the vertebral column and detects potential invasion of the epidural space or neural foramen by the tumor. Early detection of such lesions is critical in order to avoid future permanent neurological deficit.[18]

## Summary

The introduction of $^{18}$F-FDG PET/CT into the imaging algorithm of cancer patients often obviates the need to separately perform BS for assessment of the presence and extent of skeletal involvement. After therapy, disappearance of [18]F-FDG accumulation in a skeletal site is an indicator of response even in the presence of residual morphological abnormalities of the bone.


## Primary Skeletal Malignancies

Osteosarcoma is the most frequent primary skeletal malignancy in children and the second in adults, following MM. The Ewing sarcoma family of tumors is the second most frequent primary skeletal malignancy in children and young adults. Outcome of patients with sarcoma has improved following the introduction of aggressive multidrug chemotherapeutic regimens and novel surgical procedures. Optimizing the treatment approach is based on accurate tumor staging and restaging as well as early detection of recurrence.


## *[18]F-FDG PET/CT for Diagnosis of Primary Skeletal Tumors*

Although sarcomas are hypermetabolic malignancies and accumulate [18]F-FDG, the value of this imaging modality in their initial diagnosis is limited since performing [18]F-FDG PET cannot replace the need for biopsy. A study in 220 patients assessed the value of [18]F-FDG imaging and semiquantitative measurement of the tumor-to-background ratio (T/B) in grading skeletal tumors and tumorlike lesions of the bone. All but three benign tumors out of the total 220 lesions were [18]F-FDG-avid. While overall sarcomas had a significantly higher T/B, malignant and benign skeletal tumors could not be separated based on the degree of [18]F-FDG-avidity. An overlap in intensity of uptake between low-grade sarcomas and highly cellular benign skeletal lesions resulted in a sensitivity of 93% but with a specificity of 67% of [18]F-FDG imaging for differentiation of benign and malignant lesions.[19]

While [18]FDG-PET is less hampered by non-cancerous tracer uptake in benign skeletal lesions as compared with BS, highly cellular benign lesions containing histiocytic or giant cells such as osteoblastoma, brown tumor, aneurismal bone cyst, sarcoidosis, and osteomyelitis, may show increased [18]F-FDG uptake. Absence of increased tracer uptake can be associated with skeletal tumors such as plasmocytoma or low-grade chondrosarcoma.

[18]F-FDG imaging can assist in better defining the biopsy site in heterogeneous masses by guiding sampling of active tumor areas and avoiding errors due to biopsy of necrotic tumor areas.[20] Differences in time–activity curves between benign and low-grade tumors have been demonstrated when the kinetics of [18]F-FDG tumor uptake over time were investigated. This quantitative approach was, however, unable to separate low-grade sarcomas from benign lesions.[21]


## *[18]F-FDG PET/CT for Staging Primary Skeletal Tumors*

Magnetic resonance imaging (MRI) is the imaging of choice for defining the extension of the primary skeletal tumor to surrounding soft tissues as well as for estimation of tumoral infiltration into bone marrow. [18]F-FDG PET/CT is also suitable for detection of intrame-dullary tumoral involvement. Patients presenting with localized disease have a better prognosis compared to those presenting with metastatic disease. The lung is the site of the most frequent metastatic spread of sarcoma. Outcome of patients with pulmonary metastases depends primarily on the ability to remove them surgically. Pulmonary metastases may be submillimeter in size. Spiral CT is the modality of choice for detection of relatively small pulmonary metastases, superior to [18]F-FDG PET, especially in lesions smaller than 9 mm in diameter. [18]F-FDG PET may, however, assist in differentiating non-specific pulmonary nodules from metastases detected by CT in case of larger pulmonary lesions.[18]F-FDG PET may also identify unexpected extra-pulmonary metastases.[22,23]

Skeletal metastases of osteosarcoma occur in 10–20% of patients with disseminated disease. In patients with Ewing sarcoma, bone and bone marrow are the second most common metastatic sites after the lung and pleural space. Bone marrow metastases occur in almost 10% of patients and are associated with a poor prognosis. Marrow involvement is patchy, requiring multiple biopsies for accurate sampling and subsequent staging. [18]F-FDG imaging has been suggested to be a sensitive screening method for detection of skeletal metastases in patients with sarcomas.[24]

## [18]F-FDG PET/CT for Monitoring Response to Therapy

Preoperative neoadjuvant chemotherapy followed by surgical removal of the tumor is the common treatment approach in primary bone sarcomas. Although its role was assessed in only a relatively small number of patients, [18]F-FDG PET seems to be successful in monitoring response of the primary tumor to neoadjuvant chemotherapy, serving as a noninvasive surrogate marker of histological response.[22] Reduction in [18]F-FDG uptake is an indicator of a reduction in the number of residual viable tumor cells after therapy, but [18]F-FDG may also accumulate in inflammatory infiltrates resulting in overestimation of the measured tracer activity. Standard uptake value (SUV) measurements within the tumor provides a more accurate indicator of response to treatment than assessing the extent of necrosis in the tumor mass, particularly in an extensively necrotic lesion which may contain only small foci of residual viable malignant tissue. The presence of foci of viable tumor identified by PET implies a less favorable outcome. In case of Ewing sarcoma, surgical oncologists may be more willing to perform limb-sparing surgical resections in the setting of a favorable response to therapy or alternatively use radiation therapy in surgically challenging sites. Moreover, [18]F-FDG PET might be able to identify poorly responding patients earlier during the course of therapy.[25]

## Summary

An optimal imaging algorithm of musculoskeletal sarcomas at different phases during the course of the disease is based on the complementary use of CT, MRI, and [18]F-FDG imaging. MRI is the modality of choice for assessing the local extension of the primary tumor and detection of local recurrence. CT is the optimal modality for assessing the presence of pulmonary metastases, and [18]F-FDG PET is the most sensitive modality for early detection of skeletal metastases, for differentiating non-specific large pulmonary lesions from metastases, and for assessing tumor viability after therapy.

# Case Presentations

## *Case II.14.1 (DICOM Images on DVD)*

### History

An 81-year-old male presented with a pulmonary mass in the right lower lobe, diagnosed by biopsy as squamous cell carcinoma. The patient was referred to $^{18}$F-FDG PET/CT for initial staging (Fig. II.14.1A–C).

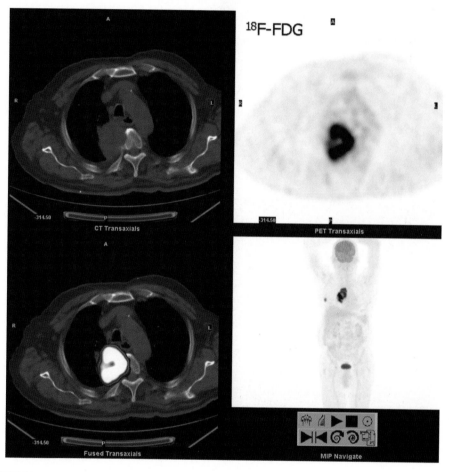

**Fig. II.14.1A**

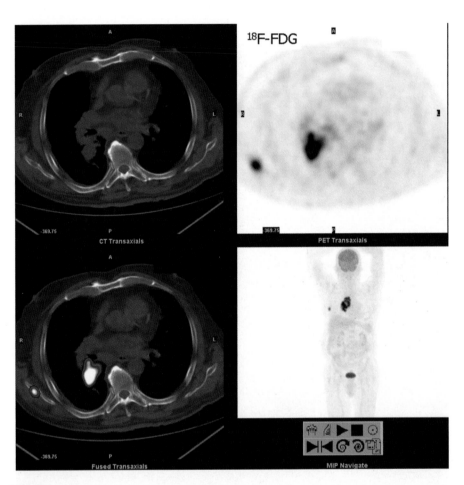

**Fig. II.14.1B**

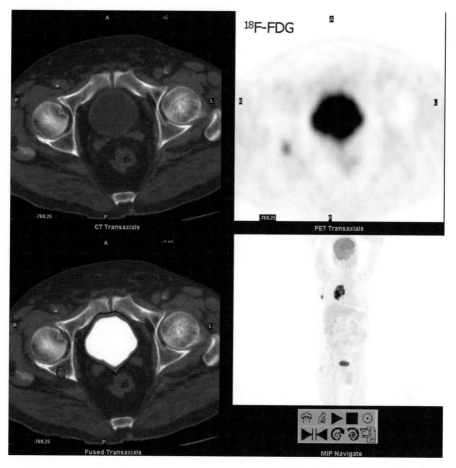

**Fig. II.14.1C**

## Findings

There is increased $^{18}$F-FDG uptake in a large mass, 75 × 58 mm in size, in the medial aspect of the lower lobe of the right lung. The tumor mass involves by continuity the lateral aspect of the T4 vertebral body (Fig. II.14.1A). In addition there is increased $^{18}$F-FDG uptake in the right scapula, with a corresponding lytic lesion on CT (Fig. II.14.1B), and in the right acetabulum with normal appearing bone on CT (Fig. II.4.1C). The lesions in the scapula and acetabulum are consistent with skeletal metastases, with the latter representing an early marrow-based lesion. Additional CT findings are seen on the DICOM images and described in the clinical report (see DVD).

## Discussion

In this patient with primary pulmonary malignancy, $^{18}$F-FDG PET/CT identifies malignant skeletal involvement both by direct extension of the primary tumor mass as well as distant metastases.

Prognosis of patients with non-small cell lung carcinoma (NSCLC) depends on stage of disease and the ability to surgically remove the entire tumor. Skeletal metastases are diagnosed at initial presentation in 3–60% of patients with NSCLC. Up to 40% of lung cancer patients with proven skeletal metastases are asymptomatic. Before the era of [18]F-FDG PET imaging, initial staging of patients with NSCLC included BS with [99m]Tc-MDP for detection of potential skeletal metastases. [18]F-FDG-PET/CT imaging has been found valuable for detection of both soft tissue and skeletal metastases, obviating the need to perform a separate BS. Moreover, [18]F-FDG imaging has been reported to be more sensitive than BS and/or CT for detection of skeletal metastases in patients with lung cancer.[26,27] In present case, in addition to a small lytic metastasis also identified by CT, increased tracer uptake has also been detected in the right acetabulum, indicating an early marrow-based metastasis identified on PET prior to the appearance of a cortical abnormality on CT.

### Diagnosis

1. Squamous cell carcinoma of the right lower lung lobe extending into the mediastinum.
2. Skeletal involvement of a thoracic vertebra by direct extension from the tumor.
3. Distant skeletal metastases.

### Clinical Report: Body [18]F-FDG PET/CT (for DVD cases only)

Indication

Initial staging of NSCLC.

History

An 81-year-old male presented with a pulmonary mass in the right lower lobe diagnosed by biopsy as squamous cell carcinoma.

Procedure

The fasting blood sugar was 104 mg/dl. [18]F-FDG (555 MBq/15 mCi) was injected intravenously and oral contrast was administered. After 85 min distribution time, reduced dose CT acquisition was performed, with 140 kV, 80 mA, 0.8s per CT rotation, a pitch of 6 and a table speed of 22.5 mm/s followed by PET acquisition over the head and neck, chest, abdomen, pelvis, and proximal femurs. The patient was positioned with arms up.

Findings

*Quality of study*: good

*Head and neck*: No sites of pathological uptake. There is physiologic distribution of [18]F-FDG in the cerebral cortex and lymphoid and glandular tissues of the neck.

*Chest*: Increased [18]F-FDG uptake is detected in a 58 × 75 mm mass located in the medial aspect of the lower lobe of the right lung, extending to the mediastinum and subcarinal region. This lesion representing the primary tumor appears to narrow the bronchus of the lower segment of the right lung. It also extends to and involves the right aspect of T4 vertebral body and the posterior pleura.

There is increased $^{18}$F-FDG uptake in subcarinal lymph nodes, up to 17 mm in size in their short axis, suspected as metastatic. Retrocaval nodes, smaller than 10 mm in diameter, are detected on CT with no increased $^{18}$F-FDG uptake.

Additional findings on chest CT include chronic fibrotic pulmonary changes, bronchiectasis in the left upper lobe, and calcifications in the left anterior descending (LAD) coronary artery.

*Abdomen and pelvis*: On CT, there is a right kidney cortical cyst (24 mm in size) and sigmoid diverticulosis.

*Musculoskeletal*: There is increased $^{18}$F-FDG uptake in the right scapula, corresponding to a small lytic lesion on CT and an additional focus of increased $^{18}$F-FDG uptake in the right acetabulum with no clear corresponding morphologic abnormality on CT. These two lesions are consistent with hematogenous metastatic spread to bone.

Additional findings on CT include a sclerotic lesion in the left iliac bone with no corresponding increased tracer uptake, most likely a bone island.

Impression

1. Increased $^{18}$F-FDG uptake in a right lower lobe pulmonary mass extending to the mediastinum and T4 vertebral body consistent with the known primary NSCLC.
2. Increased uptake in subcarinal lymphadenopathy suspected as metastatic.
3. Increased uptake in a lytic metastasis in the right scapula and in an early metastatic lesion in the right acetabulum.

## Case II.14.2

### History

A 51-year-old female presented with rising tumor markers 30 months after chemo- and radiation therapy for invasive ductal carcinoma of the left breast. She was referred to [18]F-FDG PET/CT for suspected recurrence (Fig. II.142A, B). Following this study, treatment was initiated. The patient was referred 6 months later to a follow-up [18]F-FDG PET/CT study to monitor response to therapy with Letrozole, an oral non-steroidal aromatase inhibitor (Fig. II.14.2C, D).

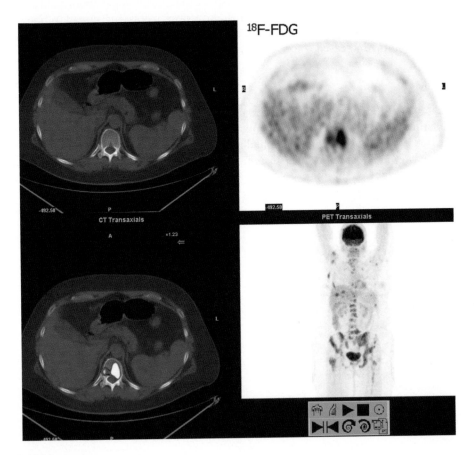

**Fig. II.14.2A**

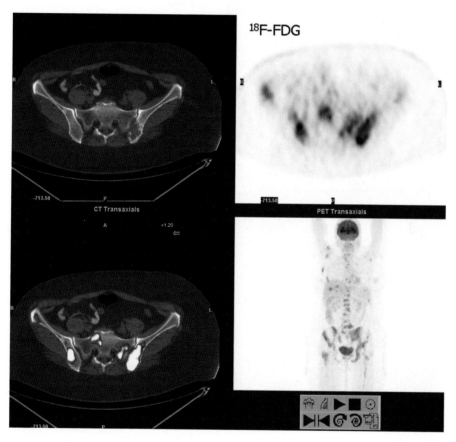

Fig. II.14.2B

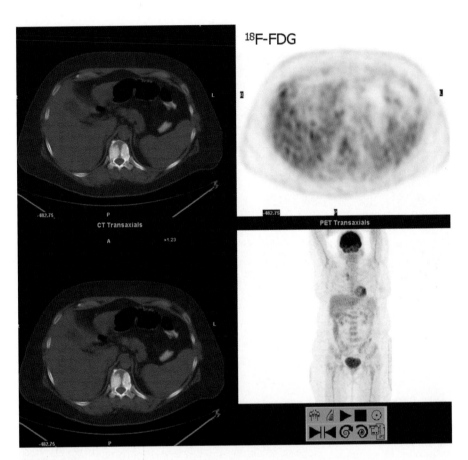

Fig. II.14.2C

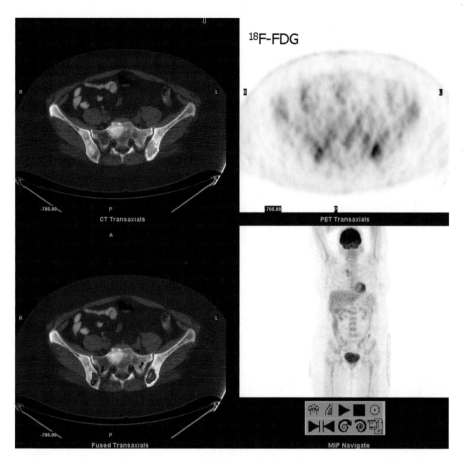

**Fig. II.14.2D**

## Findings

Increased $^{18}$F-FDG uptake is detected in multiple sites in the axial and peripheral skeleton (Fig. II.14.2A, B) including the vertebral column, pelvis, scapulae, sternum, rib cage, and femuri (maximum intensity projection (MIP) image). Figure II.14.2A illustrates the presence of a focus of increased $^{18}$F-FDG in the T11 vertebra with normal appearance on CT, representing one of the sites of early metastases. After successful therapy, sclerotic changes are detected in this location on CT while there is no longer increased uptake of $^{18}$F-FDG indicating repair (Fig. II.14.2C). In Fig. II.14.2B at the level of the pelvis, there is increased $^{18}$F-FDG uptake with no clear cortical changes in the right iliac wing and the posterior aspect of the right ilium and in the sacrum, and increased uptake in the posterior aspect of the left ilium with a corresponding large lytic lesion with cortical destruction and soft tissue mass on CT. After therapy, sclerotic changes are detected on CT in the right ilium and in the periphery of the left iliac lesions. There is also a decrease in the intensity of $^{18}$F-FDG uptake in the posterior aspect of both iliac bones indicating partial response in these sites with residual active metastatic disease (Fig. II.14.2D).

Additional findings seen on the MIP images of the baseline study include multiple foci of increased $^{18}$F-FDG uptake in the liver consistent with metastatic spread (Fig. II.14.2A, B).

## Discussion

As indicated by the $^{18}$F-FDG PET/CT findings, hepatic and skeletal metastases were responsible for the rising tumor markers in this patient. The skeleton appears to be extensively involved with many of the lesions characterized by increased uptake of $^{18}$F-FDG and normal skeletal morphology on CT, representing early, marrow-based metastases.

Skeletal metastases may develop in 30–85% of patients with breast cancer during the course of their disease. The risk for skeletal metastases increases with the stage of disease. Skeletal metastases found in patients with breast cancer may be marrow-based and/or cortical. Cortical skeletal metastases in breast cancer are predominately lytic, with blastic or mixed type lesions found in 15–20% of the patients.[6,28] BS with $^{99m}$Tc-MDP has been the most commonly used modality for detection of skeletal metastases in patients with breast cancer. Several publications have reported the superiority of $^{18}$F-FDG imaging over BS and/or conventional imaging in detecting skeletal metastases in patients with breast cancer. The most important advantage of $^{18}$F-FDG imaging is its ability to detect early marrow-based spread prior to the appearance of structural abnormalities on CT or osteoblastic activity on BS. While significantly superior to BS in detecting marrow-based, lytic, and mixed type metastases, $^{18}$F-FDG PET has a limited sensitivity for detection of blastic metastases.[29,30] Port and colleagues[31] compared the role of conventional and $^{18}$F-FDG imaging in detection of skeletal metastases in patients with high-risk, operable breast cancer. Conventional imaging studies resulted in a higher number of findings that required further tests and biopsies that ultimately had negative results (17% versus 5% for PET). In 5% of the study patients, accounting for 50% of patients with skeletal metastases, $^{18}$F-FDG PET imaging identified additional sites of disease, which affected treatment decisions.

After successful treatment, normal appearing bone or lytic lesions become sclerotic. When monitoring response of metastatic skeletal disease to therapy, CT and BS are of limited value in differentiating active disease from a repair process. $^{18}$F-FDG PET/CT is a superior imaging modality as it allows accurate separation between active disease and burnt-out metastases, when skeletal morphology remains abnormal. In a recent publication by Du and coworkers,[15] sequential PET/CT studies were performed in 408 consecutive patients with known or suspected recurrent breast cancer. $^{18}$F-FDG uptake was found to reflect the immediate tumor activity of skeletal metastases, whereas the radiographic morphologic changes varied greatly with time. In the present case, CT performed after treatment actually identified more skeletal lesions than initially. The lack of tracer uptake in these lesions on the follow-up $^{18}$F-FDG PET/CT study clarified that the "new" sclerotic lesions seen on CT represent a repair process rather than active disease, whereas increased $^{18}$F-FDG uptake at other sites indicated the presence of residual active metastatic disease.

**Diagnosis**

<u>Baseline study</u>

1. Marrow-based and cortical skeletal metastases.
2. Hepatic metastases.

<u>Follow-Up Study</u>

Partial and complete response in various skeletal metastases to treatment.

## Case II.14.3

### History

A 59-year-old male with newly diagnosed NSCLC in the left lung presented with complains of severe back pain He was referred to $^{18}$F-FDG PET/CT imaging for initial staging (Fig. II.14.3).

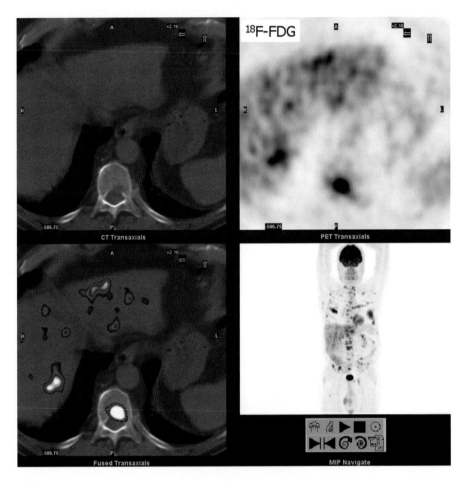

**Fig. II.14.3**

### Findings

There is increased $^{18}$F-FDG uptake in the primary lung tumor (Fig. II.14.3, MIP). There are multiple sites of increased $^{18}$F-FDG uptake in the skeleton and additional foci in the liver. At the level of the T11 vertebra, the increased $^{18}$F-FDG uptake corresponds to a lytic lesion in the posterior aspect of the vertebral body with destruction of the posterior cortex and extension into the epidural space (Fig. II.14.3).

**Discussion**

The vertebral column is the most common skeletal region involved by metastatic spread. Tumoral tissue may invade the epidural space by direct extension from adjacent bone. Early diagnosis and treatment prior to the development of permanent neurological deficit is essential for a favorable outcome.[18] As illustrated in this case, fused [18]F-FDG PET/CT images enable detection of epidural space invasion in patients with metastatic disease involving the vertebral column.

**Diagnosis**

1. Left lung NSCLC.
2. Extensive metastatic spread in the skeleton with invasion of the epidural space at T11.
3. Hepatic metastases.

## *Case II.14.4*

### History

A 46-year-old patient with newly diagnosed follicular non-Hodgkin lymphoma (NHL) was referred to $^{18}$F-FDG PET/CT for initial staging (Fig. II.14.4A–C).

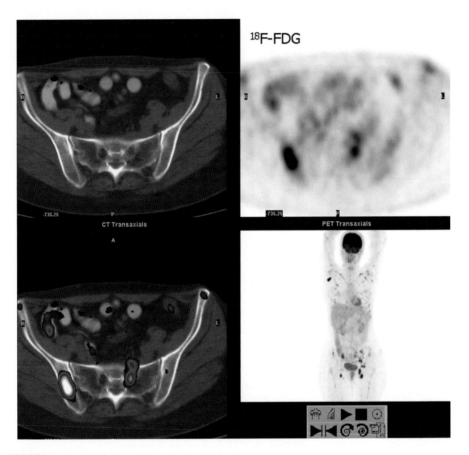

**Fig. II.14.4A**

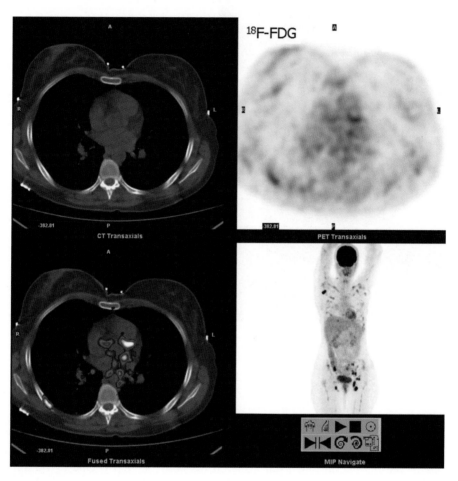

**Fig. II.14.4B**

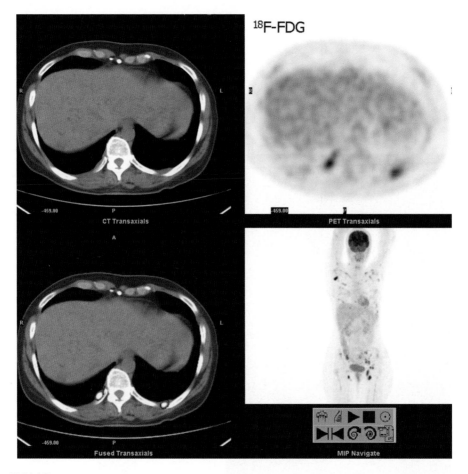

**Fig. II.14.4C**

**Findings**

There are multiple sites of nodal [18]F-FDG-avid disease, more prominent in the inguinal and right axillary regions. In addition, patchy increased [18]F-FDG uptake is detected in the peripheral and axial skeleton (as seen on MIP). One of the multiple skeletal lesions is displayed in Fig. II.14.4A. Increased [18]F-FDG uptake is detected in the posterior aspect of the right ilium, with a corresponding hyperdense intramedullar area on CT, consistent with lymphomatous marrow involvement. There is also increased uptake in the left iliacus muscle with invasion of the S1 nerve root. Figure II.14.4B illustrates increased [18]F-FDG uptake in the rib cage indicating additional sites of skeletal involvement. Figure II.14.4C illustrates the presence of increased [18]F-FDG uptake in a similar location, precisely localized by fused images to nodular pleural thickening seen on CT, consistent with extranodal soft tissue lymphomatous involvement.

**Discussion**

The incidence of bone marrow involvement in patients with lymphoma is high, varying between 25–40% in high-grade and 50–80% in patients with low-grade NHL. Marrow involvement by lymphoma has a "patchy" pattern. In contrast, diffuse increased tracer uptake is more often associated with reactive hematopoietic changes within the bone marrow or myeloid hyperplasia, mainly after chemotherapy or following G-CSF administration.[32] Pakos and colleagues[33] have published a meta-analysis of 13 studies addressing the role of [18]F-FDG PET in evaluating bone marrow infiltration in lymphoma. Sites of increased [18]F-FDG uptake in the bone marrow, which were considered false positive when compared to "blindly" performed bone marrow sampling, became true positive sites of involvement, when the site of biopsy was guided by PET findings. In 50 consecutive patients with lymphomatous involvement of the skeleton, [18]F-FDG PET/CT upstaged disease in 42% of patients as compared with the combined information of CT and "blind" marrow sampling.[34] In present case, there appears to be extensive lymphomatous involvement demonstrating the characteristic pattern of "patchy" increased uptake in the axial and peripheral skeleton. Retrospective evaluation of the CT component indicated sites of denser marrow, a finding often overlooked when CT is interpreted alone.

[18]F-FDG PET allows detection of both soft tissue and skeletal tumoral involvement, but fused PET/CT images are often necessary for accurate localization of the foci of abnormal uptake to one or both areas.[17] In present case, fused images allowed to precisely localize and differentiate suspicious foci showing a similar pattern and topography to lymphomatous involvement in a rib and to a pleural nodule.

Lymphoma tends to invade cranial and peripheral nerves as well as nerve roots. The pathogenesis of localized peripheral nerves invaded by malignant B-cells remains obscure.[35] In this patient, increased uptake was detected in the S1 neural foramen suggesting its involvement.

**Diagnosis**

1. Nodal lymphoma above and below the diaphragm.
2. Extranodal soft tissue pleural and left iliacus muscular involvement.
3. Skeletal involvement.
4. Suspected involvement of the left S1 neural foramen.

## Case II.14.5

### History

An 18-year-old male patient was referred for BS due to pain in his right shin (Fig. II.14.5A). The scintigraphic lesion found in the right tibia was biopsied, revealing bone lymphoma. The patient was referred to $^{18}$F-FDG PET/CT for initial staging 2 weeks after biopsy (Fig. II.14.5B–E).

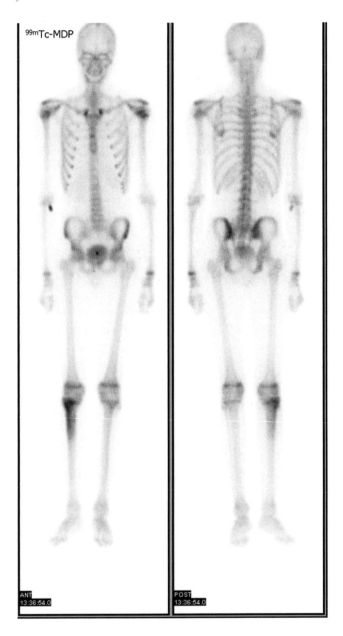

**Fig. II.14.5A**

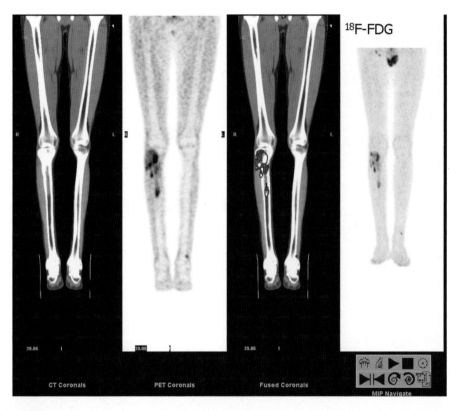

CT Coronals    PET Coronals    Fused Coronals

$^{18}$F-FDG

MIP Navigate

**Fig. II.14.5B**

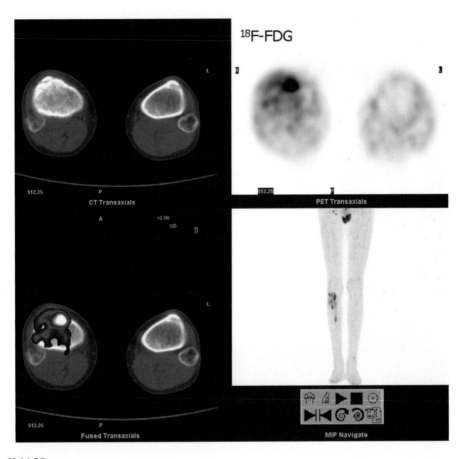

Fig. II.14.5C

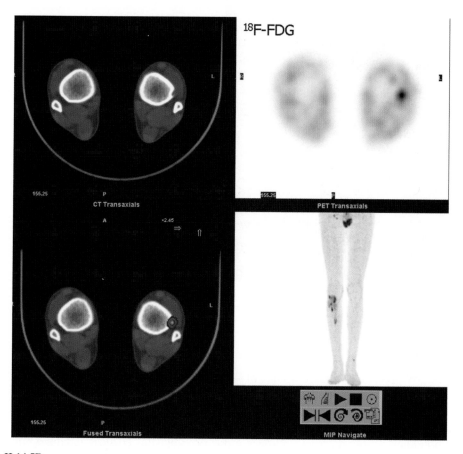

**Fig. II.14.5D**

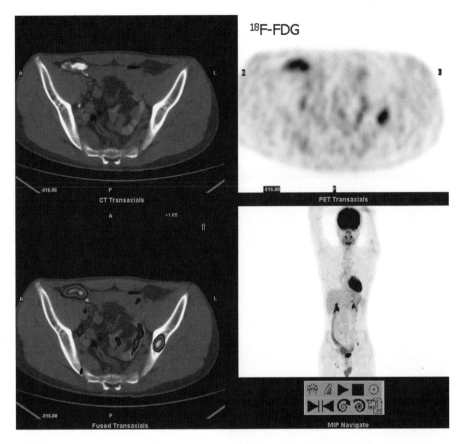

**Fig. II.14.5E**

## Findings

On planar BS, there is increased uptake of $^{99m}$Tc-MDP in the upper third of the right tibia (Fig. II.14.5A), a lesion found by biopsy to represent primary bone lymphoma.

On $^{18}$F-FDG PET/CT images, the increased uptake in the right tibia appears to be located in the intramedullary compartment and in the cortex of the right tibia, with corresponding dense marrow changes and osteoblastic cortical changes on CT (Fig. II.14.5B, C). Increased $^{18}$F-FDG uptake is also demonstrated in a small lytic lesion in the lateral aspect of the distal left tibia (Fig. II.14.5D) and in the left ilium, of normal appearance on CT (Fig. II 14.5 E). The latter two sites of lymphoma were overlooked by BS.

Increased $^{18}$F-FDG uptake is also detected in small right inguinal lymph nodes (MIP). The differential diagnosis of the focal tracer uptake in theses nodes may, however, include reactive inflammatory reaction related to the recently performed bone biopsy.

## Discussion

Primary NHL of bone is an uncommon entity. Almost all lesions are localized in long bones (particularly the femur, tibia, pelvis, and humerus), and patients present with pain and/or a palpable mass. When a skeletal lesion is found by biopsy to be NHL, it is clinically relevant to define whether this is a secondary manifestation of lymphoma or a primary bone lymphoma since extent and location of disease is essential for optimization of therapy. Patterns of primary bone lymphoma on CT include cortical erosion, radiolucent lesions, and/or sclerotic zones.[36] BS with $^{99m}$Tc-MDP allows mainly detection of the large lesions, as was the case in this patient where only the large lesion in the right tibia was detected while two other lymphoma sites were missed: a small lytic lesion in the contralateral lower limb and a marrow-based lesion in the pelvis.

## Diagnosis

1. Primary bone lymphoma involving the proximal right tibia, distal left tibia, and left iliac bone.
2. Increased uptake in inguinal lymph nodes, probably reactive after biopsy.

## *Case II.14.6*

### History

A 74 year-old male presented with monoclonal gammopathy 5 months after completion of radiation therapy for plasmocytoma in L5. He was referred to $^{18}$F-FDG PET/CT for restaging (Fig. II.14.6A, B).

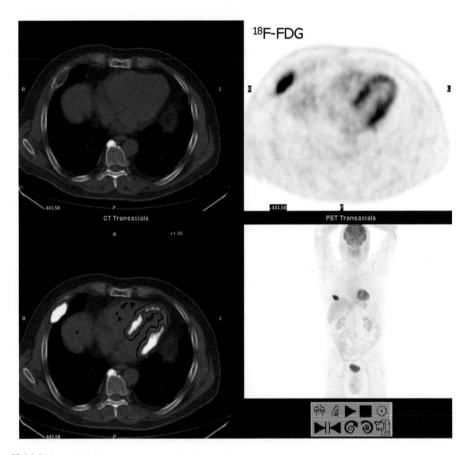

Fig. II.14.6A

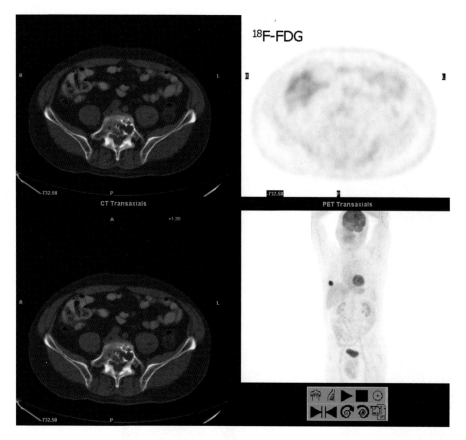

**Fig. II.14.6B**

### Findings

Increased uptake of $^{18}$F-FDG is detected in an expansile lytic lesion in the anterior aspect of the fifth right rib (Fig. II.14.6A) consistent with an active site of myeloma. In the previously irradiated L5 vertebra, mixed lytic and sclerotic cortical changes are detected on CT with no congruent increased $^{18}$F-FDG uptake, consistent with a non-active site of myeloma (Fig. II.14.6B).

### Discussion

$^{18}$F-FDG is accumulated in active sites of myeloma. $^{18}$F-FDG imaging is of value in assessing both the extent and activity of myeloma.[37,38] CT is an accurate modality for diagnosis of bone destruction. However, skeletal morphology may remain abnormal on CT even when the myeloma has been eradicated. As illustrated in this case, the use of $^{18}$F-FDG/CT allows the identification of myeloma sites and their activity status.

### Diagnosis

1. Active myeloma in the fifth right rib.
2. Post-radiotherapy inactive myeloma in L5.

## Case II.14.7 (DICOM Images on DVD)

### History

A 33-year-old male with newly diagnosed Ewing sarcoma in the right femur was referred to $^{18}$F-FDG PET/CT for initial staging (Fig. II.14.7A–D).

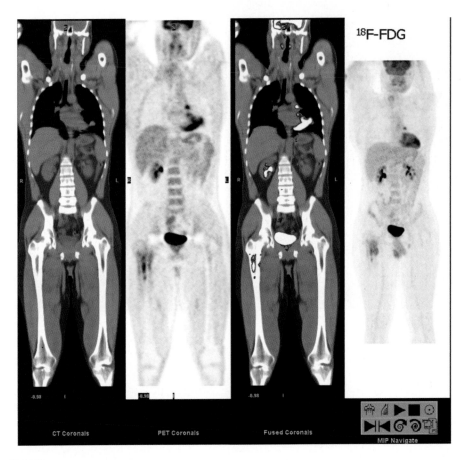

Fig. II.14.7A

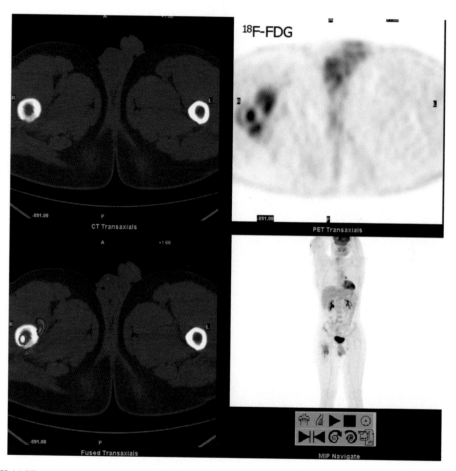

**Fig. II.14.7B**

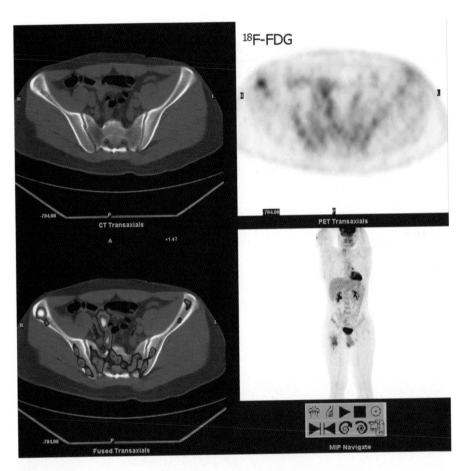

**Fig. II.14.7C**

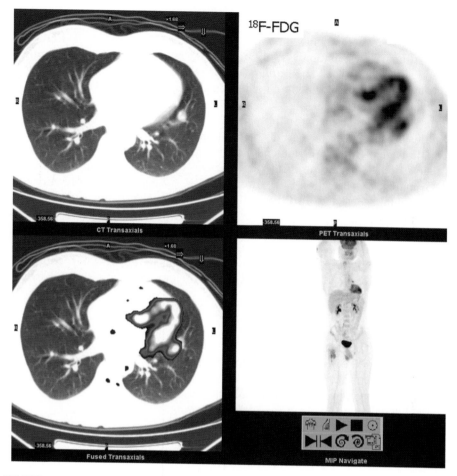

**Fig. II.14.7D**

**Findings**

Increased uptake of ${}^{18}$F-FDG is detected in the proximal right femur. The lesion is located intramedullary with hyperdense bone marrow and destructive cortical changes, mainly in the inner cortical surface, seen on CT. There is also increased ${}^{18}$F-FDG uptake in the muscles anterior and posterior to the involved bone with disappearance of the fat planes on CT (Fig. II.14.7A, B).

There is focally increased ${}^{18}$F-FDG uptake in the right iliac wing, with corresponding mixed lytic/sclerotic changes on CT, suggestive of an additional malignant skeletal site (Fig. II.14.7C). While on CT multiple pulmonary nodules are identified, only the two larger nodules show increased ${}^{18}$F-FDG uptake consistent with pulmonary metastases, one located in the lingula, 28 mm in size (Fig. II.14.7D) and another in the left lower lobe, 19 mm in diameter (not shown). There is a "hot" lymph node in the left hilum, suspicious for metastasis (not shown, see DICOM images on DVD).

## Discussion

This patient with Ewing sarcoma illustrates the potential advantages of [18]F-FDG PET/CT imaging in primary skeletal tumors resulting from the inherent whole-body imaging of soft tissues and skeleton of PET. The primary tumor is well delineated on the fused PET/CT images demonstrating involvement of the intramedullary cavity, the skeletal cortex as well as the surrounding soft tissue.

Lung is the most common organ for metastatic spread of sarcoma. Lung metastases can be, as in this patient, small, beyond the detectability range of PET. [18]F-FDG imaging can differentiate benign from malignant pulmonary nodules detected by CT when they are larger than twice the resolution of the PET system. CT is, however, more sensitive than [18]F-FDG imaging for detection of small metastases.[38] Therefore, the presence of small pulmonary nodules detected on CT should be reported even if not showing increased [18]F-FDG uptake.

In patients with Ewing sarcoma, bone and bone marrow are the second most common metastatic sites, after the lung and pleural space.[39] In this patient, an unexpected malignant skeletal site was detected on PET/CT, later confirmed by biopsy. Data on the benefit of [18]F-FDG PET/CT for detecting skeletal metastases in sarcoma patients are still very sparse.

## Diagnosis

1. Ewing sarcoma in the proximal right femur with muscular involvement.
2. Pulmonary metastases.
3. Suspected metastasis in the right iliac bone.
4. Suspected nodal involvement in the left hilar region.

## Clinical Report: Whole Body [18]F-FDG PET/CT (for DVD cases only)

Indication

Initial staging of Ewing sarcoma.

History

A 33-year-old male with biopsy-proven Ewing sarcoma in the right femur was referred to [18]F-FDG PET/CT for initial staging.

Procedure

The fasting blood sugar was 98 mg/dl. [18]F-FDG (503 MBq/13.6 mCi) was injected intravenously and oral contrast was administered. After 90 min distribution time, reduced dose CT acquisition was performed, with 140 kV, 80 mA, 0.8 s per CT rotation, a pitch of 6 and a table speed of 22.5 mm/s followed by the PET acquisition over the head and neck, chest, abdomen, pelvis, femurs, and knees. The patient was positioned with arms up.

Findings

*Quality of study*: Good

*Head and Neck*: There are no sites of pathological $^{18}$F-FDG uptake. There is physiologic tracer distribution in the cerebral cortex, the lymphoid, and glandular tissues of the neck. There is a mucous retention cyst in the right maxillary sinus.

*Chest*: Increased $^{18}$F-FDG uptake is detected in a 10 mm (short diameter) lymph node in the left suprahilar region suspicious for metastasis.

Increased $^{18}$F-FDG uptake is also detected in a 28 mm pulmonary nodule in the lingula and in a 19 mm nodule in the left lower lobe consistent with pulmonary metastases. On CT, there are at least six additional nodules in both lungs, few to 8 mm in size, with no increased tracer uptake, probably representing pulmonary metastases, below the resolution of PET.

In the anterior mediastinum, there is a small soft tissue mass with smooth contours on CT showing slightly increased $^{18}$F-FDG uptake. In view of its location and the patient's age, this is most consistent with physiologic thymic uptake.

*Abdomen and pelvis*: No abnormal findings.

*Musculoskeletal*: Increased $^{18}$F-FDG uptake is demonstrated in the proximal right femur. It appears to be located in the intramedullary part of the bone with associated dense bone marrow. Destructive cortical changes are also seen on CT, mainly in the inner cortical surface. Focal increased $^{18}$F-FDG uptake is found in the muscles anterior and posterior to the involved bone, with disappearance of the fat planes on CT. These findings are consistent with the site of the primary sarcoma. In the right iliac wing there is a focus of increased $^{18}$F-FDG uptake corresponding to mixed lytic/ sclerotic changes on CT, suggestive of an additional malignant skeletal site.

Impression

1. Primary sarcoma involving the marrow and cortex of the proximal right femur and the surrounding musculature.
2. Multiple pulmonary metastases bilaterally.
3. Suspected skeletal metastasis in the right iliac bone.
4. Suspected nodal involvement in the left hilar region.

# References

1. Roodman GD. Mechanisms of bone metastasis. *N Engl J Med* 2004;350:1655–1664.
2. Padhani A, Husband J. Bone metastases. In Husband JES, Reznek RH, (eds): *Imaging in Oncology*. Oxford, UK: Isis Medical Media Ltd., 1998: 765–787.
3. Blake GM, Park-Holohan SJ, Cook GJ, Fogelman I. Quantitative studies of bone with the use of $^{18}$F-fluoride and $^{99m}$Tc-methylene diphosphonate.*Semin Nucl Med* 2001;31:28–49.
4. Cook GJ, Fogelman I. The role of positron emission tomography in skeletal disease. *Semin Nucl Med* 2001;31:50–61.
5. Even-Sapir E. Imaging of malignant bone involvement by morphologic, scintigraphic, and hybrid modalities. *J Nucl Med* 2005;46:1356–1367.
6. Hamaoka T, Madewell JE, Podoloff DA, Hortobagyi GN, Ueno NT. Bone imaging in metastatic breast cancer. *J Clin Oncol* 2004; 22:2942–2953.
7. Liu FY, Chang JT, Wang HM, Liao CT, Kang CJ, Ng SH, Chan SC, Yen TC. [18F]fluorodeoxyglucose positron emission tomography is more sensitive than skeletal scintigraphy for detecting bone metastases in endemic nasopharyngeal carcinoma at initial staging. *J Clin Oncol* 2006;24:599–604.
8. Cook GJ, Fogelman I. The role of positron emission tomography in the management of bone metastases. *Cancer* 2000; 88:2927–2933.
9. Cook GJ, Houston S, Rubens R, Maisey MN, Fogelman I. Detection of bone metastases in breast cancer by $^{18}$FDG PET: differing metabolic activity in osteoblastic and osteolytic lesions. *J Clin Oncol* 1998;16:3375–3379.
10. Moog F, Bangerter M, Kotzerke J, Guhlmann A, Frickhofen N, Reske SN. 18-F-fluorodeoxyglucose-positron emission tomography as a new approach to detect lymphomatous bone marrow. *J Clin Oncol* 1998;16:603–609.
11. Even-Sapir E, Lievshitz G, Perry C, Herishanu Y, Lerman H, Metser U. Fluorine-18 fluorodeoxyglucose PET/CT patterns of extranodal involvement in patients with Non-Hodgkin lymphoma and Hodgkin's disease. *Radiol Clin North Am* 2007;45:697–709.
12. Durie BG. The role of anatomic and functional staging in myeloma: description of Durie/Salmon plus staging system. *Eur J Cancer* 2006;42:1539–1543.
13. Adam Z, Bolcak K, Stanicek J, Buchler T, Pour L, Krejci M, Prasek J, Neubauer J, Vorlicek J, Hajek R. Fluorodeoxyglucose positron emission tomography in multiple myeloma, solitary plasmocytoma and monoclonal gammapathy of unknown significance. *Neoplasma* 2007;54:536–540.
14. Israel O, Goldberg A, Nachtigal A, Militianu D, Bar-Shalom R, Keidar Z, Fogelman I. FDG-PET and CT patterns of bone metastases and their relationship to previously administered anti-cancer therapy. *Eur J Nucl Med Mol Imaging* 2006;33:1280–1284.
15. Du Y, Cullum I, Illidge TM, Ell PJ. Fusion of metabolic function and morphology: Sequential [18F]Fluorodeoxyglucose positron-emission tomography /computed tomography studies yield new insights into the natural history of bone metastases in breast cancer. *J Clin Oncol* 2007;25:3440–3447.
16. Kazama T, Swanston N, Podoloff DA, Macapinlac HA. Effect of colony-stimulating factor and conventional- or high-dose chemotherapy on FDG uptake in bone marrow. *Eur J Nucl Med Mol Imaging* 2005;32:1406–1411.
17. Kostakoglu L, Hardoff R, Mirtcheva R, Goldsmith SJ. PET/CT Fusion imaging in differentiating physiologic from pathologic FDG uptake. *Radiographics* 2004;24:1411–1431.
18. Metser U, Lerman H, Blank A, Lievshitz G, Bokstein F, Even-Sapir E. Malignant involvement of the spine: assessment by 18F-FDG PET/CT. *J Nucl Med* 2004;45:279–284.
19. Schulte M, Brecht-Krauss D, Heymer B, Guhlmann A, Hartwig E, Sarkar MR, Diederichs CG, Von Baer A, Kotzerke J, Reske SN. Grading of tumors and tumorlike lesions of bone: evaluation by FDG PET. *J Nucl Med* 2000;41:1695–701.
20. Pezeshk P, Sadow CA, Winalski CS, Lang PK, Ready JE, Carrino JA. Usefulness of 18F-FDG PET-directed skeletal biopsy for metastatic neoplasm. *Acad Radiol* 2006;13:1011–1015.
21. Lodge MA, Lucas JD, Marsden PK, Cronin BF, O'Doherty MJ, Smith MA. A PET study of $^{18}$FDG uptake in soft tissue masses. *Eur J Nucl Med* 1999;26:22–30.
22. Brenner W, Bohuslavizki KH, Eary JF. PET imaging of osteosarcoma. *J Nucl Med* 2003;44:930–942.
23. Cotterill SJ, Ahrens S, Paulussen M, Jürgens HF, Voûte PA, Gadner H, Craft AW. Prognostic factors in Ewing's tumor of bone: analysis of 975 patients from the European Intergroup Cooperative Ewing's Sarcoma Study Group. *J Clin Oncol* 2000;18:3108–3114.

24. Franzius C, Daldrup-Link HE, Wagner-Bohn A, Sciuk, J, Heindel WL, Jürgens H, Schober O. FDG-PET for detection of recurrences from malignant primary bone tumors: comparison with conventional imaging. *Ann Oncol* 2002;13:157–160.

25. Hawkins DS, Rajendran JG, Conrad EU 3rd, Bruckner JD, Eary JF. Evaluation of chemotherapy response in pediatric bone sarcomas by [F-18]-fluorodeoxy-D-glucose positron emission tomography. *Cancer* 2002;94:3277–3284.

26. Cheran SK, Herndon JE, Patz EF. Comparison of whole-body FDG-PET to bone scan for detection of bone metastases in patients with a new diagnosis of lung cancer. *Lung Cancer* 2004; 44:317–325.

27. Fogelman I, Cook G, Israel O, Van der Wall H. Positron emission tomography and bone metastases. *Semin Nucl Med* 2005;35:135–142.

28. Langsteger W, Heinisch M, Fogelman I. The role of fluorodeoxyglucose, 18F-dihydroxyphenylalanine, 18F-choline, and 18F-fluoride in bone imaging with emphasis on prostate and breast. *Semin Nucl Med* 2006;36:73–92.

29. Nakai T, Okuyama C, Kubota T, Yamada K, Ushijima Y, Taniike K, Suzuki T, Nishimura T. Pitfalls of FDG-PET for the diagnosis of osteoblastic bone metastases in patients with breast cancer. *Eur J Nucl Med Mol Imag* 2005;32:1253–1258.

30. Abe K, Sasaki M, Kuwabara Y, Koga H, Baba S, Hayashi K, Nakahashi N, Honda H. Comparison of 18FDG-PET with 99mTc-HMDP scintigraphy for the detection of bone metastases in patients with breast cancer. *Ann Nucl Med* 2005;19:573–579.

31. Port ER, Yeung H, Gonen M, Liberman L, Caravelli J, Borgen P, Larson S. (18)F-2-fluoro-2-deoxy-d: -glucose positron emission tomography scanning affects surgical management in selected patients with high-risk, operable breast carcinoma. *Ann Surg Oncol* 2006;13:677–684.

32. Kazama T, Faria SC, Varavithya V, Phongkitkarun S, Ito H, Macapinlac HA. FDG PET in the evaluation of treatment for lymphoma: clinical usefulness and pitfalls. *Radiographics* 2005;25:191–207.

33. Pakos EE, Fotopoulos AD, Ioannidis JP. 18F-FDG PET for evaluation of bone marrow infiltration in staging of lymphoma: A meta-analysis. *J Nucl Med* 2005;46:958–963.

34. Schaefer NG, Strobel K, Taverna C, Hany TF. Bone involvement in patients with lymphoma: The role of FDG-PET/CT. *Eur J Nucl Med Mol Imaging* 2007;34:60–67.

35. Baehring JM, Damek D, Martin EC, Betensky RA, Hochberg FH. Neurolymphomatosis. *Neuro-Oncology* 2003;5:104–115.

36. Heyning FH, Kroon HM, Hogendoorn PC, Taminiau AH, van der Woude HJ. MR imaging characteristics in primary lymphoma of bone with emphasis on non-aggressive appearance. *Skeletal Radiol* 2007;36:937–944.

37. Durie BG., Waxman AD, D'Agnolo A, Williams CM. Whole-body [18]F-FDG PET identifies high-risk myeloma. *J Nucl Med* 2002;43:1457–1463.

38. Schirrmeister H, Bommer M, Buck AK, Müller S, Messer P, Bunjes D,. Döhner H, Bergmann L, Reske S. Initial results in the assessment of multiple myeloma using F-18 FDG PET. *Eur J Nucl Med Mol Imag* 2002;29:361–366.

39. Daldrup-Link HE, Franzius C, Link TM, Laukamp D, Sciuk J, Jürgens H, Schober O, Rummeny EJ. Whole-body MR imaging for detection of bone metastases in children and young adults: comparison with skeletal scintigraphy and FDG PET. *AJR* 2001;177:229–236.

# Chapter II.15
# Pediatric Applications for PET/CT and SPECT/CT

Helen R. Nadel and Angela T. Byrne

## Introduction

Positron emission tomography/computed tomography (PET/CT) and single photon emission computed tomography/computed tomography (SPECT/CT) are becoming increasingly important imaging tools in the noninvasive evaluation and monitoring of children with known or suspected malignant diseases. The recent advent of dual-modality imaging systems has improved the diagnostic capabilities by revealing the precise anatomical localization of metabolic information and characterization of normal and abnormal structures. In addition, the use of CT transmission scanning for attenuation correction has shortened the total acquisition time for PET, which is an especially desirable attribute in pediatric imaging.[1] Hybrid imaging has been beneficial to pediatric oncology, with SPECT/CT used in the diagnosis of tumors such as neuroblastoma and in better delineating skeletal involvement in sarcomas, while PET/CT using $^{18}$F-fluorodeoxyglucose ($^{18}$F-FDG) is used in the diagnosis, staging, and response assessment of malignancies such as sarcoma, lymphoma, and solid organ tumors.

## Neuroblastoma

Neuroblastoma is the second most common abdominal neoplasm in children following Wilms' tumor and overall the third most common pediatric malignancy, after leukemia and central nervous system tumors. It accounts for almost 15% of childhood cancer fatalities, a number that reflects its aggressive nature and frequency of metastatic disease at diagnosis.[2] Most children with neuroblastoma are diagnosed between the age of 1 and 5 years, median age 2 years, with a palpable abdominal mass that may be detected as an incidental finding in an otherwise healthy child or in one who is unwell from metastatic spread of the tumor.[3] The therapeutic strategy strongly depends on initial staging with multimodality imaging. The patient is referred to surgery when possible or to chemotherapy as in the majority of the cases, as well as to bone marrow transplantation that has been recently introduced.[4] Neuroblastoma arises from the adrenal glands, the organ of Zuckerkandl, or follows the distribution of the sympathetic ganglia along the paraspinal areas from the neck to the pelvis. Ultrasonography (US) is the initial imaging modality to investigate a child or infant

H.R. Nadel (✉)
Division of Nuclear Medicine, Department of Radiology, British Columbia Children's Hospital, University of British Columbia, Vancouver, BC, Canada
e-mail: hnadel@cw.bc.ca

D. Delbeke, O. Israel (eds.), *Hybrid PET/CT and SPECT/CT Imaging*,
DOI 10.1007/978-0-387-92820-3_17, © Springer Science+Business Media, LLC 2010

with a palpable abdominal mass and provides an excellent screening procedure. Tomographic imaging for staging of a newly discovered neuroblastoma is performed with either CT or magnetic resonance imaging (MRI). Imaging with [123]I-metaiodobenzylguanidine ([123]I-MIBG) gives an excellent whole body map of the disease with high sensitivity of 88% and specificity of 99% for detection of both the primary tumor and metastases involving mainly cortical bone, bone marrow, and lymph nodes, in over 90% of patients.[5]

Since the development of hybrid SPECT/CT systems, it is possible to acquire morphologic (CT) and functional (SPECT) images in one setting following administration of [123]I-MIBG. SPECT/CT is becoming as an integral part of the diagnostic pathway following chest radiography and US in the diagnosis of neuroblastoma. SPECT/CT defines foci of physiologic tracer activity and differentiates them from malignant lesions. For example, in the abdomen, it defines physiologic bowel activity of [123]I-MIBG. In the left hemithorax it can localize diffuse [123]I-MIBG uptake to physiologic activity of the heart, which can be otherwise misinterpreted as mediastinal, sternal, or vertebral sites of disease. SPECT/CT diagnoses tumor involvement occurring adjacent to or in organs with increased physiologic [123]I-MIBG activity. In this group of pediatric patients, SPECT/CT can also differentiate between bilateral symmetric activity in the neck, shoulder girdle, or upper thorax related to physiologic muscular or brown adipose tissue uptake of [123]I-MIBG and malignant lesions such as skeletal metastases in the scapula or ribs or malignant supraclavicular lymphadenopathies.

[18]F-FDG PET is also a promising modality for diagnosis and assessment of neuroblastoma involving both the soft tissues and the skeleton. [18]F-FDG uptake is directly proportional to tumor burden and to tumor cell proliferation.[6] While primary tumors and metastases concentrate [18]F-FDG avidly before therapy, variable patterns of accumulation have been observed after treatment. [18]F-FDG imaging has been used for diagnosis, initial staging, monitoring tumor response to therapy, and assessing recurrence. Other PET radiotracers such as [18]F-fluorodopamine (F-DOPA) and [18]F-dihydroxyphenylalanine may prove useful particularly when MIBG studies are negative but, as yet, only few pediatric patients have been evaluated.[7]

## Sarcoma

Osteosarcoma is the most common primary malignant neoplasm of bone and occurs between the ages of 10 and 25. It accounts for 60% of malignant skeletal tumors in the first two decades of life, is slightly more common in males, and is usually located in the metaphysis of long bones, especially around the knee. Pain and swelling are typical presenting features. Ewing sarcoma occurs in a younger age group and is the most common skeletal in the first decade of life. While long bones are primarily affected, 25% of cases occur in the pelvis. Rhabdomyosarcoma is the most common soft-tissue sarcoma in children.

Baseline imaging of skeletal and soft-tissue sarcomas in children currently includes MRI of the primary tumor, CT of the chest in search of pulmonary metastases, and [99m]Tc-methylenediphosphonate ([99m]Tc-MDP) skeletal scintigraphy to identify metastatic disease.[8] [18]F-FDG PET/CT is becoming increasingly useful in identifying and localizing unusual sites of soft tissue and skeletal metastases not appreciated on physical examination or imaging performed during the conventional metastatic workup. It has, however, limited specificity in distinguishing between benign lymphadenopathy and malignant nodal disease.[8–10]

Evaluating response to neoadjuvant chemotherapy is crucial in the management of childhood sarcomas, particularly osteosarcoma, for which tumor response is highly predictive of patient outcome and may impact surgical planning for either amputation or limb-salvage procedures. Radiation therapy and chemotherapy may invoke significant changes in tumor viability, whereas only minimal changes in morphology are apparent on conventional imaging. [18]F-FDG PET/CT is used prior to and after local therapy in order to assess outcome. The measured standard uptake values (SUV) in sarcoma at presentation are usually above 5, and its percentage of decrease following neoadjuvant therapy is a good predictor of prognosis.[11] PET/CT is useful in the identification of unknown primary rhabdomyosarcoma and in the detection of unsuspected and unusual metastatic sites of a variety of childhood sarcomas. Its value has been demonstrated as an adjunct in monitoring response to chemo- and radiation therapy and radiofrequency ablation, and in the postoperative evaluation of these tumors.[11–15]

At the authors' institution, [18]F-FDG PET/CT for initial staging is performed using contrast-enhancement for the CT component with follow-up using non-contrast low-dose CT with 40 mAs and 80 kVp. This protocol provides diagnostic quality images with a radiation exposure that compares very favorably to other tests such as [99m]Tc-MDP skeletal scintigraphy. A caveat however is that for tumor follow-up, additional CT of the chest needs to be performed due to the propensity of sarcomas to metastasize to the lungs. As [18]F-FDG PET/CT is usually performed with the patient quietly breathing, this does not provide optimal resolution for detection of small pulmonary nodules.[16,17]

## Lymphoma

In addition to conventional imaging using CT, single-photon scintigraphy with [67]Gallium ([67]Ga) citrate has been widely used for assessment of lymphomas. [18]F-FDG imaging has gained a role in the staging and follow-up of lymphomas, largely replacing [67]Ga citrate as the functional modality of choice. In one comparative study in 26 pediatric patients with both Hodgkin disease (HD) and non-Hodgkin lymphoma (NHL), [18]F-FDG PET had a higher sensitivity and specificity of 94 and 100%, respectively, as compared to 90 and 88% for [67]Ga citrate scintigraphy and CT/MRI.[18] [18]F-FDG PET has proved useful in the staging and follow-up of HD and NHL, in particular in the more aggressive types of disease.[1,19]

Pediatric HD and NHL are usually [18]F-FDG avid malignancies at initial presentation. In most studies using [18]F-FDG imaging, patients with HD and NHL were assessed as a single group. In comparison to morphologic imaging with contrast-enhanced CT, metabolic imaging with [18]F-FDG PET has a higher specificity for staging. Another major indication for [18]F-FDG imaging is the evaluation of response after completion of therapy. In patients with residual masses, it is unclear whether these represent residual active tumor. [18]F-FDG PET has a significantly higher site- and patient-based sensitivity than [67]Ga scintigraphy for both staging and early therapy evaluation of children with lymphoma.[20,21] [18]F-FDG PET upstaged patients and changed response criteria while [67]Ga scintigraphy did not.[22] The negative predictive value (NPV) for lymphoma relapse off therapy was 89% for [18]F-FDG PET and 83% for [67]Ga scintigraphy. Several studies assessing [18]F-FDG imaging in the follow-up of pediatric lymphoma, have confirmed its high sensitivity of 95% and NPV of 100%, but cautioned on the interpretation of a positive finding during surveillance due to the low positive predictive value (PPV) of around 50% for both PET/CT and CT alone.[23,24] In a review of the current literature, the value of [18]F-FDG imaging of childhood lymphoma has been validated for staging in both HD and NHL, prior to decisions on treatment modification, and for assessment of residual masses at the end of therapy in HD.[25] The review also suggests that there may be a role for the use of [18]F-FDG imaging for radiation field planning, and for diagnosis of bone marrow involvement. Further evaluation is still necessary to clarify the role of [18]F-FDG imaging in detecting extranodal sites of disease, for assessment of response in NHL, and for defining its role in surveillance to detect relapse.

It is important to consider the potential causes of misinterpretation of [18]F-FDG PET that relate to physiologic tracer distribution in children. High [18]F-FDG uptake is typically seen in the thymus, in skeletal growth centers, and in brown adipose tissue. This can be problematic, particularly when attempting to delineate the presence of nodal lymphomatous involvement in the neck.

## Considerations on Radiation Exposure from PET/CT

PET/CT used as a combined diagnostic imaging modality in children can save both time and radiation exposure by eliminating the need for additional stand-alone imaging procedures. Because many pediatric tumors can have distant metastatic or skip disease, it is imperative to always image the whole body when performing PET/CT. However, radiation exposure from [18]F-FDG PET/CT is not trivial in the pediatric population, and standardization of PET/CT examinations is particularly important in this group of patients. Whereas many centers perform low-dose CT with lowered kVp and mAs for attenuation maps and then a separate diagnostic post-contrast acquisition, a single post-contrast diagnostic evaluation with lower kVp and mAs can serve both as the CT portion of the PET/CT study and also be used for attenuation correction.[26]

At the authors' institution, the CT portion of the PET/CT study is performed as a diagnostic stand-alone multidetector CT examination. The routine CT protocol includes acquisition with 80 kVp and 40 mAs with dose modulation. This provides diagnostic quality optimized CT examinations without the need for additional conventional "diagnostic" studies. A considerable reduction in absorbed dose is thus achieved, from 15 to 21 mSv for PET/CT using standard adult algorithms to approximately 7–9 mSv. The patient acquisition parameters and dose estimates obtained from the system are routinely recorded as part of the study parameters that are archived in the patient's file. This CT, particularly with the use of intravenous (IV) contrast, can provide adequate anatomic information when reviewed with appropriate window and level modification, using bone and soft-tissue algorithm reconstruction. Software developments of future PET/CT systems will allow even more refined protocols, tailoring the acquisition of the CT component to PET positive sites only. While the best single practice for performing [18]F-FDG PET/CT in pediatric patients is not yet established, attention is being directed to these aspects due to increasing concerns regarding radiation exposure for both the PET and CT portions of the examination and will require further prospective larger trials.[26,27]

## PET/CT Procedure and Preparation of the Pediatric Patient

Technical adaptations are often needed in pediatric patients. Regarding patient preparation, the same instructions are given to pediatric and adult patients. Patients are instructed to fast for 6 h and to refrain from strenuous exercise in the preceding 24 h. A high-protein meal the evening prior to the examination is also suggested.

Children are often fearful of needle insertion. Liberal use of topical anesthetics is encouraged and can be placed by the parents before the patient arrives at the PET facility. Pediatric patients are scheduled to arrive a minimum of 45 min prior to their expected injection time. This allows for any additional time that might be needed for the establishment of the IV site and for a delay to allow the patient to relax before the radiopharmaceutical is injected, and has virtually eliminated significant uptake in brown adipose tissue.

Conscious sedation and general anesthesia are administered when needed, usually for children 6 years of age and under. In the authors' institution, administration of all pediatric sedation as well as the use of anxiolytics is performed under the supervision of a pediatric anesthesiologist. Minimum requirements for conscious sedation would be continuous oxygen saturation monitoring and a monitored recovery period before the patient is discharged. The dose of $^{18}$F-FDG is weight-based at 5.18 MBq/kg (0.14 mCi/kg), with a minimal dose of 37 MBq (1 mCi) and maximum of 555 MBq (15 mCi). Uptake time is usually 60 min.

Since the protocol for the stand-alone multislice CT does not include oral bowel contrast, this is also not administered for the PET/CT examinations at the authors' institution. If administered, the protocol for oral contrast would be similar to that for the adult population, both for negative or positive agents. The IV contrast dose is also weight-based with 2 ml/kg, up to a maximum of 100 ml non-ionic contrast. The protocol aims for portal venous opacification. Contrast is injected with a power injector. A central venous line is not routinely used for the CT contrast injection, but an accessed central venous line is used for the administration of $^{18}$F-FDG. If a peripheral line is established for $^{18}$F-FDG and then IV contrast injection, the injection site should be remote from any anticipated disease localization. IV is administered over 50 s, and the acquisition of the images is initiated at the end of the contrast infusion.

PET and CT are both performed as craniocaudal acquisitions with the patient instructed to breathe normally. The arms are usually positioned above the head unless the child is not able to hold this position. Immobilization devices other than wraps are not generally used but may be useful to achieve less movement and better image co-registration. These immobilization devices may be beneficial in particular for transferring PET/CT data to therapy planning systems. Dual-time point studies are not routinely performed in the pediatric population, but examinations should be tailored as needed on an individual basis. The clinical report should be consistently integrated as recommended in the Society of Nuclear Medicine Procedure Guidelines for tumor imaging using $^{18}$F-FDG PET/CT.[28]

## SPECT/CT Procedure and Preparation of the Pediatric Patient

SPECT/CT with diagnostic CT can increase the specificity of the nuclear medicine procedure. This is already proved helpful when routine bone scintigraphy is compared to diagnostic CT to further localize foci of increased tracer uptake.[29] In addition, there is improved workflow efficiency if both the SPECT and CT are performed in one imaging setting. The diagnostic CT portion of SPECT/CT can also be tailored to include only the abnormal area seen on scintigraphy. Attenuation correction is not a routine problem in children and it is thus possible to limit the radiation exposure to the area of interest and thereby adhere to the As Low As Reasonably Achievable (ALARA) principle and other suggested programs in appropriately using ionizing radiation in children, and mainly as it pertains to the use of CT.[30,31]

As with PET/CT, the CT protocol parameters are the same as used for a stand-alone multislice CT. The same reconstruction algorithms for bone and soft tissue and multiplanar reformats are performed as for standard CT imaging for the area of the body or disease process to be evaluated. The use of non-ionic IV contrast for the CT portion of the SPECT/CT is performed along the same steps as discussed above for PET/CT with the usual timing of acquisition set for portal venous opacification. SPECT/CT is still not widely used in the pediatric population.

## Case Presentations

### *Case II.15.1 (DICOM Images on DVD)*

A 14-year-old male presented with a left parotid swelling and had been treated with antibiotics for what was a presumed inflammatory process without improvement. Biopsy of the left neck mass diagnosed lymphoblastic lymphoma. $^{18}$F-FDG PET/CT imaging and skeletal scintigraphy were performed for initial staging (Fig. II.15.1A–D).

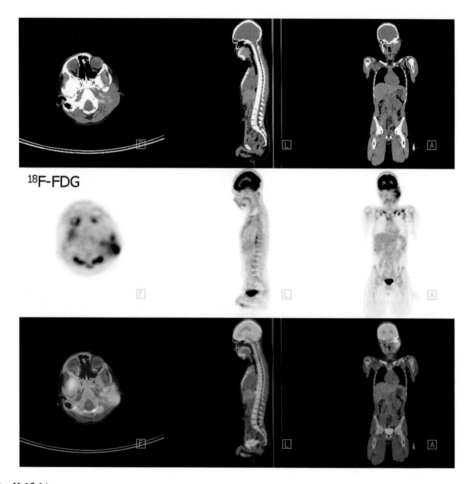

**Fig. II.15.1A**

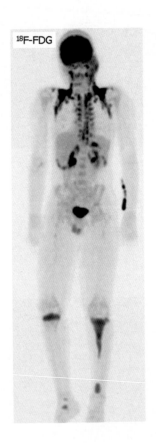

**Fig. II.15.1B**

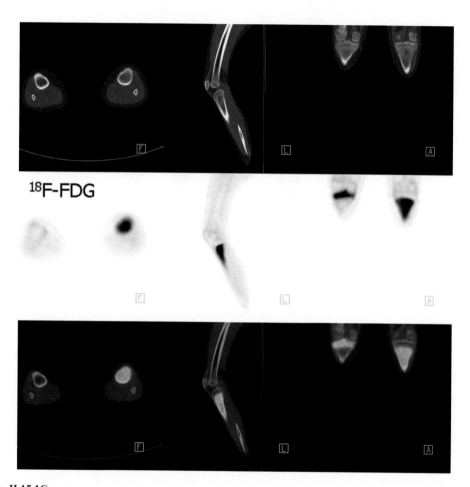

**Fig. II.15.1C**

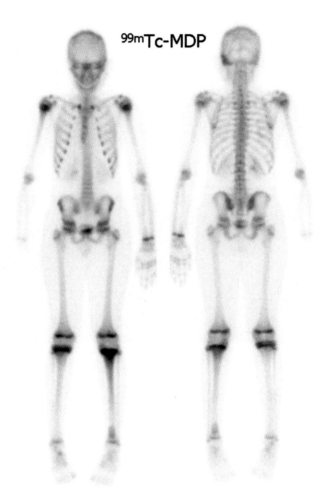

99mTc-MDP

**Fig. II.15.1D**

**Findings**

On the maximum intensity projection (MIP) image (Fig. II.15.1B) and PET/CT images
(Fig. II.15.1A), there is extensive abnormal [18]F-FDG uptake in the left side of the face and
neck corresponding to the 72 × 35 mm peritonsillar and pharyngeal mass. There is also
bilateral [18]F-FDG uptake corresponding to brown adipose tissue uptake above and below
the diaphragm. There is extensive abnormal [18]F-FDG uptake in both lower extremities,
involving the right proximal tibia and talus, the left tibia, and the left fibula (Fig. II.15.1B,
C). A bone marrow abnormality is seen on the corresponding CT in these skeletal areas
(Fig. II.15.1C). This boy had no focal complaints related to the lower extremities, and a
vague history of pain was only elicited when he was questioned about the findings. No
abnormality was seen in the abdomen or pelvis on the PET/CT images. Subsequent [99m]Tc-
MDP skeletal scintigraphy demonstrated the same pattern of skeletal lesions in the lower
extremities (Fig. II.15.1D).

## Discussion

Diagnosis of sites of lymphomatous involvement distal to the knees on the whole body [18]F-FDG PET/CT study upstaged this patient to stage IV disease. Lymphoma of the bone, whether primary or secondary, is seen in less than 10% of cases.[32–35] Many pediatric malignancies have a propensity for bone and soft-tissue involvement that is distal to the elbows and knees, an unusual occurrence in adult malignancy. In fact, tumors such as neuroblastoma, lymphoma, and leukemia may present with unexplained pain and sometimes rheumatological symptoms. The standard of care in pediatric patients is to perform whole body and not regional skeletal scintigraphy. With [18]F-FDG PET as well, it is essential to perform whole body imaging in pediatric patients.

The additional diagnostic information provided by the merged [18]F-FDG and CT imaging is particularly helpful when brown adipose tissue tracer uptake is present. While [18]F-FDG uptake in brown adipose tissue is more common in children than in adults, distribution of uptake is similar.[36–38]

## Diagnosis

B-cell lymphoblastic lymphoma, stage IV disease with left face and neck, and skeletal involvement in the lower extremities.

## Follow-up

Biopsy confirmed stage IV lymphoblastic lymphoma with skeletal involvement.

## Clinical Report: Whole Body [18]F-FDG PET/CT (for DVD cases only)

Indication

Left neck mass.

History

This 14-year-old male presented with a left parotid swelling and had been treated with antibiotics for what was a presumed inflammatory process without improvement. Biopsy of the left neck mass diagnosed lymphoblastic lymphoma. PET/CT imaging was performed for initial staging.

Procedure

Following a 6 h fast and informed consent, 240 MBq (6.5 mCi) of [18]F-FDG were administered IV in the left wrist, with some residual activity at the injection site. Prior to injection, the blood glucose level was 4.9 mmol/L. After 1 hour uptake time, low mAs non-contrast CT images for attenuation correction and co-registered PET emission images were acquired from head to toes. The images were reconstructed and displayed using a whole body format. The CT images were reviewed with soft tissue, lung, and bone window settings.

Findings

Quality of study: The image quality is good. The interpretation is difficult due to intense $^{18}$F-FDG uptake in brown adipose tissue in the neck, chest, and paraspinal regions.

Brain: within normal range

Head and neck: There is extensive abnormal increased $^{18}$F-FDG activity in the left side of the neck corresponding to a $72 \times 35$ cm peritonsillar and pharyngeal mass. There is bilateral $^{18}$F-FDG uptake corresponding to brown adipose tissue on CT, making it difficult to assess if the small lymph nodes in the right neck are $^{18}$F-FDG-avid or not.

Chest: Two subcentimeter lung nodules are seen on the CT component in the right middle lobe. Neither of them show $^{18}$F-FDG avidity, but they are beyond the limits of resolution of the PET study.

Abdomen: Two small splenic cysts are identified on the CT component with no $^{18}$F-FDG avidity.

Skeleton: There is extensive skeletal involvement in the left tibia from the proximal metaphyseal area to distally corresponding to abnormal marrow density on CT. There is also abnormal increased activity in the proximal left fibula. There is intense $^{18}$F-FDG activity in the right proximal tibial epiphysis and epiphyseal plate, corresponding to an abnormality seen on a recent skeletal scintigraphy. Being adjacent and within the epiphyseal area, it is difficult to precisely identify a definite skeletal abnormality on the corresponding CT. Two areas of abnormally increased $^{18}$F-FDG activity are seen in the anterior and posterior aspect of the right talus.


Impression

1. Abnormal $^{18}$F-FDG uptake in the left neck mass consistent with known lymphoma.
2. Questionable nodal involvement in the right cervical region, but the interpretation is complicated because of extensive uptake in brown adipose tissue.
3. Extensive skeletal involvement in the left tibia, to a lesser degree in the proximal left fibula, in the proximal right tibia and the right talus.
4. Two small pulmonary nodules seen on the CT scan below PET resolution.

## Case II.15.2

### History

This 8-year-old female presented with vague abdominal pain and subsequent hematemesis. Endoscopy revealed a pre-pyloric mass, but biopsy was inconclusive. Chest CT revealed small nodules in the lungs. The patient was referred to surgery. Partial gastrectomy was performed, and a 50 mm tumor was removed. Pathology indicated a gastrointestinal stromal tumor (GIST) with one margin not completely clear. A second nodular area was found at pathological assessment of the specimen. Because it was unclear whether the patient was disease-free after resection, $^{18}$F-FDG PET/CT was performed for restaging to assess the need for further treatment (Fig. II.15.2A–C).

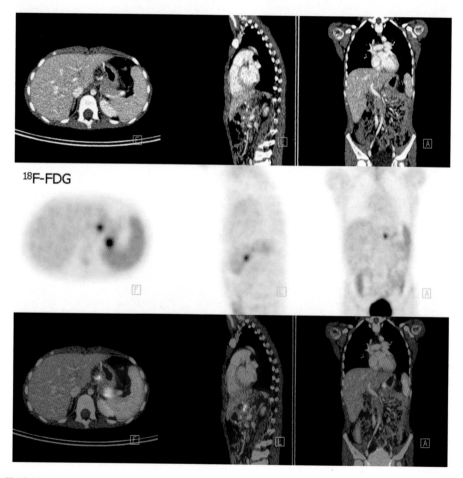

Fig. II.15.2A

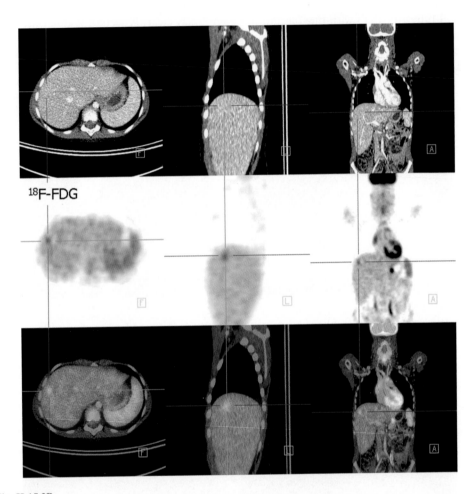

Fig. II.15.2B

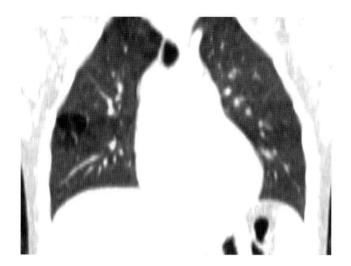

**Fig. II.15.2C**

## Findings

PET/CT performed at restaging (Fig. II.15.2A) showed two foci of abnormal [18]F-FDG activity in the left upper quadrant, located in the gastric stump, one close to the previous resection site and a second lesion along the remaining posterior gastric wall. There is also a small hepatic metastasis in addition to the gastric lesions (Fig. II.15.2B). Total gastrectomy was performed, and multiple tumor foci were found in the resected specimen. In addition, bullous changes in the right lung were demonstrated on the CT component of the study (Fig. II.15.2C). In the course of her disease, the patient has had spontaneous pneumothorax requiring chest tube insertion. No abnormal [18]F-FDG uptake was seen in the lungs. The patient was treated with Sunatinib in spite of not showing the characteristic C-kit gene mutation. On follow-up PET/CT studies, the patient showed slowly enlarging hepatic metastases but no other widespread disease.

## Discussion

Adults with GIST often have a typical mutation of the C-kit gene or the platelet-derived growth factor receptor alpha (PDGFR alpha), and this mutation makes them amenable to treatment with Imatinib or other drugs in this category. This mutation is less likely to be found in children and occurs in about 15% of pediatric patients with GIST. Thus, treatment with Imatinib-type drugs may not have the same response as in adults.[39] Children with GIST are also at risk for developing other tumors of the "Carney's triad," including paraganglioma, pulmonary chondroma, adrenocortical adenoma, and esophageal leiomyoma, at times associated with neurofibromatosis type 1 (NF1). Pediatric GIST affects girls more than boys. This patient had a similar course of disease as has been previously reported in a series of 15 children with pediatric GIST. Multifocal nodular lesions remained often undetected until evaluation of the resected specimen, and it was suggested that this may be the reason for the local recurrence in the gastric stump, which occurs more often in children than adults. This study also reported that even in the presence of a high rate of recurrence with hepatic and abdominal metastases, pediatric GIST has a more indolent course, independent of Imatinib therapy.[40]

**Diagnosis**

1. Multiple GIST tumors, metastatic to the liver.
2. Unconfirmed pulmonary chondromas.

## *Case II.15.3*

### History

This 16-year-old female had been treated 2 years prior to current examination with chemo- and radiation therapy followed by resection of an Ewing sarcoma of the L3 vertebral body. The patient underwent routine follow-up evaluation, and 2 years later a 4 mm pulmonary nodule was identified on CT. Prior to possible resection of this nodule, she underwent further studies for restaging including $^{99m}$Tc-MDP skeletal scintigraphy and $^{18}$F-FDG PET/CT imaging (Fig. II.15.3A–C).

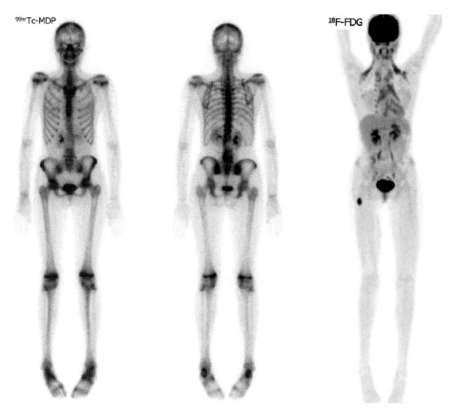

**Fig. II.15.3A**                                              **Fig.II.15.3B**

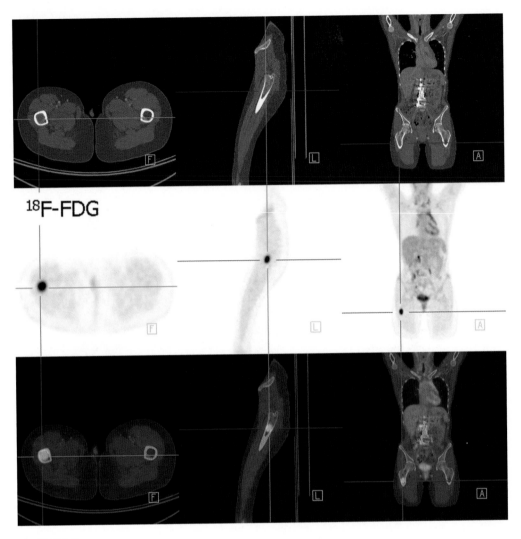

**Fig. II.15.3C**

## Findings

Planar $^{99m}$Tc-MDP skeletal scintigraphy shows an area of decreased uptake in the body of the L3 vertebra, with no other abnormalities (Fig. II.15.3A). $^{18}$F-FDG PET/CT demonstrates a focal area of abnormal tracer activity in the subtrochanteric region of the right proximal femur, localized to the bone marrow, with no associated soft-tissue mass (Fig. II.15.3B, C). The pulmonary lesion was not $^{18}$F-FDG avid and was not visualized on the non-breathhold CT component of the PET/CT study, maybe related to its small size.

## Discussion

At biopsy, the lesion in the proximal femur was confirmed to be metastatic Ewing sarcoma. A photopenic area was seen at site of the primary tumor following radiation therapy and resection. Following further chemotherapy and bone marrow transplantation, the pulmonary nodule remains stable and was not resected. The patient remains free of disease.

Many children present with metastatic Ewing sarcoma at diagnosis, and almost 50% of these patients will develop metastatic disease within 2 years of diagnosis. Metastatic disease at presentation has a poor prognosis. Skeletal metastases can develop prior to pulmonary lesions and are often silent, with no clinical symptoms.[41] Imaging efforts have been directed at identifying metastatic or recurrent disease as early as possible. [18]F-FDG imaging is helpful for response assessment and for monitoring progressive Ewing sarcoma.

Hawkins and colleagues[13] have shown that an SUV of less than 2.5 during follow-up indicated histologic response in approximately 70% of patients and was predictive of progression-free survival. Arush and colleagues[42] reported an accuracy of 77% for [18]F-FDG PET/CT in detecting metastatic Ewing sarcoma. Similar to this case, PET/CT was the only modality to detect distant disease in two patients. In one of the first articles on the use of [18]F-FDG imaging in a pediatric population, Shulkin and coworkers[43] report a patient in whom PET identified two lesions that were negative on [99m]Tc-MDP skeletal scintigraphy.

The timing of [18]F-FDG PET/CT studies in children with skeletal sarcoma is not yet standardized. Recommendations of the cooperative pediatric tumor groups, such as the Children's Oncology Group (COG), suggest the use of [18]F-FDG PET/CT at diagnosis, prior to definitive surgery, and at the end of therapy. Restaging should be directed by symptoms or findings on other imaging studies.[44]

**Diagnosis**

Ewing sarcoma with solitary skeletal metastasis.

## Case II.15.4

### History

This 9-year-old male was diagnosed with osteosarcoma of the left femur and pulmonary metastases and was treated with chemotherapy and rotationplasty. Follow-up $^{18}$F-FDG PET/CT imaging was performed 6 months after completion of chemotherapy. The patient had no complaints until 18 months after treatment when he presented with a 2-week history of lethargy, anorexia, night fevers, and fluctuating skeletal pain. Blood tests, including blood cell counts, were normal. He was treated symptomatically for a viral infection with some improvement, but persistent low-grade fever and skeletal pain remained. A $^{99m}$Tc-MDP skeletal scintigraphy was performed followed by $^{18}$F-FDG PET/CT imaging because of ongoing symptoms and the equivocal results of the bone scintigraphy (Fig. II.15.4A–D).

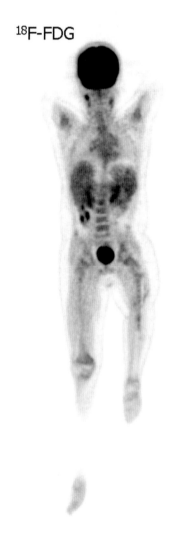

$^{18}$F-FDG

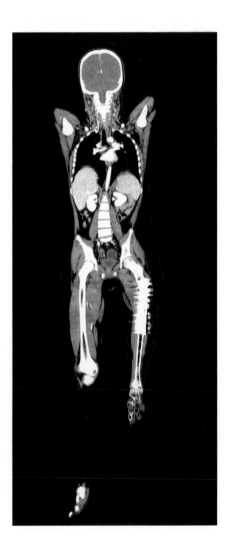

**Fig. II.15.4A**

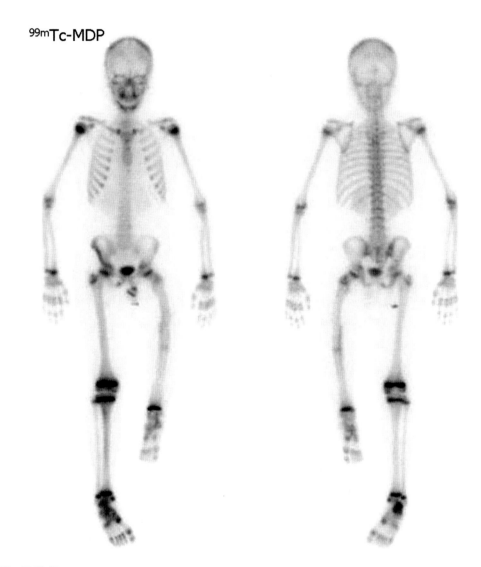

$^{99m}$Tc-MDP

**Fig. II.15.4B**

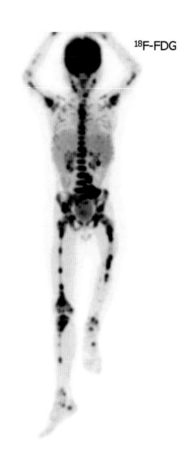

¹⁸F-FDG

**Fig. II.15.4C**

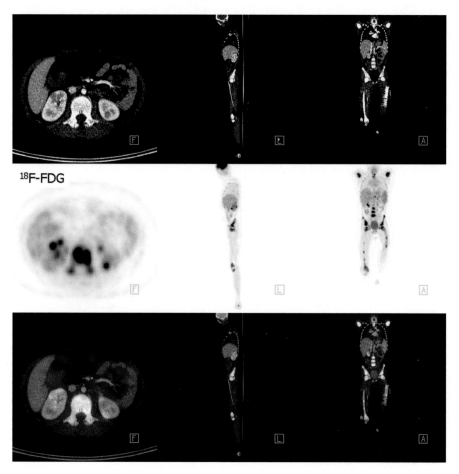

**Fig. II.15.4D**

### Findings

The first PET/CT examination showed some low-grade $^{18}$F-FDG uptake at the rotation-plasty anastamotic site but no evidence of metastatic disease (Fig. II.15.4A). The $^{99m}$Tc-MDP skeletal scintigraphy performed at the time of recurrent symptoms showed moderately increased tracer activity related to the rotationplasty, with no other focal abnormality (Fig. II.15.4B). The follow-up $^{18}$F-FDG PET/CT showed multiple foci of abnormal $^{18}$F-FDG uptake throughout the axial and appendicular skeleton. In addition, focal soft tissue $^{18}$F-FDG-avid masses were seen in the periphery of both kidneys and within bowel loops in the right lower quadrant (Fig. II.15.4C, D).

Bone marrow aspiration showed pre-B acute lymphocytic leukemia (ALL). No osteosarcoma metastases were detected. The patient was restarted on chemotherapy, suffered an early on-treatment relapse, and was referred for bone marrow transplantation.

### Discussion

This patient had a high risk, greater than 10%, of developing a second malignancy due to a 20% residual tumor after resection of the osteosarcoma and because of pulmonary metastatic disease at diagnosis. More second malignancies and more long-term sequelae of treatment for childhood cancer are being encountered in recent years due to the overall improvement in childhood survival. Therefore, major efforts in childhood cancer care are currently directed toward reducing potential long-term sequelae while maintaining the same survival statistics.

**Diagnosis**

1. ALL with skeletal, renal, and gastrointestinal tract (GIT) involvement.
2. Post-surgical changes related to previous rotationplasty for osteogenic sarcoma.

## Case II.15.5 (DICOM Images on DVD)

### History

This 4-year-old male presented with a calcified left adrenal mass and skeletal lesions consistent with stage IV neuroblastoma. [123]I-MIBG SPECT/CT was performed at presentation (Fig. II.15.5A, B). Subsequently, the patient was treated with chemotherapy, underwent resection of primary tumor in the left upper quadrant followed by autologous bone marrow transplantation and was referred for [123]I-MIBG SPECT/CT reevaluation (Fig. II.15.5C, D).

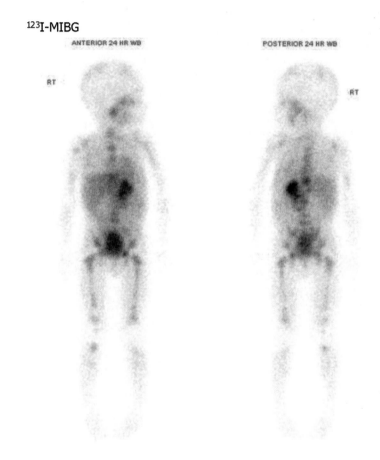

**Fig. II.15.5A**

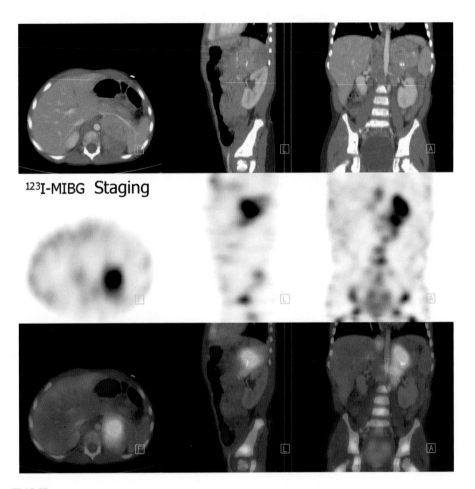

**Fig. II.15.5B**

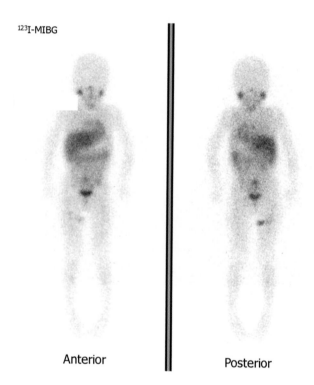

¹²³I-MIBG

Anterior                    Posterior

**Fig. II.15.5C**

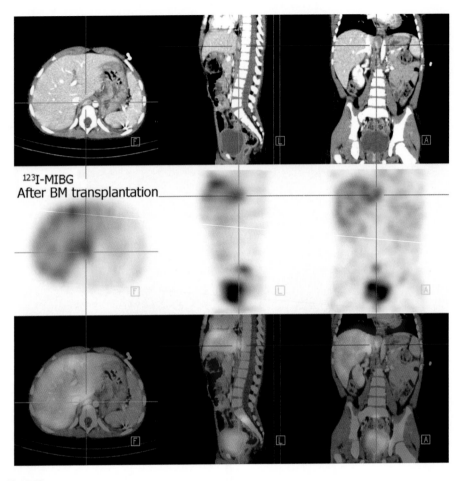

**Fig. II.15.5D**

### Findings

[123]I-MIBG SPECT/CT at presentation confirmed the presence of left upper abdominal and right retrocrural disease, and diffuse skeletal involvement (Fig. II.15.5A, B). After therapy, [123]I-MIBG SPECT/CT imaging showed persistence of right retrocrural disease and in the mid-sacrum, but the absence of disease at the primary site in the left upper quadrant (Fig. II.15.5C, D).

### Discussion

In this case, the right upper quadrant activity seen post-therapy on [123]I-MIBG SPECT alone could be mistaken for physiologic [123]I uptake that can be seen in up to 50% of cases. The addition of the CT component localizes this right upper quadrant activity to the retrocrural lesion consistent with residual disease.

**Diagnosis**

1. Stage IV neuroblastoma with residual retrocrural disease and skeletal metastasis in the sacrum after treatment.
2. Post-surgical changes in the left upper quadrant.

**Follow-up**

Biopsy confirmed stage IV neuroblastoma with residual retrocrural disease on follow-up examination after resection of the left upper quadrant tumor.

**Clinical Report: $^{123}$I-MIBG SPECT/CT (for DVD cases only)**

Indication

Calcified abdominal mass in a 4 year-old child.

History

This 4-year-old male presented with left upper quadrant mass and skeletal lesions diagnosed as stage IV neuroblastoma and was referred at initial presentation.

Procedure

The patient was premedicated with 170 mg of potassium perchlorate prior to the IV injection of 225 MBq (6 mCi) $^{123}$I-MIBG through the central line. Total body scintigraphy was obtained at 24 and 48 h including SPECT of the abdomen and pelvis. In addition, at 24 h post-injection of $^{123}$I-MIBG, contrast-enhanced CT of the abdomen and pelvis was obtained following the IV injection of 32 ml of Omnipaque 300. SPECT/CT of the abdominopelvic region was performed under sedation support provided by anesthesiology.

Findings

*Quality of study*:The quality of the study is good. A left-sided central line is in place.
*Chest*: The entire lungs have not been included in the SPECT/CT study. There is an enlarged 17 mm in diameter right retrocrural lymph node showing moderate $^{123}$I-MIBG uptake.
On the CT component there is atelectasis at the base of both lungs. No pulmonary nodules are seen at the base of the lungs.
*Abdomen*: There is intense abnormal $^{123}$I-MIBG uptake in a left upper quadrant abdominal mass. The main bulk of the $^{123}$I-MIBG-avid mass extends up to the midline. Its boundaries are the celiac axis medially, splenic vessels anteriorly, and the spleen laterally. It extends posteriorly to but does not involve the ribs.
On the CT component, there is a moderately enlarged right para-aortic lymph node at the mid-level of the mass, with no $^{123}$I-MIBG uptake. The left adrenal is not visualized. The right adrenal is of normal appearance. The pancreas is not involved by the mass. The celiac axis and other vessels are not compressed by the mass. The liver and spleen are normal. There is no ascites. There is mild left hydronephrosis, and the kidney is compressed by the mass and displaced slightly laterally and posteriorly. The

right kidney appears normal with no hydronephrosis. The kidneys are not involved by the mass.

*Skeleton*: There is diffuse abnormal skeletal [123]I-MIBG uptake corresponding to patchy sclerotic changes on CT at multiple levels in the pelvis and spine diffusely.

Impression

1. [123]I-MIBG-avid left upper quadrant heterogeneous mass with calcification arising from the left adrenal gland.
2. [123]I-MIBG-avid right retrocrural adenopathy.
3. Right para-aortic lymphadenopathy that is not [123]I-MIBG-avid.
4. Diffuse [123]I-MIBG avid skeletal disease.

## Case II.15.6

### History

A 4-year-male with neurodevelopmental delay presented with swelling of the right foot but with no fever and negative radiographs. Three phase skeletal scintigraphy including SPECT/CT of the feet and repeat radiography of the calcaneus were performed in search of focal skeletal abnormalities (Fig. II.15.6A–E).

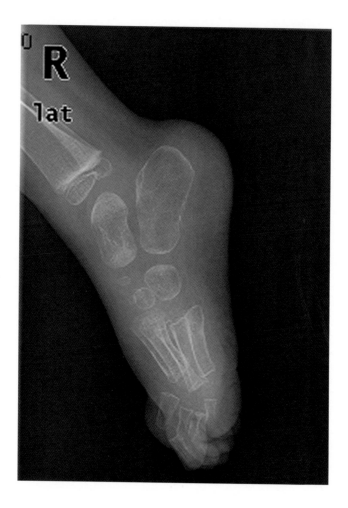

**Fig. II.15.6A**

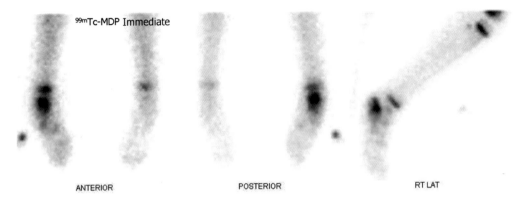

ANTERIOR POSTERIOR RT LAT

Fig. II.15.6B

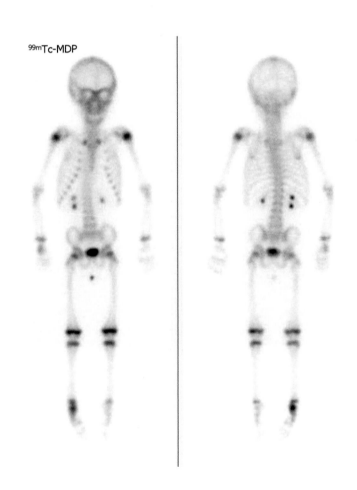

Fig. II.15.6C

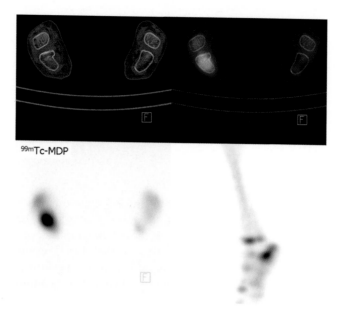

**Fig. II.15.6D**

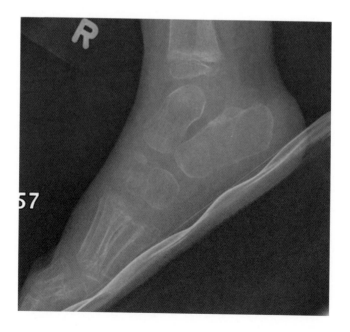

**Fig. II.15.6E**

**Findings**

Initial radiographic examination of the foot was normal (Fig. II.15.6A). Three-phase skeletal scintigraphy following the injection of $^{99m}$Tc-MDP demonstrates hyperemia on blood pool images (Fig. II.15.6B) and delayed increased activity in the right heel (Fig. II.15.6C). Because radiographs were initially normal, a SPECT/CT was then performed and showed a focal buckle fracture corresponding to the area of increased tracer activity (Fig. II.15.6D). Subsequent repeat radiograph also confirmed the buckle fracture of the right calcaneus (Fig. II.15.6E).

**Discussion**

Skeletal scintigraphy can be a very sensitive screening examination to localize a specific site of pain but with rather low specificity. Results of skeletal scintigraphy should be correlated with conventional radiographs when possible. If these radiographs do not demonstrate an abnormality, a limited CT done at the same time as the SPECT examination improves diagnostic accuracy. At the authors' institution, SPECT/CT is performed in a majority of skeletal scintigraphy involving extremities and in all cases with symptoms suggestive of disease involving the axial skeleton.

As with PET/CT imaging, all pediatric patients undergoing skeletal scintigraphy should have some form of whole body imaging. Regional skeletal scintigraphy is not routinely performed in children. However, unlike PET/CT, a complete correlative SPECT/CT acquisition is not necessary, and the CT component should be limited to a field of view as small as necessary to define the scintigraphic abnormality or to further evaluate regional clinical complaints. The SPECT/CT report should include assessment of both parts of the examination in an integrated report.

**Diagnosis**

Occult calcaneal stress fracture.

# References

1. Jadvar H, Connolly LP, Fahey FH, Shulkin BL. PET and PET/CT in pediatric oncology. *Semin Nucl Med* 2007;37:316–331.
2. Kushner BH. Neuroblastoma: A disease requiring a multitude of imaging studies. *J Nucl Med* 2004;45:1172–1188.
3. Hiorns MP, Owens CM. Radiology of neuroblastoma in children. *Eur Radiol* 2001;11:2071–2081.
4. Lonergan GJ, Schwab CM, Suarez ES, Carlson CL. Neuroblastoma, ganglioneuroblastoma, and ganglioneuroma: Radiologic-pathologic correlation. *Radiographics* 2002;22:911–934.
5. Boubaker A, Bischof Delaloye A. Nuclear medicine procedures and neuroblastoma in childhood. Their value in the diagnosis, staging and assessment of response to therapy. *Q J Nucl Med* 2003;47:31–40.
6. Papaioannou G, McHugh K. Neuroblastoma in childhood: Review and radiological findings. *Cancer Imaging* 2005;5:116–127.
7. Ilias I, Pacak K. Diagnosis and management of tumors of the adrenal medulla. *Horm Metab Res* 2005;37:717–721.
8. McCarville MB, Christie R, Daw NC, Spunt SL, Kaste SC. PET/CT in the evaluation of childhood sarcomas. *AJR Am J Roentgenol* 2005;184:1293–1304.
9. Tateishi U, Yamaguchi U, Seki K, Terauchi T, Arai Y, Kim EE. Bone and soft-tissue sarcoma: preoperative staging with fluorine 18 fluorodeoxyglucose PET/CT and conventional imaging. *Radiology* 2007;245:839–847.
10. Volker T, Denecke T, Steffen I, Misch D, Schönberger S, Plotkin M, Ruf Y, Furth C, Stöver B, Hautzel H, Henze G, Amthauer H. Positron emission tomography for staging of pediatric sarcoma patients: Results of a prospective multicenter trial. *J Clin Oncol* 2007;25:5435–5441.
11. Bredella MA, Caputo GR, Steinbach LS. Value of FDG positron emission tomography in conjunction with MR imaging for evaluating therapy response in patients with musculoskeletal sarcomas. *AJR Am J Roentgenol* 2002;179:1145–1150.
12. Hawkins DS, Rajendran JG, Conrad EU 3rd, Bruckner JD, Eary JF. Evaluation of chemotherapy response in pediatric bone sarcomas by [F-18]-fluorodeoxy-D-glucose positron emission tomography. *Cancer* 2002;94:3277–3284.
13. Hawkins DS, Schuetze SM, Butrynski JE, Rajendran JG, Vernon CB, Conrad III EU, Eary JF. [18F]Fluorodeoxyglucose positron emission tomography predicts outcome for Ewing sarcoma family of tumors. *J Clin Oncol* 2005;23:8828–8834.
14. Iagaru A, Masamed R, Chawla SP, Menendez LR, Fedenko A, Conti PS. F-18 FDG PET and PET/CT evaluation of response to chemotherapy in bone and soft tissue sarcomas. *Clin Nucl Med* 2008;33:8–13.
15. Schuetze SM, Rubin BP, Vernon C, Hawkins DS, Bruckner JD, Conrad III EU, Eary JF. Use of positron emission tomography in localized extremity soft tissue sarcoma treated with neoadjuvant chemotherapy. *Cancer* 2005;103:339–348.
16. Franzius C, Juergens KU, Vormoor J. PET/CT with diagnostic CT in the evaluation of childhood sarcoma. *AJR Am J Roentgenol* 2006;186:581; author reply 581–582.
17. Iagaru A, Chawla S, Menendez L, Conti PS. 18F-FDG PET and PET/CT for detection of pulmonary metastases from musculoskeletal sarcomas. *Nucl Med Commun* 2006;27:795–802.
18. Mody RJ, Bui C, Hutchinson RJ, Frey KA, Shulkin BL. Comparison of (18)F Flurodeoxyglucose PET with Ga-67 scintigraphy and conventional imaging modalities in pediatric lymphoma. *Leuk Lymphoma* 2007;48:699–707.
19. Miller E, Metser U, Avrahami G, Dvir R, Valdman D, Sira LB, Sayar D, Burstein Y, Toren A, Yaniv I, Even-Sapir E. Role of 18F-FDG PET/CT in staging and follow-up of lymphoma in pediatric and young adult patients. *J Comput Assist Tomogr* 2006;30:689–694.
20. Juweid ME. 18F-FDG PET as a routine test for posttherapy assessment of Hodgkin's disease and aggressive non-Hodgkin's lymphoma: Where is the evidence? *J Nucl Med* 2008;49:9–12.
21. Juweid ME, Stroobants S, Hoekstra OS, Mottaghy FM, Dietlein M, Guermazi A, Wiseman GA, Kostakoglu L, Scheidhauer K, Buck A, Naumann R, Spaepen K, Hicks RJ, Weber WA, Reske SN, Schwaiger M, Schwartz LH, Zijlstra JM, Siegel BA, Cheson BD. Use of positron emission tomography for response assessment of lymphoma: consensus of the Imaging Subcommittee of International Harmonization Project in Lymphoma. *J Clin Oncol* 2007;25:571–578.
22. Hines-Thomas M, Kaste SC, Hudson MM, Howard SC, Liu WA, Wu J, Kun LE, Shulkin BL, Krasin MJ, Metzger ML. Comparison of gallium and PET scans at diagnosis and follow-up of pediatric patients with Hodgkin lymphoma. *Pediatr Blood Cancer* 2008;51:198–203.

23. Meany HJ, Gidvani VK, Minniti CP. Utility of PET scans to predict disease relapse in pediatric patients with Hodgkin lymphoma. *Pediatr Blood Cancer* 2007;48:399–402.

24. Rhodes MM, Delbeke D, Whitlock JA, Martin W, Kuttesch JF, Frangoul HA, Shankar S. Utility of FDG-PET/CT in follow-up of children treated for Hodgkin and non-Hodgkin lymphoma. *J Pediatr Hematol Oncol* 2006;28:300–306.

25. Shankar A, Fiumara F, Pinkerton R. Role of FDG PET in the management of childhood lymphomas – case proven or is the jury still out? *Eur J Cancer* 2008;44:663–673.

26. Nadel HR, Shulkin BL. Pediatric positron emission tomography-computed tomography protocol considerations. *Semin Ultrasound CT MR* 2008;29:271–276.

27. Almusa OR, Daly B, Shreve P. Protocol considerations for positron emission tomography. *Semin Ultrasound CT MR* 2008;29:251–262.

28. Delbeke D, Coleman RE, Guiberteau MJ, Brown ML, Royal HD, Siegel BA, Townsend DW, Berland LL Parker JA, Hubner K, Stabin MG, Zubal J, Kachelriess M, Cronin V, Holbrook S. Procedure guideline for tumor imaging with 18F-FDG PET/CT 1.0. *J Nucl Med* 2006;47:885–895.

29. Nadel HR. Bone scan update. *Semin Nucl Med.* 2007;37:332–339.

30. Brenner DJ, Hall EJ. Computed tomography-an increasing source of radiation exposure. *N Engl J Med* 2007;357:2277–2284.

31. Goske MJ, Applegate KE, Boylan J, Butler PF, Callahan MJ, Coley BD, Farley S, Frush DP, Hernanz-Schulman M, Jaramillo D, Johnson ND, Kaste SC, Morrison G, Strauss KJ, Tuggle N. The 'Image Gently' campaign: increasing CT radiation dose awareness through a national education and awareness program. *Pediatr Radiol* 2008;38:265–269.

32. Rademaker J. Hodgkin's and non-Hodgkin's lymphomas. *Radiol Clin North Am* 2007;45:69–83.

33. Karadeniz C, Oguz A, Citak EC, Uluoglu O, Okur V, Demirci S, Okur A, Aksakal N. Clinical characteristics and treatment results of pediatric B-cell Non-Hodgkin lymphona patients in a single center. *Pediatr Hematol Oncol* 2007;24:417–430.

34. Haddy TB, Keenan AM, Jaffe ES, Magrath IT. Bone involvement in young patients with non-Hodgkin's lymphoma: Efficacy of chemotherapy without local radiotherapy. *Blood* 1988;72:1141–1147.

35. Durr HR, Muller PE, Hiller E, Maier M, Baur A, Jansson V, Refior H. Malignant lymphoma of bone. *Arch Orthop Trauma Surg* 2002;122:10–16.

36. Wehrli NE, Bural G, Houseni M, Alkhawaldeh K, Alavi A, Torigian DA. Determination of age-related changes in structure and function of skin, adipose tissue, and skeletal muscle with computed tomography, magnetic resonance imaging, and positron emission tomography. *Semin Nucl Med* 2007;37:195–205.

37. Yeung HW, Grewal RK, Gonen M, Schoder H, Larson SM. Patterns of (18)F-FDG uptake in adipose tissue and muscle: a potential source of false-positives for PET. *J Nucl Med* 2003;44:1789–1796.

38. Cohade C, Osman M, Pannu HK, Wahl RL. Uptake in supraclavicular area fat ("USA-Fat"): description on 18F-FDG PET/CT. *J Nucl Med* 2003;44:170–176.

39. Janeway KA, Liegl B, Harlow A, Le C, Perez-Atayde A, Kozakewich H, Corless CL, Heinrich MC, Fletcher JA. Pediatric KIT wild-type and platelet-derived growth factor receptor alpha-wild-type gastrointestinal stromal tumors share KIT activation but not mechanisms of genetic progression with adult gastrointestinal stromal tumors. *Cancer Res* 2007;67:9084–9088.

40. Prakash S, Sarran L, Socci N, DeMatteo RP, Eisenstat J, Greco AM, Maki RG, Wexler LH, LaQuaglia MP, Besmer P, Antonescu CR. Gastrointestinal stromal tumors in children and young adults: A clinicopathologic, molecular, and genomic study of 15 cases and review of the literature. *J Pediatr Hematol Oncol* 2005;27:179–187.

41. Nadel HR. Nuclear oncology in children. In Freeman LM (ed): *Nuclear medicine annual*. New York: Raven Press, 1996:143–193.

42. Arush MW, Israel O, Postovsky S, Militianu D, Meller I, Zaidman I, Even Sapir A, Bar-Shalom R. Positron emission tomography/computed tomography with 18fluoro-deoxyglucose in the detection of local recurrence and distant metastases of pediatric sarcoma. *Pediatr Blood Cancer* 2007;49:901–905.

43. Shulkin BL, Mitchell DS, Ungar DR, Prakash D, Dole MG, Castle VP, Hernandez RJ, Koeppe RA, Hutchinson RJ. Neoplasms in a pediatric population: 2-[F-18]-fluoro-2-deoxy-D-glucose PET studies. *Radiology* 1995;194:495–500.

44. Meyer S, Nadel HR, Marina N, Womer RB, Brown KL, Eary JF, Gorlick R, Grier HE, Randall RL, Lawlor ER, Lessnick SL, Schomberg PJ, Kailo MD. Imaging guidelines for children with Ewing Sarcoma and Osteosarcoma: A report from the Children's Oncology Group Bone Tumor Committee. *Pediatr Blood Cancer* 2008;51:163–170.

# Part III
# Other Clinical Applications

# Chapter III.1
# Cardiac Hybrid Imaging (PET/CT and SPECT/CT): Assessment of CAD

Gabriel Vorobiof, Zohar Keidar, Sharmila Dorbala, and Marcelo F. Di Carli

## Introduction

The field of nuclear cardiology is witnessing a rapid growth in the installed base of hybrid single-photon emission computed tomography (SPECT)/computed tomography (CT) and positron emission tomography (PET)/CT scanners. Although the CT component in the original hybrid SPECT/CT scanners was conceived only as a tool for performing attenuation correction (AC), this is now rapidly evolving into a multi-detector CT configuration that allows acquisition of diagnostic anatomic information including coronary calcium scoring (CCS) and coronary CT angiography (CCTA). A similar evolution has occurred with PET/CT devices. Original scanners were designed only for oncologic imaging and fitted with single- or two-slice CT scanners.[1] However at present 16-slice and higher CT configuration is common across all manufacturers. The objective of this chapter is to provide the reader with a case-based teaching file that will illustrate the potential applications, strengths, and limitations of hybrid cardiac imaging with SPECT/CT and PET/CT. The discussion will be focused on the use of hybrid imaging for evaluation of patients with known or suspected coronary artery disease (CAD).

## Imaging Protocols for Hybrid Cardiac Imaging

While the basic principles for cardiac imaging protocols are similar, there are marked workflow differences between hybrid SPECT/CT and PET/CT that largely relate to the type of radiopharmaceuticals that are used as well as fundamental differences in the acquisition of images. The following sections will describe the most common clinical protocols.

### CT Imaging for Hybrid Cardiac SPECT/CT and PET/CT

#### Attenuation Correction

The most basic use of CT in hybrid scanners is to position the heart in the field of view (topogram or scout) and to acquire a transmission scan to create an attenuation map for subsequent AC. The transmission scan consists of a low-dose CT scan covering the region

G. Vorobiof (✉)

Department of Cardiovascular Imaging, Yale University, New Haven, CT, USA

e-mail: gabriel.vorobiof@yale.edu

D. Delbeke, O. Israel (eds.), *Hybrid PET/CT and SPECT/CT Imaging*,
DOI 10.1007/978-0-387-92820-3_18, © Springer Science+Business Media, LLC 2010

of the heart. It provides a high-quality attenuation map by scaling the Hounsfield Units (HU) to the photon energy of the radiotracer.[2] The map of attenuation coefficients is further smoothed to match the resolution of the perfusion image. During iterative reconstruction of the acquired projections, the a priori CT information can be incorporated to provide an attenuation-corrected perfusion image. Alternatively, for filtered backprojection reconstructions, AC methods such as the modified Chang algorithm may be used.[3] It is important to understand that acquisition parameters for CT-based transmission imaging vary with the configuration of the CT scanner and clinical protocol. However, the general settings utilized in most clinics for CT transmission imaging, independent of the manufacturer, include

(1) slow gantry rotation speed (e.g., 1 s/revolution) combined with a relatively high pitch (e.g., 0.5–0.6:1);
(2) a non-gated scan;
(3) a high tube potential (e.g., 140 kVp) and a low tube current (~10–20 mA);
(4) CT acquisition obtained during tidal expiration breath-hold or shallow breathing.

It is generally accepted that the rest and stress perfusion images should each be corrected with its own dedicated transmission scan due to known changes in cardiac and pulmonary volumes during pharmacologic stress especially with vasodilators.

The AC of cardiac SPECT images is not universally applied and remains an open question, related in part to a relative paucity of peer-reviewed studies proving its clinical value. When properly applied, AC of cardiac SPECT improves the diagnostic accuracy, increases the reporting physician's confidence, reduces inter- and intra observer variability, and improves sensitivity in diagnosis of multi-vessel disease, being also associated with a better cost-to-benefit ratio.[4] AC is mandatory for PET imaging. AC obtained from an external radioactive source ($^{68}$Ge, $^{137}$Ce) and with an X-ray source from CT have yielded similar diagnostic accuracies.[5]

## Diagnostic CT

One advantage of hybrid scanners is their ability to collect diagnostic cardiac CT data; namely CCS and CCTA.[6] The minimum CT configuration for CCS is 6 slices (500 ms gantry rotation) and 16 slices for CCTA. Most vendors are currently offering 64-slice devices. Protocols for gated CT with or without contrast are vendor specific. There are a few important considerations when planning hybrid studies, especially for combining myocardial perfusion scintigraphy (MPS) and CCTA in the same setting. Because of the fact that beta blockers used for heart rate control before the CCTA study may interfere with the maximal response to stress (i.e., exercise, vasodilators, and dobutamine), the workflow requires careful planning. Most centers conducting hybrid studies perform the CCTA after the stress MPS.

The radiation dose to the patient from a hybrid study can be quite high. Careful consideration should be therefore given to the indication for the study as well as the clinical utility of the integrated dataset. The radiation dose can be reduced by one of the following steps:

(1) PET perfusion imaging using $^{13}$N-ammonia;
(2) rest–stress $^{99m}$Tc protocols that deliver lower doses than dual isotope (rest $^{201}$Thallium, stress $^{99m}$Tc) studies; and
(3) acquiring the CCTA study using electrocardiogram (ECG) dose modulation whenever possible.

Newer technology such as the step-and-shoot acquisition mode for CT will enable to significantly reduce radiation dose to approximately 2–3 mSv.[7]

## Cardiac SPECT/CT

MPS with SPECT is performed using $^{99m}$Tc-labeled flow tracers, which can be used in single or two-day protocols depending on the patient characteristics and laboratory logistics, or $^{201}$Thallium chloride.[8] Myocardial viability can be assessed with immediate and delayed $^{201}$Thallium studies.[8] Stress SPECT studies are performed following physical exercise or pharmacologic means (e.g., adenosine, dipyridamole, adenosine$_{2a}$ agonists, or dobutamine). Typically, in a same day, single isotope protocol, rest MPS is performed 60–90 min after injection of 370 MBq (10 mCi) $^{99m}$Tc-labeled Sestamibi or Tetrofosmin. Stress electrocardiography-gated MPS is performed using 1110 MBq (30 mCi) of the same radiotracer injected at peak ergometric or pharmacologic stress. Both the rest and stress SPECT studies are followed by a low-dose CT scan for AC. Fusion of the segmented coronary artery tree obtained from CCTA data combined with 3D myocardial perfusion images obtained from SPECT is consecutively generated using a software package.

## Cardiac PET/CT

Myocardial perfusion PET is currently performed with either $^{82}$Rubidium or $^{13}$N-ammonia as perfusion agents, while myocardial viability imaging uses $^{18}$F-Fluoro-2-deoxyglucose ($^{18}$F-FDG) as a tracer of metabolism.

### Emission Imaging

Different acquisition modes can be used: ECG-gated, static (single-frame), dynamic (or multi-frame), and list mode. The *ECG-gated acquisition mode* is the most common clinical approach. Imaging begins 90–120 s after $^{82}$Rubidium, or 3–5 min after $^{13}$N-ammonia injection, to allow for clearance of radioactivity from the lungs and blood pool. The scan duration is approximately 5 or 20 min, respectively, for $^{82}$Rubidium or $^{13}$N-ammonia.[6] Both the rest and stress images are gated. This allows for assessment of left ventricular ejection fraction and volumes, and offers the additional advantage of quantifying peak-stress gating for the evaluation of ischemic wall motion abnormalities or global stunning.

The *static (or single frame) acquisition mode* is identical to the ECG-gated mode except that the data are collected without an ECG trigger and is used only for patients with arrhythmias where cardiac gating cannot be confidently achieved. In the *dynamic (or multi-frame) acquisition mode*, imaging begins with the bolus administration of the radiotracer and the data are collected in pre-determined frames of variable length throughout the acquisition. The advantage of this approach is the ability to quantify myocardial blood flow (in ml/min/g). Its main disadvantage is the need to perform a separate radionuclide injection to obtain ECG-gated images from which to assess cardiac function, especially when using $^{82}$Rubidium.

With the availability of faster and more powerful computers, *list mode* has become the ideal mode of data acquisition because it allows multiple image reconstructions (i.e., summed, ECG-gated, and multi-frame or dynamic) for a comprehensive physiologic examination of the heart. This approach, however, generates large data sets that can be taxing on computer memory and reconstruction time. Image acquisition can be performed either by 2D or 3D methods. 2D methods involve leaving the lead septa between the PET camera detectors in place, which results in a lower number of overall counts but less random and scattered counts. Many of the current PET scanners allow only 3D imaging, thereby requiring careful optimization of radiotracer dose and acquisition mode.

As with SPECT, stress testing for myocardial perfusion PET imaging can be performed most common with pharmacologic means (e.g., adenosine, dipyridamole, selective adenosine$_{2a}$ agonists, or dobutamine) or with exercise.[9] The latter is easier with $^{13}$N-ammonia because of its physical half-life of $\sim$10 min than with $^{82}$Rubidium, which has a physical half-life of 76 s.

## Quality Control of Cardiac Hybrid Imaging

Performing good quality cardiac PET/CT or SPECT/CT imaging is technically demanding, and, thus, familiarity with key quality control steps is crucial to optimize clinical results. Quality control includes routine inspection of the transmission and emission data and the transmission–emission alignment. The emission data need to be carefully evaluated for the adequacy of count density. Physicians should be familiar with the recognition of reconstruction artifacts and identification of patient motion. One of the most common sources of artifacts in hybrid cardiac imaging is the misalignment between the transmission and emission images caused by patient motion or respiratory mismatch between nuclear and CT data.[10] Cases III.1.1 and III.1.2 illustrate this common problem. A more detailed description of routine maintenance, calibration, and quality control of hybrid scanners is provided in Chapter 1.

## Clinical Applications of Cardiac Hybrid Imaging

### Diagnosis of CAD Using Cardiac Hybrid Imaging

The diagnostic performance of myocardial perfusion SPECT and PET as well as CCTA has been extensively documented. For SPECT, the average sensitivity for detecting >50% angiographic stenosis is 87%, whereas the average specificity is 73%.[11] Of note, most of the published data come from series without attenuation correction. With the use of attenuation correction methods (not necessarily CT based), the specificity improves especially among patients undergoing exercise stress testing.[11]

For PET, the average weighted sensitivity for detecting at least one coronary artery with >50% stenosis is 90%, whereas the average specificity is 89%. The corresponding average positive (PPV) and negative predictive values (NPV) are 94 and 73%, respectively, and the overall diagnostic accuracy is 90%.[12]

For CCTA, the average weighted sensitivity for detecting at least one coronary artery with >50% stenosis is 94%, whereas the average specificity is 77%. The corresponding average PPV and NPV are 84 and 87%, respectively, and the overall diagnostic accuracy is 89%.[12]

On the other hand, there is growing and consistent evidence documenting the potential added value of the hybrid imaging approach. Recent data from multiple laboratories using either sequential (CCTA followed by SPECT)[13–16] or hybrid imaging (SPECT/CT or PET/CT)[17–20] suggest that the PPV of CCTA for identifying coronary stenoses producing objective evidence of stress-induced ischemia is suboptimal (Chart III.1.1). Hybrid imaging provides a simple and accurate integrated measure of the effect of anatomic stenoses on coronary resistance and tissue perfusion, thereby optimizing selection of patients who may ultimately benefit from revascularization. Cases III.1.3 and III.1.4 illustrate the complementary value of the integrated imaging approach.

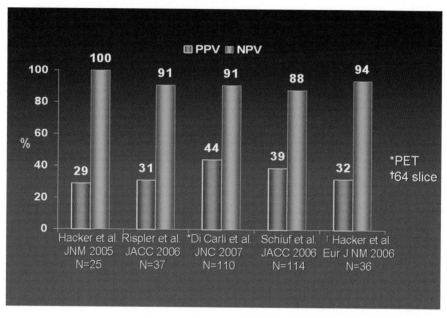

**Chart III.1.1** Frequency of inducible ischemia by myocardial perfusion imaging in territories supplied by stenosis >50% on CT coronary angiography. (Modified with permission Wolters Kluwer from Di Carli and Hachamovitch[12])

## Risk Assessment Using Cardiac Hybrid Imaging

The potential to acquire and quantify rest and stress myocardial perfusion (in mL/min/g and derive estimates of coronary vasodilator reserve) and CT information from a single hybrid imaging study opens the door to expand the prognostic potential of stress imaging. Recent data suggest that quantification of CCS at the time of stress myocardial perfusion PET imaging using a hybrid approach can enhance risk predictions in patients with suspected CAD.[21] In a consecutive series of 621 patients undergoing stress PET imaging and CCS in the same clinical setting, risk-adjusted analysis demonstrated a stepwise increase in cardiac event rates with increasing levels of CCS for any level of perfusion abnormality in patients with and without evidence of ischemia on PET MPS (Chart III.1.2). The annualized event rate in patients with normal PET MPS and no CCS was substantially lower than among those with normal PET MPS and a CCS ≥1,000. Likewise, the annualized event rate in patients with ischemia on PET MPS and no CCS was lower than among those with ischemia and a CCS ≥1,000. These findings suggest an improved risk

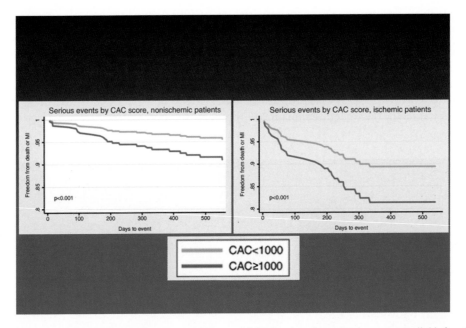

**Chart III.1.2** Cox proportional hazards regression model for freedom from death or myocardial infarction (MI) adjusted for age, sex, symptoms, and conventional CAD risk factors in patients without ischemia (*left panel*) and with ischemia (*right panel*). (Reproduced with permission of Wolters Kluwer from Schenker et al.[21])

stratification by incorporating information on the anatomic extent of atherosclerosis as compared to conventional models using myocardial perfusion alone. This may serve as the rational basis for personalizing the intensity and goals of medical therapy in a more cost-effective manner.

As an adjunct to PET perfusion imaging, CCTA may expand the opportunities to identify patients at greater risk of adverse cardiovascular events. Recent limited data suggest that quantification of the extent and severity of CAD by CCTA can provide estimates of risk similar to those obtained with invasive coronary angiography.[22] Case III.1.5 illustrates the complementary value of the integrated imaging approach for assessing prognosis.

### Guiding Management of CAD Using Cardiac Hybrid Imaging

Cardiac hybrid imaging will play in future a potential significant clinical role due to its ability for optimizing and personalizing management decisions. The importance of stress perfusion imaging in the integrated strategy is the ability to provide noninvasive estimates of jeopardized myocardium. Cardiac hybrid imaging, either with SPECT/CT or PET/CT, will be able to identify which patients may benefit from revascularization, thus differentiating high-risk patients with extensive scar versus those with extensive ischemia. The advantages of this approach are clear – avoidance of unnecessary catheterizations that expose patients to risk and the potential for associated cost savings.[23]

The cardiac hybrid imaging approach may also facilitate identification of patients without flow-limiting disease (i.e., normal perfusion) who have extensive, albeit subclinical, CAD. Recent data from multiple laboratories suggest that as many as 50% of patients with normal stress perfusion imaging may show extensive, non-flow limiting coronary athero-sclerosis with both calcified and non-calcified plaques.[14,17] While these patients with extensive atherosclerosis do not require revascularization in the absence of ischemia, they are at higher risk of adverse events,[21,24,25] and thus more aggressive medical therapy is probably warranted. Cases III.1.3 through III.1.6 also illustrate the complementary value of the integrated imaging approach for management decisions.

## Conclusions

Innovation in noninvasive cardiovascular imaging such as hybrid PET/CT and SPECT/CT is rapidly advancing our ability to image in great detail the structure and function of the heart and coronary vessels. By providing quantitative information about myocardial perfusion and metabolism concurrent with coronary and cardiac anatomy, hybrid imaging offers a comprehensive noninvasive tool for the evaluation of the burden of atherosclerosis and its physiologic consequences in the coronary arteries and the myocardium. This integrated platform for assessing anatomy and biology allows for translating advances in molecularly targeted imaging into humans. The goals of future investigation will be to refine these technologies, establish standard protocols for image acquisition and interpre-tation, address the issue of cost-effectiveness, and validate a range of clinical applications in large-scale clinical trials.

## Case Presentations

### *Case III.1.1*

#### History

This is a 52-year-old asymptomatic male with no history or risk factors for ischemic heart disease (height − 5.77 feet/176 cm, weight − 163 pounds/74 kg, body mass index (BMI) − 23.9). The patient had a positive stress test during routine checkup and was referred to rest/stress MPS for further cardiac assessment (Fig. III.1.1A–C).

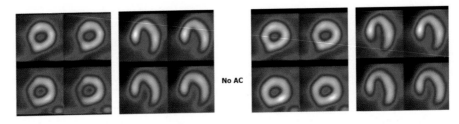

No AC

**Fig. III.1.1A**

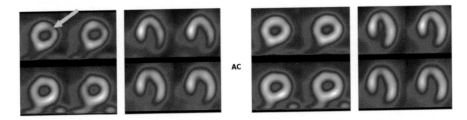

AC

**Fig. III.1.1B**

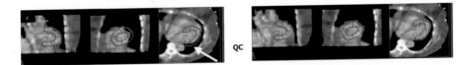

QC

**Fig. III.1.1C**

#### Protocol

One day-single isotope protocol SPECT MPS was acquired. The patient performed tread-mill exercise according to the Bruce protocol (12 min, 13 mets, achieved 88% of the target heart rate). $^{99m}$Tc-sestamibi, 370 MBq (10 mCi), was injected for rest and 1,110 MBq (30 mCi) for gated stress MPS SPECT. The study was performed using a SPECT/CT scanner with low-dose CT used for AC (Fig. III.1.1A = SPECT without AC, Fig. III.1.1B = SPECT with AC, Fig. III.1.1C = quality control for registration).

## Findings

Non-corrected SPECT slices (Fig. III.1.1A left column, upper row – stress, bottom row – rest) demonstrate normal cardiac perfusion. AC-SPECT slices (Fig. III.1.1B left column, upper row – stress, bottom row – rest) show mild decreased perfusion to the antero-lateral wall (arrow). Assessment of SPECT/CT registration maps for the stress study (Fig. III.1.1C, left column) shows a 2 pixel ventral misregistration between SPECT cardiac perfusion contours and the anatomic left ventricle on CT (arrow).

Following manual re-registration AC and non-corrected SPECT slices (Fig. III.1.1A,B right column) show normal myocardial perfusion at rest and stress. SPECT/CT re-registration maps for the stress study (Fig. III.1.1C right column) confirm the now accurate registration between SPECT and CT.

## Discussion

This case illustrates the importance of routine quality control of the transmission and emission data and the transmission–emission alignment.

## Diagnosis

1. Normal myocardial perfusion SPECT study.
2. Mild decreased uptake in the antero-lateral wall on AC SPECT slices due to misregistration between the SPECT and CT component of the study.

## *Case III.1.2*

### History

A 52-year-old female with hypertension and a family history of CAD was referred for a PET MPS due to complaints of chronic atypical chest discomfort (Fig. III.1.2A,B).

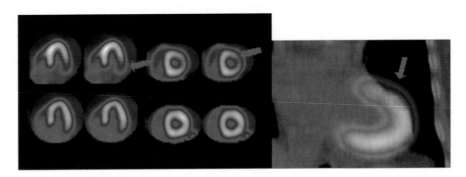

**Fig. III.1.2A**

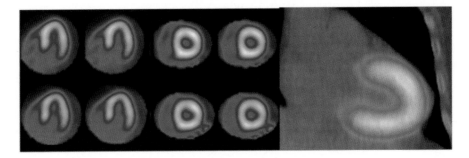

**Fig. III.1.2B**

### Protocol

A single-day rest–stress $^{82}$Rubidium PET was performed. The patient underwent vasodilator stress with dipyridamole (140 μg/kg/min, 0.56 mg/kg total dose, infusion duration 4 min). PET acquisition was performed using a hybrid PET/CT scanner with a 64-slice CT used for AC and CCS (Fig. III.1.2A – PET with AC, Fig. III.1.2B – PET with AC with re-alignment of transmission/emission images).

### Findings

An apparent medium-sized perfusion defect of moderate intensity is noted in the basal- and mid-antero-lateral wall, with complete reversibility at rest. Inspection of the registration maps reveals misregistration of PET and CT images (arrow, Fig. III.1.2A). Following the application of a software for shifting and re-alignment of images (Fig. III.1.2B), adequate registration has been achieved with disappearance of perfusion defects, as demonstrated on the reconstructed MPS images.

**Discussion**

Misregistration of transmission and emission images due to patient motion can degrade image quality and produce reversible perfusion defects in the anterior or antero-lateral walls. Inspection of the registration maps has to be performed routinely to eliminate erroneous interpretation of PET/CT studies. Potential solutions to the problem of misregistration include acquisition of the emission scan de novo or application of a specialized shifting software for accurate alignment of transmission and emission images.

**Diagnosis**

1. Normal myocardial perfusion PET study.
2. Mild decreased uptake in the antero-lateral wall on AC PET slices due to misregistration.

## Case III.1.3

### History

This is a 61-year-old male with a history of multivessel CAD, 12 years after coronary artery bypass graft surgery including saphenous vascular grafts (SVG) to marginal and right coronary arteries, and left internal mammary artery (LIMA) bypass to the left anterior descending (LAD) artery. A number of years after surgery, stents were placed in the LIMA and in the native LAD. The patient presented with non-ST elevation myocardial infarction and was referred for evaluation before discharge from the hospital (Fig. III.1.3A–C).

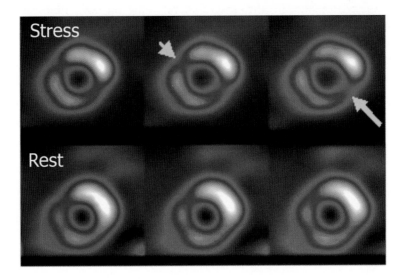

**Fig. III.1.3A**

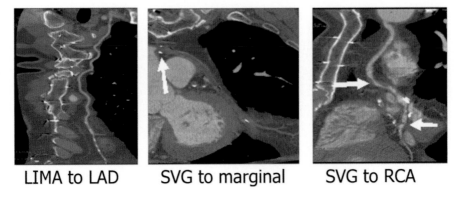

LIMA to LAD      SVG to marginal      SVG to RCA

**Fig. III.1.3B**

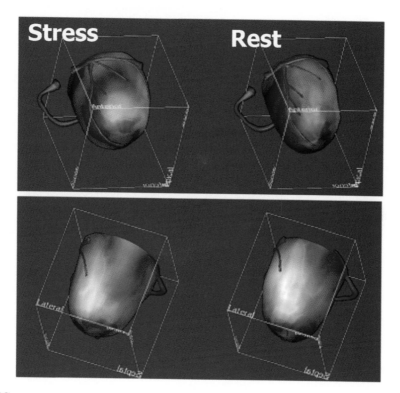

**Fig. III.1.3C**

## Protocol

One day-single isotope protocol SPECT-MPS study was acquired. $^{99m}$Tc-sestamibi, 370 MBq (10 mCi), was injected for rest and 1,110 MBq (30 mCi) for gated stress MPS-SPECT. The patient underwent pharmacological stress using dipyridamole (140 µg/kg/min, 0.56 mg/kg total dose, infusion duration 4 min). SPECT acquisition was performed using a SPECT/CT scanner with a 64-slice CT for AC, CCS, and CCTA (Fig. III.1.3A–C).

## Findings

AC-SPECT slices (Fig. III.1.3A, upper row – stress, bottom row – rest) show a reversible perfusion defect in the infero-lateral segment (arrow) and a fixed perfusion defect in the antero-septal segment (arrowhead). CCTA (Fig. III.1.3B left – LIMA, center – SVG to marginal artery, right – SVG to right coronary artery (RCA)) shows a patent LIMA to LAD, an occluded SVG to marginal artery (middle, arrow), and two severe stenoses in the SVG to RCA (right, arrows). Fused images (Fig. III.1.3C left – stress, right – rest) demonstrate the relationship between the ischemic and infarcted territories on SPECT and the occluded and stenotic vessels on CT.

## Discussion

This case illustrates the complementary value of the integrated imaging approach.

**Diagnosis**

1. Hemodynamically significant lesion in the territory of the RCA related to stenosis in SVG to RCA.
2. Antero-septal scar tissue in the territory of the occluded SVG to marginal artery.

**Follow-Up**

On coronary catheterization, there was a 90% stenosis in the proximal SVG to the RCA. Total occlusion was found in the SVG to marginal and the native LAD, marginal, and RCA. Based on the data provided by SPECT/CT, an intraluminal stent was inserted to the SVG. The patient was asymptomatic for a follow period of 8 months.

## *Case III.I.4*

### History

This is a 52-year-old male with a history of diabetes mellitus and hyperlipidemia. The patient underwent coronary catheterization with insertion of an intraluminal stent to a 90% LAD stenosis 7 years prior to current study. Two years later, he complained again of chest pain. Repeat coronary angiography showed normal arteries. The patient presented with typical chest pain (Fig. III.1.4A–C).

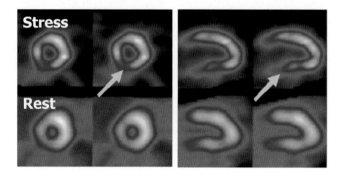

**Fig. III.1.4A**

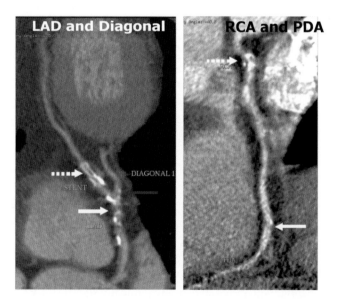

**Fig. III.1.4B**

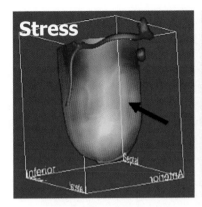 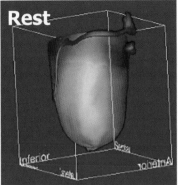

**Fig. III.1.4C**

## Protocol

One day-dual isotope protocol myocardial perfusion SPECT study was acquired. A dose of [201]Thallium of 129 MBq (3.5 mCi) was injected for rest and 888 MBq (24 mCi) [99m]Tc-Sestamibi for gated stress MPS. The patient underwent pharmacological stress using dipyridamole (140 μg/kg/min, 0.56 mg/kg total dose, duration of infusion 4 min). Image acquisition was performed using a SPECT/CT scanner with 16-slice CT for AC, CCS, and CCTA.

## Findings

AC-SPECT slices (Fig. III.1.4A, upper row – stress, bottom row – rest) show a reversible perfusion defect involving the inferior wall (arrows). CCTA (Fig. III.1.4B. left – LAD and diagonal, right – RCA and posterior descending artery (PDA)) shows a calcified plaque causing severe stenosis in the proximal RCA and additional stenosis in the PDA (right, arrows). Additional severe stenoses are demonstrated in a lesion located at an LAD bifurcation, proximal to a patent stent, as well as in the proximal part of the first diagonal artery (left, arrows). Fused images (Fig. III.1.4C, left – stress, right – rest) demonstrate the relationship between the ischemic territory on SPECT and the stenotic lesions on CT (arrow). The Agaston CCS was 422.

## Discussion

This is another case illustrating the complementary value of the integrated imaging approach.

## Diagnosis

1. Inferior wall ischemia indicating the hemodynamically significant RCA lesion.
2. Stenotic lesions in LAD with no hemodynamic changes in its territory of blood supply.

**Follow-Up**

Based on the information provided by the SPECT/CT data, a repeat therapeutic coronary angiography was performed. A stent was inserted at the level of the stenotic lesion in the RCA. The patient has no clinical complaints and is free of cardiac events for a follow-up of 12 months.

# Case III.1.5

## History

A 55-year-old female patient with no prior history of CAD presented for evaluation of new onset angina pectoris (Fig. III.1.5A,B).

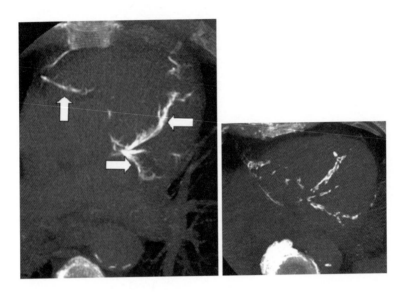

Fig. III.1.5A

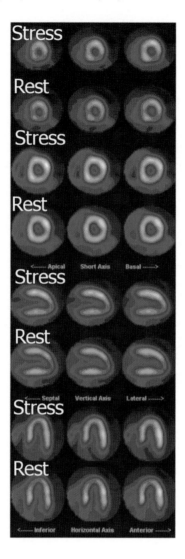

**Fig. III.1.5B**

### Protocol

A single-day rest–stress $^{82}$Rubidium PET was performed. The patient underwent vasodilator stress with dipyridamole (140 µg/kg/min, 0.56 mg/kg total dose, infusion duration 4 min). PET acquisition was performed using a PET/CT scanner with a 64-slice CT used for AC and CCS (Fig. III.1.5A = CCS and Fig. III.1.5B = PET).

### Findings

There is a high burden of total coronary calcium (CCS = 2,417) on the CT (Fig. III.1.5A) in all three major coronary arteries (arrows), which has been shown to correlate well with total atherosclerotic disease burden and less well with the presence of focal coronary artery stenosis. The PET MPS (Fig. III.1.5B) demonstrates normal myocardial distribution of the radiotracer with no evidence for reversible ischemic defects.

## Discussion

Recent data seem to suggest that, in patients with a high CCS, the risk of a hard event is significantly reduced in the presence of normal myocardial perfusion. Potential false-negative PET results are associated with high-risk features suggestive of extensive CAD in the presence of so-called "balanced ischemia." Quantification of myocardial perfusion may represent the solution to exclude the presence of extensive coronary disease in this clinical setting.

## Diagnosis

CCS >1,000 with no evidence of ischemia on MPS PET.

## Case III.1.6

### History

This 65-year-old male patient with multiple risk factors for CAD was referred for further evaluation of stable angina pectoris (Fig. III.1.6).

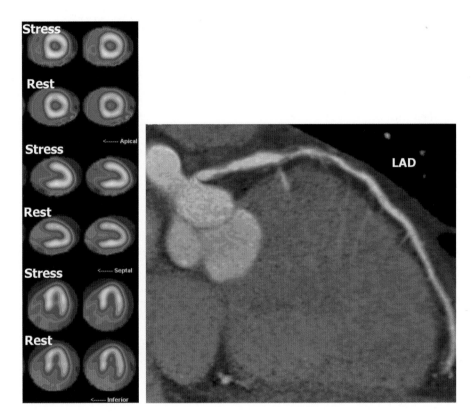

**Fig. III.1.6**

## Protocol

A single-day rest–stress $^{82}$Rubidium PET was performed. The patient underwent vasodilator stress with dipyridamole (140 µg/kg/min, 0.56 mg/kg total dose, infusion duration 4 min). PET acquisition was performed using a hybrid PET/CT scanner with a 64-slice CT used for AC and CCTA (Fig. III.1.6-left PET, right-CCTA of the LAD).

### Findings

The PET MPS (Fig. III.1.6, left) reveals normal radiotracer distribution with no evidence for stress-induced perfusion defects. However, CCTA (Fig. III.1.6, right) demonstrates moderate atherosclerotic stenosis in the mid-LAD as well as in the RCA (not shown).

## Discussion

The functional significance of even severe CAD on CCTA does not necessarily translate into downstream myocardial ischemia. At present, CCTA has limited ability to provide information regarding the risk of future adverse clinical events.

## Diagnosis

Moderate stenosis in the RCA with normal PET MPS.

# References

1. Beyer T, Townsend DW, Brun T, Kinahan PE, Charron M, Roddy R, Jerin J, Young J, Byars L, Nutt R. A combined PET/CT scanner for clinical oncology. *J Nucl Med* 2000;41:1369–1379.

2. O'Connor MK, Kemp B, Anstett F, Christian P, Ficaro EP, Frey E, Jacobs M, Kritzman JN, Pooley RA, Wilk M. A multicenter evaluation of commercial attenuation compensation techniques in cardiac SPECT using phantom models. *J Nucl Cardiol* 2002;9:361–376.

3. Stone CD, McCormick JW, Gilland DR, Greer KL, Coleman RE, Jaszczak RJ. Effect of registration errors between transmission and emission scans on a SPECT system using sequential scanning. *J Nucl Med* 1998;39:365–373.

4. Garcia EV. SPECT attenuation correction: an essential tool to realize nuclear cardiology's manifest destiny. *J Nucl Cardiol* Jan 2007;14:16–24.

5. Sampson UK, Dorbala S, Limaye A, Kwong R, Di Carli MF. Diagnostic accuracy of rubidium-82 myocardial perfusion imaging with hybrid positron emission tomography/computed tomography in the detection of coronary artery disease. *J Am Coll Cardiol* 2007;49:1052–1058.

6. Di Carli MF, Dorbala S, Meserve J, El Fakhri G, Sitek A, Moore SC. Clinical myocardial perfusion PET/CT. *J Nucl Med* 2007;48:783–793.

7. Earls JP, Berman EL, Urban BA, Curry CA, Lane JL, Jennings RS, McCulloch CC, Hsieh J, Londt JH. Prospectively gated transverse coronary CT angiography versus retrospectively gated helical technique: improved image quality and reduced radiation dose. *Radiology* 2008;246:742–753.

8. Di Carli MF, Dorbala S. Detection and evaluation of coronary artery disease with myocardial perfusion-gated SPECT imaging. In St. John Sutton MG RJ (ed): *Clinical cardiovascular imaging: A companion to Braunwald's heart disease*. Philadelphia: Elsevier Saunders, 2004; 115–125.

9. Chow BJ, Beanlands RS, Lee A, DaSilva J, deKemp R, Alkahtani A, Ruddy T. Treadmill exercise produces larger perfusion defects than dipyridamole stress N-13 ammonia positron emission tomography. *J Am Coll Cardiol* 2006;47:411–416.

10. Gould KL, Pan T, Loghin C, Guha A, Sdringola S. Frequent diagnostic errors in cardiac PET/CT due to misregistration of CT attenuation and emission PET images: a definitive analysis of causes, consequences, and corrections. *J Nucl Med* 2007;48:1112–1121.

11. Klocke FJ, Baird MG, Lorell BH et al. ACC/AHA/ASNC guidelines for the clinical use of cardiac radionuclide imaging – executive summary: a report of the American College of Cardiology/American Heart Association Task Force on Practice Guidelines (ACC/AHA/ASNC Committee to Revise the 1995 Guidelines for the Clinical Use of Cardiac Radionuclide Imaging). *J Am Coll Cardiol* 2003;42:1318–1333.

12. Di Carli MF, Hachamovitch R. New technology for noninvasive evaluation of coronary artery disease. *Circulation* 2007;115:1464–1480.

13. Hacker M, Jakobs T, Matthiesen F, Vollmar C, Nikolaou K, Becker C, Knez A, Pfluger T, Reiser M, Hahn K, Tiling R. Comparison of spiral multidetector CT angiography and myocardial perfusion imaging in the noninvasive detection of functionally relevant coronary artery lesions: First clinical experience. *J Nucl Med* 2005;46:1294–1300.

14. Schuijf JD, Wijns W, Jukema JW, Atsma D, de Roos A, Lamb H, Stokkel M, Dibbets-Schneider P, Decramer I, De Bondt P. Relationship between noninvasive coronary angiography with multi-slice computed tomography and myocardial perfusion imaging. *J Am Coll Cardiol* 2006;48:2508–2514.

15. Gaemperli O, Schepis T, Kalff V, Namdar M, Valenta I, Stefani L, Desbiolles L, Leschka S, Husmann L, Alkadhi H, Kaufmann PA. Validation of a new cardiac image fusion software for three-dimensional integration of myocardial perfusion SPECT and stand-alone 64-slice CT angiography. *Eur J Nucl Med Mol Imaging* 2007;34:1097–1106.

16. Gaemperli O, Schepis T, Valenta I, Husmann L, Scheffel H, Duerst V, Eberli FR, Luscher TF, Alkadhi H, Kaufmann PA. Cardiac image fusion from stand-alone SPECT and CT: Clinical experience. *J Nucl Med* May 2007;48:696–703.

17. Di Carli MF, Dorbala S, Curillova Z, Kwong R, Goldhaber S, Rybicki F, Hachamovitch R. Relationship between CT coronary angiography and stress perfusion imaging in patients with suspected ischemic heart disease assessed by integrated PET-CT imaging. *J Nucl Cardiol* 2007;14:799–809.

18. Rispler S, Keidar Z, Ghersin E, Roguin A, Soil A, Dragu R, Litmanovich D, Frenkel A, Aronson D, Engel A. Integrated single-photon emission computed tomography and computed tomography coronary angiography for the assessment of hemodynamically significant coronary artery lesions. *J Am Coll Cardiol* 2007;49:1059–1067.

19. Delbeke D, Keidar Z, Kronenberg MW, Churchwell K, Brenner R, Patton JA, Rispler S, Israel O, Sandler MP. Integrated rest/stress myocardial perfusion SPECT (MPS) and 64-slice coronary CTA: Impact on management in patients with intermediate likelihood of CAD. Annual meeting of SNM, June 14–18, 2008, New Orleans, LA. *J Nucl Med* 2008; 49 (suppl 1):205P

20. Hacker M, Jakobs T, Hack N, Nikolaou K, Becker C, von Ziegler F, Knez A, König A, Klauss V, Reiser M, Hahn K, Tiling R. Sixty-four slice spiral CT angiography does not predict the functional relevance of coronary artery stenoses in patients with stable angina. *Eur J Nucl Med Mol Imaging* 2007;34:4–10.

21. Schenker MP, Dorbala S, Hong EC, Rybicki FJ, Hachamovitch R, Kwong RY, Di Carli MF. Interrelation of coronary calcification, myocardial ischemia, and outcomes in patients with intermediate likelihood of coronary artery disease: A combined positron emission tomography/computed tomography study. *Circulation* 2008;117:1693–1700.

22. Min JK, Shaw LJ, Devereux RB, Okin P, Weinsaft J, Russo D, Lippolis N, Berman D, Callister T. Prognostic value of multidetector coronary computed tomographic angiography for prediction of all-cause mortality. *J Am Coll Cardiol.* 2007;50:1161–1170.

23. Shaw LJ, Hachamovitch R, Berman DS, Marwick TH, Lauer MS, Heller GV, Iskandrian AE, Kesler KL, Travin MI, Lewin HC, Hendel RC, Borges-Neto S, Miller DD, and for the Economics of Noninvasive Diagnosis (END) Multicenter Study Group. The economic consequences of available diagnostic and prognostic strategies for the evaluation of stable angina patients: an observational assessment of the value of precatheterization ischemia. Economics of Noninvasive Diagnosis (END) Multicenter Study Group. *J Am Coll Cardiol* 1999;33:661–669.

24. Budoff MJ, Shaw LJ, Liu ST, Weinstein S, Mosler T, Tseng P, Flores F,. Callister T, Raggi P, Berman D. Long-term prognosis associated with coronary calcification: observations from a registry of 25,253 patients. *J Am Coll Cardiol* 2007;49:1860–1870.

25. Greenland P, Bonow RO, Brundage BH et al. ACCF/AHA 2007 clinical expert consensus document on coronary artery calcium scoring by computed tomography in global cardiovascular risk assessment and in evaluation of patients with chest pain: a report of the American College of Cardiology Foundation Clinical Expert Consensus Task Force (ACCF/AHA Writing Committee to Update the 2000 Expert Consensus Document on Electron Beam Computed Tomography) developed in collaboration with the Society of Atherosclerosis Imaging and Prevention and the Society of Cardiovascular Computed Tomography. *J Am Coll Cardiol* 2007;49:378–402.

# Chapter III.2
# Hybrid Imaging of Benign Skeletal Diseases

**Einat Even-Sapir, Hedva Lerman, Gideon Flusser, and Arye Blachar**

## $^{99m}$Tc-MDP SPECT/CT

$^{99m}$Tc-methylene diphosphonate ($^{99m}$Tc-MDP) is the most commonly used bone radio-pharmaceutical for scintigraphic assessment of skeletal abnormalities. The compound, an analogue of pyrophosphate, is chemisorbed onto bone surface. Its uptake depends on local blood flow and bone turnover. As little as 5–10% change in lesion to normal bone uptake ratio is required to detect pathology on skeletal scintigraphy (BS) preceding their detection on plain radiographs or computed tomography (CT) by 2–18 months.[1] Based on these characteristics, BS with $^{99m}$Tc-MDP is highly sensitive for the detection of various benign skeletal abnormalities associated with increased bone turnover including trauma, osteomyelitis, osteoporosis, metabolic skeletal disease, degenerative changes, etc. When performing the conventional BS procedure, two-dimensional planar images are acquired over the entire body in the anterior and posterior projection. With the introduction of single photon emission computed tomography (SPECT), it became apparent that this technique improves the diagnostic accuracy of BS for detection of bone pathology. SPECT increases the detectability rate of skeletal lesions by 20–50% compared to planar BS and allows side-by-side comparison with other tomographic techniques such as CT and magnetic resonance imaging (MRI).[2] The benefit of SPECT in accurate localization of increased tracer uptake is especially prominent in skeletal regions with complex architecture such as the spine, pelvis, or skull.[3] Better localization of lesions by SPECT improves the specificity of BS in differentiating benign from malignant lesions located in the thoracic and lumbar vertebral column, as different disease processes tend to involve different parts of the vertebra, which can be precisely identified by SPECT.[4] However, although differentiation between malignant and benign etiology can be achieved, final diagnosis still requires morphologic characterization.[5] The high sensitivity of BS results in a high rate of incidental findings, which are not necessarily related to the patient's clinical presentation. Fusion of SPECT and CT data may be obtained by co-registration of images of separately performed SPECT and CT studies using software packages.[6] SPECT/CT hybrid systems that are now available allow same-session morphologic characterization of scintigraphic lesions.[3] Depending on the system used, the CT component of the hybrid device may be either single- or multislice low-dose, reduced-dose, or full-dose spiral CT.

E. Even-Sapir (✉)
Department of Nuclear Medicine, Tel Aviv Sourasky Medical Center, Tel Aviv University, Tel Aviv, Israel
e-mail: evensap@tasmc.health.gov.il

D. Delbeke, O. Israel (eds.), *Hybrid PET/CT and SPECT/CT Imaging*,
DOI 10.1007/978-0-387-92820-3_19, © Springer Science+Business Media, LLC 2010

Horger and colleagues[7] have used a hybrid system with a low-dose single slice CT (140 kV, 2.5 mA) for classification of skeletal lesions in 47 patients with known malignant disease who had 104 abnormal scintigraphic lesions on BS. Fused SPECT/CT data allowed accurate classification of 85% of the lesions as benign or malignant, compared to 36% on SPECT alone. Using the same system, this group has also evaluated the contribution of SPECT/CT for diagnosis and localization of skeletal infection. SPECT/CT was compared to BS (including three-phase planar and SPECT stand-alone data) and to visual fusion of SPECT with data of additional CT, X-ray, or MRI studies. Sensitivity of stand-alone BS or fused with CT was 78%. However, the specificity of BS was 50% compared with 86% for SPECT/CT. The limited specificity of BS was due mainly to the presence of non-infectious skeletal pathology such as fracture or previous surgery, which is also associated with increased $^{99m}$Tc-MDP uptake and difficult to differentiate from infection, mainly low grade. SPECT/low-dose CT reduced the false-positive rate as well as the number of equivocal results. The differential diagnosis between reactive osteitis and osteomyelitis requires that scintigraphic data be correlated with morphological patterns of the skeletal lesion. Osteitis is characterized by increased soft tissue uptake on dynamic images, only mild tracer uptake on delayed BS images, and no evidence of clear cortical abnormality on CT. Osteomyelitis is characterized by hyperperfusion on the early dynamic images, and increased uptake on delayed images, reflecting the high skeletal turnover, and typical anatomical changes compatible with skeletal infection on CT, such as cortical bone erosion, periosteal elevation, osteolysis, or sequestration. Low-dose CT may be insufficient for early identification of the above-described changes and thus cannot replace the need for correlation of scintigraphic findings with a full-dose diagnostic CT. Correlating SPECT data with diagnostic MRI or full-dose CT yielded the highest sensitivity, reaching 100%.[8]

Using a hybrid system combining a dual-head gamma camera with 4-slice low-dose CT (140 kV, 2.5 mA), Even-Sapir and colleagues[9] assessed the role of SPECT/CT in 76 consecutive non-oncologic patients with non-specific scintigraphic findings, which required further correlation with morphologic data. SPECT/CT was of clinical added value in 89% of patients. In 58% of the patients, the morphological data obtained by the low-dose multislice CT allowed the authors to reach the final diagnosis, thus obviating the need to perform additional imaging. In an additional 30% of the patients, an optimized diagnostic workup was based on SPECT/CT findings, which guided the authors toward the use of diagnostic full-dose CT, MRI, or labeled leukocytes scintigraphy as the most appropriate imaging modality for further assessment. Low-dose CT has also been used as a gateway for accurate co-registration with full-dose CT, when it is performed separately.

Römer and coworkers[10] have assessed the role of SPECT/CT in cancer patients with indeterminate skeletal lesions requiring further workup for definite diagnosis using a hybrid system that combines a gamma camera and a spiral diagnostic CT with an acquisition protocol including 130 kV, 0.8 s rotation time, $2 \times 2.5$ mm collimation, with a tube current reduced to 40 mA to minimize radiation exposure. The decision to perform reduced-dose rather than full-dose spiral CT was based on previous studies, which showed that the inherent high contrast between normal and abnormal bone allows for accurate identification of skeletal pathology even by reduced-dose CT.[11] SPECT/CT was able to clarify more than 90% of indeterminate SPECT findings. In 63% of cases, these indeterminate scintigraphic lesions correlated with a benign process on CT, mainly of degenerative etiology, while metastases were identified on CT as corresponding to 29% of the unclear lesions on BS.[10]

The scope of the study by Utsunomiya and colleagues[12] was also to differentiate between benign and malignant skeletal lesions identified on BS. They compared the diagnostic confidence of side-by-side interpretation of CT and SPECT data with that of fused SPECT/CT images obtained in a single setting using a system that combines a dual-head gamma camera with a multi-detector diagnostic CT and acquired a full-dose CT with 120 kV, 140 mA, 0.7 s per rotation, 2.5 mm collimation, and 5 mm reconstruction. Their results showed that fused images allowed for a better differentiation of benign from malignant lesions compared to side-by-side reading, with a higher degree of confidence. Metastatic foci, which were overlooked on separate interpretation of scintigraphy and CT were identified on fused images.

Assessment of the added value of fusion of SPECT and CT in cancer patients with unclear skeletal findings was also the scope of a study by Strobel and coworkers.[13] Data of separately performed SPECT and full-dose CT were fused using a software package, and correct anatomic fusion was possible for all patients by bringing internal anatomic landmarks into agreement. Similar to the results of Utsunomiya and colleagues,[12] the highest degree of confidence in diagnosis was obtained by fused images. The authors commented that fusion of separately performed studies using software packages was time consuming, a relevant argument in daily routine practice. However, its advantage was to allow fusion of SPECT and CT performed in different settings or at separate locations, obviating the need to expose the patient to additional radiation.[13]

McDonald and coworkers[14] fused SPECT and CT in 37 patients with back pain clinically attributable to facet joint disease. Transaxial CT images were transferred in DICOM format. Image fusion was successfully performed in all patients, and the image quality allowed definitive localization of the "hot" lesion in all cases. In contrast to SPECT alone, SPECT/CT allowed precise localization to L4/5 versus L5/S1. In patients with solitary lesions, localized anesthetic blockade led to complete, even if temporary, pain resolution. Clinical data on the use of SPECT/CT in diagnosis of skeletal abnormalities are accumulating. As noted earlier, most studies published so far have investigated the role of SPECT/CT in differentiating benign from malignant skeletal lesions, with data on the use of SPECT/CT in solely non-malignant clinical condition being scarce. It should be kept in mind that in non-oncologic patients the radiation exposure resulting from adding CT to the scintigraphic study needs to be clinically justified. Whereas cancer patients will at some point have CT as part of the imaging algorithm of their oncologic disease, the quality of CT required for fusion with SPECT in order to reach diagnosis in non-oncologic skeletal diseases is yet to be determined.

# $^{18}$F-Fluoride PET/CT

$^{18}$F-Fluoride is a highly sensitive bone-seeking positron emission tomography (PET) tracer used for detection of skeletal abnormalities. The uptake mechanism of $^{18}$F-Fluoride resembles that of $^{99m}$Tc-MDP with better pharmacokinetic characteristics, including faster blood clearance and twofold higher uptake in bone. Uptake of $^{18}$F-Fluoride reflects blood flow and bone remodeling.[1] $^{18}$F-Fluoride imaging has been performed mainly for assessment of bone involvement in various malignant diseases. Although the mechanism of uptake of $^{18}$F-Fluoride depends on bone turnover, it is very sensitive for detecting not only osteoblastic metastases but also of lytic lesions. This may be explained by the fact that even when considered "pure lytic," these lesions have minimal osteoblastic activity, which can be detected by [18]F-Fluoride PET.[15,16] [18]F-Fluoride is, however, not tumor specific and often requires correlation with CT for accurate interpretation. The use of novel hybrid PET/CT systems has significantly improved the specificity of [18]F-Fluoride imaging as the CT component of the study allows morphologic characterization of the functional lesion and accurate differentiation between benign lesions and metastases.[17,18]

Most data on the role of [18]F-Fluoride PET in benign conditions are based on assessment of quantitation and evaluation of [18]F-Fluoride kinetics. Quantitative [18]F-Fluoride PET imaging allows regional characterization of metabolic skeletal diseases including Paget, osteoporosis, and renal osteodystrophy, as well as monitoring their response to therapy. [18]F-Fluoride imaging is a valuable diagnostic tool for assessment of viability of bone grafts, early prediction of fracture nonunion, and diagnosis of osteonecrosis.[19]

Only few studies assess the role of [18]F-Fluoride PET in non-oncologic indications. Recent studies evaluated the role of [18]F-Fluoride imaging in assessment of back pain in children and young adults using either PET or PET/CT.[20,21] In addition to accurate diagnosis of the cause of back pain, [18]F-Fluoride imaging had a high negative predictive value. Patients with negative [18]F-Fluoride imaging did not require medical intervention.[20]

Even-Sapir and colleagues[19] performed [18]F-Fluoride PET/CT in 82 patients with a suspected non-oncologic skeletal abnormality, mainly with skeletal pain, but also for assessment of vertebral fusion and of viability of free fibular flaps. [18]F-Fluoride PET/CT was of value in identifying clinically relevant skeletal lesions overlooked when CT was interpreted alone. Fusion of [18]F-Fluoride PET with CT was beneficial in assessing the integrity of bones with complicated structure.

Radiation exposure of patients performing [18]F-Fluoride studies is in the same range as that for [99m]Tc-MDP. The CT acquisition protocol used by Even-Sapir and colleagues[19] for [18]F-Fluoride PET/CT imaging is associated with radiation doses of 7.3 mGy (0.730 rads) in adults and 10.5 mGy (1.05 rads) in a 10-year-old patient. Reduction in exposure can be achieved by decreasing the CT acquisition parameters to 120 kV and/or 40 mA.

In spite of the high performance of [18]F-Fluoride PET/CT in diagnosis of skeletal abnormalities, issues of price and availability still limit its use to selected patients.[15,16]

# [18]FDG PET/CT

[18]F-Fluorodeoxyglucose ([18]FDG) PET imaging is used mainly in oncology. It has been shown to accurately identify malignant involvement of the skeleton even in early stages when the disease is confined to the marrow, prior to the presence of cortical lesions. [18]FDG PET is limited to a lesser degree than [99m]Tc-MDP BS by uptake in benign skeletal lesions. However, increased skeletal [18]FDG uptake is not specific for tumoral involvement. Highly cellular benign lesions containing histiocytic or giant cells may also be associated with increased [18]FDG PET uptake, such as osteoblastoma, brown tumor, aneurismal bone cyst, sarcoidosis, radionecrosis, or skeletal infection. It is assumed that the predominant energy supply of monocyte/macrophage-derived cells or fibroblasts, which play a major role in the host response to injury and infection, is by intracellular glucose metabolism.[22] Uptake in benign

skeletal lesions may be incidentally identified in cancer patients and can be differentiated by their morphologic CT patterns from malignant involvement of the bone, thus avoiding false-positive upstaging of the disease.[23]

Data on the role of [18]FDG PET imaging in assessment of skeletal pathology in patients without cancer are accumulating, mainly for suspected musculo-skeletal infection. Various studies have assessed the role of [18]FDG-PET imaging and recently of [18]FDG PET/CT imaging in patients with suspected chronic osteomyelitis, in osteomyelitis in immuno-compromised patients or after trauma, in patients with diabetic foot, infected joint prosthesis, or inflammatory joint diseases.[3,23–27] The role of hybrid imaging in infection and inflammation is the scope of Chapter III.3.

## Summary

Imaging of benign skeletal abnormalities is a common indication for skeletal scintigraphy. [99m]Tc-MDP and [18]F-Fluoride, a bone-seeking PET tracer, are highly sensitive for detection of skeletal abnormalities associated with high bone turnover. The detection of increased focal uptake in the skeleton, which is non-specific and may be found in a large variety of etiologies, often warrants further correlation with morphologic imaging, mainly CT, for definitive diagnosis.[18]FDG-PET imaging is used primarily in oncologic patients in whom the detection of focal increased [18]FDG uptake in the bone may suggest the presence of malignant skeletal involvement. However, the tracer is also not tumor specific and increased uptake may also be associated with benign skeletal abnormalities. Integrated systems combining SPECT or PET and CT have been recently introduced in the routine practice, allowing for automatic generation of fused images on which each lesion is characterized by its tracer uptake and morphologic appearance.

## Case Presentations

## *Case III.2.1*

### History

A 42-year-old male was referred for $^{99m}$Tc-MDP BS for low-back pain. No abnormality was identified in the spine or pelvis; however, incidental increased uptake was identified in the mid-left tibia. The lesion was further assessed by planar and SPECT/4-slice low-dose CT (140 kV, 2.5 mA) (Fig. III.2.1A, B).

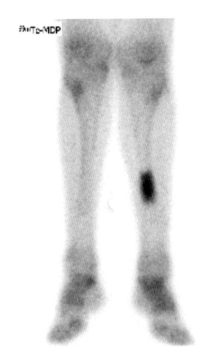

**Fig. III.2.1A**

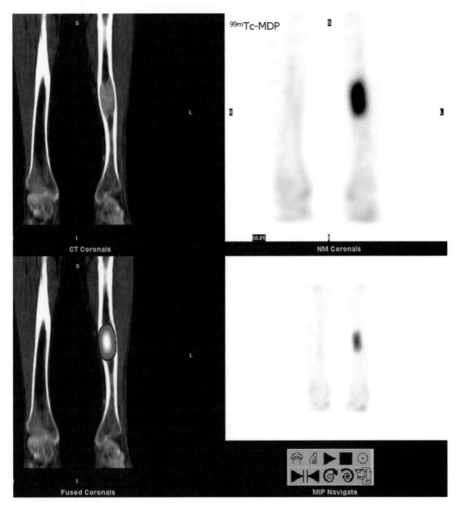

**Fig. III.2.1B**

**Findings**

Increased uptake is detected in the mid-shaft of the left tibia (Fig. III.2.1A). On low-dose CT, the scintigraphic finding corresponds in location with an intramedullary lesion showing ground-glass appearance with skeletal expansion, suggestive of fibrous dysplasia (Fig. III.2.1B).

**Discussion**

Fibrous dysplasia is a common benign developmental anomaly of the bone, in which normal bone marrow is replaced by fibro-osseous tissue. It can be confined to a single bone or show a multifocal distribution in the skeleton. Patients with fibrous dysplasia are as a rule asymptomatic, with the lesion being incidentally found, as in the present case. On CT, fibrous dysplasia shows a typical ground-glass appearance and on $^{99m}$Tc-MDP BS increased tracer uptake.[28]

BS is highly sensitive for detection of skeletal pathology and often detects unexpected lesions that require further correlation with CT. SPECT/CT allows for the morphological and scintigraphical characterization of lesions in the same setting.

## Diagnosis

Incidentally found fibrous dysplasia in the left tibia.

## Case III.2.2

### History

A 25-year-old male was referred for $^{99m}$Tc-MDP BS for assessment of pain in the left knee. Planar images and SPECT/single slice low-dose CT images of the knees are illustrated (Fig. III.2.2A, B).

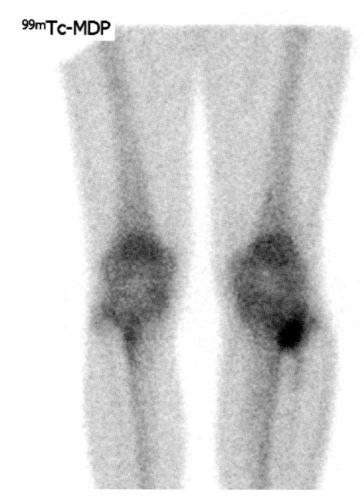

**Fig. III.2.2A**

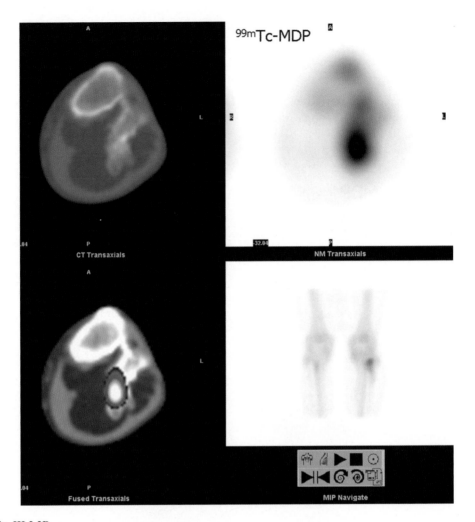

**Fig. III.2.2B**

## Findings

Planar images demonstrate increased $^{99m}$Tc-MDP uptake in the left tibio-fibular region (Fig. III.2.2A). SPECT/low-dose CT of this region indicates that the focus of increased uptake is located in an ossification extending from the fibula and is surrounded by a hypodense soft tissue mass with fat attenuation (Fig. III.2.2B). The findings are highly suggestive of parosteal ossifying lipoma.

## Discussion

Following the $^{99m}$Tc-MDP BS, MRI of the left knee validated the suggested diagnosis of parosteal lipoma. An osseous localization of lipoma is unusual, accounting for only 0.3% of all cases. Three types of osseous lipomas have been described with respect to their relation to the bone: intraosseous, cortical, and parosteal, the latter being very rare, with attachment to the external surface of the bone, mainly adjacent to long bones. The proximity of lipoma often causes pathological changes such as hyperostosis of the adjacent bone, as was the case of our patient.[29]

**Diagnosis**

Parosteal ossifying lipoma in the left fibula.

## Case III.2.3 (DICOM Images on DVD)

### History

A 33-year-old male was referred for $^{99m}$Tc-MDP BS for severe long-standing pain in the sacral area. Findings on planar BS, SPECT/4-slice low-dose CT, 140 kV, 2.5 mA CT, and registered image of SPECT with contrast-enhanced full-dose CT are illustrated (Fig. III.2.3A–C).

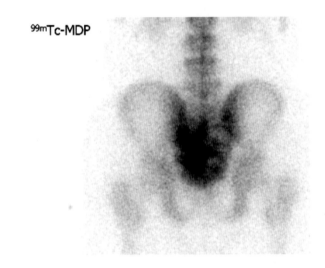

**Fig. III.2.3A**

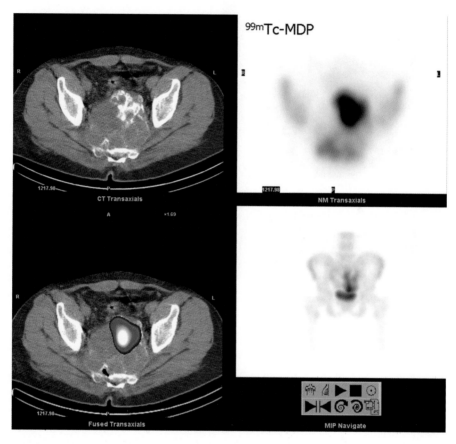

**Fig. III.2.3B**

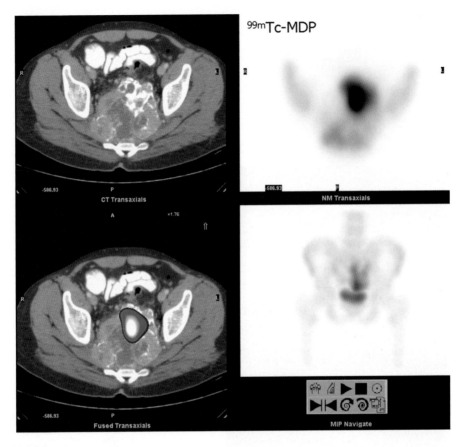

**Fig. III.2.3C**

**Findings**

Posterior planar view of the pelvis demonstrates inhomogenous uptake in the sacrum, mainly on the left (Fig. III.2.3A). As indicated by SPECT, the area of intense uptake appears to be located in soft tissue in the presacral region. The fused SPECT/low-dose CT image demonstrates destructive changes in the sacral bone and a large inhomogenous soft tissue mass with hypodense lesions and areas of gross calcification extending into the presacral space (Fig. III.2.3B). The high-intensity increased uptake seen in the left pelvis corresponds in location with the soft tissue calcifications identified in the left aspect of the pelvic mass (Fig. III.2.3B).

Based on the SPECT/low-dose CT findings, which were highly suggestive of giant cell tumor or chordoma, the patient was referred for a contrast-enhanced full-dose CT. The low-dose CT was further used as a gateway for registration of SPECT with the separately performed full-dose CT (Fig. III.2.3C) using an automatic image-based rigid registration software. The heterogeneous enhancement pattern of the mass as well as the presence of low-density regions was better appreciated on the diagnostic CT, increasing the confidence that giant cell tumor was the diagnosis.

## Discussion

Pain in the sacral region may be caused by various benign and malignant lesions. Benign lesions include giant cell or neurogenic tumor, fracture, and infection, while malignant lesions include primary bone sarcoma, lymphoma, plasmacytoma, and chordoma.[30]

Giant cell tumor is the second most common primary sacral tumor after chordoma. It is locally aggressive and rarely metastasizes. Approximately 5–10% of giant cell tumors are malignant. The typical pattern of giant cell tumors is that of a lytic, destructive process, often eccentrically located, with an adjacent soft tissue mass, heterogeneous in appearance due to the presence of hemorrhage and necrosis as illustrated in this case.[31] CT-guided biopsy of the mass was performed, and the diagnosis of giant cell tumor was histologically proven. The tumor was initially embolized followed by surgical resection.

## Diagnosis

Giant cell tumor of the sacral bone and presacral region.

## Clinical Report: Whole-Body Planar $^{99m}$Tc-MDP and SPECT/Low-Dose CT of the Pelvis (for DVD cases only)

Indication

Pain in the posterior pelvis.

History

A 33-year-old male was referred for $^{99m}$Tc-MDP BS for severe long-standing pain in the sacrum area.

Procedure

Planar BS of the entire skeleton was performed 2 h after the IV injection of 925 MBq (25 mCi) $^{99m}$Tc-MDP followed by SPECT/low-dose CT of the pelvis. SPECT/CT was performed using a hybrid system that incorporates a dual-head camera and a low-dose, four 5 mm slice thickness CT. SPECT was performed in H mode, with a matrix size of 128, an angle step of 6°, and a time per frame of 16 s. CT was acquired with 140 kV and a current of 2.5 mA.

Findings

*Quality of study*: Good

Increased uptake is detected in the pelvis. On planar images, there is inhomogeneity in the uptake in the sacral area. However, on the SPECT images, the intense uptake is located anterior to the sacrum.

On SPECT/low-dose CT of the pelvis, destructive changes in the sacral bone and a large soft tissue mass extending into the presacral space are demonstrated. The mass is inhomogenous presenting hypodense lesions and areas of gross calcification. The area of increased uptake in the left pelvis corresponds to the soft tissue calcifications identified in the left aspect of the pelvic mass.

There are no other remarkable lesions in the skeleton.

Impression

The findings are highly suggestive of giant cell tumor of the sacral bone and presacral region.

## *Case III.2.4 (DICOM Images on DVD)*

### History

A 13-year-old female was referred to $^{18}$F-Fluoride PET/CT imaging due to severe back pain, one-and-a-half years after being treated for osteomyelitis in the left ankle (Fig. III.2.4A–D).

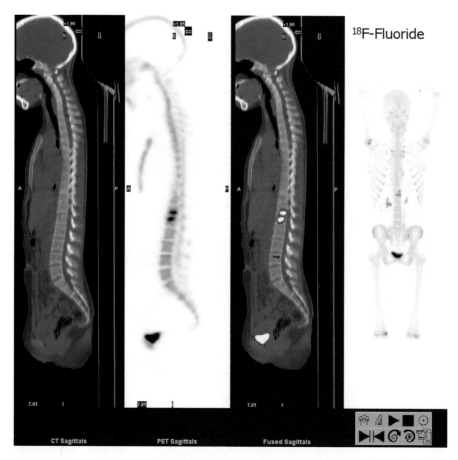

**Fig. III.2.4A**

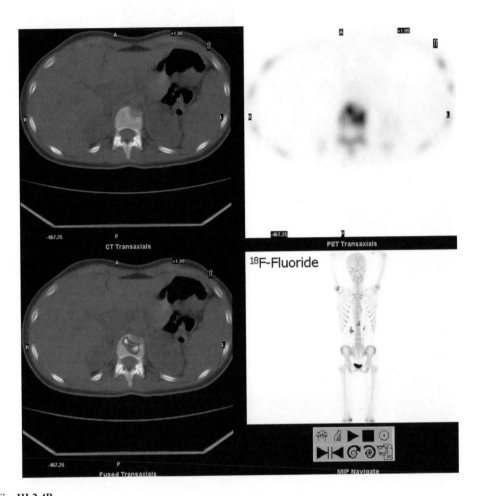

**Fig. III.2.4B**

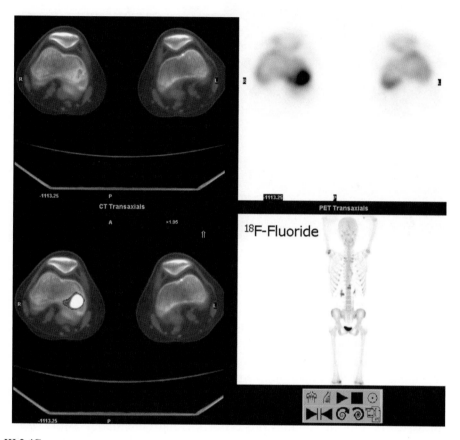

**Fig. III.2.4C**

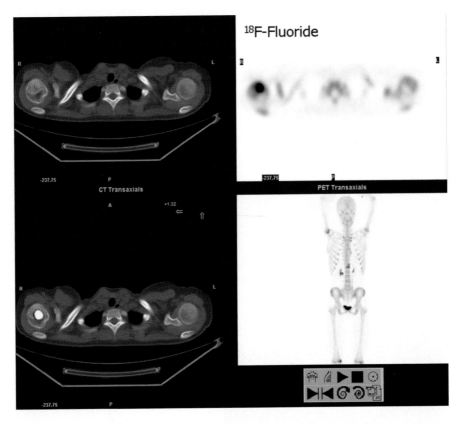

**Fig. III.2.4D**

**Findings**

There is increased tracer uptake in the body of two adjacent vertebrae, T12 and L1 (Fig. III.2.4A). CT demonstrates irregularity of the disc space and lytic lesions with sclerosis in their periphery, corresponding to the scintigraphic lesions (Fig. III.2.4B). Similar findings are seen in the right medial femoral condyle (Fig. III.2.4C) and in the head of the right humerus (Fig. III.2.4D). Additional focal sites of increased uptake corresponding to subtle morphologic changes in the spine of the right scapula, the anterior aspect of T10, the spinous process of L2, and the anterior aspect of the left lateral femoral condyle are seen only retrospectively on CT (see DVD).

**Discussion**

The child presented with complaints of severe back pain. Multifocal skeletal lesions were identified by $^{18}$F-Fluoride PET/CT. Some of the lesions showed subtle morphological changes on CT, found only with the guidance of $^{18}$F-Fluoride, a highly sensitive tracer for detection of skeletal abnormalities. Histological assessment of one of the lesions was considered to be necessary for diagnosis. The lesion located in the right knee was chosen for biopsy, which showed findings consistent with chronic osteomyelitis. The patient was diagnosed with chronic recurrent multifocal osteomyelitis (CRMO).

CRMO is a severe form of chronic nonbacterial osteomyelitis occurring mainly in children and adolescents. It is characterized by a prolonged, fluctuating course with recurrent episodes of skeletal pain over several years. Histopathological and laboratory findings are non-specific, and bacterial culture is negative. CRMO is often diagnosed by exclusion of bacterial infections and malignancy. The disease is probably more common than originally thought. Due to its multifocal nature, patients with suspected or diagnosed CRMO are referred for $^{99m}$Tc-MDP BS or total-body MRI in order to assess the extent of disease. Clinically occult lesions are often present, as in this patient. Lesions of CRMO can occur throughout the skeleton. As illustrated in present case, spinal lesions are characterized by erosion of the vertebral endplates with adjacent sclerosis resembling the appearance of spondylo-discitis.[32,33]

There are no previously published data on the use of $^{18}$F-Fluoride PET in CRMO. The small size of some of the lesions identified by $^{18}$F-Fluoride in present case suggests that $^{18}$F-Fluoride PET is a good imaging modality for detection of the true extent of CRMO.

**Diagnosis**

CRMO in the thoracic and lumbar spine, femuri, right humerus, and scapula.

**Clinical Report: Whole-Body $^{18}$F-Fluoride-PET/CT**

Indication

Severe back pain.

History

A 13-year-old female was referred for $^{18}$F-Fluoride PET/CT due to severe back pain 18 months after being treated for osteomyelitis of the left ankle.

Procedure

An hour after the IV injection of 185 MBq (5 mCi) $^{18}$F-Fluoride reduced-dose CT of the axial skeleton, lower limbs up to the knees, and upper limbs up to the elbows was acquired with the following protocol: 140 kV, 80 mA, 0.8 s per CT rotation, a pitch of 6, and a table speed of 22.5 mm/s. PET was then acquired over the same areas with 3 min acquisition time per each bed position.

Findings

*Quality of study*: good.

*Spine*: Increased uptake is detected in the body of two adjacent vertebrae, T12 and L1. On CT, there is irregularity of the disc space and lytic lesions with sclerosis in their periphery, corresponding to the scintigraphic abnormalities. On CT, the skeletal lesions are accompanied by a thin prevertebral soft tissue density. There are additional focal sites of increased uptake corresponding to subtle morphologic changes (lucency) in the spine of the right scapula, anterior aspect of T10, spinous process of

L2, and the anterior aspect of the left lateral femoral condyle, seen only retrospectively on CT.

*Chest*: Increased $^{18}$F-Fluoride uptake is seen in the spine of the right scapula corresponding to mixed lytic/sclerotic changes on CT.

*Upper limbs*: Increased uptake of $^{18}$F-Fluoride is seen in the head of the right humerus with a corresponding lucent area on CT.

*Lower limbs*: Increased uptake of $^{18}$F-Fluoride is seen in the right medial femoral condyle with a corresponding lytic lesion surrounded by some sclerosis. Similar findings, less prominent, are detected in the anterior aspect of the left lateral femoral condyle.

Impression

Multifocal skeletal lytic/sclerotic lesions showing increased $^{18}$F-Fluoride uptake. Multifocal osteomyelitis and malignant spread are the main differential diagnoses.

## Case III.2.5

### History

A 22-year-old male with Hodgkin's disease, 25 months after completion of chemotherapy, with no clinical or laboratory evidence of disease, was referred for routine follow-up $^{18}$F-FDG-PET/CT imaging. A year prior to the study, the patient underwent right hip joint replacement due to avascular necrosis of the femoral head. The images shown are those of the knee areas (Fig. III.2.5A, B).

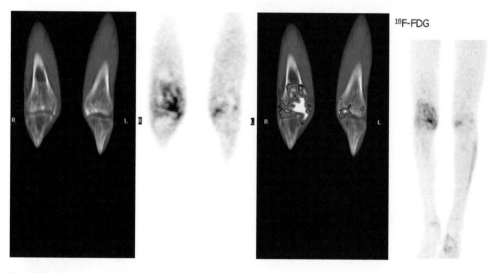

Fig. III.2.5A

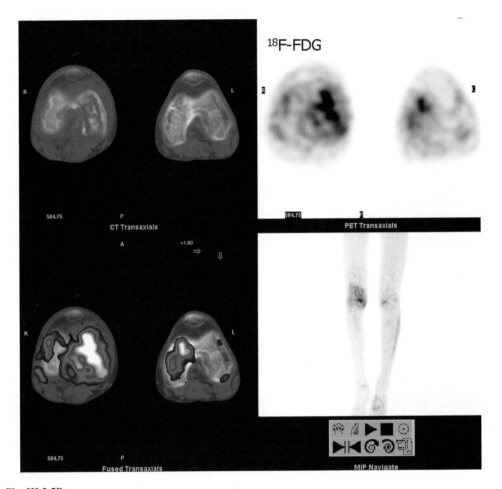

<sup>18</sup>F-FDG

**Fig. III.2.5B**

**Findings**

Increased $^{18}$F-FDG uptake around both knees, more prominent on the right, is demonstrated. The uptake appears to be located in the articular surface of the femoral condyles, mainly the medial, as well as the metaphysis, and in the articular surface of the tibia. CT demonstrates mixed lucent and sclerotic areas with a linear component, consistent with osteonecrosis (Fig. III 2.5A, B).

**Discussion**

This case illustrates a non-malignant skeletal abnormality – osteonecrosis – which may be associated with increased uptake of $^{18}$F-FDG in its active phase. Osteonecrosis (or infarction) may be idiopathic or associated with a variety of risk factors, most common alcohol abuse, or systemic antineoplastic and glucocorticosteroid treatment, as was the case in this patient. Osteonecrosis represents areas of dead trabecular bone. Its repair begins at the junction of the necrotic and viable bone, extending into the necrotic segment.[34–37] Inflammatory cells may reactively infiltrate the lesion during the pathogenesis and repair of osteonecrosis, probably contributing to the increased uptake of $^{18}$F-FDG, as described in several case reports.[38,39]

In the context of cancer patients, increased $^{18}$F-FDG uptake in bone infarction should be differentiated from malignant skeletal involvement. The diagnosis of osteonecrosis may be suggested by its periarticular location and the detection of corresponding morphologic changes on CT, which can differentiate between bone infarction and metastases. The present case diagnosis of osteonecrosis in both knees was validated by MRI, and the patient subsequently underwent right knee replacement.

**Diagnosis**

Osteonecrosis in both knees.

# References

1. Blake GM, Park-Holohan SJ, Cook GJ, Fogelman I. Quantitative studies of bone with the use of 18F-fluoride and 99mTc-methylene diphosphonate. *Semin Nucl Med* 2001;31:28–49.
2. Gates GF. SPECT bone scanning of the spine. *Semin Nucl Med* 1998;28:78–94.
3. Horger M, Bares R. The role of single-photon emission computed tomography/computed tomography in benign and malignant bone disease. *Semin Nucl Med* 2006;36:286–294.
4. Even-Sapir E, Martin RH, Barnes DC, Pringle CR, Iles SE, Mitchell MJ. Role of SPECT in differentiating malignant from benign lesions in the lower thoracic and lumbar vertebrae. *Radiology* 1993;187:193–198.
5. Hamaoka T, Madewell JE, Podoloff DA, Hortobagyi GN, Ueno NT. Bone imaging in metastatic breast cancer. *J Clin Oncol* 2004;22:2942–2953.
6. Even-Sapir E. Imaging of malignant bone involvement by morphologic, scintigraphic, and hybrid modalities. *J Nucl Med* 2005; 46:1356–1367.
7. Horger M, Eschmann SM, Pfannenberg C, Vonthein R, Besenfelder H, Claussen CD, Bares R. Evaluation of combined transmission and emission tomography for classification of skeletal lesions. *AJR* 2004;183:655–661.
8. Horger M, Eschmann SM, Pfannenberg C, Storek D, Vonthein R, Claussen CD, Bares R. Added value of SPECT/CT in patients suspected of having bone infection: preliminary results. *Arch Orthop Trauma Surg* 2007;127:211–221.
9. Even-Sapir E, Flusser G, Lerman H, Lievshitz G, Metser U. SPECT/multislice low-dose CT: A clinically relevant constituent in the imaging algorithm of non-oncologic patients referred for BS. *J Nucl Med* 2007;48:319–324.
10. Römer W, Nomayr A, Uder M, Bautz W, Kuwert T. SPECT-guided CT for evaluating foci of increased bone metabolism classified as indeterminate on SPECT in cancer patients. *J Nucl Med* 2006; 47:1102–1106.
11. Horger M, Claussen CD, Bross-Bach U, Vonthein R, Trabold T, Heuschmid M, and Pfannenberg C. Whole-body low-dose multidetector row-CT in the diagnosis of multiple myeloma: an alternative to conventional radiography. *Eur J Radiol* 2005;54:289–297.
12. Utsunomiya D, Shiraishi S, Imuta M, Tomiguchi S, Kawanaka K, Morishita S, Awai K, Yamashita Y. Added value of SPECT/CT fusion in assessing suspected bone metastasis: comparison with scintigraphy alone and nonfused scintigraphy and CT. *Radiology* 2006;238:264–271.
13. Strobel K, Burger C, Seifert B, Husarik DB, Soyka JD, Hany TF. Characterization of focal bone lesions in the axial skeleton: performance of planar BS compared with SPECT and SPECT fused with CT. *AJR* 2007;188:467–474.
14. McDonald M, Cooper R, Wang MY. Use of computed tomography-single-photon emission computed tomography fusion for diagnosing painful facet arthropathy. Technical note. *Neurosurg Focus* 2007;15:22:E2.
15. Langsteger W, Heinisch M, Fogelman I. The role of 18F-fluorodeoxyglucose, 18F-dihydroxyphenyla-lanine, 18F-choline, and 18F-fluoride in bone imaging with emphasis on prostate and breast. *Semin Nucl Med* 2006;36:73–92
16. Schirrmeister H. Detection of bone metastases in breast cancer by positron emission tomography. *Radiol Clin North Am* 2007;45:669–676.
17. Even-Sapir E, Metser U, Flusser G, Zuriel L, Kollender Y, Lerman H, Lievshitz G, Ron I, Mishani E. Assessment of malignant skeletal disease: Initial experience with 18F-fluoride PET/CT and comparison between 18F-fluoride PET and 18F-fluoride PET/CT. *J Nucl Med* 2004; 45:272–278
18. Even-Sapir E, Metser U, Mishani E, Lievshitz G, Lerman H, Leibovitch I. The detection of bone metastases in patients with high-risk prostate cancer: 99mTc-MDP planar BS, single- and multi-field-of-view SPECT, 18F-fluoride PET, and 18F-fluoride PET/CT. *J Nucl Med* 2006; 47:287–297.
19. Even-Sapir E, Mishani E, Flusser G, Metser U. 18F-Fluoride positron emission tomography and positron emission tomography/computed tomography. *Semin Nucl Med* 2007;37:462–469.
20. Ovadia D, Metser U, Lievshitz G, Yaniv M, Wientroub S, Even-Sapir E. Back pain in adolescents: assessment with integrated 18F-fluoride positron-emission tomography-computed tomography. *J Pediatr Orthop* 2007;27:90–93.
21. Lim R, Fahey FH, Drubach LA, Connolly LP, Treves ST. Early experience with fluorine-18 sodium fluoride bone PET in young patients with back pain. *J Pediatr Orthop* 2007;27:277–282.
22. Dimitrakopoulou-Strauss A, Strauss LG, Heichel T, Wu H, Burger C, Bernd L, Ewerbeck V. The role of quantitative $^{18}$F-FDG PET studies for the differentiation of malignant and benign bone lesions. *J Nucl Med* 2002;43:510–518.

23. Metser U, Even-Sapir E. Increased (18)F-fluorodeoxyglucose uptake in benign, non-physiologic lesions found on whole-body positron emission tomography/computed tomography (PET/CT): Accumulated data from four years of experience with PET/CT. *Semin Nucl Med* 2007;37:206–222.
24. Hartmann A, Eid K, Dora C, Trentz O, von Schulthess GK, Stumpe KD. Diagnostic value of 18F-FDG PET/CT in trauma patients with suspected chronic osteomyelitis. *Eur J Nucl Med Mol Imaging* 2007;34:704–714.
25. Keidar Z, Militianu D, Melamed E, Bar-Shalom R, Israel O. The diabetic foot: initial experience with 18F-FDG PET/CT. *J Nucl Med* 2005;46:444–449.
26. Beckers C, Jeukens X, Ribbens C, André B, Marcelis S, Leclercq P, Kaiser MJ, Foidart J, Hustinx R, Malaise MG. (18)F-FDG PET imaging of rheumatoid knee synovitis correlates with dynamic magnetic resonance and sonographic assessment as well as with the serum level of metalloproteinase-3.*Eur J Nucl Med Mol Imaging* 2006; 33:275–280.
27. Mahfouz T, Miceli MH, Saghafifar F, Stroud S, Jones-Jackson L, Walker R, Grazziutti ML, Purnell G, Fassas A, Tricot G, Barlogie B, Anaissie E. 18F-fluorodeoxyglucose positron emission tomography contributes to the diagnosis and management of infections in patients with multiple myeloma: A study of 165 infectious episodes. *J Clin Oncol* 2005; 23:7857–7863.
28. Kransdorf MJ, Moser RP Jr, Gilkey FW. Fibrous dysplasia. *Radiographics* 1990;10:519–537.
29. Val-Bernal JF, Val D, Garijo MF, Vega A, González-Vela MC. Subcutaneous ossifying lipoma: case report and review of the literature. *J Cutan Pathol* 2007;34:788–792.
30. Peh WC, Koh WL, Kwek JW, Htoo MM, Tan PH. Imaging of painful solitary lesions of the sacrum. *Australas Radiol* 2007;51:507–515.
31. Diel J, Ortiz O, Losada RA, Price DB, Hayt MW, Katz DS. The sacrum: pathologic spectrum, multimodality imaging, and subspecialty approach. *Radiographics* 2001;21:83–104.
32. Jurriaans E, Singh N, Finlay K, Friedman L. Imaging of chronic recurrent multifocal osteomyelitis. *Radiol Clin North Am* 2001;39:305–327.
33. Jurik AG. Chronic recurrent multifocal osteomyelitis. *Semin Musculoskelet Radiol* 2004;8:243–253.
34. Sawicka-Zukowska M, Kajdas L, Muszynska-Roslan K, Krawczuk-Rybak M, Sonta-Jakimczyk D, Szczepanski T. Avascular necrosis – an antineoplastic-treatment-related toxicity: the experiences of two institutions. *Pediatr Hematol Oncol* 2006;23:625–629.
35. Enrici RM, Anselmo AP, Donato V, Santoro M, Tombolini V. Avascular osteonecrosis in patients treated for Hodgkin's disease. *Eur J Haematol* 1998;61:204–209.
36. Cruess RL. Osteonecrosis of bone. Current concepts as to etiology and pathogenesis. *Clin Orthop Relat Res* 1986;208:30–33.
37. Mont MA, Jones LC, Hungerford DS. Nontraumatic osteonecrosis of the femoral head: Ten years later. *J Bone Joint Surg Am* 2006;88:1117–1132.
38. Grigolon MV, Delbeke D. F-18 FDG uptake in a bone infarct: a case report. *Clin Nucl Med* 2001;26:613–614.
39. Sohn MH, Jeong HJ, Lim ST, Song SH, Yim CY. FDG uptake in osteonecrosis mimicking bone metastasis on PET/CT images. *Clin Nucl Med* 2007;32:496–497.

# Chapter III.3
# Infectious and Inflammatory Diseases

Christopher J. Palestro, Zohar Keidar, and Charito Love

## Introduction

The detection and localization of inflammation and infection with nuclear medicine techniques has been studied for nearly half a century. The most commonly performed procedures are skeletal (for osteomyelitis), [67]Ga citrate, and in vitro labeled leukocyte scintigraphy. Positron emission tomography (PET) with [18]F-fluorodeoxyglucose ([18]F-FDG) also has proved to be useful, and its role in imaging inflammation and infection will undoubtedly increase in the future. Radiotracers, regardless of whether they are single-photon- or positron-emitting agents, primarily reflect function. Only gross anatomic details can be inferred from radionuclide images. The anatomic details that can be critical to differentiating physiologic from pathologic processes often are lacking. Integrating scintigraphic and anatomic images can significantly improve diagnostic confidence and test accuracy for the assessment of infectious and inflammatory processes.[1]

## Radionuclide Procedures

### Skeletal Scintigraphy

Skeletal scintigraphy is performed with [99m]Tc-labeled diphosphonates, usually methylene diphosphonate (MDP). Tracer uptake is dependent on blood flow and rate of new bone formation. When done for suspected osteomyelitis, three-phase skeletal scintigraphy usually is performed. It is widely available, relatively inexpensive, and easily performed. Skeletal scintigraphy is extremely sensitive, can be positive within 2 days after onset of symptoms, and has an accuracy of more than 90% in bones not affected by underlying conditions. Abnormalities on skeletal scintigraphy reflect the rate of new bone formation in general, not infection specifically, and, in the setting of violated bone, the test is less specific and therefore less useful.[2]

C.J. Palestro (✉)
Albert Einstein College of Medicine of Yeshiva University, Bronx, NY, USA; Division of Nuclear Medicine and Molecular Imaging, North Shore Long Island Jewish Health System, Manhasset and New Hyde Park, Bronx, NY, USA
e-mail: palestro@lij.edu

D. Delbeke, O. Israel (eds.), *Hybrid PET/CT and SPECT/CT Imaging*,
DOI 10.1007/978-0-387-92820-3_20, © Springer Science+Business Media, LLC 2010

# $^{67}$Gallium Scintigraphy

$^{67}$Gallium ($^{67}$Ga) citrate has been used for localizing infection for nearly 40 years. Several factors govern the uptake of this tracer in inflammation and infection. About 90% of circulating $^{67}$Ga is in the plasma, and nearly all of it is bound to transferrin. Increased blood flow and increased vascular membrane permeability result in increased delivery and accumulation of transferrin-bound $^{67}$Ga at sites of infection and inflammation. $^{67}$Ga also binds to lactoferrin, which is present in high concentrations in inflammatory foci. Direct bacterial uptake has been observed in vitro. Siderophores, low molecular weight chelates produced by bacteria, are $^{67}$Ga avid. The siderophore–gallium complex is presumably transported into the bacterium, where it remains until phagocytosed by macrophages. Some $^{67}$Ga may be transported bound to leukocytes, but it is important to note that even in patients with few or no circulating white cells, the test remains sensitive.

Imaging usually is performed 18–72 h after injection of 185–370 MBq (5–10 mCi) $^{67}$Ga citrate. The normal biodistribution of $^{67}$Ga, which can be variable, includes bone, bone marrow, liver, urinary and gastrointestinal tract, and soft tissues. Once the mainstay of nuclear medicine infection imaging, primary indications for $^{67}$Ga citrate imaging at the present time include fever of unknown origin (FUO), opportunistic infection, spinal osteomyelitis, pulmonary inflammatory conditions, granulomatous diseases including tuberculosis and sarcoidosis, and interstitial nephritis.[3]

# Labeled Leukocyte Scintigraphy

Although a variety of in vitro leukocyte-labeling techniques have been used, the most commonly employed procedures use $^{111}$In-oxine and $^{99m}$Tc-exametazime (hexamethylpropyleneamine oxime, HMPAO). The labeling process takes about 2–3 h, involves withdrawal of blood from the patient, separation of leukocytes from other blood elements, labeling of the cells, and finally reinjection of the labeled cells. The usual dose of $^{111}$In-oxine-labeled leukocytes is 10–18.5 MBq (0.3–0.5 mCi) and the usual dose of $^{99m}$Tc-exametazime-labeled leukocytes is 185–370 MBq (5–10 mCi).[3]

Labeled white cell uptake depends on intact chemotaxis, the number and types of cells labeled, and the cellular response in a particular condition. The labeling of white cells, now a routine procedure, does not affect their chemotactic response. A total white count of at least 2000/mL is needed to obtain diagnostically useful images. In the average clinical setting, the majority of leukocytes labeled are neutrophils, and the procedure is most useful for identifying neutrophil-mediated inflammatory processes, such as bacterial infections. The procedure is less useful for those illnesses in which the predominant cellular response is other than neutrophilic, such as tuberculosis.[3]

Regardless of whether leukocytes are labeled with $^{111}$In or $^{99m}$Tc, images obtained shortly after injection are characterized by intense pulmonary activity, which clears rapidly and is probably due to leukocyte activation during labeling, which impedes their movement through the pulmonary vascular bed, prolonging their passage through the lungs.[3]

At 24 h after injection, the usual imaging time for $^{111}$In-labeled leukocytes, the normal distribution of activity is limited to the liver, spleen, and bone marrow. Advantages of the $^{111}$In label, in addition to a constant biodistribution, include a very stable label, with little elution from leukocytes. The 67 h physical half-life of $^{111}$In allows for delayed imaging, which is useful for musculoskeletal infection. There is another advantage to the use of

[111]In-labeled leukocytes in musculoskeletal infection. These patients often require bone or marrow scintigraphy, which can be performed while the patient's cells are being labeled, as simultaneous dual isotope acquisitions, or immediately after completion of the labeled leukocyte study. Disadvantages of the [111]In label include a low photon flux and less than ideal photon energies for imaging. This is an important consideration when contemplating tomographic imaging.[3]

The normal biodistribution of [99m]Tc-exametazime-labeled leukocytes is more variable than that of [111]In-labeled white cells. In addition to the reticuloendothelial system, activity is also normally present in the urinary tract, large bowel (within 4 h after injection), and occasionally the gallbladder.

Advantages of [99m]Tc-labeled white cells include the ability to detect abnormalities within a few hours after injection and a photon energy that is optimal for imaging using current instrumentation, which is important for tomographic imaging. Disadvantages include genitourinary tract and colonic activity. The time interval between injection of [99m]Tc-exametazime-labeled leukocytes and imaging varies with the indication. Imaging usually is performed within a few hours after injection.[3] The instability of the label and the short half-life of [99m]Tc are relative disadvantages when delayed 24 h imaging is needed. When indicated, [99m]Tc-labeled bone marrow scans can be performed 24 h later.[3]

In vitro labeled scintigraphy is the modality of choice for imaging infection (except for spinal osteomyelitis) in the immunocompetent population.[3]

# [18]F-FDG Imaging

[18]F-FDG is transported into cells via glucose transporters and phosphorylated to [18]F-2'-FDG-6 phosphate, but it is not metabolized. Cellular uptake of [18]F-FDG is related to the cellular metabolic rate and to the number of glucose transporters. Activated leukocytes demonstrate increased glucose transporter expression, and the affinity of glucose transporters for deoxyglucose presumably is increased by circulating cytokines and growth factors.[4]

[18]F-FDG has several potential advantages over conventional nuclear medicine tests. Results are available within 1 to 2 h after tracer administration. Physiologic[18]F-FDG uptake in most normal organs, except for the heart, brain, and urinary tract, is quite low, resulting in relatively high target to background ratios. Bone marrow has a low glucose metabolism under physiological conditions, which may facilitate the distinction of inflammatory cellular infiltrates from hematopoietic marrow. Degenerative bone changes usually show only faintly increased [18]F-FDG uptake compared to infection. [18]F-FDG PET has a distinctly higher spatial resolution than images obtained with single photon emitting tracers. [18]F-FDG itself is also less expensive than combined labeled leukocyte/bone marrow/bone scans. The exquisite sensitivity of the test makes [18]F-FDG especially useful in FUO, an entity with diverse etiologies. In addition to tumor and infection, vasculitis, thromboembolic disease, sarcoidosis, and chronic granulomatous disease, all of which can present as FUO, are associated with increased [18]F-FDG uptake.[4-7]

[18]F-FDG imaging is quite sensitive for detecting focal infection, with a negative predictive value of about 90%. [18]F-FDG imaging has proven to be sensitive for detecting infected prosthetic vascular grafts, mycotic aneurysms, lung abscesses, and intraabdominal infections.[7] [18]F-FDG imaging also is playing an increasingly important role in diagnosing musculoskeletal infection, especially in the setting of previous trauma and metallic implants. [18]F-FDG uptake in uninfected fractures rapidly normalizes, thus facilitating the differentiation between fracture and infection.[6]

## Case Presentations

### *Case III.3.1*

#### History

This 11-year-old male with acute lymphoblastic leukemia presented with *Escherichia coli* septicemia, 3 weeks of fever, which had not responded to antibiotic therapy, and with no localizing signs or symptoms. $^{67}$Ga SPECT/CT was performed (Fig. III 3.1A, B).

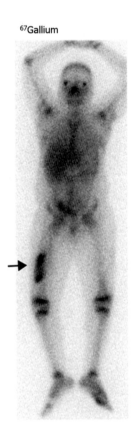

**Fig. III.3.1A**

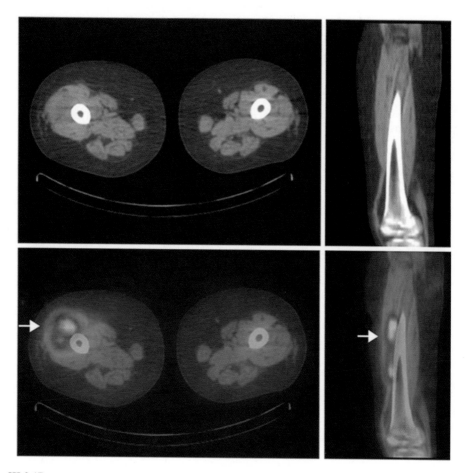

**Fig. III.3.1B**

### Findings

The anterior whole-body image (Fig. III.3.1A), performed 24 h after intravenous administration of 150 MBq (4 mCi) $^{67}$Ga citrate, shows an area of increased tracer uptake in the right mid-thigh (arrow). The transaxial (left) and sagittal (right) SPECT/CT images (Fig. III.3.1B) demonstrate that the abnormal uptake is confined to a hypodense region in the lateral aspect of the quadriceps muscle (arrows) and does not involve the bone.

### Discussion

The right thigh abnormality on the $^{67}$Ga scintigraphy is obvious. Its precise location to bone or soft tissue, however, is not. The CT component of the test confirms that the abnormality is confined to the soft tissues. Several investigations, using various tracers, have shown the value of SPECT/CT for differentiating soft tissue from skeletal infection. As part of a larger investigation, Bar-Shalom and colleagues[8] reviewed the results of SPECT/CT in 32 patients suspected of having osteomyelitis, including 21 who underwent

$^{67}$Ga imaging. SPECT/CT was contributory in 48% of the 21 patients. The principal contributions of SPECT/CT were precise anatomic localization and delineation of the extent of the infectious process after its scintigraphic detection.

## Diagnosis

Right quadriceps abscess.

## Case III.3.2

### History

Ten months after undergoing reconstructive jaw surgery, including a mandibular bone graft, this 37-year-old male developed left facial swelling and tenderness. He had no systemic signs of infection. $^{67}$Ga citrate scintigraphy was performed (Fig. III.3.2A, B).

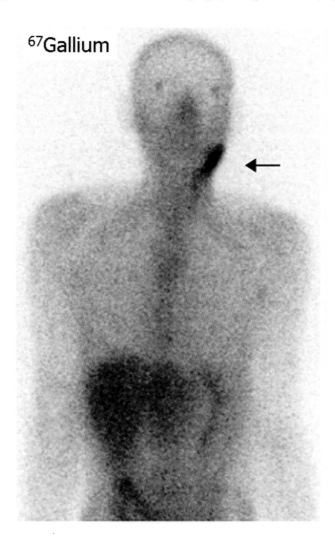

**Fig. III.3.2A**

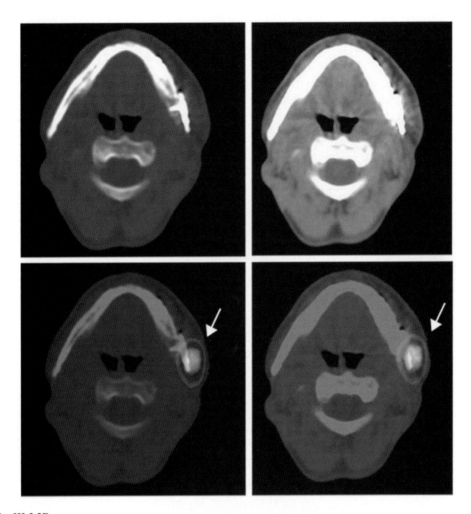

**Fig. III.3.2B**

**Findings**

The anterior whole-body scan (Fig. II.3.2A) obtained 24 h after injection of 185 MBq (5 mCi) [67]Ga citrate shows an area of increased tracer uptake in the left side of the face and neck (arrow). Transaxial SPECT/CT images (Fig. III.3.2B) demonstrate that the abnormal tracer uptake involves the soft tissues of the upper left neck and face as well as the posterior aspect of the bone graft (arrows).

**Discussion**

The value of [67]Ga citrate imaging for infection of the skull and skull base is well documented. The anatomy of the skull is complex, however, making tracer localization, even with SPECT, difficult. Moschilla and colleagues[9] explored the use of $^{67}$Ga citrate SPECT/ CT in focal infections involving the skull and skull base. These investigators found that the addition of morphologic imaging improved both accuracy and diagnostic confidence.

**Diagnosis**

1. Soft tissue abscess
2. Osteomyelitis of the bone graft

## Case III.3.3

### History

This 20-year-old female with a history of vasculitis, steroid-related diabetes mellitus, and a non-healing ulcer along the lateral aspect of the left ankle underwent planar $^{99m}$Tc-MDP and $^{111}$In-labeled leukocyte SPECT/CT imaging for suspected osteomyelitis (Fig. III.3.3A–C).

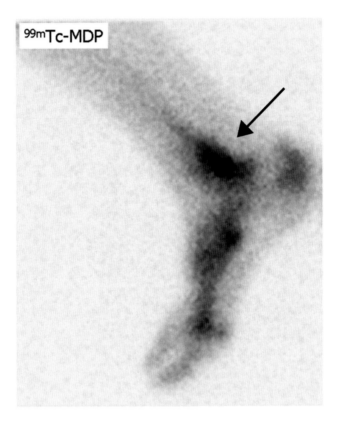

**Fig. III.3.3A**

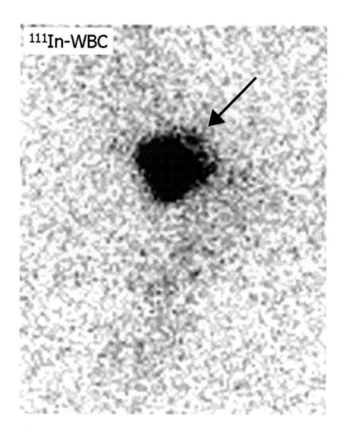

**Fig. III.3.3B**

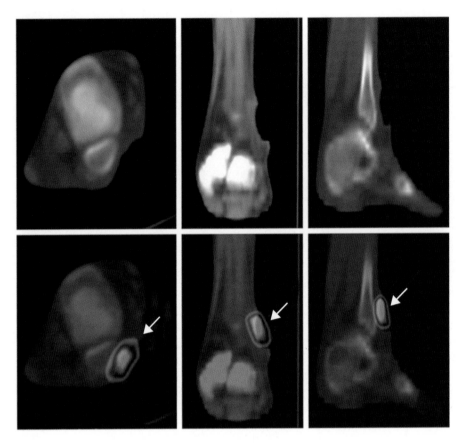

**Fig. III.3.3C**

### Findings

Planar skeletal scintigraphy (Fig. III.3.3A) performed 4 h after injection of 875 MBq (23 mCi) $^{99m}$Tc-MDP shows intense tracer uptake in the left fibula. Planar $^{111}$In-labeled leukocyte image (Fig. III.3.3B) shows intense tracer uptake in the postero-lateral aspect of the left ankle (arrow), although it is not possible to determine whether this uptake involves soft tissue, bone, or both. The $^{111}$In-labeled leukocyte SPECT/CT (Fig. III.3.3C) demonstrates that the abnormality is confined to a large deep ulcer in the soft tissues (arrows), adjacent to, but not involving, the fibula.

### Discussion

Skeletal scintigraphy is extremely sensitive, but as this case illustrates, it is not specific for osteomyelitis, and complementary labeled leukocyte imaging is frequently performed.[2] Labeled leukocyte images are relatively count poor, especially when $^{111}$In is the radiolabel, with few or no anatomic landmarks.[2] Differentiating soft tissue from skeletal uptake can be challenging, particularly in the distal extremities. Several recent publications confirm the incremental value of SPECT/CT in patients with musculoskeletal infection. Horger and coworkers[10] compared SPECT/CT to three-phase skeletal imaging, including SPECT, in 31 patients suspected of having skeletal infection. Nine patients had osteomyelitis. The sensitivities of the three-phase skeletal scintigraphy and SPECT/CT both were 78%. The specificity of SPECT/CT was significantly higher (86 versus 50%, $p < 0.05$). These investigators found that the CT component of the test improved specificity by excluding active skeletal infection and by identifying abnormalities other than infection, responsible for increased tracer uptake.

As part of a larger investigation, Bar-Shalom and colleagues[8] reviewed the results of SPECT/CT in 32 patients suspected of having osteomyelitis, including 11 who underwent [111]In-labeled leukocyte imaging. SPECT/CT was contributory in 55% of the 11 patients. Filippi and coworkers[11] evaluated [99m]Tc-exametazime-labeled leukocyte scintigraphy with and without SPECT/CT in 28 patients, including 13 with orthopedic implants, suspected of having musculoskeletal infection. They reported an accuracy of 64% for scintigraphy (including SPECT) alone and of 100% for SPECT/CT. Fused images significantly changed the interpretation of the study in 36% of the patients. The improved localization of the labeled white cells enabled by the CT component of the test resulted in the exclusion of osteomyelitis in seven patients and provided a more precise delineation of the extent of infection in three patients. SPECT/CT did not contribute additional information in patients with negative planar scans. Horger and colleagues[12], using a [99m]Tc-labeled anti-granulocyte antibody, evaluated the role of SPECT/CT in 27 patients with a history of trauma and superimposed skeletal infection. The accuracy of scintigraphy (including SPECT) alone was 59%, while that of SPECT/CT was 97%. SPECT/CT was especially useful for distinguishing soft tissue infection from osteomyelitis in the appendicular skeleton. Interobserver agreement was stronger for SPECT/CT (k=1.0) than for scintigraphy alone (k=0.68).

**Diagnosis**

Soft tissue infection lateral aspect of the left ankle.

## Case III.3.4

### History

This 51-year-old diabetic female presented with fever, weakness, and severe mid-back pain radiating to the right and, based on a chest x-ray, was diagnosed with pneumonia. She did not respond to antibiotic therapy and was referred for $^{67}$Ga citrate SPECT/CT imaging to identify other sites of infection (Fig. III.3.4A, B).

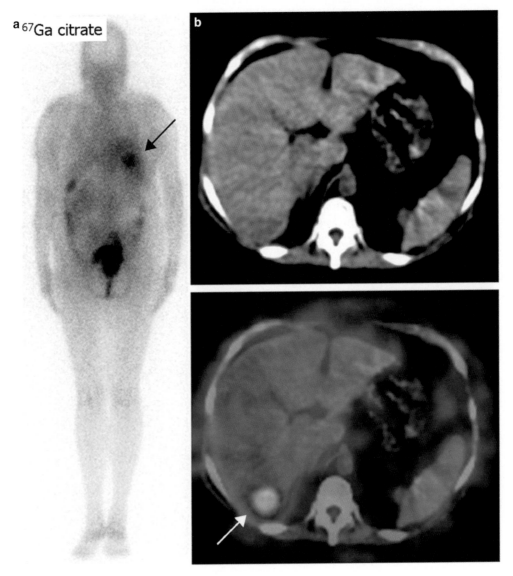

Fig. III.3.4A, B

**Findings**

The posterior whole-body image (Fig. III.3.4A) performed 24 h after injection of 185 MBq (5 mCi) $^{67}$Ga citrate shows a focal area of increased tracer accumulation in the right lower thorax/upper abdomen (arrow). SPECT/CT (Fig. III.3.4B) localizes the abnormality to a hypodense region (arrow) in the upper posterior aspect of the right lobe of the liver.

**Discussion**

This case illustrates the value of contemporaneous morphologic imaging in localizing a scintigraphically identified abnormality, which in this patient could be pulmonary, supra- or subdiaphragmatic, or intrahepatic in location. Bar-Shalom and colleagues[8] studied SPECT-CT in 82 patients for various indications. Thirteen patients underwent $^{67}$Ga citrate imaging for FUO and thirteen for soft tissue infection. Among these 26 patients SPECT/CT contributed important information in 27%, including 4 with FUO and 3 with soft tissue infection. The main value of SPECT/CT was the improved anatomical localization of an infectious process and the delineation of the extent of infection after its diagnosis on scintigraphy.

**Diagnosis**

Hepatic abscess.

## *Case III.3.5*

### History

This 53-year-old diabetic male, who had recently undergone amputation of the first right toe, developed purulent drainage and an abscess in the right forefoot, which did not respond to antibiotics or hyperbaric oxygen therapy. He was referred for evaluation for suspected osteomyelitis. [18]F-FDG PET/CT imaging was performed (Fig. III.3.5A–C).

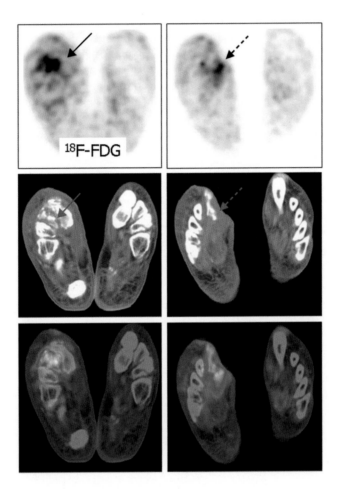

**Fig. III.3.5**

### Findings

The patient's fasting blood glucose level at the time of injection of 222 MBq (6 mCi) [18]F-FDG was 260 mg/dL. Transaxial PET images (Fig. III.3.5 top row), performed about 1 h after tracer injection, show areas of intense [18]F-FDG uptake in the mid (solid arrow) and medial (broken arrow) regions of the distal right forefoot. It is not possible to determine if this uptake is confined to the soft tissues or involves the bone. On the CT component (Fig. III.3.5 center row) of the examination, there is destruction of the right medial cuneiform bone (solid arrow) and the right first metatarsal (broken arrow). The fused images (Fig. III.3.5 bottom row) confirm that the two abnormal foci of [18]F-FDG uptake correspond to the areas of osseous destruction seen on the CT.

## Discussion

Diabetes mellitus affects about 5% of the U.S. population. The most common complication in the diabetic fore foot is the mal perforans ulcer, accounting for more than 90% of all cases of diabetic pedal osteomyelitis. Many patients with pedal osteomyelitis present without systemic illness and lack obvious clinical signs and symptoms, other than an ulcer. Establishing the diagnosis of osteomyelitis in the presence of contiguous soft tissue infection or altered bony anatomy often is difficult. Laboratory tests such as circulating white cell count, erythrocyte sedimentation rate, and C-reactive protein are of limited value. Imaging studies, both morphological and functional, are part of the diagnostic evaluation. The current radionuclide gold standard for diagnosing diabetic pedal osteomyelitis is labeled leukocyte imaging, with an accuracy of about 80%.[2] A major limitation to this test, however, is the poor resolution of the images, making it difficult, even in the larger bones of the mid and hind foot, to differentiate soft tissue from skeletal infection.

At the present time, there are few data about the use of [18]F-FDG PET and PET/CT in diabetic pedal osteomyelitis. Höpfner and colleagues[13] reported that [18]F-FDG PET reliably differentiated osteomyelitis from the neuropathic joint and from nonspecific soft tissue infection. More recently, Schwegler and coworkers[14] reported that, in a series of 21 diabetic patients, [18]F-FDG PET detected only two of seven cases of pedal osteomyelitis. The accuracy of the test was adversely affected by motion artifact and limited spatial resolution due to the small size of the structures being imaged. Keidar and colleagues[15] studied [18]F-FDG PET/CT in 14 diabetic patients with 18 suspected sites of pedal osteomyelitis. PET, CT, and fused images were independently evaluated for diagnosis and localization of foci of infection. Additional information provided by PET/CT about localization of the infection to bone or soft tissue was recorded. [18]F-FDG PET detected 14 sites of infection in ten patients. It was not possible on the basis of PET alone to localize the abnormal uptake to bone or soft tissue. PET/CT localized eight foci in four patients, to bone and excluded osteomyelitis in five sites in five patients. One site of mildly increased [18]F-FDG uptake was localized on PET/CT to an area of diabetic osteoarthropathy.

## Diagnosis

1. Osteomyelitis of the right medial cuneiform bone
2. Osteomyelitis of the right first metatarsal bone

## Case III.3.6

### History

This 65-year-old male with a history of severe atherosclerotic vascular disease underwent numerous revascularization procedures including an aorto-bifemoral bypass, two right femoro-popliteal bypass grafts, left femoro-popliteal and a fem–fem bypass graft. The patient presented with fever, right thigh swelling, and local pain and underwent $^{18}$F-FDG PET/CT for suspected graft infection (Fig. III.3.6A–C).

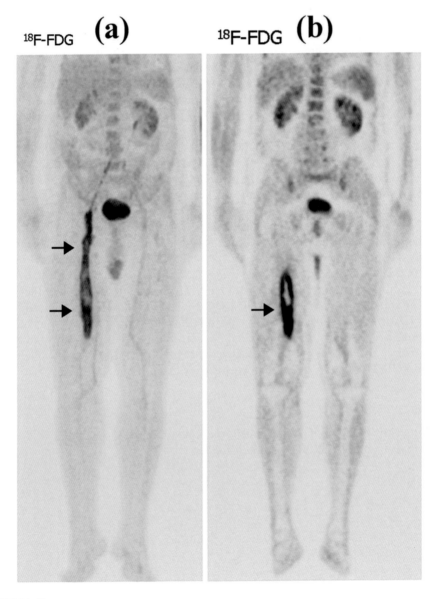

**Fig. III.3.6A, B**

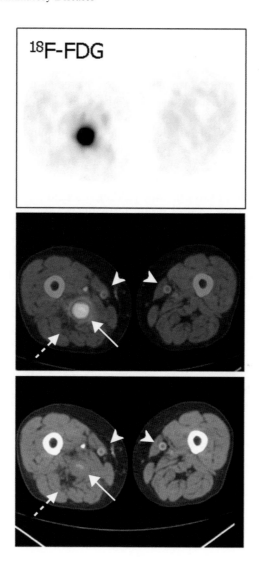

**Fig. III.3.6C**

## Findings

The patient's fasting blood glucose level was 100 mg/dL at the time of injection of 518 MBq (14 mCi) [18]F-FDG. Imaging was performed about 90 min later. Maximal intensity projection (MIP) image (Fig. III.3.6A) and coronal PET image (Fig. III.3.6B) show a linear area of intense [18]F-FDG activity along the medial aspect of the right thigh (arrows). Transaxial PET/CT images through the mid-thigh (Fig. III.3.6C) localize the increased [18]F-FDG uptake to the original right femoro-popliteal bypass graft (solid arrow) surrounded by a hypodense area of soft tissue swelling (broken arrow). The uninfected vascular grafts (arrowheads) do not concentrate [18]F-FDG.

**Discussion**

Although the rate of infection following placement of a prosthetic vascular graft is less than 5%, morbidity and mortality range from about 20 to 75% when present. Radionuclide studies, especially labeled leukocyte imaging, often are used in the diagnostic workup of this entity.[3] Initial reports about the value of [18]F-FDG PET and PET/CT for diagnosing vascular graft infection are promising.[16–18] Keidar and colleagues[18] evaluated [18]F-FDG PET/CT in the diagnosis of prosthetic vascular graft infection in 39 patients, with 69 vascular grafts. Forty of the 69 grafts were suspected of being infected, including 38 patients with possible infection in one graft and one patient with possible infection of two grafts. Fifteen grafts in this series were infected. [18]F-FDG PET/CT was true positive in 14, false negative in one, and false positive in two, yielding a sensitivity and specificity of 93 and 91%, respectively. Both false positive results were due to infected hematomas adjacent to the graft. In the one false negative study, uptake was localized to soft tissues adjacent to the infected graft. The precise localization of [18]F-FDG uptake provided by PET/CT enabled the accurate differentiation between graft and soft tissue infection.

Similar results have been reported using labeled leukocyte SPECT/CT imaging for prosthetic vascular graft infection. Bar-Shalom and colleagues[8] reported that, among 24 patients who underwent labeled leukocyte imaging for possible vascular graft infection, SPECT CT contributed additional information in 67%.

**Diagnosis**

Infected right femoro-popliteal graft.

## Case III.3.7A (DICOM Images on DVD)

### History

This is a 10-year-old female with a history of general malaise and intermittent fever over several months, with no localizing signs or symptoms. Laboratory tests, plain x-rays, and ultrasound were noncontributory, and the patient was referred for further evaluation with $^{18}$F-FDG PET/CT (Fig. III.3.7Aa,b).

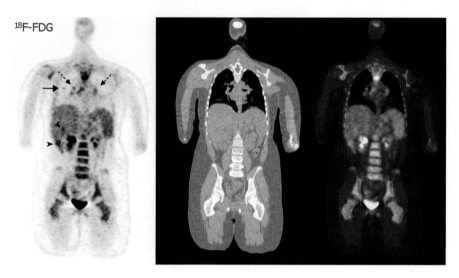

**Fig. III.3.7Aa**

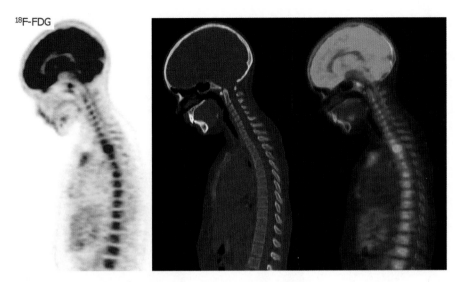

**Fig. III.3.7Ab**

## Findings

The patient's fasting blood glucose level was 85 mg/dL at the time of injection of 370 MBq (10 mCi) $^{18}$F-FDG. Imaging was performed about 60 min later. A representative coronal image (Fig. III.3.7Aa) demonstrates hypermetabolic foci in the right lung (solid arrow), both hilar regions (broken arrows), and in the liver (arrowheads). There is focal intense hypermetabolism in an upper thoracic vertebra, approximately T3, which is best appreciated in the sagittal image (Fig. III.3.7Ab).

## Diagnosis

Biopsy demonstrated non-Hodgkin's lymphoma.

## Clinical Report: Body $^{18}$F-FDG PET/CT (for DVD cases only)

History

This is a 10-year-old female with history of general malaise and intermittent fever over several months, with no localizing signs or symptoms. Laboratory tests, plain x-rays, and ultrasound were noncontributory, and the patient was referred for further evaluation with $^{18}$F-FDG PET/CT.

Procedure

The patient fasted for more than 4 h and had a normal blood glucose level (86 mg/dL) prior to $^{18}$F-FDG injection. PET acquisition was performed using a PET/CT scanner with a low-dose CT used for anatomical correlation and attenuation correction. Oral contrast was used. PET emission images were started approximately 60 min after IV injection of

370 MBq (10 mCi) of $^{18}$F-FDG and covered the area from the vertex of the skull to the knees.

Findings

> *Quality of Study*: The quality of the study is good. There is physiologic distribution of the radiopharmaceutical in the brain and myocardium.
>
> *Head and neck*: There is symmetrically increased uptake in the tonsillar regions bilaterally (maximum standardized uptake values (SUV) on the right is 8.9, on the left is 8.4).
>
> *Chest*: There is a focus of mildly increased uptake in the right paratracheal region, maximum SUV 3.3, with no corresponding abnormality on the CT portion of the study. There are multiple hypermetabolic foci in both lungs, corresponding to multiple lung nodules, mostly in the periphery, on the CT component. As a reference, a left upper lobe nodule has a maximum SUV of 4.6, a right mid-lung nodule has a maximum SUV of 1.6, and a right lower lobe nodule has a maximum SUV of 1.6. Several other pulmonary nodules are seen on the transmission CT scan, not $^{18}$F-FDG avid but also below the limits of resolution of the system.
>
> There is mildly increased uptake in the hilar regions bilaterally (maximum SUV is 3.3 on the left and 3.0 on the right) with no obvious abnormality on the noncontrast CT component of this study. There is physiologic $^{18}$F-FDG activity in the rest of the mediastinum and in the axillary regions.
>
> *Abdomen*: There are foci of increased $^{18}$F-FDG uptake in the midline of the mid-abdomen (maximum SUV 5.8) and in the periportal region (maximum SUV 5.3), which correspond to poorly defined soft tissue masses and lymphadenopathy on the CT component of the test. There is focally increased activity in the cecal region (maximum SUV 8.8) with no corresponding abnormality on the CT. There are several small foci of increased $^{18}$F-FDG uptake in the liver (maximum SUV ranging from 3.2 to 5.0) with no corresponding abnormalities identified on the CT component of this study. The right collecting system and ureter are prominent.
>
> *Pelvis*: There is mild hypermetabolism in the right inguinal region (maximum SUV 2.3) corresponding to a lymph node with a fatty hilum on CT.
>
> *Musculoskeletal System*: There is focal, intense hypermetabolism in an upper thoracic vertebra, approximately T3, (maximum SUV 11.5), with no corresponding abnormality on the CT component of the study. The remainder of the osseous structures are unremarkable.

Impression

1. Hypermetabolic foci in T3 vertebra, both lungs, right paratracheal region, both hila, the liver, and periportal and mesenteric lymph nodes. Findings are most suggestive of a malignant process and biopsy should be considered.
2. Nonspecific cecal tracer uptake. Clinical correlation and colonoscopic evaluation, as clinically indicated, are recommended.
3. Prominent right collecting system and ureter. Diuretic renography can be performed if indicated.
4. Symmetrical hypermetabolism in the tonsillar regions, probably inflammatory.

## Case III.3.7B

### History

This 48-year-old male with insulin-dependent diabetes mellitus presented with 3 weeks of fever and general malaise without any localizing signs or symptoms. Laboratory and imaging investigations including microbial and virological assays, chest and abdomen CT, and abdominal ultrasound were noncontributory, and the patient was referred for further evaluation with $^{18}$F-FDG PET/CT imaging (Fig. III.3.7B).

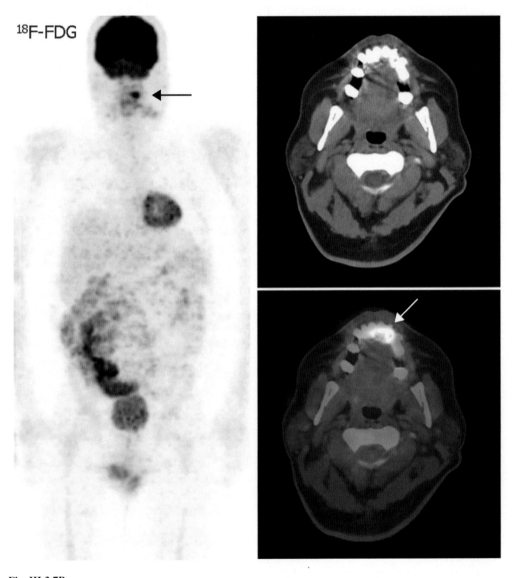

**Fig. III.3.7B**

**Findings**

The patient's fasting blood glucose level was 67 mg/dL at the time of injection of 205 MBq (5.5 mCi) $^{18}$F-FDG. Imaging was performed about 90 min later. MIP image (Fig. III.3.7B left) shows focal $^{18}$F-FDG uptake in the region of the left jaw (arrow). Transaxial CT and fused images (Fig. III.3.7B right) localize the abnormality to the maxilla (arrow).

**Diagnosis**

Dental abscess.

**Follow-Up**

The patient underwent extraction of three teeth, and the fever resolved within a few days.

## Case III.3.7C

### History

Within a few days after undergoing an uncomplicated live-donor renal transplant, this 21-year-old female developed fever and septicemia. The patient failed to respond to appropriate antibiotic therapy, and $^{18}$F-FDG-PET/CT imaging was performed (Fig. III.3.7Ca,b,c).

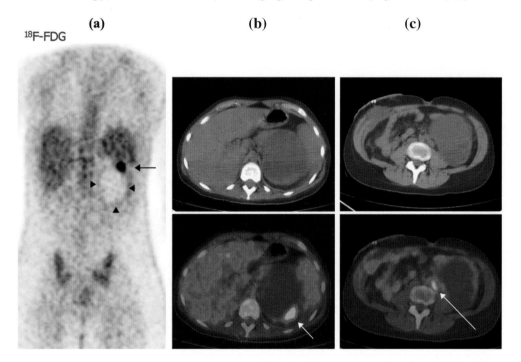

**Fig. III.3.7Ca,b,c**

## Findings

The patient's fasting blood glucose level was 97 mg/dL at the time of injection of 235 MBq (6.3 mCi) [18]F-FDG. Imaging was performed about 90 min later. Representative coronal PET image (Fig. III.3.7Ca) shows an area of intense [18]F-FDG focus (arrow) just below the spleen. This focus is just above a large hypometabolic region (arrowheads). Transaxial CT and fused images (Fig. III.3.7Cb) localize this focus to the upper margin of a very large hydronephrotic left kidney (arrow). Transaxial CT and fused images (Fig. III.3.7 Cc) at the level of L3 demonstrate hypermetabolism in a paravertebral lymph node measuring $16 \times 8$ mm (arrow).

## Diagnosis

Infected left renal cyst.
Reactive lymph node

## Follow-Up

Pus was drained percutaneously from the cyst, the patient underwent a course of antibiotic therapy and recovered.

## Discussion for Cases III.3.7A, B, and C

Fever of unknown (undetermined) origin, or FUO, usually is defined as an illness of at least 3 weeks duration, with several episodes of fever exceeding 38.3°C, and no diagnosis after an appropriate inpatient or outpatient evaluation. There are numerous causes of FUO. Infection accounts for about 20–30% and tumor for about 10% of the cases. Other etiologies include thromboembolic disease, collagen, vascular or granulomatous disease, cerebrovascular accidents, and drug fever. Identifying the source of FUO often is difficult, and radionuclide studies are an important part of the diagnostic evaluation of this entity. Labeled leukocyte imaging is more sensitive in the acute setting, whereas [67]Ga citrate may be more sensitive in the chronic setting, and the selection of the procedure is sometimes governed by the duration of the illness. Because the etiologies of the FUO are so diverse, some individuals prefer the sensitive, but nonspecific [67]Ga citrate as the initial radionuclide study. Regardless of which study is performed first, however, it may take several days before both procedures are completed.[3]

The use of [18]F-FDG poses no such problems. Like [67]Ga citrate, though not specific, [18]F-FDG is sensitive, which is an important consideration when investigating an entity with diverse etiologies. Furthermore, the short half-life of [18]F does not delay the performance of any additional radionuclide studies that might be contemplated. Several investigations confirm the value of [18]F-FDG PET in the workup of the patient with FUO.[19–23] Blockmans and colleagues[20] evaluated 58 patients with FUO and reported that [18]F-FDG PET was helpful in 41% of cases. Forty of the patients underwent [67]Ga citrate imaging and in this subgroup [18]F-FDG PET was helpful in 35% of the cases as compared to [67]Ga citrate that was helpful in 25%. [18]F-FDG PET compared therefore favorably with and could replace [67]Ga citrate imaging in this population. Meller and coworkers[21] prospectively evaluated the utility of [18]F-FDG PET using a coincidence camera in 20 patients with FUO and found that [18]F-FDG imaging had a sensitivity of 84% and specificity of 86% for identifying the source of the FUO. In a subgroup of 18 patients who also underwent [67]Ga scintigraphy, [18]F-FDG was more sensitive (81%) and specific (86%) than $^{67}$Ga citrate (67% sensitivity, 78% specificity). Bleeker-Rovers and colleagues[22] evaluated 35 patients with FUO. $^{18}$F-FDG PET was clinically helpful in 37% of the cases. The sensitivity and specificity of the test were 93% and 90%, respectively. The positive predictive value of the test was 87%, and the negative predictive value was 95%.

Initial data suggest that the high predictive value of a negative $^{18}$F-FDG PET study makes it very unlikely that a morphological origin of the fever will be identified if the $^{18}$F-FDG-PET study is negative. Should future investigations confirm these data, it is entirely possible that $^{18}$F-FDG PET/CT may become the initial, and perhaps the only imaging study needed in the patient with FUO.[22,23]

## *Case III.3.8 ( DICOM Images on DVD )*

### History

This 51-year-old female with a history of lung cancer had recently completed chemotherapy and radiation. She had fallen about 3 months previously and was complaining of persistent low-back pain. Laboratory values, except for a slightly elevated erythrocyte sedimentation rate, were unremarkable. She was referred for $^{99m}$Tc-MDP SPECT/CT (Fig. III.3.8A, B) and $^{18}$F-FDG PET/CT (Fig. III.3.8C) to evaluate for metastatic disease and possible spinal osteomyelitis.

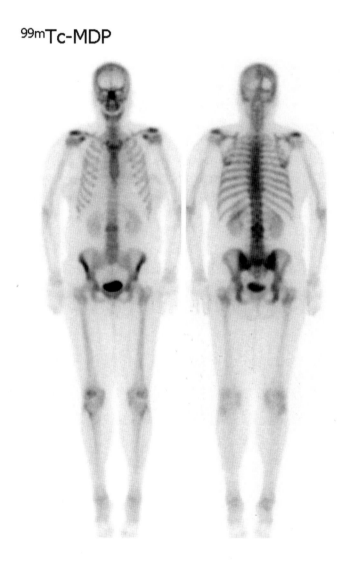

**Fig. III.3.8A**

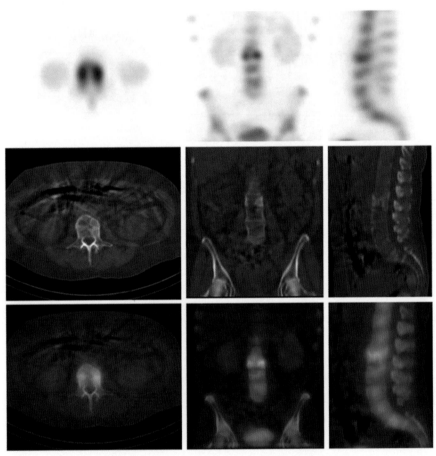

**Fig. III.3.8B**

## $^{18}$F-FDG

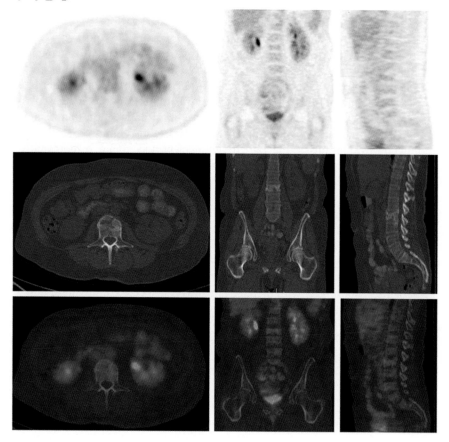

**Fig. III.3.8C**

### Findings

Anterior and posterior whole-body skeletal images (Fig. III.3.8A) demonstrate increased uptake in the mid-lumbar spine. On SPECT/CT (Fig. III.3.8B), the abnormal uptake is localized to L3, which is fractured.

The patient's fasting blood glucose level was 88 mg/dL at the time of injection of 518 MBq (14 mCi) of $^{18}$F-FDG. Imaging was performed about 60 min later. Representative $^{18}$F-FDG PET/CT images (Fig. III.3.8C) show homogeneous tracer uptake throughout the lumbar spine, including the sclerotic L3 fracture.

### Discussion

$^{18}$F-FDG PET has generated considerable interest as an alternative to conventional radionuclide imaging in the evaluation of osteomyelitis, with sensitivities of more than 95% and specificities ranging from 75 to 99% having been reported. In contrast to skeletal scintigraphy, $^{18}$F-FDG uptake appears to normalize rapidly following surgical and traumatic fractures.[6,24-26] In a retrospective study of 14 patients who had traumatic or surgical fractures within 3 months prior to imaging, only six had abnormally increased [18]F-FDG uptake.[24] In the group of patients with fractures or surgery more than 3 months prior to [18]F-FDG-PET, only one showed abnormally increased uptake and had biopsy-proven osteomyelitis at the fracture site. In a subgroup of patients with recent spinal compression fractures or spinal surgery, all scans were negative, including the patients in whom the interval between the fracture and [18]F-FDG PET imaging was brief. In another series, none of the patients with fractures 4–12 months old had abnormally increased [18]F-FDG uptake.[25] In another study, reactive changes in aseptic fracture non-union showed only faint uptake that could be clearly distinguished from osteomyelitis.[27]

Radionuclide evaluation of the patient with suspected spinal osteomyelitis usually involves combined bone/[67]Ga citrate imaging.[18]F-FDG PET is a promising alternative for diagnosing this entity and as accurate as [67]Ga citrate imaging for diagnosing spinal osteomyelitis.[28-31] It may be especially useful for distinguishing true infectious spondylodiscitis from severe granulation-type degenerative disc disease, a differentiation that is not always easily made with magnetic resonance imaging (MRI).[29] One group of investigators reported that [18]F-FDG PET was superior to MRI in patients who had a history of surgery and suffered from high-grade infection in combination with paravertebral abscess formation and in those with low-grade spondylitis or discitis.[30]

In 57 patients, including 27 with metallic hardware, suspected of having spinal infection after spinal surgery, the sensitivity, specificity, and accuracy of [18]F-FDG PET were 100, 81, and 86%, respectively. The positive predictive value was 65%, and the negative predictive value was 100%. The authors concluded that spinal infection can be excluded when the [18]F-FDG PET study is negative.[31]

**Diagnosis**

Healing traumatic L3 vertebral fracture.

**Clinical Report: Body [18]F-FDG PET/CT and [99m]Tc-MDP SPECT/CT (for DVD cases only)**

This 51-year-old female with a history of lung cancer had recently completed chemotherapy and radiation to the left upper lung. She had fallen about 3 months previously and was complaining of low back pain. Laboratory values, except for a slightly elevated erythrocyte sedimentation rate, were unremarkable. She was referred for a skeletal scintigraphy and [18]F-FDG PET/CT to evaluate for metastatic disease and possible spinal osteomyelitis.

Protocol

[99m]Tc-MDP SPECT/CT: The patient underwent imaging about 2 h after intravenous injection of 925 MBq (25 mCi) [99m]Tc-MDP. SPECT/CT of the lumbar spine was performed using a SPECT/CT scanner with a low-dose CT used for anatomical localization and attenuation correction.

[18]F-FDG-PET/CT: The patient fasted for more than 4 h and had a normal blood glucose level (88 mg/dL) prior to [18]F-FDG injection. The PET acquisition was performed using a PET/CT scanner with a low-dose CT used for anatomical correlation and attenuation correction. Oral contrast was used. PET emission images were started approximately

60 min after IV injection of 518 MBq (14 mCi) of $^{18}$F-FDG and covered the area from the base of the skull to the mid-thighs.

Findings

> *Skeletal SPECT/CT*: The quality of the study is good. There is focally increased radionuclide accumulation corresponding to a fracture involving L3. There is physiologic distribution of radiotracer in the remainder of the osseous structures. Both kidneys are visualized and are symmetric in appearance.
>
> $^{18}$*F-FDG-PET/CT*: The quality of the study is good.
>
> *Head and neck*: Post-craniotomy changes are seen in the right parietal region. There is normal $^{18}$F-FDG activity in the remainder of the visualized head and neck.
>
> *Chest*: There is diffusely increased uptake in the left upper lung (maximum SUV 6.1), which corresponds to a large area of parenchymal consolidation with air bronchograms identified on the CT. There is physiologic tracer activity in the mediastinum and both axillary regions.
>
> *Abdomen*: There is physiologic tracer activity in the liver, spleen, kidneys, and bowel.
>
> *Pelvis*: There is physiologic tracer activity in the urinary bladder and soft tissues of the pelvis and thighs.
>
> *Musculoskeletal System*: There is physiologic tracer activity throughout the imaged osseous structures. The L3 fracture identified on the CT component is not hypermetabolic. $^{18}$F-FDG uptake in this vertebra is indistinguishable from that in the adjacent vertebrae.

Impression

1. Diffuse hypermetabolism in left upper lung likely representing post-radiation changes. Close clinical follow-up is suggested.
2. Traumatic fracture L3.
3. No evidence of osteomyelitis.

# References

1. Bunyaviroch T, Aggarwal A, Oates ME. Optimized scintigraphic evaluation of infection and inflammation: role of single-photon emission computed tomography/computerized tomography fusion imaging. *Sem Nucl Med* 2006; 36:295–311.
2. Palestro CJ, Love C. Radionuclide imaging of musculoskeletal infection: coventional agents. *Semin Musculoskelet Radiol* 2007;11:335–352.
3. Love C, Palestro CJ. Radionuclide imaging of infection. *J Nucl Med Tech* 2004;32:47–57.
4. Love C, Tomas MB, Tronco GG, Palestro CJ. Imaging infection and inflammation with [18]F-FDG-PET. *RadioGraphics* 2005;25:1357–1368.
5. Vos FJ, Bleeker-Rovers CP, Corstens FH, Kullberg BJ, Oyen WJ.FDG-PET for imaging of non-osseous infection and inflammation. *Q J Nucl Med Mol Imag* 2006;50:121–130.
6. Strobel K, Stumpe KD. PET/CT in musculoskeletal infection. *Semin Musculoskelet Radiol* 2007;11:353–364.
7. Bleeker-Rovers CP, Vos FJ, Corstens FH, Oyen WJ. Imaging of infectious diseases using [18F] fluorodeoxyglucose PET. *Q J Nucl Med Mol Imaging* 2008;52:17–29.
8. Bar-Shalom R, Yefremov N, Guralnik L, Keidar Z, Engel A, Nitecki S, Israel O. SPECT/CT using [67]Ga and [111]In-labeled leukocyte scintigraphy for diagnosis of infection. *J Nucl Med* 2006; 47:587–594.
9. Moschilla G, Thompson J, Turner JH. Co-registered Gallium-67 SPECT/CT imaging in the diagnosis of infection and monitoring treatment. *World J Nucl Med* 2006; 5:32–39.
10. Horger M, Eschmann SM, Pfannenberg C, Storek D, Vonthein R, Claussen CD, Bares R. Added value of SPECT/CT in patients suspected of having bone infection: preliminary results. *Arch Orthop Trauma Surg* 2007;127:211–221.
11. Filippi L, Schillaci O. Tc-99m HMPAO-labeled leukocyte scintigraphy for bone and joint infections. *J Nucl Med* 2006;47:1908–1913.
12. Horger M, Eschmann SM, Pfannenberg C, Storek D, Vonthein R, Dammann F, Claussen CD, Bares R. The value of SPET/CT in chronic osteomyelitis. *Eur J Nucl Med Mol Imaging* 2003;30:1665–1673.
13. Höpfner S, Krolak C, Kessler S, Tiling R, Brinkbäumer K, Hahn K, Dresel S. Preoperative imaging of Charcot neuroarthropathy in diabetic patients: comparison of ring PET, hybrid PET, and magnetic resonance imaging. *Foot Ankle Int* 2004;25:890–895.
14. Schwegler B, Stumpe KD, Weishaupt D, Strobel K, Spinas GA, von Schulthess GK, Hodler J, Böni T, Donath MY. Unsuspected osteomyelitis is frequent in persistent diabetic foot ulcer and better diagnosed by MRI than by 18F-FDG PET or 99mTc-MOAB. *J Intern Med* 2008;263:99–106.
15. Keidar Z, Militianu D, Melamed E, Bar-Shalom R, Israel O. The diabetic foot: initial experience with [18]F-FDG-PET/CT. *J Nucl Med* 2005;46:444–449.
16. Keidar Z, Engel A, Nitecki S, Bar SR, Hoffman A, Israel O. PET/CT using 2-deoxy-2-[18F]fluoro-D-glucose for the evaluation of suspected infected vascular graft. *Mol Imaging Biol* 2003;5:23–25.
17. Fukuchi K, Ishida Y, Higashi M, Tsunekawa T, Ogino H, Minatoya K, Kiso K, Naito H. Detection of aortic graft infection by fluorodeoxyglucose positron emission tomography: comparison with computed tomographic findings. *J Vasc Surg* 2005;42:919–925.
18. Keidar Z, Engel A, Hoffman A, Israel O, Nitecki S. Prosthetic vascular graft infection: the role of [18]F-FDG-PET/CT. *J Nucl Med* 2007; 48:1230–1236.
19. Lorenzen J, Buchert R, Bohuslavizki KH. Value of FDG PET in patients with fever of unknown origin. *Nucl Med Commun* 2001;22:779–783.
20. Blockmans D, Knockaert D, Maes A. De Caestecker J, Stroobants S, Bobbaers H, Mortelmans L. Clinical Value of [[18]F]fluoro-deoxyglucose positron emission tomography for patients with fever of unknown origin. *Clin Infect Dis* 2001;32:191–196.
21. Meller J, Altenvoerde G, Munzel U, Jauho A, Behe M, Gratz S, Luig H, Becker W. Fever of unknown origin: prospective comparison of [[18]F]FDG imaging with a double-head coincidence camera and [67]Ga citrate SPET. *Eur J Nucl Med* 2000;27:1617–1625.
22. Bleeker-Rovers CP, de Kleijn EMHA, Corstens FHM, van der Meer JWM, Oyen WJG. Clinical Value of FDG PET in patients with fever of unknown origin and patients suspected of focal infection or inflammation. *Eur J Nucl Med Mol Imaging* 2004; 31:29–37.
23. Bleeker-Rovers CP, Vos FJ, de Kleijn EM, Mudde AH, Dofferhoff TS, Richter C, Smilde TJ, Krabbe PF, Oyen WJ, van der Meer JW. A prospective multicenter study on fever of unknown origin: the yield of a structured diagnostic protocol. *Medicine* 2007;86:26–38.

24. Zhuang H, Sam JW, Chacko TK, Duarte PS, Hickeson M, Feng Q, Nakhoda KZ, Guan L, Reich P, Altimari SM, Alavi A. Rapid normalization of osseous FDG uptake following traumatic or surgical fractures. *Eur J Nucl Med Mol Imaging* 2003;30:1096–1103.

25. De Winter F, Van de Wiele C, Vogelaers D, De Smet K, Verdonk R, Dierckx RA. Flourine –18 flourodeoxyglucose-positron emission tomography: a highly accurate imaging modality for the diagnosis of chronic musculoskeletal infections. *J Bone Joint Surg* 2001;83-A:651–660.

26. Guhlmann A, Brecht-Krauss D, Suger G, Glatting G, Kotzerke J, Kinzl L, Reske SN.Chronic osteomyelitis: detection with FDG PET and correlation with histopathologic findings. *Radiology* 1998;206:749–754.

27. Hartmann A, Eid K, Dora C, Trentz O, von Schulthess GK, Stumpe KDM. Diagnostic value of [18]F-FDG PET/CT in trauma patients with suspected chronic osteomyelitis. *Eur J Nucl Med Mol Imaging* 2007;34:704–714.

28. Palestro CJ, Love C, Miller TT. Imaging of musculoskeletal infections. Best Practice & Research. *Clin Rheumatol* 2006;20:1197–1218.

29. Stumpe KD, Zanetti M, Weishaupt D, Hodler J, Boos N, von Schulthess GK. FDG positron emission tomography for differentiation of degenerative and infectious endplate abnormalities in the lumbar spine detected on MR imaging. *Am J Roentgenol* 2002; 179:1151–1157.

30. Gratz S, Dorner J, Fischer U, Behr TM, Béhé M, Altenvoerde G, Meller J, Grabbe E, Becker W. 18F-FDG hybrid PET in patients with suspected spondylitis. *Eur J Nucl Med Mol Imaging* 2002; 29:516–524.

31. De Winter F, Gemmel F, Van de Wiele C, Poffijn B, Uyttendaele D, Dierckx R. 18-fluorine fluorodeoxyglucose positron emission tomography for the diagnosis of infection in the postoperative spine. *Spine* 2003;28:1314–1319.

# Subject Index

D. Delbeke, O. Israel (eds.), *Hybrid PET/CT and SPECT/CT Imaging,*
DOI 10.1007/978-0-387-92820-3, © Springer Science+Business Media, LLC 2010

Printed in the United States of America

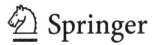 Springer